Essentials of Rhinology

Hitesh Verma • Alok Thakar
Editors

Essentials of Rhinology

BYWORD
BOOKS™

Springer

Editors
Hitesh Verma
Department of Otorhinolaryngology
All India Institute of Medical Sciences
New Delhi
India

Alok Thakar
Department of Otorhinolaryngology
All India Institute of Medical Science
New Delhi
India

ISBN 978-981-33-6283-3 ISBN 978-981-33-6284-0 (eBook)
https://doi.org/10.1007/978-981-33-6284-0

Jointly published with Byword Books

This Springer imprint is published by the registered company Springer Nature Singapore Pte Ltd.
The registered company address is: 152 Beach Road, #21-01/04 Gateway East, Singapore 189721, Singapore

Foreword

Rhinology has been perhaps the most rapidly involving subspecialty in oto-rhinolaryngology over the last few decades. *Essentials of Rhinology* is an up-to-date and excellently illustrated text on the subject which captures the essence of contemporary rhinology. As a multi-author book, led by the team of Dr. Hitesh Verma and Dr. Alok Thakar at AIIMS New Delhi, it brings together the experience of many recognized pioneers and experts from the Indian subcontinent.

The book expands its scope beyond the conventional by including sections on rhinological instruments, biofilms, packing materials, surgical cavity management, open transcranial skull base surgery, and a detailed description of complications and their management. Authors from allied specialties have contributed to sections on diagnostic microbiology, intervention radiology, and nuclear medicine in sino-nasal diseases. Controversies are covered in a comprehensive and balanced manner.

My congratulations to the editors in compiling this excellent textbook on the subject. It serves both as a textbook on fundamental aspects of the subject and as a reference guide for the recent advancements in the field.

Naresh Panda
Department of Otolaryngology
PGIMER
Chandigarh, India

Preface

The nose is an amazing organ. It undertakes humidification, filtration, and heat exchange of inhaled air. It communicates with the four pairs of paranasal sinuses to enable vocal resonance, allow spacing for the brain and eyes, and enable protection of these structures from trauma. The exact dynamics relating to its contribution of inspiratory and expiratory resistance in respiration and ventilatory physiology and sleep disordered breathing are yet not fully apparent. Rhinology has benefited enormously from recent improved diagnostic tools and refinement of surgical techniques. The field of rhinology has matured and evolved in the last two decades, but it does seem that there is yet some way to go for its complete understanding.

This book is an attempt to capture the state of current knowledge in the subject. It focuses on the basic principles of diagnosis and treatment, and supplements on these with recent developments. Sections from allied specialties including microbiology, nuclear medicine, and interventional radiology are designed to enable integrated care. Sinusitis, as the most common clinical entity encountered by the practicing rhinologist, is discussed in detail, and lessons from the past regarding the practice of non-endoscopic external sinus procedures in current times are well covered.

We would hope and expect that the book shall provide rhinologists with a template for contemporary care for their patients and also enable a basic understanding of principles so as to be able to evaluate and adopt newer developments as they become available.

New Delhi, India

Hitesh Verma
Alok Thakar

Contents

About the Editors

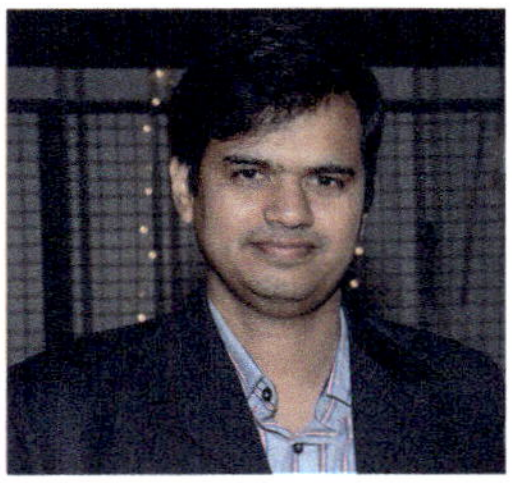

Hitesh Verma MBBS (SMS Medical College, Jaipur), MS (PGIMER), DNB, MBA (IGNOU), is working as Associate Professor of Otorhinolaryngology, All India Institute of Medical Sciences, New Delhi. The focus of his work has been on rhinology and skull base surgery, sleep surgery, and airway surgeries. Dr. Hitesh's research has included three funded research projects and more than 70 research publications. He has also received gold medal and Junior Consultant Award by the Indian Rhinology and Delhi AOI society.

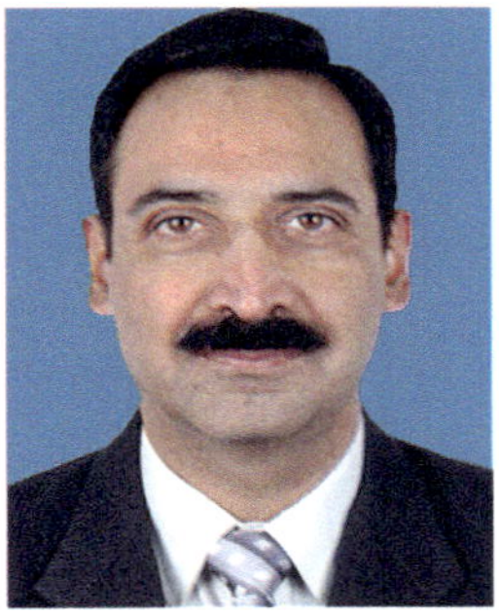

Alok Thakar MBBS (AIIMS), MS (AIIMS), DNB, DLO (London), FRCS (Edinburgh), is the Professor and Head of Otorhinolaryngology, All India Institute of Medical Sciences, New Delhi. He worked as a Specialist Registrar and a Skull Base Fellow-Commonwealth Fellow in the UK. Dr. Thakar's research includes 11 funded research projects, more than 250 research publications, with 2200 citations, and 2 patent applications. He has also received Shakuntala Amir Chand Award by the ICMR and a Gold Medal by the NES Society of India.

List of Contributors

Abha Kumari ENT, Command Hospital, Kolkata, West Bengal, India
e-mail: abhak12@gmail.com

Abhishek Gugliani ENT, AIIMS, Jodhpur, Rajasthan, India
e-mail: abhishekgugliani@gmail.com

Amit Kesari Neurootology, SGPGIMS, Lucknow, UP, India
e-mail: amitkeshri2000@yahoo.com

Amit Shanker ENT, Brighton and Sussex University Hospital NHS, Brighton, UK
e-mail: shankarpgi22@yahoo.com

Anand Pendakur Allergy Asthma ENT Clinic, Bangalore, Karnataka, India
e-mail: pendakur.anand@gmail.com

Anandita Gupta ENT, Army College of Medical Sciences, New Delhi, India
e-mail: anandita0508@gmail.com

Anchal Kakkar Pathology, AIIMS, New Delhi, India
e-mail: aanchalkakkar@gmail.com

Anindya Nayak ENT, AIIMS, Bhubaneswar, Odisha, India
e-mail: anindaa_nayak30690@yahoo.in

Ankur Goyal Radiology, AIIMS, New Delhi, India
e-mail: ankurgoyalaiims@gmail.com

Alok Thakar Department of ENT, AIIMS, New Delhi, India
e-mail: drathakar@gmail.com

Anoop Singh ENT, AIIMS, New Delhi, India
e-mail: anoop.aiims1@gmail.com

Anupam Kanodia ENT, AIIMS, New Delhi, India
e-mail: kanodiaanupam@gmail.com

Arulalan Mathialagan Neurootology, SGPGIMS, Lucknow, UP, India
e-mail: arulalan87@gmail.com

Arvind K. Kairo ENT, AIIMS, New Delhi, India
e-mail: arvindkairo@yahoo.com

Ashu Seith Bhalla Radiology, AIIMS, New Delhi, India
e-mail: ashubhalla1@yahoo.com

Avni Jain ENT, ESIC Medical College Faridabad, Faridabad, Haryana, India
e-mail: avanijain87@hotmail.com

Bharti Devnani Radiotherapy, AIIMS, New Delhi, India
e-mail: bhartidevnani@gmail.com

Darwin Kaushal ENT, AIIMS, Jodhpur, Rajasthan, India
e-mail: drdarwin.aiims@gmail.com

David Victor Kumar Irugu ENT, AIIMS, New Delhi, India
e-mail: irugudavid72kumar@rediffmail.com

Debesh Bhoi Anaesthesiology, Pain Medicine and Critical Care, AIIMS, New Delhi, India
e-mail: debeshbhoi@gmail.com

Deepali Jain Pathology, AIIMS, New Delhi, India
e-mail: deepalijain76@gmail.com

Gagandeep Singh Microbiology, AIIMS, New Delhi, India
e-mail: drgagandeep@gmail.com

Ganakalyan Behera ENT, AIIMS, Bhopal, MP, India
e-mail: drganakalyan@gmail.com

Gaurav Gupta ENT, SP Medical College, Bikaner, Rajasthan, India
e-mail: drgauravgupta24@gmail.com

Gopica Kalsotra ENT, GMC, Jammu, India
e-mail: drgopikapgimer@gmail.comm

Gurbax Singh ENT, GGS Medical College and Hospital, Faridkot, Punjab, India
e-mail: drgurbax@gmail.com

Gyan Nayak ENT, PGIMER, Chandigarh, India
e-mail: gyani.nayak@gmail.com

Harpreet Kocher ENT, Yatharth Superspeciality Hospital, Greater Noida, UP, India
e-mail: hpskochar@gmail.com

Hitender Gautam Microbiology, AIIMS, New Delhi, India
e-mail: drhitender@gmail.com

Hitesh Verma ENT, AIIMS, New Delhi, India

Department of ENT, AIIMS, New Delhi, India
e-mail: drhitesh10@gmail.com

Immaculata Xess Microbiology, AIIMS, New Delhi, India
e-mail: immaxess@gmail.com

Jaini Lodha ENT, Seven Hills Hospital, Andheri East Mumbai, Maharashtra, India
e-mail: jainilodha@gmail.com

K. Davraj ENT, KMC, Manipal, Karnataka, India
e-mail: deardrdr@gmail.com

Kapil Sikka ENT, AIIMS, New Delhi, India
e-mail: kapil_sikka@yahoo.com

Kranti Bhawna ENT, AIIMS, Patna, Bihar, India
e-mail: bhavana.kranti@gmail.com

Kshitiz Charya Indus Hospital, Mohali, Punjab, India
e-mail: charaya.k@gmail.com

Kuldeep Thakur ENT, AIIMS, New Delhi, India
e-mail: drkuldeep70@gmail.com

M. Ravi Sankar Neurootology, SGPGIMS, Lucknow, UP, India
e-mail: drravisankarpgi@gmail.com

Manish Gupta ENT, MMIMSR, MMU, Ambala, Haryana, India
e-mail: manishgupta1217@gmail.com

Manju Silu ENT, SP Medical College, Bikaner, Rajasthan, India
e-mail: manjusilu35@gmail.com

Mohnish Grover ENT, SMS Medical College, Jaipur, Rajasthan, India
e-mail: drmohnish.aiims@gmail.com

Mayank Yadav ENT, SHKM GMC, Nalhar, Nuh, Haryana, India
e-mail: drmayankyadav@yahoo.co.in

Nagesh Tangirala Anaesthesiology, Pain Medicine and Critical Care, AIIMS, New Delhi, India
e-mail: nag947@gmail.com

Namrita Mahmi Department of ENT, AIIMS, New Delhi, India
e-mail: namritamehmi@gmail.com

Nikhil Singh ENT, AIIMS, Raipur, Chhattisgarh, India
e-mail: doc.niks03@gmail.com

Nitin Gupta ENT, GMCH, Chandigarh, India
e-mail: nitinent123@gmail.com

Nitin M. Nagarkar ENT, AIIMS, Raipur, Chhattisgarh, India
e-mail: nmnent63@gmail.com

Pankuri Mittal Department of ENT, AIIMS, New Delhi, India
e-mail: mamc.pankhuri@gmail.com

Pooja D. Nayak ENT, SP Medical College, Bikaner, Rajasthan, India
e-mail: poomahe2007@gmail.com

Pradip Kumar Tiwari ENT, NIGRIMS, Shillong, Meghalaya, India
e-mail: dr.pradiptiwari@gmail.com

Prateek Sharma ENT, AIIMS, New Delhi, India
e-mail: drprateeksharma.mamc@gmail.com

Preetam Chappity ENT, AIIMS, Bhubaneswar, Odisha, India
e-mail: drcpreetam@aiimsbhubaneswar.edu.in

Prity Sharma ENT, AIIMS, Bhubaneswar, Odisha, India
e-mail: sharmaprity21@gmail.com

R. S. Virk ENT, PGIMER, Chandigarh, India
e-mail: virkdoc@hotmail.com

Raja Pramanik Medical Oncology, Dr.B.R.A-IRCH, AIIMS, New Delhi, India
e-mail: drrajapramanik@gmail.com

Rajesh Kumar Meena Neurosurgery, AIIMS, New Delhi, India
e-mail: drrajeshmeena165@gmail.com

Rakesh Kumar ENT, AIIMS, New Delhi, India
e-mail: winirk@hotmail.com

Ramesh S. Doddamani Neurosurgery, AIIMS, New Delhi, India
e-mail: drsdramesh@gmail.com

Ravneet Singh ENT, GMCH, Chandigarh, India
e-mail: ravneetrverma@gmail.com

Ripu Daman Arora ENT, AIIMS, Raipur, Chhattisgarh, India
e-mail: neelripu@gmail.com

Rohit Verma ENT, DMC, Ludhiana, Punjab, India
e-mail: rohitaiims@yahoo.co.in

Rupa Mehta ENT, AIIMS, Raipur, Chhattisgarh, India
e-mail: rmehta0409@yahoo.com

Sanjeev Bhagat ENT, Rajindra Hospital Patiala, Patiala, Punjab, India
e-mail: sbent224@gmail.com

Saurav Sarkar ENT, AIIMS, Bhubaneswar, Odisha, India
doc.sauravsarkar@gmail.com

Shamim Ahmed Shamim Nuclear Medicine, AIIMS, New Delhi, India
e-mail: sashamim2002@gmail.com

Shashank Nath Singh ENT, SMS Medical College, Jaipur, Rajasthan, India
e-mail: drshashanknathsingh@gmail.com

Shashikant Paul ENT, JIPMER, Pondicherry, India
e-mail: drshashikantpol@gmail.com

Sheetal Kumari ENT, GMC, Jammu, India
e-mail: gphonshashetal@gmail.com

Shitanshu Sharma ENT, SMS Medical College, Jaipur, Rajasthan, India
e-mail: shsharma811@gmail.com

Smita Manchanda Radiology, AIIMS, New Delhi, India
e-mail: smitamanchanda@gmail.com

Smriti Panda Department of ENT, AIIMS, New Delhi, India
e-mail: smriti.panda.87@gmail.com

Sonu Kumari Agrawal Microbiology, AIIMS, New Delhi, India
e-mail: drhitender@gmail.com

Suman Bhasker Radiotherapy, AIIMS, New Delhi, India
e-mail: drsumanbhasker@gmail.com

Sunil Kumar ENT, LHMC, New Delhi, India
e-mail: suku321@rediffmail.com

Suresh Mani ENT, CMC, Vellore, Tamil Nadu, India
e-mail: msuresh.doc@gmail.com

Surya Prakash Vadlamani Medical Oncology, Dr.B.R.A-IRCH, AIIMS, New Delhi, India
e-mail: vadlamanisuryaprakash@gmail.com

Tanmaya Kataria ENT, SMS Medical College, Jaipur, Rajasthan, India
e-mail: tanmayakataria@gmail.com

Vaibhav Saini ENT, AIIMS, Bhatinda, Punjab, India
e-mail: drvaibhavsaini@gmail.com

Vikas Gupta ENT, AIIMS, Bhopal, MP, India
e-mail: vikasmsent@gmail.com

Vishal Sharma ENT, Rajindra Hospital Patiala, Patiala, Punjab, India
e-mail: drvishalsharma2@gmail.com

Zareen Lynrah ENT, NIGRIMS, Shillong, Meghalaya, India
e-mail: zareenalynrah@gmail.com

Endoscopic Anatomy and Surgery

1

Hitesh Verma, Smita Manchanda, Sunil Kumar, Vaibhav Saini, Debesh Bhoi, Nagesh Tangirala, Abha Kumari, and Anandita Gupta

Contents

H. Verma (✉)
ENT, AIIMS, New Delhi, India
e-mail: drhitesh10@gmail.com

S. Manchanda
Radiology, AIIMS, New Delhi, India

S. Kumar
ENT, LHMC, New Delhi, India

V. Saini
ENT, AIIMS, Bhatinda, Punjab, India

D. Bhoi · N. Tangirala
Anaesthesiology, Pain Medicine and Critical Care, AIIMS, New Delhi, India

A. Kumari
ENT, Command Hospital, Kolkata, West Bengal, India

A. Gupta
ENT, Army College of Medical Sciences, New Delhi, India

H. Verma, A. Thakar (eds.), *Essentials of Rhinology*, https://doi.org/10.1007/978-981-33-6284-0_1

1.1 Part A: Anatomy of Nasal Cavity and Paranasal Sinuses

The nasal cavity is the initial entry point in the airway. It extends from anterior nares to posterior choana. Pneumatized air spaces within facial bones are known as paranasal sinuses. They converse with the nasal cavity at various levels. The frontal sinus is the supraorbital airspace within the frontal bone which comes in the superior relationship of the nasal cavity and it drains into the middle meatus via frontal recess. The maxillary sinus is the airspace inside the maxilla bone which communicates with the middle meatus via ethmoid infundibulum. Ethmoid air cells are located within the nasal cavity just below the skull base from agger nasi cells till anterior wall of the sphenoid sinus. The sphenoid sinus is the airspace of the body of the sphenoid and it lies in the superior relationship of the nasopharynx. The nasal placode and mesenchymal processes around the primitive mouth develop nose. A primitive nasal cavity develops by fusion of maxillary process of the first brachial arch with the medial nasal process and frontonasal process. Choana is derived by a split of bucconasal membrane which separates the primitive oral cavity from the nasal cavity. The nasal cavity is divided into two half by fusion of septum with palatine process of both sides. Failure of fusion or split of these processes will present as congenital anomalies like cleft lip, cleft palate, choanal atresia, etc. The vestibule is the initial part of the nasal cavity which extends from the external opening till the nasal valve. The vestibule is a line by the skin with vibrissae, sweat, and sebaceous gland. The nasal cavity proper is the remaining part of the nasal cavity which is a line by pseudo-stratified columnar epithelium. The anatomy of the nose and paranasal sinuses is very complex. The detailed knowledge of anatomical variation is the foremost thing to overcome complications of surgery. The lateral nasal wall contains three to four projections which are known as turbinates [1].

A. **Inferior Turbinate:** Inferior turbinate is a separate bone with an irregular surface. It is the largest turbinate of the nasal cavity (Fig. 1.1).
B. **Middle Turbinate**
   1. In the sagittal plane, it attaches with cribriform plate at the junction of the vertical and horizontal lamina (Fig. 1.1). Inadvertent pooling of middle turbinate can lead to cribriform plate injury and iatrogenic CSF leak. The collection of air within the lower free part of the middle turbinate is known as concha bullosa (Fig. 1.1).

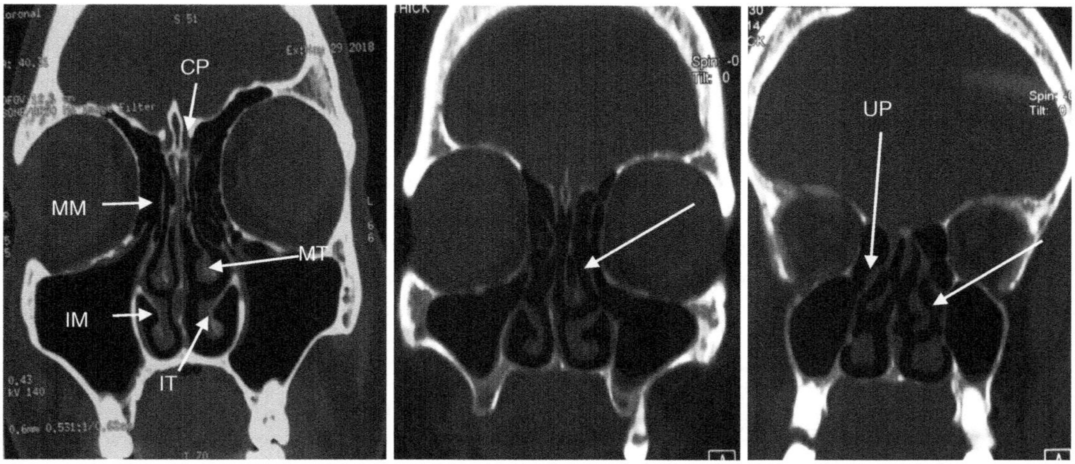

Fig. 1.1 NCCT PNS orbit (Coronal cuts) is showing inferior turbinate (IT), inferior meatus (IM) middle turbinate (MT), middle meatus (MM), and cribriform plate (CP). The central picture is depicting bullosa of MT (white arrow) and the right side picture is showing paradoxical MT with uncinate process attachment on middle turbinate

2. In frontal and horizontal plane it attached with lamina papyracea. It is known as ground lamella. Ground lamella divides ethmoid air cells into anterior and posterior ethmoid cells. Lamina papyracea is thin at the site of attachment so that unintentional pooling of turbinate can leads to orbital fat prolapse.
3. Normally middle turbinate is concave on the middle meatus side. Paradoxical turbinate is the convex presentation of middle turbinate which reduces the volume of middle meatus (Fig. 1.1). Minimum inflammation in the middle meatus can affect the drainage of anterior sinuses significantly.

Meatus is the part of the nasal cavity which is present deep and lateral to the turbinate. Sphenoethmoidal recess and supreme meatus are present medial to superior turbinate (Fig. 1.7). Inferior meatus is the largest and it is present along the entire length of the inferior turbinate. Nasolacrimal duct opening locates at anterior third and posterior two-third junction of the inferior turbinate. Genu is the part of inferior meatus which locates just below and posterior to the nasolacrimal duct opening. Surgical window to reach the floor of the maxillary sinus in endoscopic surgery, in ancient surgery like Proof puncture and for inferior meatal antrostomy (2 × 1 cm) is performed at genu because lateral wall bone is thinnest in this area. The middle meatus is the space present lateral to the middle turbinate. It contains the uncinate process, hiatus semilunaris, bulla ethmoidalis, and ethmoid infundibulum (Fig. 1.2). Anterior ethmoid air cells, maxillary, and frontal sinuses drains into middle meatus. Middle turbinate along with its contents is known as osteomeatal complex (Fig. 1.2).

Superior meatus is the smallest meatus. It is located between the middle and superior turbinate and posterior ethmoid cells lies within it. Sphenoethmoid recess is the space above and behind the superior meatus. Posterior ethmoid cells and sphenoid sinus drains into it.

C. **Uncinate Process**

It is a boomerang shape of two-dimensional structure. It attaches laterally with the lacrimal bone and inferiorly with the inferior turbinate. Superiorly, the uncinate process has three different kinds of attachments. In 70–80% cases, it attaches with the lamina papyracea and allows the drainage of the frontal sinus into the middle meatus. Recess terminalis is the blind sac formed by the attachment of the uncinate process with the lamina papyracea. Skull base and middle turbinate are two other attachments and it allows the drainage of the frontal sinus into ethmoid infundibulum (Fig. 1.1). The presence of the frontoethmoidal cells may be responsible for the upper attacment of the uncinate process. Hiatus semilunaris inferior is the space between the free posterior edge of the uncinate process and bulla ethmoidalis (Fig. 1.2). It allows the drainage of the ethmoid infundibulum into the middle meatus.

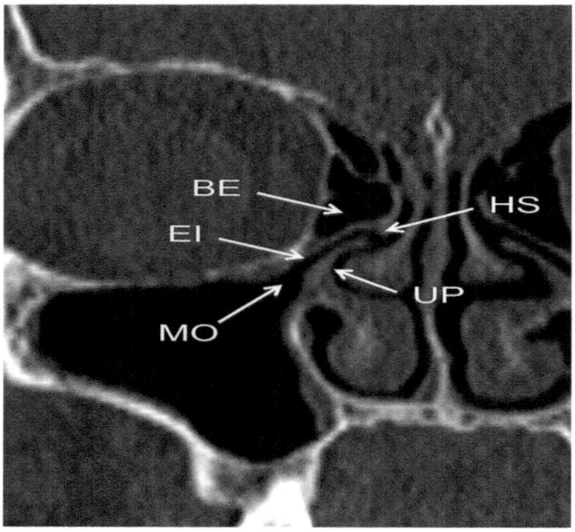

Fig. 1.2 Osteomeatal Complex. Components of osteomeatal unit are maxillary ostium (MO), ethmoidal infundibulum (EI), uncinate process (UP), hiatus semilunaris (HS), and bulla ethmoidalis (BE)

D. **Ethmoid Infundibulum**
It is a three dimensional space. It is bounded anteriorly by the uncinate process, posteriorly by the bulla ethmoidalis, medially by the uncinate process medial surface (Fig. 1.2). It communicates with middle meatus via hiatus semilunaris inferior. Superiorly, it is either end as recess terminalis or it continues with frontal recess, when the uncinate process attaches with the middle turbinate and the skull base.

1.1.1 Ethmoid Cells

Ethmoid air cells are 3–18 in number. It is broadly divided into anterior and posterior by the ground lamella. The anatomical variations are seen more in and around anterior ethmoid cells.

1. Agger Nasi Cells
   (a) Anterior most ethmoidal cells locate over the lacrimal bone (Fig. 1.3). It lies anterior and superior to the axilla of the middle turbinate.

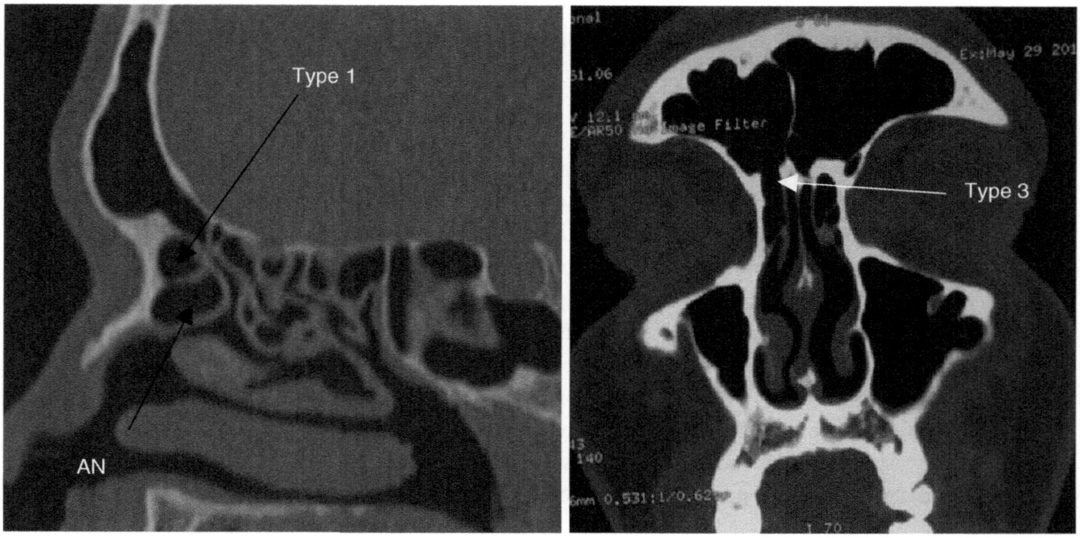

Fig. 1.3 The NCCT PNS orbit (sagittal cut) is depicting type 1 Frontoethmoidal air cells. The coronal cut is depicting type 3 frontoethmoidal cell

2. Frontal Cells

   Frontal cells (frontoethmoidal cells, anterior ethmoid cells) are present in a 20–41% population (Fig. 1.3). It is classified into four types [2].
   (a) Type 1 (most common)—single cell above the agger nasi cells (Fig. 1.3)
   (b) Type 2- the tier of cells above
   (c) Type 3 (least common)—large cell protruding more than 50% within frontal sinus (Fig. 1.3)
   (d) Type 4 is found in the frontal sinus. Sometime extended pneumatization of the bulla ethmoidalis can presented as isolated cell in the frontal sinus. Saggital section is the useful tool to differentiate both type of cells

   Frontal bullar cell is the single cell above bulla ethmoidalis and it may extend anteriorly into frontal sinus. Its infection can affect the drainage of the frontal sinus by narrowing the frontal recess area.
3. Bulla Ethmoidalis

   It is the largest anterior ethmoid air cells (Fig. 1.2). It drains into the middle meatus. Well pneumatized bulla ethmoidalis reaches upto skullbase and ground lamella. Lateral sinus (suprabullar cell) is the air space found above the bulla ethmoidalis when it is not extent till the skullbase. Retrobullar recess is the space between the bulla ethmoidalis and ground lamella. Hiatus semilunaris superior is the medial communication of the retrobullar recess with the middle meatus. Torus ethmoidalis is the terminology used for nonpneumatized bulla ethmoidalis. Pneumatized bulla ethmoidalis is three types
   (a) Simple bulla-single cavity
   (b) Compound bulla—two–three compartments communicated at hiatus semilunaris
   (c) Complex bulla—two–three compartments communicated at hiatus semilunaris, ethmoid infundibulum
4. Heller cell
   (a) It is an infraorbital anterior ethmoid cell. It can affect the drainage of the maxillary sinus by narrowing its outflow tract.

   Posterior ethmoid cells are the cells present behind the ground lamella of the middle turbinate. It extends posteriorly till the anterior face of the sphenoid sinus. It drains into the nasal cavity by superior meatus or by sphenoethmoidal recess. Onodi cell is the posterior extension of the posterior ethmoid cell over the sphenoid sinus. The optic nerve runs very close to the lateral wall of the Onodi cell. Fovea ethmoidalis is the part of skull bone present over ethmoid cells. Fovea ethmoidalis is found higher when the ratio of the vertical height of ethmoid air cells with a vertical height of maxillary sinus or orbit is more than 50% and when skull base angle with the horizontal lamina of the cribriform plate is more than 55°. In such cases chances of injury to the skull base is more at fovea ethmoidalis region.

Frontal recess is bound anteriorly by the uncinate process, laterally by lamina papyracea, medially by middle turbinate. The posterior boundary is the anterior face of the bulla ethmoidalis or lateral sinus in the superior part. It continues inferiorly with the ethmoid infundibulum or the middle meatus, which depends on the superior attachment of the uncinate process (Fig. 1.4).

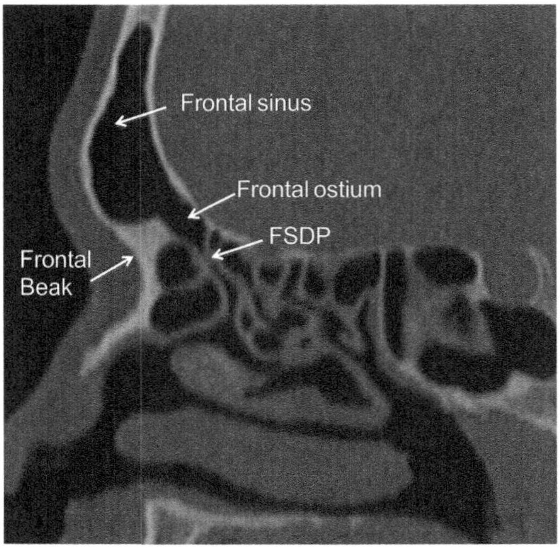

Fig. 1.4 Depicting frontal sinus and frontal beak at the level of the frontal ostium. The frontal sinus is above the frontal beak and the frontal sinus drainage pathway (FSDP) is below the beak

1.1.2 Frontal Sinus

Frontal sinus dimensions are 24 × 20 × 12 mm with a volume of 6–7 ml. It develops from the embryonic infundibulum at frontal recess superior part during the 16th week of intrauterine life. The frontal sinuses are absent at birth and reach their full size by the end of puberty. The anterior edge of the frontal sinus ostia is formed by the frontal beak and the posterior edge by the skull base. Ostia is the narrowest part of the frontal outflow tract. Frontal sinus is an asymmetrically paired sinus with scalloping margins which may loss in the frontal sinus chronic diseases e.g mucocele. The anterior wall is thicker than the posterior wall (Fig. 1.4).

1.1.3 Maxillary Sinus

Maxillary sinus is also known as the antrum of Highmore. It is pyramidal in shape. It is the largest paranasal sinus with a volume of approximately 10 ml. Maxillary sinus ostium is lying high in the medial wall which opens into the ethmoid infundibulum (Fig. 1.2). Maxillary sinus ostium is 2–3 mm oval structure. It is not visible on routine nasal endoscopy as the ostium is covered by the uncinate process. Anterior and posterior accessory maxillary sinus ostium are found at membranous fontanelle. they are visible on endoscopic examination. Accessory ostium is round and it is present in up to 43% of cases. The lining epithelium is the pseudo stratified ciliated columnar epithelium and it is known as Schneiderian membrane.

1.1.4 Anterior Ethmoid Artery

It is the largest branch of the ophthalmic artery. It runs in the orbit between the superior oblique and medial rectus muscles. It enters into the nasal cavity via the anterior ethmoid foramen and runs in the ethmoid roof 1–2 mm behind the anterior end of bulla ethmoidalis. The anterior ethmoid foramen is present 24 mm deep to anterior lacrimal crest. Anterior ethmoid artery runs out of fovea ethmoidalis in the nasal cavity in 8–10% of cases. The radiological sign for the nasal cavity entry point is visible in the form of a point (Kennedy nipple) the radiological features for intranasal course of anterior ethmoid artery are Keros 3 cribriform plate, presence of supraorbital cell or wide antero-posterior width of frontal recess and more than 2 cm length of cribriform plate (Fig. 1.5).

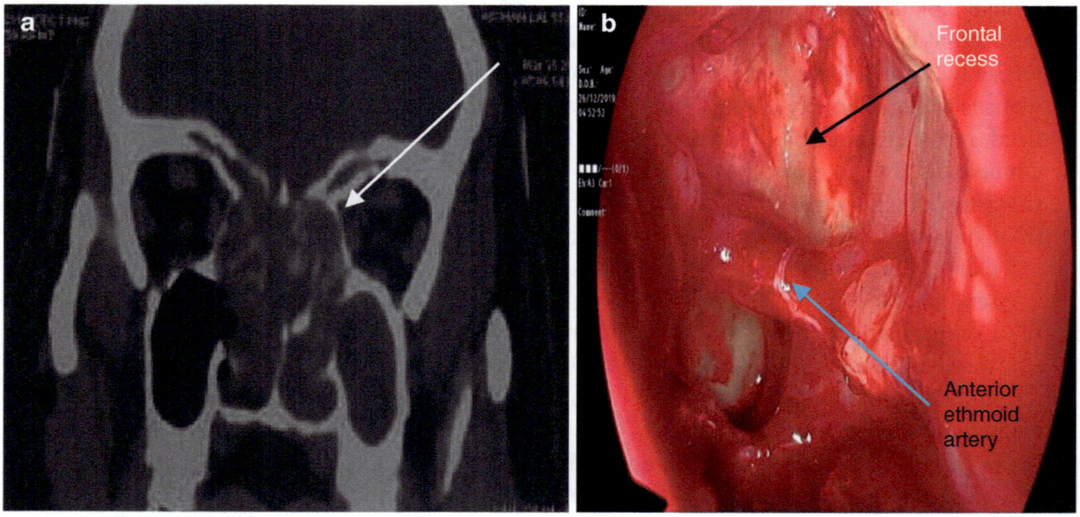

Fig. 1.5 (**a**) NCCT PNS orbit is showing bilateral soft tissue density in the nose and paranasal sinus. Anterior ethmoid artery enter site is depicted by the arrow. (**b**) Post operative endoscopic picture is showing the intranasal anterior ethmoid artery

1.1.5 Sphenopalatine Artery

It is the largest terminal branch of third part of maxillary artery and it supplies a major part of the nasal cavity and paranasal sinuses. It originates within the pterygopalatine fossa region and it enters into the nose via the sphenopalatine foramen. Foramen lies just deep to the posterior-most attachment of middle turbinate. The presence of the anterior bony crest in the middle meatus close to posterior end of middle turbinate is the landmark for endoscopic surgery (see Chap. 9).

1.1.6 Cribriform Plate

It is made up of the horizontal medial part (lamina cribrosa) and vertical lateral part (Fig. 1.6). Crista galli is the thick upward middle projection on the lamina cribrosa. Olfactory nerve comes out via the perforators in the lamina cribrosa. Flax cerebri attaches with the crista galli and the olfactory bulb and tract lie above lamina cribrosa. Keros classification is based on the depth of olfactory fossa (height of vertical lamina). Type 1 is when the depth of the olfactory fossa varies from 1 to 3 mm. In this risk of injury to the cribriform plate is less but the height if the skull base is less so that the risk of injury is more in fovea ethmoidalis (bone of skull base over ethmoid air cells). Type 2 is when the depth of olfactory fossa varies from 4 to 7 mm. It is the most common keros type. Type 3 is when the depth of olfactory fossa is more than 8 mm and it is least common. Type 3 is more associated with skull base injury at the cribriform plate area. The thickness of the vertical lamina is 0.2 mm. The thickness reduces with increasing height of vertical lamina [3]. The thickness is 0.05 mm at the entry point of the anterior ethmoid artery. It is the weakest part of the vertical lamina [4].

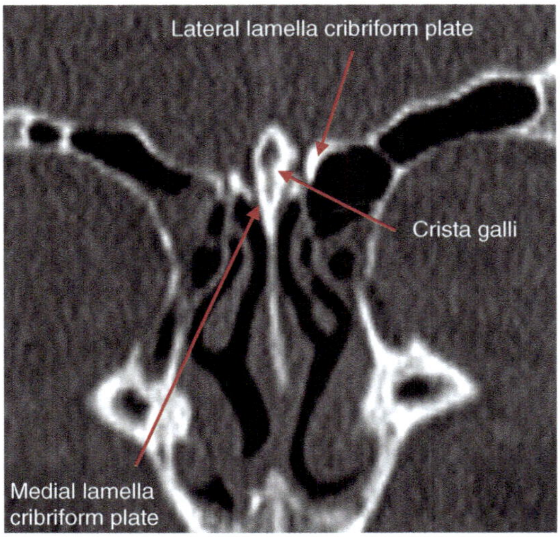

Fig. 1.6 Crista galli is a thick upward projection on lamina cribrosa. The olfactory fossa is bounded by lateral lamella of cribriform plate laterally, medial lamella of cribriform plate inferiorly, and crista galli medially

1.1.7 Sphenoid Sinus

Sphenoid sinus dimension is 22 × 20 × 22 mm. Sphenoid sinus ostia is present 7 cm from the anterior nasal spine at 30° angle. Other landmarks for ostium are 1–1.5 cm above choana and 5 mm from the septum. Pneumatized sphenoid sinus can show bluish hue when the skull base is exposed. The skull base is concave whereas it is convex over sphenoid sinus anterior wall. Conchal, presellar, and sellar are types of pneumatization. In the conchal type, the sphenoid sinus is either nonpneumatized or minimally pneumatized and it is the rarest type of pneumatization. Seller is the most common subtype. The protrusion of the internal carotid artery (ICA) in the lateral wall ranges from 8% to 70% in different studies (Fig. 1.7). ICA dehiscence ranges from 3% to 30% and it is more common with the sellar type of pneumatization. Accessory pneumatization is more commonly seen in the sellar type. Optic canal dehiscence is documented from 4% to 30% (Fig. 1.7). The presence of accessory sphenoid septa ranges from 10% to 80% and it is more common on the right side. It can inserts on the carotid canal and optic canal in 6–26% of cases [5]. Inadvertent injury to accessory septa can lead to the internal carotid artery or optic nerve injury so that whenever required, accessory septum must be drilled.

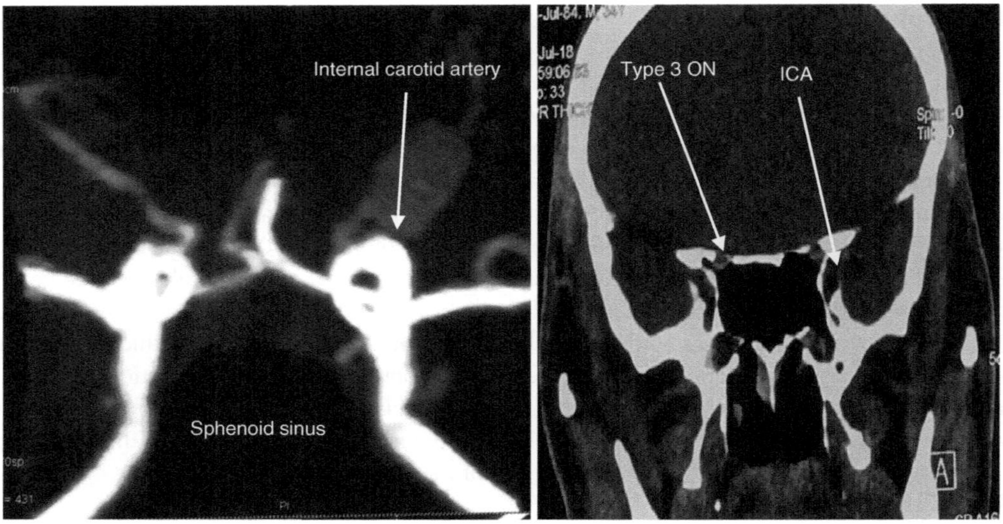

Fig. 1.7 CT angiography is depicting the relationship of internal carotid artery with sphenoid sinus. The right picture is showing relationship of the internal carotid artery and optic nerve and the optic canal is dehiscent on both sides

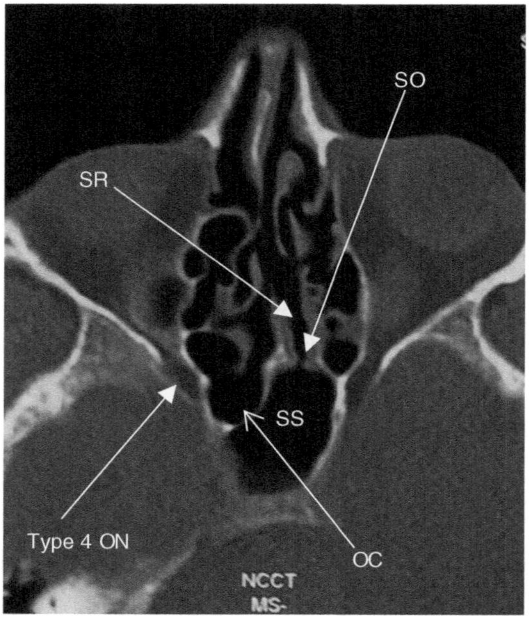

Fig. 1.8 Optic nerve (ON) is visible in lateral relation with the left side Onodi cell (OC). Sphenoid ostia (SO) is demarked on the right side which communicates with a sphenoethmoidal recess (SR)

1.1.8 Optic Nerve Relationship with Paranasal Sinuses

The optic nerve runs in the lateral wall of the sphenoid sinus and Onodi cell (Fig. 1.8). It is classified into four different types. Type 1 is when no indentation visible in the lateral wall on the sphenoid sinus. Type 2 is when indentation visible in the lateral wall on the sphenoid sinus. Type 3 is when the optic canal is within the sphenoid sinus. Type 4 is when the optic canal is present adjacent to the posterior ethmoid and sphenoid sinus.

1.2 Part B: Local Anesthesia and Regional Blocks in Nasal Surgery

The detailed preoperative evaluation is very much important to attain the healthiest patient. It helps in reducing perioperative morbidity and mortality to a significant extent. The cardiovascular and respiratory system needs more attention to overcome the possibility of complication during surgery under local anesthesia (LA). Routine laboratory investigations like hemogram, electrolytes, ECG, and chest X-ray are part of the basic preoperative workup for surgery. Pre-existing acute and chronic medical illnesses needs stabilization. Cardiovascular illnesses require detail preoperative evaluation and intra- operative monitoring by the anesthetist. Proper consent and good preoperative medication are requiring to obtain excellent intraoperative patient's cooperation. Daycare surgery and minor operations can be performed under local anesthesia and regional block. It is also administered for the procedure in general anesthesia as part of preoperative preparation to get good local vasoconstriction and postoperative pain control. The outcome of surgery under local anesthesia is based on detailed knowledge of anatomy and injection techniques. Sensory innervations of the nose are supplied by the branches of the trigeminal nerve (V). The external nose is supplied by branches of the trigeminal nerve (supratrochlear, infratrochlear, anterior ethmoid nerve) and maxillary nerve (branches of the infraorbital nerve). The internal nose is supplied by anterior and posterior ethmoid nerves, sphenopalatine, and greater palatine nerve. Local anesthetic drugs act by reversible blocking or inhibiting conduction at nerve endings by blocking the inflow of sodium ions via the nerve membrane. These agents are applied at mucosa or in the neighborhood of peripheral nerve endings. Commonly used drugs are lidocaine, prilocaine, bupivacaine, ropivacaine, cocaine, etc. Cocaine is out of use because of its high toxicity profile and addictive potential. The action of local anesthetic depends on the following parameters.

1. Diffusion, water solubility, and penetration in tissue, potency, etc.
2. Protein binding ability.
3. Ionized drugs are more diffusible at the nerve ending and have a faster onset of action. Inflamed tissue has poor drug penetration by decreasing local tissue pH. Sodium bicarbonate increases potency by increasing the pH at the inflamed nerve ending site.
4. Local anesthetic drugs can cause vasodilatation except for cocaine and lignocaine. Administration of adrenaline reduces drug absorption and increases the duration of action.

The amount of doses that need to be administered is depending on listed parameters.

1. Smallest effective dose
2. Addition of adrenaline
3. 1 cc of sodium bicarbonate in every 9 ml of LA would increase potency and reduce the burning sensation

Lignocaine is a heat-stable and autoclavable local anesthetic drug. The duration of action is 1 h for injectable preparation and it can extend to 2–3 h by the accumulation of adrenaline. The infiltrative form comes in 0.5–1.5% formulation. The dose of lignocaine (0.5%) without adrenaline is 3 mg/Kg body weight with maximum safe administrative dose is 200 mg in healthy adults whereas lignocaine with adrenaline is 7 mg/kg body weight. The maximum dose is 500 mg in healthy adult. 2% viscous, 4% solution, and 10% spray are the lignocaine preparations for topical anesthesia with maximum safe limit is 200 mg. Mucosal surface anesthesia is required to prepare the nose prior to the application of injection [6]. The action lasts till 20 min. Bupivacaine is more potent than lignocaine and it comes only in injection form [7]. The dose without adrenaline (0.5%) is 2 mg/Kg body weight and the maximum safe limit is 175 mg/dose whereas with adrenaline, the dose is 2.5 mg/kg body weight and the maximum safe limit is 225 mg/dose. It is generally used for regional nerve block because of its long duration of action. Other drugs like prilocaine and amethocaine are less effective than lignocaine. For adrenaline, the dose is 0.01 mg/kg with maximum safe limit is 0.5 mg in healthy adults and 1: 200,000 is required for surgical procedure.

The toxicity profile can vary from redness at the application site to multi-organ failure [8]. An allergic reaction is relatively rare and the common ones are rashes, bronchospasm, etc. so preoperative sensitivity should be done for all cases planned under LA. The cardiac effect is hypotension and circulatory collapse. The neurological side effect can be classified into three stages.

1. Early stage—local anesthetics can cross the blood brain barrier. It depresses inhibitory cortical activity and presents with symptoms of light-headedness, tinnitus, visual changes, slurred speech, dizziness, etc.
2. Late stage—If proper resuscitative methods are not taken than symptoms like drowsiness,

disorientation, seizure, loss of consciousness, etc. can develop.

3. Respiratory distress, severe hypoxia occurs if proper resuscitative measures are not taken.

The therapeutic measures for mild to moderate levels of toxicity are the administration of 100% oxygenation. Anesthetist and resuscitation cart should be warranted if muscle twitching and convulsion occur. The commonly used technique for the regional block is mentioned below.

(a) **Moffett's technique**—The original Moffett's solution was 2 ml cocaine 8%, 2 ml sodium bicarbonate 1%, 1 ml 1:1000 adrenaline. Modified Moffett's solution is prepared by 4% xylocaine (6 ml) with 1: 100,000 adrenaline. It is poured in each nostril, in drop by drop form in a hyperextended position (Proetz position) of the neck. The drops are dispensing along the superior most part of lateral wall of the vestibule to block the sphenopalatine nerve (Fig. 1.9).
(b) **For nasal packing**—Self-prepared cotton pledgets or commercially available non-absorbable packs can be used. They are soaked in 4% lignocaine solution with adrenaline. One pack is kept along the floor of the nasal cavity. The second is above first one and encroaching in the middle meatus. Third one is at the frontal recess area for 10–20 minutes. Periodic suctioning over the throat is required to prevent aspiration during surgery as pharyngeal mucosa gets anesthetized.

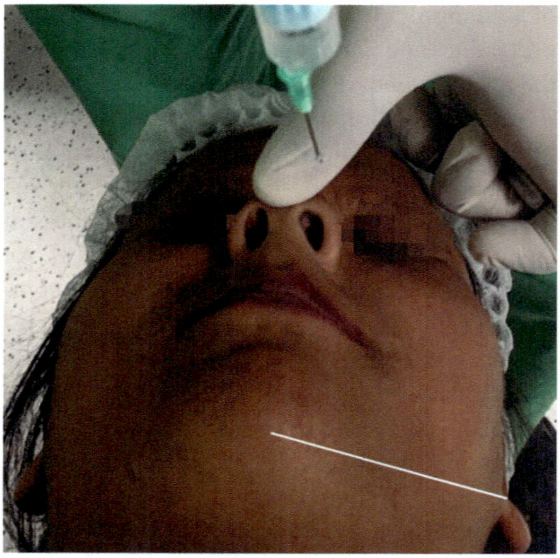

Fig. 1.9 The white line is showing chin and the external auditory canal is in the same line. The needle is pointed towards the supero-lateral part of the vestibule (Courtesy—Dr. Hitesh Verma, Associate Professor, AIIMS, New Delhi, India)

(c) **For endoscopic surgery**—First block is applied at the uppermost part of the middle turbinate and at the axilla of the middle turbinate to anasthetise the anterior ethmoid neurovascular tissue and infraorbital neurovascular tissue. It can be blocked by external route as mentioned in nasociliary (anterior ethmoid) block. The second injection is applied to block the sphenopalatine neurovascular tissue (Fig. 1.10). It is performed by administration of drug at the posterior-most part of the middle meatus just inferior to the middle turbinate and above choana.
(d) **For rhinoplasty**—Local anesthetic is applied at columella over the tip, in between and around the dome of lower lateral cartilage, at the rim of lower lateral cartilage. The quantity is varying from 0.1 to 0.3 ml with 26 gage needle to prevent distortion of anatomy. For intercartilaginous incision, LA is injected at limen nasi in the subperichondrial plane. For osteotomies, LA is injecting inside and outside of the frontal process of the maxilla in the sub-periosteal plane.

Nerve blocks—It is required for the therapeutic purpose only. The various kind of blocks require for nasal surgeries are mentioned subsequently [9].

A. **Frontal Nerve Block**

It is required for the median forehead flap. Supraorbital and supratrochlear divisions of frontal nerve exit through supraorbital foramen and supply frontal scalp and forehead, medial part of the upper eyelid, and root of the nose. Supraorbital foramen can easily be palpated along the medial orbital rim. It is

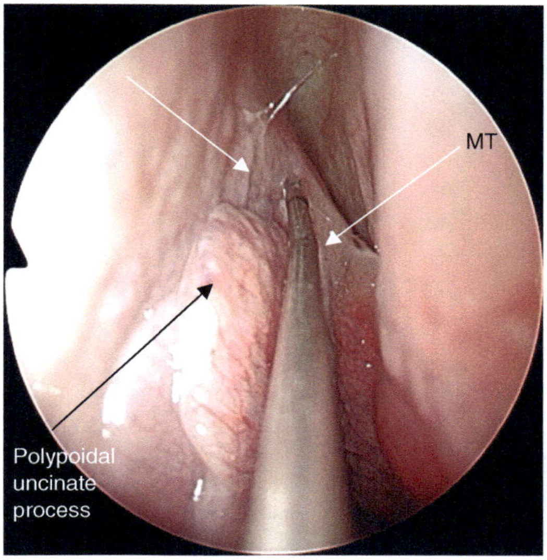

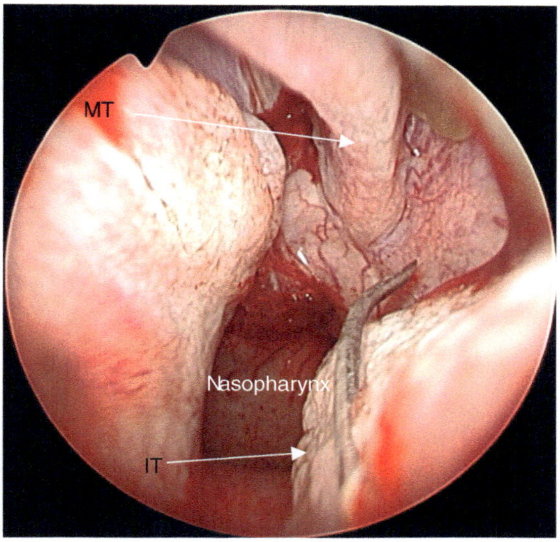

Fig. 1.10 Both figures are representing the site of local infiltration for the anterior ethmoid and the sphenopalatine neurovascular structure. *MT* middle turbinate, *IT* inferior turbinate (Courtesy—Dr. Hitesh Verma, Associate Professor, AIIMS, New Delhi, India)

2 cm from the midline in adults. Series of injections from central to medial brow block frontal nerve branches. After the injection, firm pressure is applied for better anesthetic spread and prevention of ecchymosis.

B. **Infraorbital Nerve Block**

It can be blocked by two routes: Extraoral and intraoral

1. Extraoral route: A longitudinal line is drawn along the pupil, another horizontal line along the ala of the nose. At the point of intersection, the needle is advanced in lateral-to-medial direction, as the foramen is directed medially and caudally.
2. Intraoral approach:-The needle is inserted into the canine fossa and the finger is kept over the infraorbital foramen to assess the proper location of the needle tip. 1–3 mL of local anesthetic is injected after negative aspiration (Fig. 1.11).

C. **Nasociliary Nerve (Anterior Ethmoid Nerve) Block**

It is blocked at the anterior ethmoidal foramen. A 26 G needle was inserted 1–1.5 cm above the medial canthus halfway between the palpebral fold and the eyebrow. The needle is directed forward and medially till it reaches the bony roof of the orbit. At a depth of 1.5–2 cm, the needle is at the level of the anterior ethmoidal foramen. 1–2 ml of local anesthetic solution is infiltrated (Fig. 1.12).

D. **Greater Palatine Nerve Block**

Greater palatine nerve supplies the lower part of the septum and floor of the nasal cavity. Greater palatine foreman is located 1 cm medial to second/third molar or 1.4–1.5 cm lateral to the maxillary suture line. The needle is inserted 0.5–1 cm and 1 cc of local anesthetic is applied (Fig. 1.13).

E. **Sphenopalatine Nerve Block**

Two approaches are recommended: Intraoral and intranasal approach.

1. Intraoral approach: Palpate the greater palatine foramen intraorally just medial to the second/third molar 5–7 mm anterior to the posterior margin of the hard palate. A needle bent 45° and advanced 2 cm in greater palatine foreman and 1–2 ml injected.
2. Intranasal approach: The nerve is blocked by injecting anesthetic solution near the

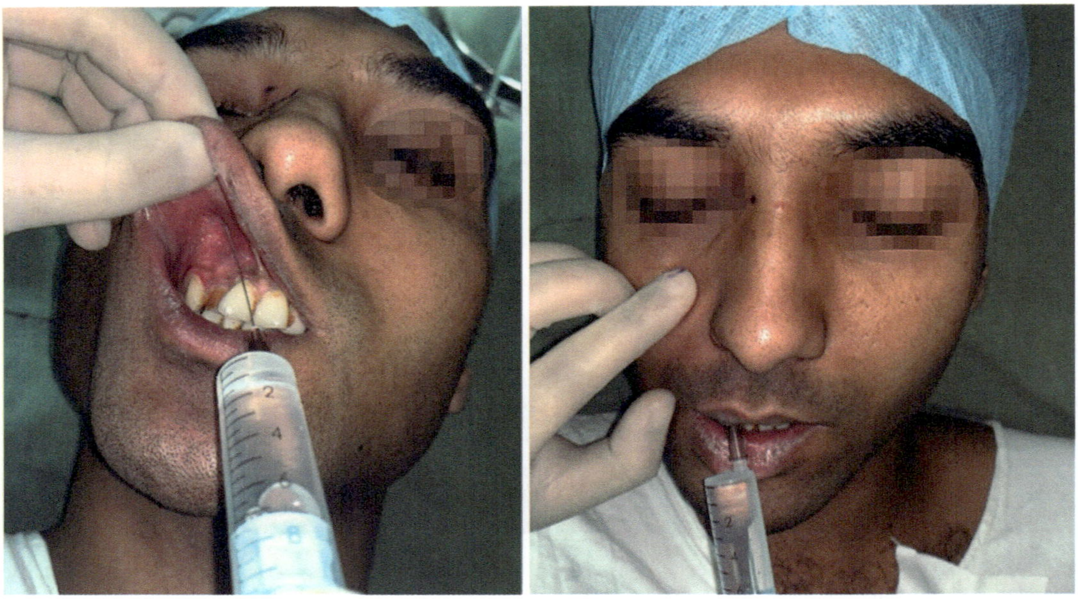

Fig. 1.11 Intraoral approach for infraorbital nerve block (Courtesy—Dr. Hitesh Verma, Associate Professor, AIIMS, New Delhi, India)

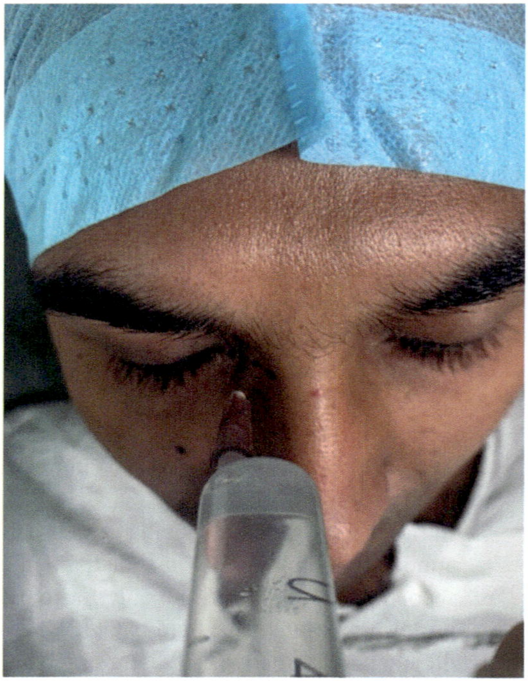

Fig. 1.12 Blue dotted line is marked from the inner canthus. 26 G needle is inserted 1 cm above the line (Courtesy—Dr. Hitesh Verma, Associate Professor, AIIMS, New Delhi, India)

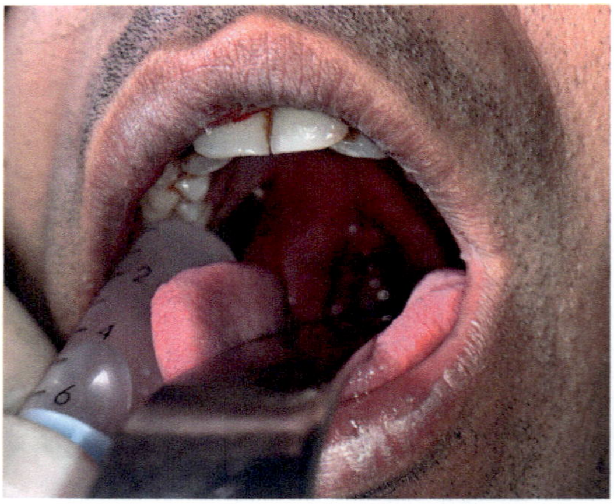

Fig. 1.13 The site of local infiltration is corresponding to the second and third molar for greater palatine nerve block (Courtesy—Dr. Hitesh Verma, Associate Professor, AIIMS, New Delhi, India)

sphenopalatine foramen region, near the posterior attachment of middle turbinate [10] (Fig. 1.10). Alternatively, cotton tipped soaked in the local anesthetic solution can be placed in the region and kept for 5–10 min (Sluder's) method.

F. **Maxillary Nerve Block**

The techniques for maxillary nerve block are external approcah, high tuberosity approach and greater palatine canal approach.

1. External approach—Needle is inserted just below the zygomatic arch at the midway of the coronoid and the condylar process of the mandible. It is inserted at the right angle to the skin till pterygoid plates are palpable. Local anasthetic is injected after minimal withdrawal of needle. The needle is pushed anteriorly towards the eye to reach the pterygopalatine fossa. 5 cc of the anesthetic drug is injected.
2. High tuberosity approach—Three centimeter insertion of the needle is done in the upper gingivobuccal sulcus at the level of second molar at 45° angle. 2 cc of the drug is needed to block maxillary nerve. For posterior superior nerve block, the needle is inserted at 2 cm depth.
3. Greater palatine canal approach—The needle is inserted till 3 cm depth in the greater palatine canal and 1.5–2 cc drug needs to be injected (Fig. 1.13).

Advantages of LA

1. Patient is conscious
2. Maintain airway
3. Smooth recovery
4. Less monitoring, less postoperative care, less expensive
5. Less pain medication required

Disadvantages of LA

1. Less operable time
2. Experience required
3. Accidental intravenous administration can induce generalized toxicity

Satisfactory application of the local anesthesia technique is the utmost requirement for the surgical execution, patient cooperation [11].

1.3 Part C: General Anesthesia

Endoscopic sinus surgery (ESS) is the primary approach used today for the surgical treatment of most of the rhinological illnesses e.g. chronic sinusitis, nasal polyposis. The surgical management of juvenile nasopharyngeal angiofibroma (JNA) has also got revolutionized with nasal endoscopic approaches; however, the extensive vascularity and vital structures nearby pose significant challenges for surgery as well as anesthesia [12]. Preoperative optimization including angioembolization of feeding vessel in high-grade JNA lessens the perioperative complications related to extensive blood loss. General anesthesia or TIVA maintaining a lower acceptable blood pressure (hypotensive anesthesia) is preferred. The anesthetic techniques should address specific concerns like stable hemodynamics during surgery, effective management of blood loss, adequate analgesia, and smooth emergence. A good perioperative multimodal analgesia is associated with better emergence.

1.3.1 Preoperative Concerns

The possibility of difficult airway should be assessed, which might be because of the distorted face due to swelling of the cheek, trismus, or inferior displacement of the soft palate by the bulk of tumor. Specifically in cases of JNA of higher grade, embolization of the terminal branches of the internal maxillary artery should ideally be done 24–48 h before surgery. Adequate blood and blood products should be cross-matched. Premedication is done with anxiolytic (benzodiazepine), the night before and morning on the day of surgery. Perioperative steroid administration is done to decrease mucosal edema and improve endoscopic visibility during surgery.

1.3.2 Anesthesia Technique

General anesthesia or Total Intravenous Anesthesia (TIVA) with oral cuffed endotracheal tube is preferred in such cases. In the case of FESS laryngeal mask airways (LMA) have also been used successfully by experienced anesthesiologists. Two large-bore (16 gauze is preferred) IV cannulas are secured and one is preferentially placed in the lower limb great saphenous vein, as the site is most easily accessed after positioning and placing the anesthesia workstation at the foot end. Routine American Society of Anesthesiologist (ASA) standard monitoring (electrocardiogram, plethysmography, and noninvasive blood pressure) is done. In case of JNA, invasive blood pressure monitoring is done by securing radial artery, anterior tibial, or dorsalis pedis artery so that beat to beat blood pressure can be monitored, and also serial blood gas sampling can be done at frequent interval. Peripherally inserted central catheter (PICC) is inserted through the antecubital vein preferably, as the neck is not accessible. It can be used for central venous pressure (CVP) monitoring and vasopressor administration if needed, as there is the anticipation of significant blood loss and hemodynamic instability. However in cases with intracranial extension, the subclavian vein is chosen for cannulation. Central venous access is often required for the infusion of irritant medications (concentrated potassium chloride) or vasoactive agents, certain diagnostic or therapeutic radiologic procedures, and in any patient for whom peripheral access is not possible. For cases with intracranial extension, N2O should be used cautiously or avoided as there is the chance of increase in ICP, although hyperventilation, barbiturates, benzodiazepines, or narcotics can attenuate the effects. In these cases, hypotensive anesthesia is also avoided, as it might impair the cerebral perfusion, because of swelling and rise in ICP. The airway is secured with cuffed endotracheal tube (South Pole Ring Adair Elwin or Armored tube) preferred over standard tube after muscle relaxant [13].

Patients with difficult airways require video laryngoscope or fiberoptic bronchoscope intervention for securing the airway. These should be explained to the patient in preoperative visit and informed consent should be taken. Positive end expiratory pressure (PEEP) is avoided. Throat packing with roller gage is done to reduce the blood contamination of the airway and at the end of surgery, it should be removed after thorough suctioning. Normothermia is maintained by infusing warm fluids through the hotline and also by the use of warming blankets. The urinary bladder is catheterized, so that hourly urine output of around 0.5–1 ml/kg can be maintained with adequate volume resuscitation. Local anesthetic with vasoconstrictor (1:100,000 adrenaline or phenylephrine drops) is either instilled topically or infiltrated. However caution should be applied in patients with hypertension, coronary artery disease as systemic absorption of these drugs causes hypertension, tachycardia, and arrhythmias. Ideally, the dose of phenylephrine should not exceed 4 drops of 0.25% preparation (0.5 mg) in adults or 20 mcg/kg in children upto 25 kg of body weight. If hypertension is severe after local vasoconstriction, direct vasodilator or α_2—antagonists are administered. Cough and straining during light plane increase the bleeding, so adequate depth of anesthesia is very essential. Blood loss is managed with crystalloids, colloids, packed red blood cells, fresh frozen plasma, and platelets.

1.3.3 Hypotensive Anesthesia

Deliberate decrease of systemic blood pressure below 20% of normal or maintenance of systolic blood pressure 85–90 mmHg with mean arterial blood pressure (MAP) at 60 ± 5 mmHg helps to provide a dry surgical field by decreasing the oozing and blood loss [9]. This can be achieved with reverse Trendelenburg position at 30 degrees with flexed knees. For maintenance of higher minimum alveolar concentration, (MAC) isoflurane or other inhalational agent is required. Total intravenous anesthesia is possible with propofol and fentanyl or remifentanil with the added advantage of decrease of sympathetic response during intubation or surgical stimulation. α-agonists such as clonidine and dexmedetomidine infusion decreases the central sympathetic outflow, thereby helps to induce controlled hypotension. It also decreases the requirement of anesthetic agent. Nitroglycerine and sodium nitroprusside infusion, by vasodilatation reduce the peripheral vascular resistance. Beta-blockers like esmolol, labetalol, or metoprolol, and calcium channel blockers also help to maintain hypotension. Magnesium sulfate infusion also helps to induce hypotension and helps to reduce blood loss, however, it might prolong the anesthesia emergence time [14].

1.3.4 Acute Normovolemic Hemodilution

It can be used as a technique for blood conservation strategies. After induction of anesthesia, blood is withdrawn upto a limit of 7 g% hemoglobin, and subsequently, crystalloids and colloids are infused to maintain the blood volume. Intraoperative red blood cell salvage is not done as there is chance of contamination by nasal flora. Blood loss is carefully estimated by counting the number of gauze pieces used and from the suction bottle. End tidal CO2 is maintained to prevent any hypercarbia or hypocapnia. Normothermia is maintained for the proper functioning of platelets and coagulation factors.

1.3.5 Juvenile Nasopharyngeal Angiofibroma with Intracranial Extension

Patients with Radkowski Grade III tumors are usually require combined approach with the neurosurgery team. Intraoperative blood loss is an predicting factor for better Glasgow Outcome scale, so these cases should be planned with multidisciplinary approach involving the neurosurgeon, intervention radiologist, and anesthesiologist, so that there will be minimal blood loss and stable hemodynamics perioperatively [12, 15]. Such cases are kept intubated and put on mechanical ventilatory support to maintain the end tidal carbon dioxide (EtCO2), as hypercarbia can cause cerebral vasodilatation and subsequent rise in intracranial pressure (ICP). The extensiveness of the surgery with massive blood loss, postoperative mechanical ventilation with intensive care unit (ICU) stay should be explained in informed consent.

1.3.6 Emergence from Anesthesia

Smooth recovery of anesthesia is warranted to prevent any straining and bleeding. The throat pack is removed after suctioning of the oral cavity and it is better to do under either direct laryngoscope or video laryngoscope. Postnasal space should be carefully evaluated to remove any blood clots. Administration of esmolol or lignocaine prevents extubation response. Decompression of the stomach with an orogastric tube should be performed prior to extubation to remove the blood clots, which is a predisposing factor for postoperative nausea and vomiting. In cases with massive blood loss or high-grade JNA with intracranial extension, patients are kept intubated and mechanically ventilated to avoid any rise of ICP by hypercarbia. Dexamethasone is administered 0.1 mg/kg to decrease airway edema by surgical trauma. Extubation should be done in controlled environment with adequate hemostasis, stable coagulation status, and hemodynamics [16].

1.3.7 Postoperative Concerns

Patients should be kept in closed observation with monitoring of vitals. Postoperative hemogram should be done to ensure adequate replacement of blood loss.

For Nausea and Vomiting:

- The presence of blood in the stomach, inflammation of the uvula and throat and the occasional use of opioids for pain control is contributing factors. Intraoperatively ondansetron and dexamethasone are administrated as a prophylactic measure.

Postoperative Pain:

- The expected postoperative pain from FESS may range from mild to moderate and is due to surgical trauma as well as nasal packing. Oral acetaminophen and an NSAID/cyclo-oxygenase 2 inhibitor usually provide safe and effective analgesia. Encourage the patient to breathe through the mouth due to the presence of nasal packing. The patient should have counseled in the preoperative visit.

1.3.8 Emergency Surgical Intervention

Sometimes there is postoperative orbital hematoma or might be progressive deterioration of vision warranting a relook for hemostasis. In such situation airway is secured by rapid sequence intubation with anticipation of blood in the oral cavity and difficult mask ventilation. The wide bored suction catheter should be kept ready during securing of airway. Invasive monitoring is continued in the perioperative period. Arterial blood gas analysis should be done to know the current hematocrit, lactate levels, and electrolytes. Sometimes patients with JNA present with epistaxis in the causality, which might be resistant to traditional compression or vasoconstrictor drops. Such cases need emergency embolization and subsequent diagnostic procedures, so that excision can be planned. In such cases with epistaxis, the airway is secured by rapid sequence induction followed by intubation with cuffed endotracheal tube.

1.4 Part D: FESS

Chronic rhinosinusitis is defined as inflammation of the nose and paranasal sinuses which generally lasts for more than 3 months. It is characterized by two or more symptoms, one of which is either nasal discharge or blockage/obstruction/congestion along with the presence or absence of either facial pain or reduction of the sense of smell. Treatment of CRS mostly involves medical therapy with surgery reserved for those cases where symptoms persist in spite of adequate medical therapy. Functional Endoscopic Sinus Surgery (FESS) aims to restore mucociliary function by restoring physiologic sinus ventilation and drainage. A proper diagnosis of the condition by thorough history, clinical examination, Endoscopy, imaging is necessary. Correct knowledge of the endoscopic anatomy, its variations, and steps of surgery aids in the successful outcome of the surgery. With advances in better understanding of disease and the introduction of newer antibiotics along with better endoscopes, the treatment of CRS has greatly revolutionized. Among the various options available for surgery it may range from Mini FESS, i.e., middle meatal antrostomy and anterior ethmoidectomy to full FESS with the opening of frontal, sphenoid, and complete ethmoidectomy. More recent advances have come like balloon sinus dilatation to the use of high-powered drills and computer navigation system. The use of the appropriate surgical technique will depend on proper evaluation of disease, its extent, and the expertise available. Here in this chapter, we would briefly discuss the steps of FESS, with emphasis on various techniques, complications, and recent advances.

1.4.1 Diagnostic Endoscopy

A careful diagnostic endoscopy is the key for successful diagnosis and planning for surgery. It is of two types anterior to posterior (**Messerklinger** technique) and posterior to anterior (Wigand technique). In anterior to posterior, it consists of three passes. In first Pass, The 0° endoscope (or 30° endoscope) passes along the floor of the nasal cavity between the inferior turbinate and septum. The structures studied are nasal septum, inferior turbinate and inferior meatus, nasal cavity anterior and inferior to the middle turbinate, posterior choana, posterior wall and roof of the nasopharynx, eustachian tube, fossa of Rosenmueller, and nasolacrimal duct. In second Pass, The scope passes medial to the middle turbinate. Structures studied are the space medial to middle turbinate, anterior face of sphenoid sinus, sphenoid ostium, superior turbinate and meatus, sphenoethmoidal recess. In third Pass, it is done to examine the contents of the middle meatus (Fig. 1.14). The scope is gently

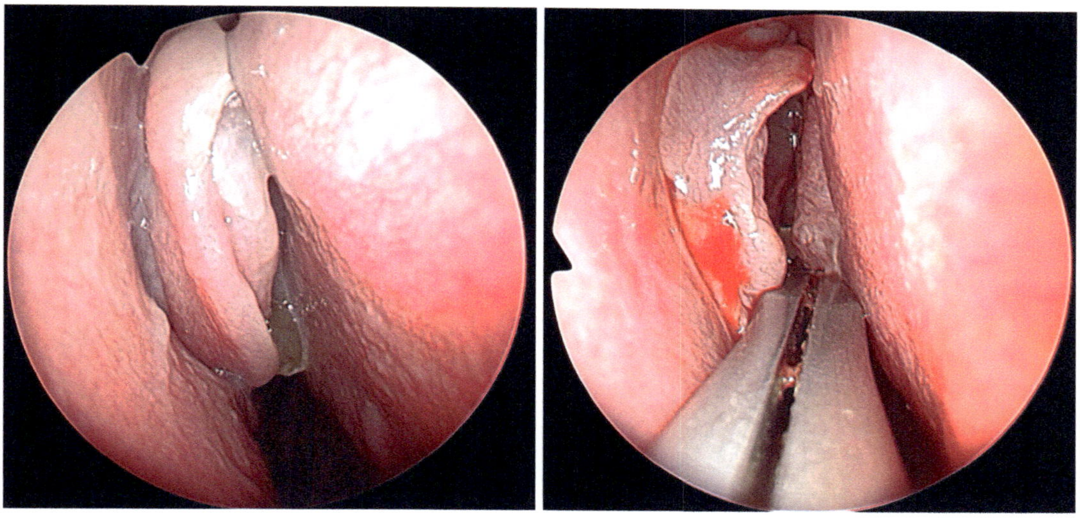

Fig. 1.14 Diagnostic nasal endoscopy is showing right polypoidal uncinate process with polyp in middle meatus is visible after removal of polyps (Courtesy—Dr. Hitesh Verma, Associate Professor, AIIMS, New Delhi, India)

passed into the middle meatus, the adjacent lateral nasal wall. The structures studied are middle turbinate, uncinate process, ethmoid bulla, ground lamella, and any variations or pathological process [17]. Wigand approach (posterior to anterior) is the diagnostic technique in revision surgery. It starts from choana then the identification of sphenoid ostia and follows skull base in retrograde fashion.

1.4.2 FESS Techniques and Steps

The classification of ESS based on the extent of surgery (Japanese Rhinologic Society, 2013)

- Type I removal of the ostiomeatal complex;
- Type II single-sinus procedure
- Type III polysinus procedure
- Type IV pansinus procedure
- Type V the extended procedure beyond the sinus wall

Uncinectomy is the first step in FESS. The technique of doing uncinectomy by various methods depends on surgeons' training and personal preference [18].

1. *Traditional Method/Anterior to Posterior*
   It was first described by Messerklinger. It starts with identification of the anterior attachment of the uncinate. It is first incised off the lateral wall using sickle knife/freer's elevator, then incision is extended to release it from its anterior attachment to the lacrimal bone (Fig. 1.15). It can be dangerous by injuring to lamina papyracea resulting in prolapse of orbital fat. To overcome complications of orbital injury in lateralized/contracted UP in traditional method and NLD injury in swing door approach, two more approaches are futher introduced.
   (a) *Uncinectomy Through the Anterior Nasal Fontanelle*
   Anterior fontanelle is membranous structure located between the lower and middle concha. It separates the maxillary sinus and the nasal cavity only by the mucosa. This approach allows complication free maxillary sinus exposure in selected cases.
   (b) *Uncinectomy Through Posterior Fontanelle*
   The posterior fontanelle is located between the tails of the middle and inferior turbinate, behind the hiatus semilunaris, and

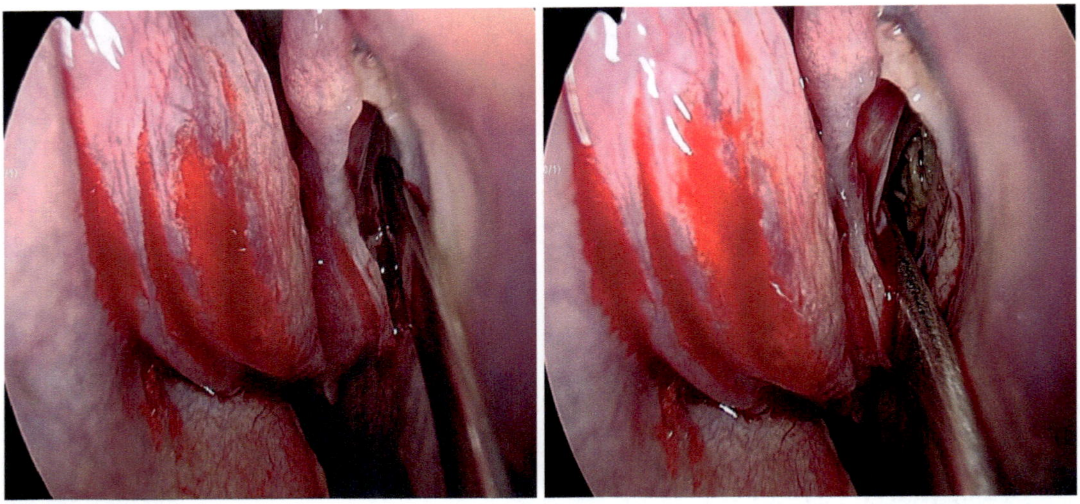

Fig. 1.15 Freer's elevator is used for antero-posterior uncinectomy. Ethmoid infundibulum is opened and fungal muck is visible through maxillary sinus ostia (Courtesy—Dr. Hitesh Verma, Associate Professor, AIIMS, New Delhi, India)

under the ethmoid bulla. It is mainly composed of soft tissue as a part of the medial wall of the maxillary sinus. It is identified, as an iatrogenic opening. The wide antrostomy is performed by combining uncinectomy and removal of medilal wall of maxillary sinus.

2. *Swing Door Technique (retrograde uncinectomy)*
   Retrograde uncinectomy is initiated by identifying the posterior edge of uncinate process (Fig. 1.16). The retrograde uncinate window is made with small backbiting forceps. The uncinate process is removed inferiorly. The uncinate is swung forward using the ball probe and then removed with blakesley forceps. The advantage is less risk of injury to orbit but it can damage nasolacrimal duct when it runs in the free medial wall of the maxilla.

Middle meatal antrostomy is performed by the identification of maxillary sinus ostium, at the same level of inferior edge of the middle turbinate. The opening is widened posteriorly and inferiorly by removing mucosa [19]. If accessory ostia have previously been identified, surgical window and accessory ostium should be interconnected to avoid a subsequent recirculation phenomenon.

Maxillary sinusotomy is of four types (Fig. 1.17):

1. Infundibulotomy (uncinectomy): Removal of the uncinate process, preserving the mucosa of the natural maxillary ostium. The superior attachment of the uncinate can be left intact.
2. Type I—Enlarging the natural maxillary ostium posteriorly by less than 1 cm.
3. Type II—Antrostomy is opened 2 cm posteriorly and inferiorly.
4. Type III—Antrostomy is opened up to the posterior wall of maxillary antrum. anteriorly to the lacrimal sac, and inferiorly to the base of the inferior turbinate.

The natural ostium of bulla ethmoidalis lies postero-medial to the anterior face. It can be located using ball probe or curette. Anterior ethmoidectomy is initiated at antero-inferior part of bulla to avoid orbital and anterior ethmoid artery injury [20]. Bullectomy can be done by placing J curette in retrobullar recess followed by anterior fracture of bulla (Fig. 1.18). Anterior ethmoid artery generally runs intracranially but in 10% of cases, it can be found in suprabullar recess so one has to be careful using microdebrider to avoid injury to artery (Fig. 1.5). The anterior ethmoid artery is 1–2 mm posterior to

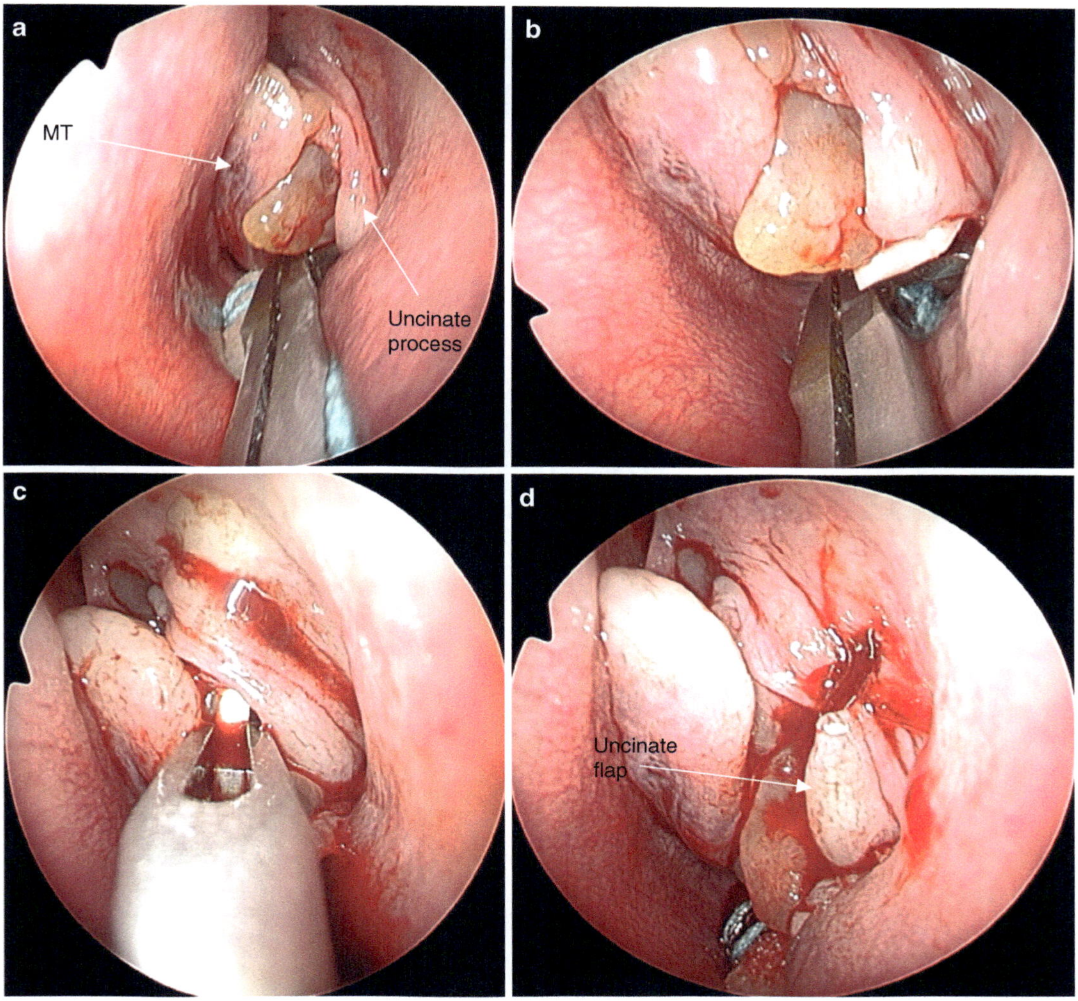

Fig. 1.16 (**a**) and (**b**) is showing site of lower cut in posterior to anterior technique. (**c**) is showing site of upper cut which can be vary in the relationship of exposure needed. (**d**) is showing uncinate flap generated after both cuts (Courtesy—Dr. Hitesh Verma, Associate Professor, AIIMS, New Delhi, India)

the superior limit of the anterior wall of the bulla ethmoidalis. The distance between the artery and the middle turbinate axilla is 17–20 mm. Mini-ESS is performed by uncinectomy and opening of the bulla with preservation of 3 or 4 mm of the anterior and inferior edge of the bulla. If a posterior ethmoidectomy is required. Complete anterior ethmoidectomy should be done.

For post ethmoidectomy, ground lamella is perforated in infero-medial quadrant (Fig. 1.19). It minimizes the risk of injury to the skull base or lamina papyracea.

The preservation of vertical sagittal and horizontal lateral attachment is required to maintain the stability of middle turbinate. Few situations where partial or total resection of the middle turbinate is necessary are

- Concha Bullosa
- Polypoidal middle turbinate
- Lateralized Atrophic Middle Turbinate
- Lateral displacement of the middle turbinate with narrowing of the frontal recess to create the wide exposure in extended endoscopic appraoches

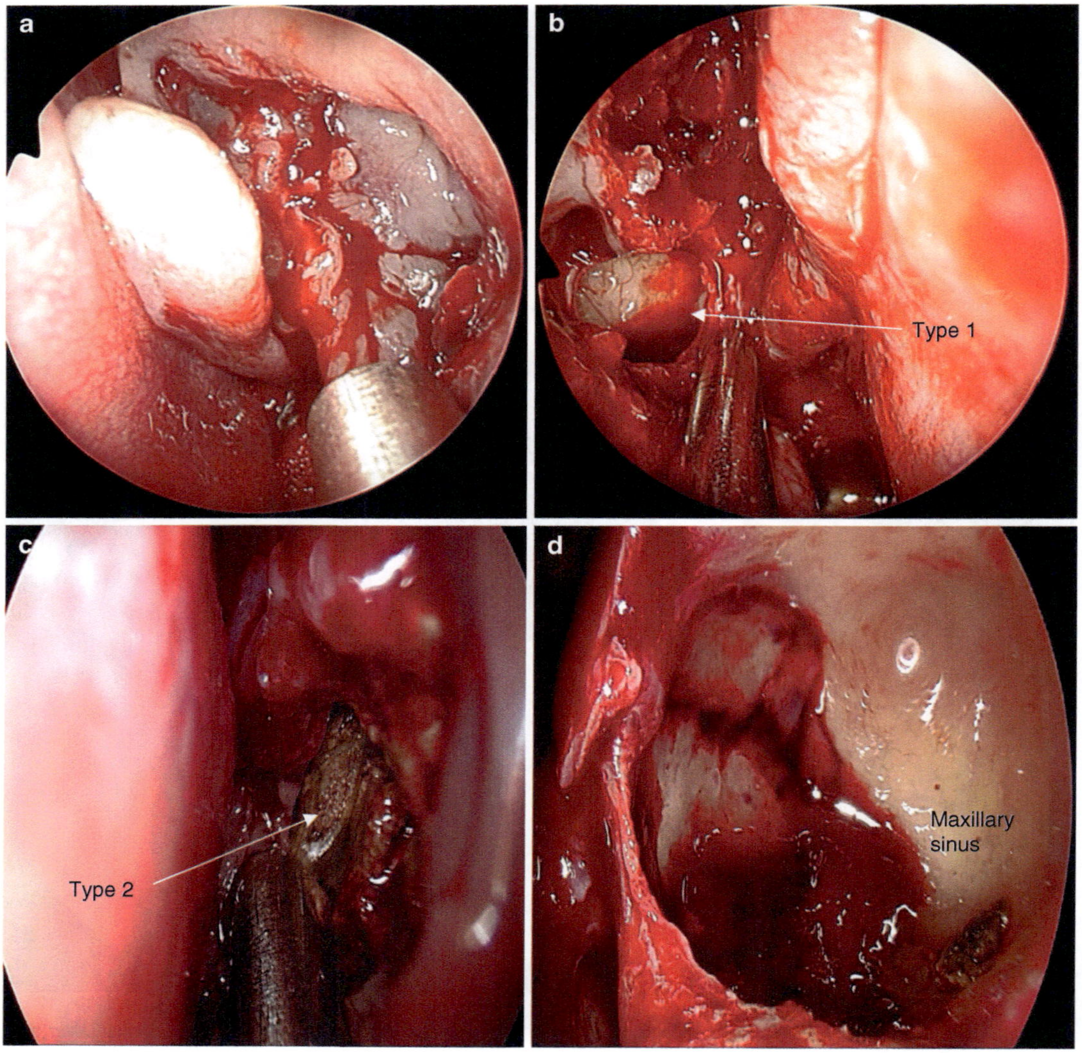

Fig. 1.17 (**a**) is representing view after complete uncinectomy. (**b**) is showing visibility of maxillary sinus after type 1 enlargement. Figure (**d**) is showing inside view of the maxillary sinus after type 3 enlargement (Courtesy—Dr. Hitesh Verma, Associate Professor, AIIMS, New Delhi, India)

The detail study of preopertive radiology helps in mapping the anatomy of posterior ethmoid sinus, presence of Onodi cell, and course of optic nerve.

Surgery of Frontal Sinus—Three distinct philosophies for surgical management of chronic rhinosinusitis affecting the frontal sinus and frontal recess is proposed by P J Wormald [21].

1. Minimal Invasive Sinus Technique (MIST)—Frontal sinusitis is developed secondary to refactory anterior ethmoid disease. Inferior uncinectomy and anterior ethmoidectomy is performed to clear the frontal recess. Clearance of disease in the ostiomeatal complex allows resolution of disease in the frontal sinus and frontal recess.
2. Frontal sinusitis is formed due to frontal recess involvement. Complete uncinectomy, anterior ethmoidectomy with removal of agar nasi and frontoethmoid cells is performed to clear the outflow tract of frontal sinus.

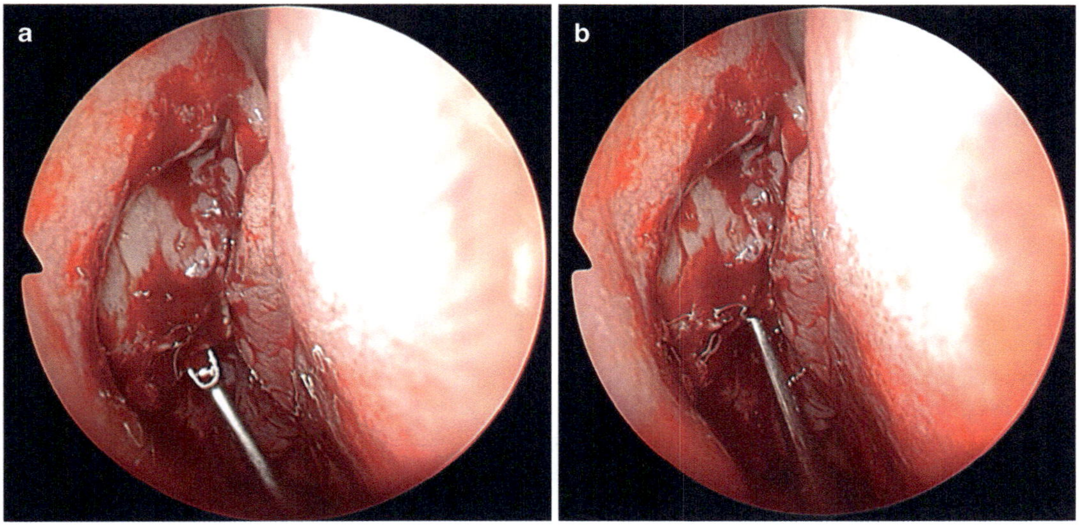

Fig. 1.18 The instrument is indicating site of entry in bulla ethmoidalis. J curette is placed in retrobullar recess for postero-anterior bullectomy (Courtesy—Dr. Hitesh Verma, Associate Professor, AIIMS, New Delhi, India)

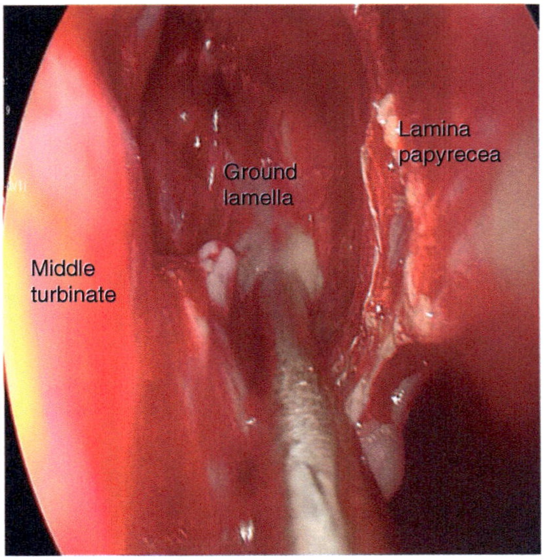

Fig. 1.19 The suction tip is indicating site of entry in posterior ethmoid after anterior ethmoidectomy in the left nasal cavity (Courtesy—Dr. Hitesh Verma, Associate Professor, AIIMS, New Delhi, India)

3. Complete exteriorization of cells of osteomeatal complex with wide frontal sinusotomy is indicated in refractory frontal sinusitis.

Instruments and techniques require viewing of frontal Sinus are listed here.

1. HRCT (nose and paranasal sinuses)- 1 mm cuts are prepared to assess the antero-posterior (AP) diameter of frontal recess, type of frontoethmoidal cells, degree of pneumatization frontal sinus. Bony remodeling and scarring of frontal outflow tract in revision surgery needs mapping and scarring created by previous surgery in frontal recess. Two-dimensional CT Scans in coronal, parasagittal, and axial planes are used to create a three-dimensional picture of the anatomy of the frontal recess.
2. Angled endoscopes are required to see the frontal sinus.
3. Axillary flap technique—It starts by removal of the anterior wall of the agger nasi cell. The flap is created by making incision 8 mm above the axilla of middle turbinate and brings 8 mm forward, turned down vertically 1–1.5 cm, and turned back under the axilla on to the roof of the middle turbinate. The mucosal flap is based medially on middle turbinate and is replaced at the end of the procedure to cover the raw exposed bone to prevent granulation and fibrosis formation. Direct examination of frontal sinus is possible after the removal of frontal beak.
4. Frontal sinus mini-trephination (mentioned in the chapter on frontal sinus).

5. Computer-aided surgery (CAS, or image guidance surgery), radiological probing (C arm) are helpful in localizing frontal sinus in difficult cases.

    1. Extensive nasal polyposis
    2. Revision surgery
    3. Distorted endoscopic anatomy
    4. Extended endoscopic or open procedures

Endoscopic management of frontal sinus diseases is classified by Draf into three types [22].

- Type-1 is Simple Drainage (DRAF1)—It is characterized by complete removal of the anterior ethmoid cells and uncinate process and obstructive frontal cells inferior to frontal ostium. The indication is limited frontal sinusitis with intractable ethmoid sinusitis.
- Type-2 Extended Drainage (DRAF 2)—It is subdivided into type IIa and IIb approaches. In type 2a, complete removal of the floor of frontal sinus from lamina papyracea to middle turbinate is performed. In type 2b, frontal sinus floor is removed from the lamina papyracea till the nasal septum. The indications are complicated frontal sinusitis, muco or pyocele, and benign tumour extending into the frontal sinus.
- Type-3 Endonasal median Drainage (DRAF 3)—Entire floor of both side of frontal sinus is removed. The limit is from one side lamina papyracea to the other side (Fig. 1.20). The indications are revision surgery, intractable frontal sinusitis and polyposis in ciliary dysfunction syndromes (Kartagener's syndrome, mucoviscidosis, etc.) and benign and malignant tumour.

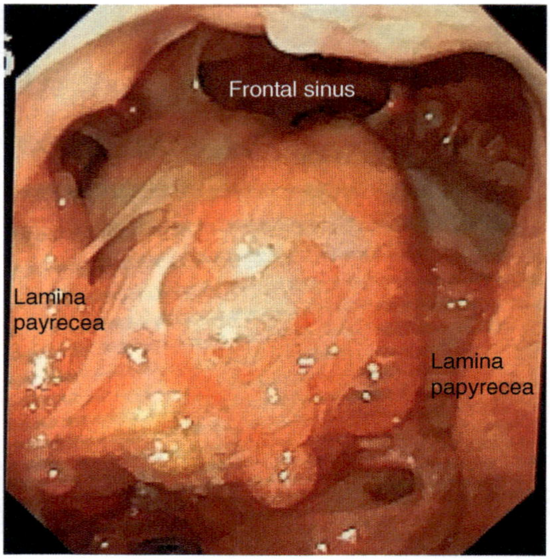

Fig. 1.20 The postoperative cavity after DRAF 3 procedure (Courtesy—Dr. Hitesh Verma, Associate Professor, AIIMS, New Delhi, India)

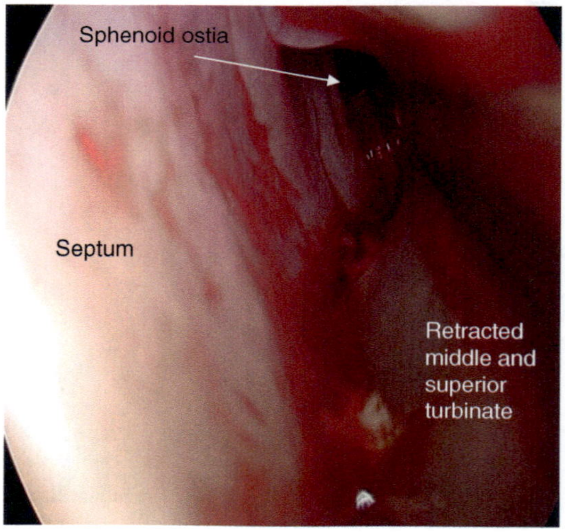

Fig. 1.21 The figure is depicting sphenoid ostia in the left nasal cavity after lateralization of middle and superior turbinate (Courtesy—Dr. Hitesh Verma, Associate Professor, AIIMS, New Delhi, India)

Sphenoid sinus is the posterior-most sinus and the landmarks for sphenoid sinus ostium and sphenoid sinus are (Fig. 1.21):

1. Ten–fifteen millimetre above the upper end of bony posterior choanae.
2. Maxillary ridge is an imaginary line between the medial and inferior wall of the orbit and it extends backwards from the upper border of the maxillary ostium. Sphenoid sinus is lying below it and ethmoid cell above it.
3. Seven centimeter from anterior nasal spine at 30° angle superiorly.
4. Four–five millimetre lateral to septum.
5. Sphenoid sinus floor is not visible whereas posterior ethmoid sinus floor is always in view.

The sphenoid sinus can be accessed by medial route (medila to middle turbinate) and lateral route (lateral to middle turbinate) after ethmoidectomy transethmoid approach. In intermediate approach, the lower half of superior turbinate is removed to get access in the sinus. The sinus ostium is lies half the distance between the superior and inferior border on the anterior wall of the sphenoid. Sinus ostium is gently widened in infero-medial direction in the intial step of widening to examine the spehnoid sinus lateral wall structures and to prevent inadvertent injury to perisinus structures. Posterior nasal branch of sphenopalatine artery may injure during inferior widening which can be prevented by pushing mucosa inferiorly before removing the bony wall. Caution to be taken for the posterior attachment of intersphenoid septa and accessory septa. Natural dehiscence of the optic nerve and internal carotid artery is always keep in mind while removing disease and violating septas. Onodi cell is the posterior extension of posterior ethmoid cells over the sphenoid sinus and the optic nerve may be seen in its lateral wall [23]. Onodi cell is present above the imaginory line passes from the roof of maxillary sinus.

Robot-Assisted Surgery (RAS)
The robotic guidance system facilitates manipulation in the surgical field and full visualization of the face of the anterior skull base. It is hands-free semi-automated endoscope guidance for advanced applications in surgery of the paranasal sinuses and the anterior skull base [24]. The literature is emerging on it.

Simulation/Three-Dimensional Tracking
It has been used for surgical training but the lack of practicality and haptic feedback limits widespread use. Three-dimensional printing has revolutionized simulation, providing high-resolution models for patient-specific anatomy [25].

Navigation and Image-Guided Surgery
The system uses computerized tracking devices to monitor the position of endoscopic instruments in conjuction to the patient's anatomical landmarks. The location of these instruments is tracked by the machine with fitted navigation probe. The machine displayed images in all planes corresponding to the pateints anatomy prepared from prefeeded radiology (CT and/or MRI) in the system. The Indications are

1. Revision sinus surgery
2. Distorted surgical anatomy
3. Extensive nasal polyposis
4. Pathology involving the skull base

1.4.3 NASAL POLYP and FESS

- Functional endoscopic sinus suergery (FESS) is indicated for complicated sinusitis and chronic sinusitis with or without nasal polyposis, failed maximum medical management. FESS aims to improve sinus ventilation and drainage as well as removing polyps. The extent of surgery varies with the extent of disease, the surgeon's individual practice, and available technology.

1.4.4 AFRS and FESS

- Surgery is usually the first-line treatment for the management of AFRS. The goal of surgery is wide opened sinus ostium with complete removal of fungal muck and allergic mucin.

1.4.5 ESS in Pediatric Age Group

The Role of ESS is limited in pediatric chronic rhinosinusitis. It should be considered after a period of medical management (and/or adenoidectomy) and after exclusion of underlying pathologies. If required, ESS should be limited to up to disease extent.

Absolute indications for ESS in children

- Complicated sinusitis
- Nasal polyposis
- Mucocoeles or mucopyocoeles
- Fungal rhinosinusitis

1.4.6 Balloon Sinuplasty

Balloon Sinuplasty technology uses a flexible, balloon catheter to open up the blocked sinus ostium, by inflation with a calibrated pressure gauge. When the sinus balloon is inflated optimally, it gently restructures the sinus ostium by inducing micro-fractures and bony displacement around the occluded ostium, thus circumferentially widening the walls of the ostium, while maintaining the integrity of the sinus mucosal lining around the ostium. The indication is chronic sinusitis limited mostly to ostial obstruction of the frontal, maxillary, and sphenoidal sinuses, with near-normal middle meatal integrity [26]. The advantages are

1. Preservation of the normal anatomy of the vital ostiomeatal complex, while precisely focusing on the occluded sinus ostium and the diseased sinus cavity beyond it.
2. Reduction in the invasiveness of the intervention, hospital stay, recovery time, postoperative debridement, postoperative medications, and office follow-up visits.

1.4.7 Conclusion

- Endoscopic sinus surgery is a remarkably safe and effective procedure. The knowledge of three-dimensional anatomies of sinuses, anatomical landmarks, and its variations is essential for the successful outcome.

1.5 Part E: Packing Materials for Nose and Paranasal Sinuses

Nasal mucosa has a rich vascular supply deriving branches both from the internal and external carotid artery system. Epistaxis is one of the commonest presentations in the accident and emergency room. It is seen in all age groups including the elderly patients who often have other co-morbid conditions. A non-specialist may be required to do the initial management, therefore a stepwise algorithm should be available in emergency to minimize complications and in patient admission. Nasal bleeds can be either anterior or posterior. Mostly anterior bleeds can be managed with cauterization of the bleeding point after identification using either a headlight or an endoscope. Cauterization can be done either using silver nitrate (chemical cautery) or bipolar diathermy (electrical cautery). Traditionally nasal packing has been used in the emergency setting for control of bleeding, though with the availability of endoscopes which allows better visualization of bleeding point, it is less preferred. Hemostatic nasal packing is rarely required for anterior bleeds unless the bleeding and coagulation profile of the patient is deranged [27]. Whereas the source of posterior nasal bleeds is not easily identifiable in an emergency setting and may require nasal packing for emergent control of bleeding. Packing of the nose and para nasal sinuses may also be required in postoperative setting. Availability of various packing materials has made nasal packing less traumatic and unpleasant. Also use of some newer materials prevents nasal synechiae, hence preferred in the postoperative setting [28]. Other conditions requiring nasal packing include endoscopic sinus surgery, septal surgery, turbinate reduction, and reduction of nasal fractures. Though significant hemorrhage post-surgery is rare, small quantity of blood oozing out from the surgical site can cause significant anxiety to the patient.

The aim of this chapter is to introduce the reader to various such materials available and guide them about their utility and usage.

1.5.1 Uses of Nasal Packing

- Provision of hemostasis in cases of nasal surgery or epistaxis
- Intranasal support to bony or cartilaginous dorsum, nasal septum, middle turbinate, or mucosal surfaces
- Prevention of mucosal adhesions
- Induces hemostasis
- Tamponade effect
- Provision of moist environment for mucosal healing
- Steroid or antibiotic impregnation may achieve better surgical outcomes

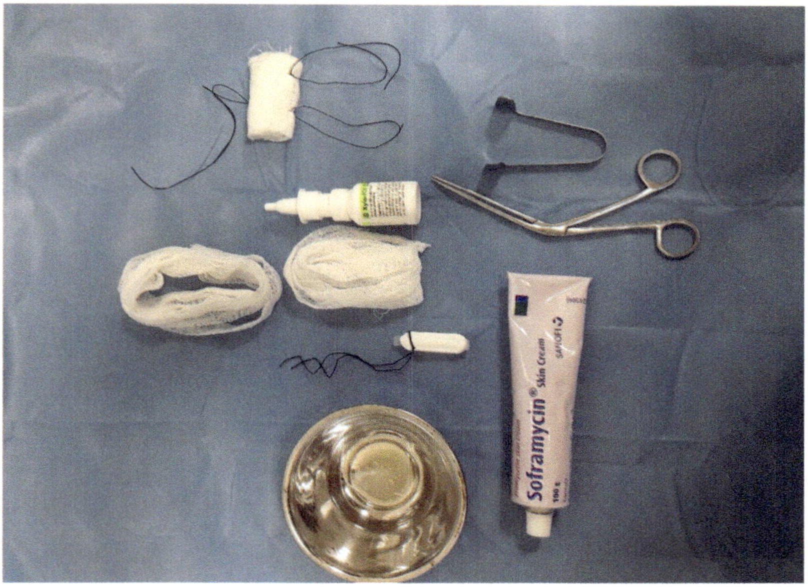

Fig. 1.22 Anterior and posterior nasal pack preparation

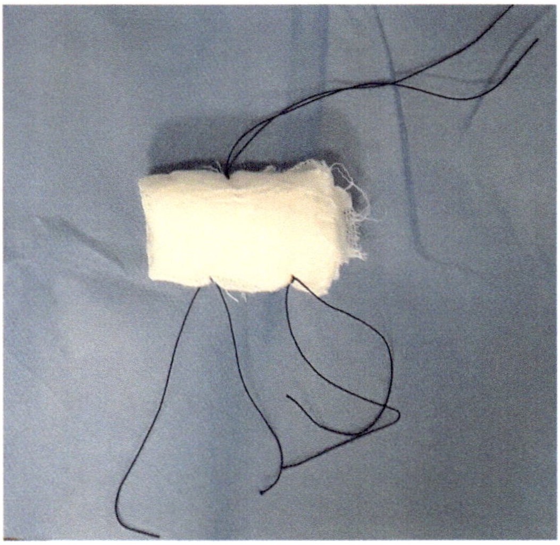

Fig. 1.23 Posterior nasal pack

1.5.2 Types of Nasal Packing Material

Traditional nasal packing is prepared from ribbon gauge. The anterior and posterior nasal packs are prepared differently for control of bleeding. Anterior packing consists of ribbon gauze of around a meter length soaked in antibiotic ointment or bismuth iodine paraffin paste (BIPP) and placed in the nasal cavity in layers.

Figure 1.22 shows the preparation required for placing ribbon gauze in the anterior nasal cavity. Posterior nasal packs are prepared using roller gauze to which tapes (or threads) are attached. Two rubber catheters are inserted through the right and left nasal cavities. The tapes on the posterior nasal pack are tied to the loose end of the rubber catheter. The pack is then pulled through the oropharynx in the posterior nasal cavity by withdrawing the rubber catheters through the nasal cavities. The tapes are then tied to each other over the columella over a small strip of gauze piece placed in between to prevent pressure necrosis. Though uncomfortable and requires experience for placement, it achieves good control of posterior epistaxis (Fig. 1.23).

In unexperienced hands, it can cause more traumas to the delicate nasal mucosa and aggravate bleeding especially in patients with coagulopathy. Choice of packing material used depends upon the inherent practice of the surgeon, cost, and availability. Both absorbable and non-absorbable materials are available.

1.5.3 Non-Absorbable Nasal Packs

Hydroxylated Polyvinyl Acetate Packs (PVA) Commonly used is Merocel which is

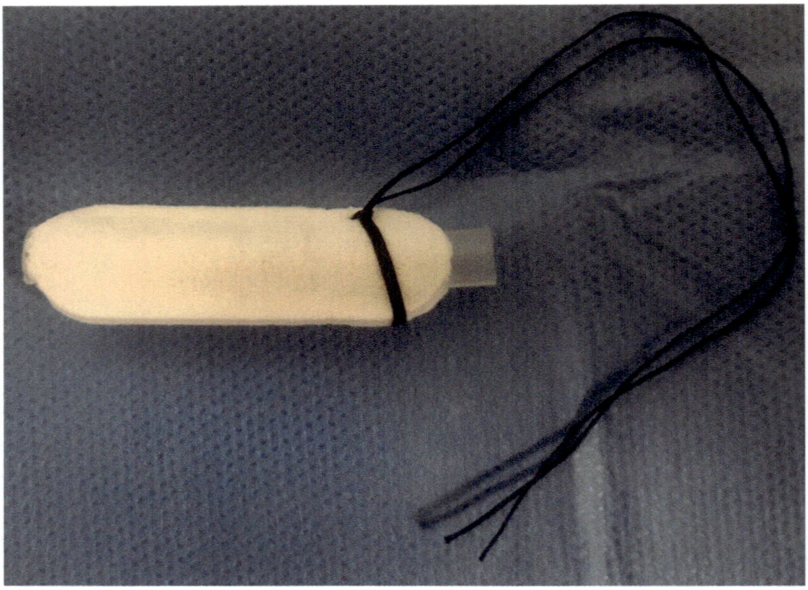

Fig. 1.24 Polyvinyl acetate nasal pack (Merocel)

available both with and without an external polyethylene coating (Fig. 1.24). Other PVA packs are Netcell packs. These compressed, dehydrated sponges are undergo expansion due to in situ rehydration with blood and nasal fluids and achieve hemostasis through tamponade. Increased localization of clotting factors is achieved which facilitates coagulation. Merocel packs laminated with polyethylene film are less adhesive to the surrounding nasal mucosa and thus less traumatic and painful during removal [29].

Rapid Rhino Device Nasal device consisting of inflatable polyvinylchloride nasal balloon with a carboxymethyl cellulose (CMC) infused hemostatic exterior to which an inflatable pilot cuff is attached (Fig. 1.25). Moist CMC forms a hydrocolloid gel and upon inflation with air conforms itself to the nasal cavity. It facilitates coagulation and provides a moist environment for the healing of traumatized nasal tissues. The pilot cuff is used to maintain a steady intranasal pressure to achieve compression for hemostasis and intranasal separation of tissues. It provides high volume and low-pressure tamponade on the nasal mucosa. Device models both with and without airway are available for control of unilateral and bilateral epistaxis and vary from 4.5 cm to 9 cm in length.

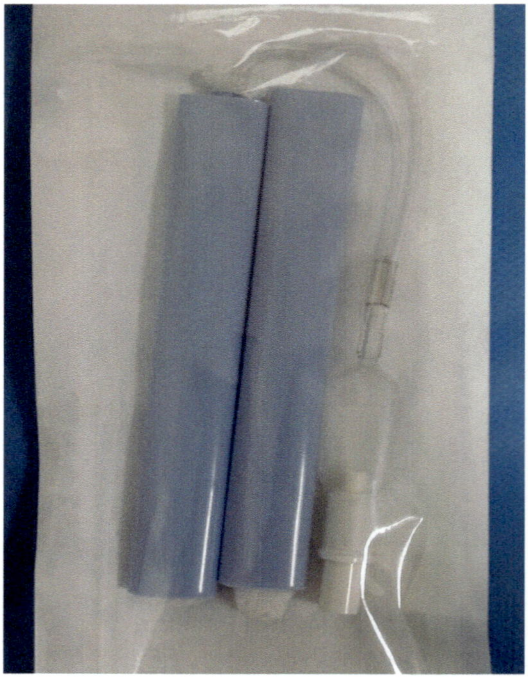

Fig. 1.25 Rapid Rhino device for bilateral nasal packing

Pain and bleeding during removal are minimized as hydrocolloid gel formed on the exterior makes only gentle contact with the nasal tissues without any adherence.

Algosteril It is a calcium alginate nasal pack that has both hemostatic and wound healing properties. It absorbs sodium ions within the nasal cavity and transforms into a hydrophilic sodium alginate gel which allows mucosal healing without adhering to it. It provides moist environment which facilitates epithelial regeneration. The calcium ions are discharged locally and facilitate the coagulation process. It also stimulates local platelet aggregation. Though it can be left in situ, removal becomes difficult due to fragmentation of the pack if kept beyond 24–48 h.

Petroleum Jelly Impregnated Gauze Strips These can cause hemostasis, however, pressure necrosis of mucosa, granuloma formation, bleeding upon removal have been reported.

Balloon Catheter Device It is specially designed device made of medical-grade silicone for control of anterior and posterior bleeding. The smaller balloon is inflated for control of posterior epistaxis and the larger balloon for anterior epistaxis. Normal saline is preferred for inflation of balloon as air leaks out through the silicon bulb thereby releasing the tamponade effect. The volume of normal saline used for inflation depends upon the pressure required for the tamponade of vessels. An integrated airway in the device provides a channel for breathing making them more acceptable to the patient. A Foley's catheter of size 12 F or 14 F can be used for posterior epistaxis control when such specialized devices are not available (Fig. 1.26). Overinflation of posteriorly placed balloon can cause inferior displacement of soft palate resulting in gagging and problems with deglutition. Mucosal necrosis is more common as compression is over a larger surface area rather than direct compression of bleeding vessels. All patients with posterior packs require in patient admission for observation as posterior pack displacement can cause fatal airway obstruction, adequate pain relief, and monitoring of oxygenation. Broad-spectrum antibiotic cover to prevent toxic shock syndrome and rhinosinusitis should also be started.

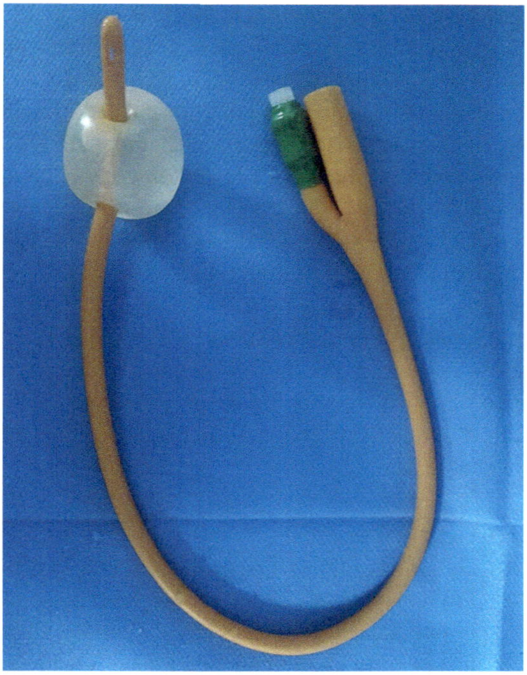

Fig. 1.26 Foley's catheter inflated with saline used for tamponade effect in the posterior choana

Advantages of Non-Absorbable Packs Insertion requires minimal training and thus preferred in an emergency setting. Benefits other than hemostasis include—prevention of formation of septal hematoma, synechiae, stabilization of septal cartilage, and middle turbinate [30].

Disadvantages of Non-Absorbable Packs Use of these packs requires in patient admission and antibiotic cover. Considerable pain, nasal blockade, and sleep disturbance occurs when these packs are in situ. Discomfort and bleeding during removal are often reported. Other problems encountered are—damage to the nasal mucosa, allergic reaction, and sinus infection. Toxic shock syndrome has also been reported when these packs are used without the antibiotic cover.

1.5.4 Absorbable Nasal Packs

Hyaluronic Acid (HA) Products (Merogel) It is a polymer consisting of esterified hyaluronic acid. Upon hydration, it transforms into a gel-like state within 24–48 h, provides hemostasis, keeps the mucosal surfaces apart, and provides a moist environment for healing [31, 32]. It is available both as a nasal foam stent and injectable nasal gel. A hybrid product consisting of HA (20%) and collagen (80%) also available. It has been found to induce osteoneogenesis in animal models which may not be a favored outcome in operated nasal cavities. Hyaluronan hydrogel is a recently available agent in this group and has shown better epithelialization in postoperative setting.

Collagen Derived Products These are derived from bovine or porcine collagen. They expand upon contact with blood to provide tamponade effect and activate coagulation cascade. They are available as:

(a) Gelatin film.
(b) Gelfoam which is its sponge form (Fig. 1.27).
(c) FloSeal—It is a viscous gel prepared by combining gelatin granules with human thrombin just prior to use and applied topically with an applicator. Easy bedside preparation, good hemostasis, less chances of re-bleeding, no requirement of antibiotic cover or hospital admission, and better acceptance by the patients favor its use over standard nasal packing in emergency setting. Due to incorporation into the healing mucosa, adhesion formation has been noted with its use [33].

Fibrin Glue It is a surgical sealant consisting of pooled human origin coagulation products. It is prepared by combining thrombin (bovine origin) reconstituted with calcium chloride and fibrinogen (lyophilized pooled human concentrate). It activates the coagulation cascade and attaches firmly to nasal tissues providing hemostasis. It causes minimal inflammation, granulation tissue formation, and crusting [34].

Biopolymers Synthetic and Natural Biopolymers Are Available:

1. **Synthetic Biopolymers**
   Nasopore—These are biodegradable, biologically inert fragmenting foam made of polyurethane that absorbs water and blood. Hemostasis is due to the compressive properties of polyurethane. It keeps the edematous mucosal surfaces apart during the initial healing phase thus preventing adhesion formation and provides adequate structural support. It starts to dissolve within days and can be suctioned from the nasal cavity after a few days [35].
   Polyethylene Glycol—It is a Thermosensitive product. It forms a hydrogel barrier in the operated nasal cavity which lasts for a week and prevents adhesion formation.

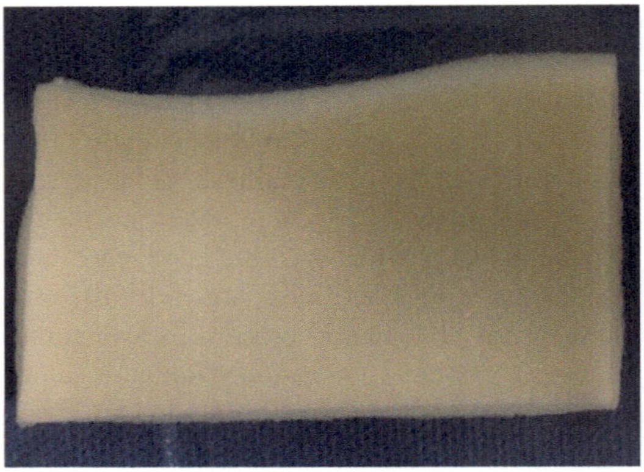

Fig. 1.27 Gelfoam, a sponge form of gelatin

2. **Natural Biopolymers**
   Carboxymethyl Cellulose (CMC) Nasal Dressings. Various CMC based products available are
   (a) Rapid Rhino Nasastent—5 cm intranasal splint which can be cut to the desired size and placed in the nasal cavity.
   (b) Rapid Rhino Sinu-Knit—a mesh-like fabric of CMC (Fig. 1.28).
   (c) Injectable Stammberger Sinu Foam—dry CMC fiber within a syringe which after contact with sterile water forms viscous foam that can be inserted into the nose.

Upon hydration with sterile water CMC turns into a hydrocolloidal gel which eventually drains out via the natural drainage pathway within ten days or can be removed with suction aspiration. The dense gel provides a moist hydrocolloid physical barrier which prevents postoperative bleeding and adhesions. Antibiotic ointments or any other liquids such as saline should be avoided as the gel formation and hemostatic properties get inhibited [36].

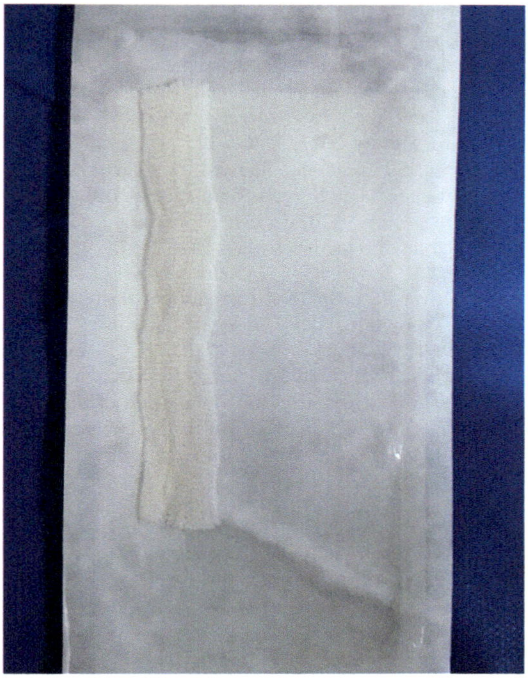

Fig. 1.28 Rapid Rhino Sinu-Knit—a mesh-like fabric of CMC

Oxidized Regenerated Cellulose It promotes platelet aggregation. It is preferably used for hemostasis in deeper regions of the nasal cavity which are difficult to access for direct vessel control. It creates an acidic environment which causes platelet activation and prevents bacterial growth. Resorption is prolonged and favors the formation of granulation tissue and adhesions.

Microporous Polysaccharide Beads These are derived from purified potato starch. These are available as an injectable powder consisting of spheres ranging from 10 to 200 μm. Due to porosity it extracts the fluid from the blood and increases the local concentration of platelets and coagulation factors.

Chitostan It is a hemostatic agent that is deacetylised polysaccharide derived from shellfish chitin. It is known to possess anti-fungal and anti-bacterial properties. It prevents adhesion formation by inhibiting fibroblast growth. It is available as aerosol and gel form.

Due to fragmentation, these absorbable nasal packs are easily removed using suction aspiration after 7–10 days thus cause less irritation of the inflamed nasal mucosa. Retention beyond 10 days may increase the chances of synechiae formation as the fragmented parts may get incorporated into the healing mucosa and facilitate epithelialization between the middle turbinate and lateral nasal wall [31]. Other benefits of absorbable packs include—increased patient comfort due to lack of feeling of nasal pressure, nasal blockade and headache, better mucosal healing. As formal removal is not required pain, discomfort, and bleeding associated with removal of non-absorbable packs are avoided.

References

1. Stemmberger H, Kennedy DW. Paranasal sinuses: anatomic terminology and nomenclature. Ann Otol Rhinol Laryngol. 1995;104:7–16.
2. Bent JP, Cuilty-Siller C, Kuhn FA. The frontal cell as a cause of frontal sinus obstruction. Am J Rhinol. 1994;8:185–91.
3. Gera R, Mozzanica F, Karligkiotis A, Preti A, Bandi F, Gallo S, Schindler A, Bulgheroni C, Ottaviani F, Castelnuovo P. Lateral lamella of the cribriform plate, a keystone landmark: proposal for a novel classification system. Rhinology. 2018;56(1):65–72.
4. Kainz J, Stammberger H. The roof of the anterior ethmoid; a place of least resistance in the skull base. Am J Rhinol. 1989;4:191–9.
5. Elwany S, Yacout YM, Talaat M, El-Nahaas M, Gunied A. Surgical anatomy of the sphenoid sinus. J Laryngol. 1983;97:227–41.
6. Wei S, Yu-Han Z, Wei-Wei J, Hai Y. The effects of intravenous lidocaine on wound pain and gastrointestinal function recovery after laparoscopic colorectal surgery. Int Wound J. 2020;17(2):351–62. https://doi.org/10.1111/iwj.13279.
7. Yilmaz AH, Ziypak E, Ziypak T, Aksoy M, Adanur S, Kocakgol H, Demirdogen SO, Polat O. Comparison of the effect of lidocaine versus a lidocaine-bupivacaine combination in a periprostatic nerve block undergoing transrectal ultrasound-guided prostate biopsy: a double-blind randomized controlled trial. Curr Urol. 2016;9(3):153–8.
8. McAlvin JB, Reznor G, Shankarappa SA, Stefanescu CF, Kohane DS. Local toxicity from local anesthetic polymeric microparticles. Anesth Analg. 2013;116(4):794–803.
9. Moskovitz JB, Sabatino F. Regional nerve blocks of the face. Emerg Med Clin North Am. 2013;31(2):517–27.

10. DeMaria S Jr, Govindaraj S, Chinosorvatana N, Kang S, Levine AI. Bilateral sphenopalatine ganglion blockade improves postoperative analgesia after endoscopic sinus surgery. Am J Rhinol Allergy. 2012;26(1):e23–7.
11. Beeson WH. The nasal septum. Otolarvngol Oin North Atli. 1997;20:743–67.
12. Ahmad R, Ishlah W, Azilah N, Rahman JA. Surgical management of juvenile nasopharyngeal angiofibroma without angiographic embolization. Asian J Surg. 2008;31(4):174–8.
13. Simpson P. Perioperative blood loss and its reduction: the role of the anaesthetist. Br J Anaesth. 1992;69(5):498–507.
14. Petrozza PH. Induced hypotension. Int Anesthesiol Clin. 1990;28(4):223–9.
15. Khanna P, Br R, Resident S, Sinha R. Anaesthetic management of endoscopic resection of juvenile nasopharyngeal angiofibroma: our experience and a review of the literature. South Afr J Anaesth Analg. 2013;19(6):314–20.
16. Bennett J, Haynes S, Torella F, Grainger H, McCollum C. Acute normovolemic hemodilution in moderate blood loss surgery: a randomized controlled trial. Transfusion. 2006;46(7):1097–103. https://doi.org/10.1111/j.1537-2995.2006.00857.x.
17. Kim DH, Seo Y, Kim KM, Lee S, Hwang SH. Usefulness of nasal endoscopy for diagnosing patients with chronic rhinosinusitis: a meta-analysis. Am J Rhinol Allergy. 2020;34(2):306–14. https://doi.org/10.1177/1945892419892157.
18. Puranik V, El-Sheikha A. Uncinectomy: Stammberger or swing-door technique? Eur Arch Otorhinolaryngol. 2007;264(10):1151–5.
19. Kim HJ, Ahn JC, Hong SN, et al. Posterior fontanelle approach for uncinectomy and middle meatal antrostomy in endoscopic sinus surgery. Laryngoscope. 2016;126:1311–4.
20. Schaefer SD, Li JC, Chan EK, Wu ZB, Branovan DI. Combined anterior-to-posterior and posterior-to-anterior approach to paranasal sinus surgery: an update. Laryngoscope. 2006;116(4):509–13.
21. Wormald PJ. Three dimensional building block approach to understanding the anatomy of the frontal recess and frontal sinus. Oper Tech Otolaryngol Head Neck Surg. 2006;17:2–5.
22. Weber R, Draf W, Kratzsch B, Hosemann W, Schaefer SD. Modern concepts of frontal sinus surgery. Laryngoscope. 2001;111(1):137–46.
23. Weber RK, Hosemann W. Comprehensive review on endonasal endoscopic sinus surgery. GMS Curr Top Otorhinolaryngol Head Neck Surg. 2015;14:Doc08. https://doi.org/10.3205/cto000123.
24. Friedrich DT, Sommer F, Scheithauer MO. An innovate robotic endoscope guidance system for transnasal sinus and skull base surgery: proof of concept. J Neurol Surg B. 2017;78:466–72.
25. Barber SR, Jain S, Son YJ. Virtual Functional Endoscopic Sinus Surgery Simulation with 3D-Printed Models for Mixed-Reality Nasal Endoscopy. Otolaryngol Head Neck Surg. 2018;159(5):933–7.
26. Zalzal HG, Makary CA, Ramadan HH. Long-term effectiveness of balloon catheter sinuplasty in pediatric chronic maxillary sinusitis. Ear Nose Throat J. 2019;98(4):207–11.
27. Melis A, Karligkiotis A, Bozzo C, Machouchas N, Volpi L, Castiglia P, et al. Comparison of three different polyvinyl alcohol packs following functional endoscopic sinus surgery. Laryngoscope. 2015;125:1067–71.
28. Douglas R, Wormald PJ. Update on epistaxis. Curr Opin Otolaryngol Head Neck Surg. 2007;15:180–3.
29. Wang YP, Wang MC, Chen YC, Leu YS, Lin HC, Lee KS. The effects of Vaseline gauze strip, Merocel, and Nasopore on the formation of synechiae and excessive granulation tissue in the middle meatus and the incidence of major postoperative bleeding after endoscopic sinus surgery. J Chin Med Assoc. 2011;74:16–21.
30. Verim A, Seneldir L, Naiboglu B, Karaca CT, Kulekci S, Toros SZ, et al. Role of nasal packing in surgical outcome for chronic rhinosinusitis with polyposis. Laryngoscope. 2014;124:1529–35.
31. Massey CJ, Singh A. Advances in absorbable biomaterials and nasal packing. Otolaryngol Clin N Am. 2017;50(3):545–63.
32. Valentine R, Wormald PJ, Sindwani R. Advances in absorbable biomaterials and nasal packing. Otolaryngol Clin N Am. 2009;42(5):813–28.
33. Chandra RK, Conley DB, Kern RC. The effect of FloSeal on mucosal healing after endoscopic sinus surgery: a comparison with thrombin-soaked gelatin foam. Am J Rhinol. 2003;17(1):51–5.
34. Iqbal IZ, Jones GH, Dawe N, Mamais C, Smith ME, Williams RJ, et al. Intranasal packs and haemostatic agents for management of adult epistaxis: systematic review. J Laryngol Otol. 2017;131:1065–92.
35. Weber RK. Nasal packing and stenting. Laryngorhinootologie. 2009;88(Suppl 1):139–55.
36. Kastl KJ, Betz CS, Siedek V, Leunig A. Effect of carboxymethylcellulose nasal packing on wound healing after functional endoscopic sinus surgery. Am J Rhinol Allergy. 2009;23:80–4.

Rhinoplasty Anatomy and Procedures

2

Arvind K. Kairo, Saurav Sarkar, Anindya Nayak, Prateek Sharma, and Rakesh Kumar

Contents

2.1 Part A: External Nasal Anatomy, Aesthetics and Photography

The external nose is pyramidal in shape. The root is continuing with the forehead and the apex is formed by a nasal tip. The nasal dorsum is part of the nose located in between the root and nasal tip. Dorsum elevation is slightly behind the line from nasion to tip defining point in female whereas in the male it is at the line. Nasal ala is the lower lateral surface of the external nose which is formed by alar cartilage and supportive tissue. Dome is the anterior projecting segment of lower lateral cartilage and anatomically, it is formed by the junction

A. K. Kairo · P. Sharma · R. Kumar (✉)
ENT, AIIMS, New Delhi, India
e-mail: winirk@hotmail.com

S. Sarkar · A. Nayak
ENT, AIIMS, Bhubaneswar, Odisha, India

H. Verma, A. Thakar (eds.), *Essentials of Rhinology*, https://doi.org/10.1007/978-981-33-6284-0_2

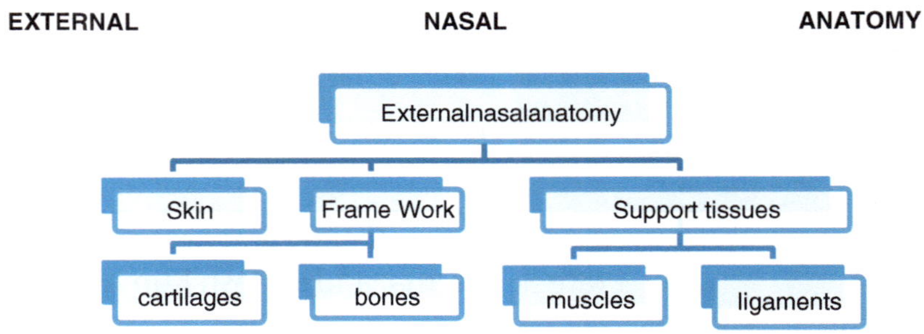

Fig. 2.1 The chart is showing various parts involve in the built-up of the nose

of middle and lateral crural of lower lateral cartilage [1, 2]. External nasal soft tissue anatomy can be divided into parts for easy understanding, i.e. skin, framework and supporting tissues (Fig. 2.1). Skin is separated from underlying bone and cartilage by four layer of tissue; the external most is the superficial fatty layer follow by the fibromuscular layer and deep fatty layer. Periosteum/perichondrium is the last layer that separates the skin from underlying bone/cartilage. The surgical plane is created deep to the perichondrium as blood supply for nasal framework runs in the deep fatty layer. The soft triangle is part of the nostril apex where outer dermis is in direct contact with the inner dermis without any deep tissue. Bony framework is the upper framework and it is formed by contribution of the nasal bone, frontal process of maxilla, and part of the frontal bone. The anterior nasal spine is a projection formed at the anterior most part of the intermaxillary suture line. Cartilaginous framework is formed by two alar and one septal cartilage. Septal cartilage is hooked in the midline by the maxillary crest. Nasal valve (10°–15°) is formed by anterior most end of the inferior turbinate, alar nasi (junction of upper and lower cartilage) and septum. In this chapter, surgically relevant and concise anatomy is given along with how to document and analyse the pre and postoperative changes.

Skin: For aesthetics, it is divided into subunits. These subunits are dorsum, lateral walls, tip and the alar region. Scar of any subunit should see as part of that subunit and should be dealt with accordingly. The thickness of the skin over the nasal dorsum is not even and its thickness keeps changing. It is mobile and thinner in the upper two-third part of the nose and adherent and thicker over the lower one-third part, thinnest at the junction of upper one-third and lower two-third. Thinner skin makes underlying anatomy more visible thus more precision is required in such patients. Postoperative results of the rhinoplasty surgery also depend on the thickness of the skin. When the patient has thick skin, slight imperfection can be hidden beneath the thick skin whereas thinner skin can show slight unevenness but results are not that much visible as visible in thin skin (Fig. 2.2).

Support Tissues

Overlying skin is attached to underlying bone and cartilage by different ligaments and other soft tissues like fat and muscle. If ligaments are severed during surgery, it should be mended at the end of the surgery. If the surgeon forgets this step then the stability of the dorsum will be compromised. Other soft tissue is subcutaneous fat, dermo-cartilaginous ligament (ligament of Pitanguy) and muscles. Eight nasal muscles have been described. Out of these, only two muscles, procerus and nasalis, are in a position to impact the nasal profile.

Blood Supply

Dorsum of the nose is very vascular especially in the central part where there is rich anastomosis of bilateral blood supplies. Unlike the major part of the face, it gets supplies from both external and internal carotid artery. The blood supply is from anterior ethmoids, dorsal nasal, columellar branches from superior labial and dorsal nasal artery from the angular artery. Columellar

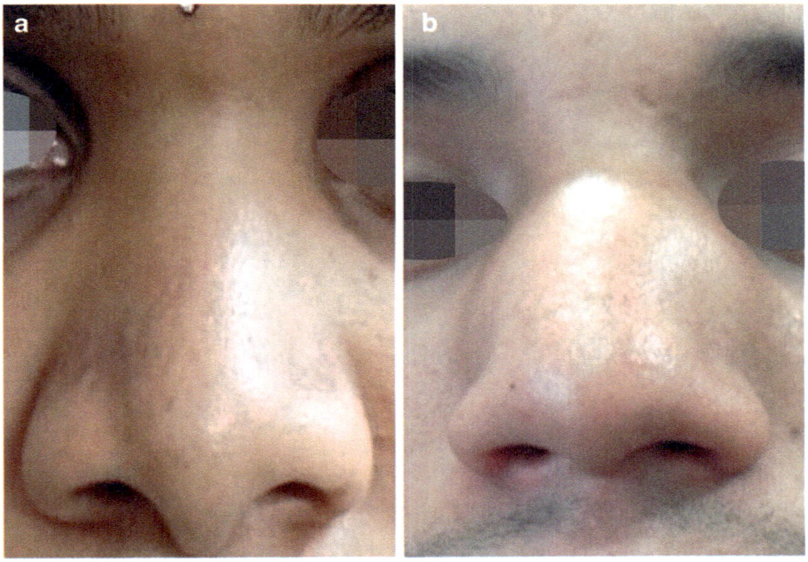

Fig. 2.2 The clinical photograph is showing the thin (**a**) and thick (**b**) skin types of patients. Figure (**b**) is showing wide nose in the middle and lower third whereas (**a**) it is in the normal range. (Courtesy—Dr. Hitesh Verma, Associate Professor, AIIMS, New Delhi, India)

branches and dorsal nasal arteries are anastomosis to form arcades over the dorsum of the nose. These arcades get damaged by excessive removal of soft tissue from dorsum.

Nerve Supply

Nerve supply follows the embryological origin of the area. The major part of the dorsum is supplied by first branch of the trigeminal nerve (ophthalmic) for sensory innervation. Some part of the lateral wall and the inner lining second branch of the trigeminal nerve (mandibular). For motor innervation, the facial nerve is a supplier. Dorsal nasal skin up to the tip is derived from branches of the trigeminal nerve (from branches of the supratrochlear and anterior ethmoidal nerve, branch of the ophthalmic nerve). The infraorbital nerve may also contribute branches to the lateral nasal walls, columella and vestibule. For endonasal mucosa—branches come from sphenopalatine ganglion.

Frame Work

The external nasal framework is divided into three nasal vaults [1, 2].

1 Upper one-third (Bony Vault)—It is formed by paired nasal bone and part of the frontal process of the maxilla (Fig. 2.3). Nasion is a midline point over the frontonasal suture line just superior to the root of the nose. Rhinion is the anterior tip at the end of the nasal bone suture line. Bony vault is narrowest and thickest at the intercanthal level. It requires osteotomies for correction.
2 Middle one-third (Upper Cartilaginous Vault)—Upper lateral cartilage is the main content in the middle vault. An area of tight synchondrosis between the bony and upper cartilaginous vault along with its attachment to the dorsal septum is known as key stone area (Fig. 2.3). Overlap of lower lateral cartilage with upper lateral cartilage is known as the scroll area (Fig. 2.3). Attachment of upper lateral cartilage with the dorsal septum forms the internal nasal valve, which can be improved by using spreader graft.
3 Lower one-third (Lower Cartilaginous Vault)—It is comprised of alar cartilage which is divided into three parts as medial, intermediate and lateral crural (Fig. 2.3). It is an essential part of the tip and its projection. Tip support is assessed by Tip recoil phenomenon. Tardy described nasal tip support mechanisms in major and minor groups
   (a) Major Tip Support

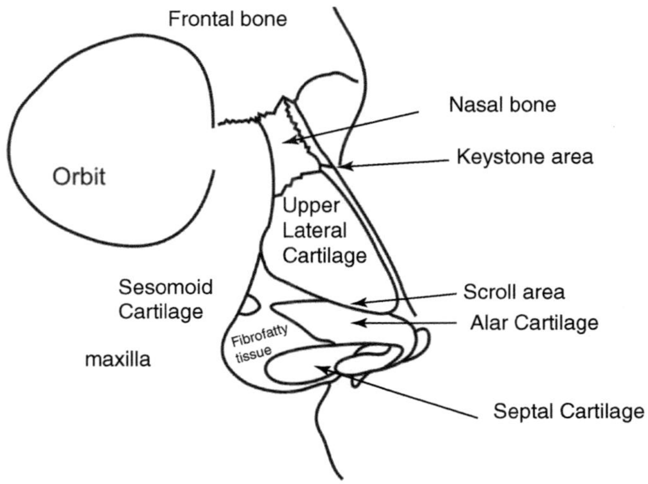

Fig. 2.3 The line diagram is depicting the nasal framework and facial division in both planes (vertical and horizontal)

(i) Size, shape and resilience of the lower lateral cartilages
(ii) Attachment of the medial crural footplate to the caudal septum
(iii) Scrolled attachment of the cephalic margins of the lower lateral cartilages to the caudal margin of the upper lateral cartilages

(b) Minor Tip Support
(i) Dorsal septum
(ii) Interdomal ligaments
(iii) Membranous septum
(iv) Anterior nasal spine
(v) Attachment of the lower lateral cartilages to the skin–soft tissue envelope
(vi) Lateral crural attachment to the pyriform aperture

Nostril is divided into three types (cheek, labial and tube) based on the relationship of nostril floor with ala base. Medial crus of further divided into columellar and foot segment. The width of the columella is affected by the intrinsic shape of cartilage, amount of soft tissue and posterior caudal edge of septal cartilage (Fig. 2.4). Asymmetric parallel, flare and straight symmetry are paring patterns of the medial and middle crux. Columella skin flap must rise in full depth to maintain the symmetry of the medial crux at the end of the operation. Anatomically middle crus is further divided into domel and lobular segment. Domel segment is thin, delicate and narrowest part of the entire alar arch. Convex, box and concave are the type of domel segment shape. Angulations, the position with other dome and thickness of overlying skin affect the shape of the nasal tip [1]. Nasal supports are essential in maintaining the normal nasal airway, as excessive resection of intermediate crura for pinching effect leads to nasal airway obstruction.

2.1.1 Photography and Analysis

Photographs are important for pre-operative analysis, documentation and for comparing postoperative results. Photographs should cover the full face (hairs to chin). Recently, computer software's are available for rhinoplasty. They are useful for planning surgery, for explanation purposes and postoperative outcome assessment (Table 2.1).

1. *Ratios*—Facial ratios can be defined to assess harmony in facial features. Following are few of common ratios
   (a) *Rule of fifths*—face can be divided vertically into five equal parts equal to the size of length from medial cantus to lateral cantus (Fig. 2.5).

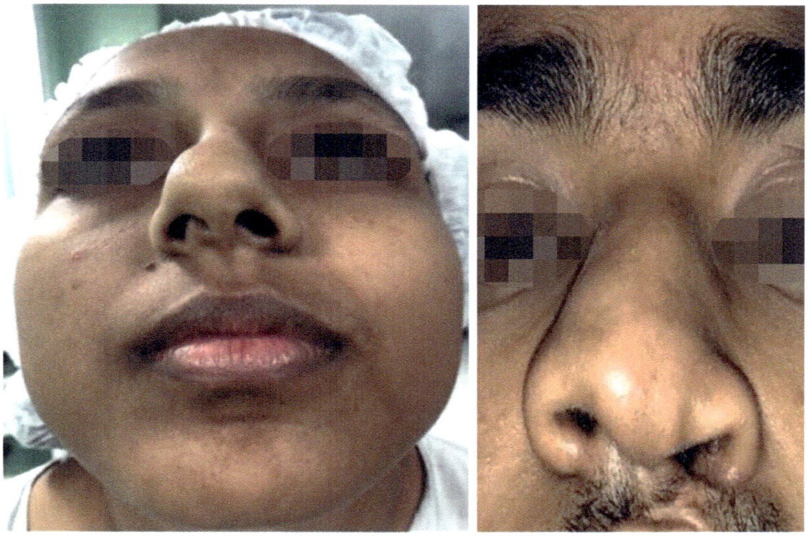

Fig. 2.4 Caudal septal deviation and asymmetry in the curvature of ala affects the width of columella (Courtesy—Dr. David Victor Kumar Irugu, Associate Professor, AIIMS, New Delhi)

Table 2.1 Computer software's for aesthetic assessment for rhinoplasty [3]

Computer softwares	Pros	Cons
www.facetouchup.com	Online Cosmetic digital image editing Software Also on Android Free	Cannot calculate different angles
Adobe Photoshop Software	Proportionate measurement angular relationship Easily available	Require more skills to use
Alter image	Cosmetic digital image editing software Dental simulation also present	Expensive
Mirror suite	Cosmetic digital image editing software Easy to measure distances, angles, proportions Colour and orientation can be matched 3D version is also available	Expensive

(b) *Rule of thirds*—face can be divided horizontally into three equal parts equal to the size of length from glabella to nasal tip (Fig. 2.5).

(c) *Golden ratio*—Fibonacci ratio or 'divine proportion'—Consider a line is divided into two parts (A and B) where A is smaller than B. The golden ratio (ϕ) is when A/B = (A + B)/A = 1.618. If nose width is 1 than length is 1.618.

2. Angles

(a) *Nasolabial angle* (Fig. 2.6)—it is the angle between a line running from columella to line between the base of the columella to mentum in lateral view. In the male, it is 90°–95° and in the female 95°–110°.

(b) *Nasomental angle*—it is angle in between lines from nasal dorsum to tip and from tip to pogonion. It is in between 120°–130°.

(c) *Nasofacial angle*—it is in between lines from nasal dorsum and nasion to pogonion. It is around 30°–35°.

(d) *Naso-frontal angle* (Fig. 2.6)—it is the intersection of tip nasion and glabella and it is around 130°.

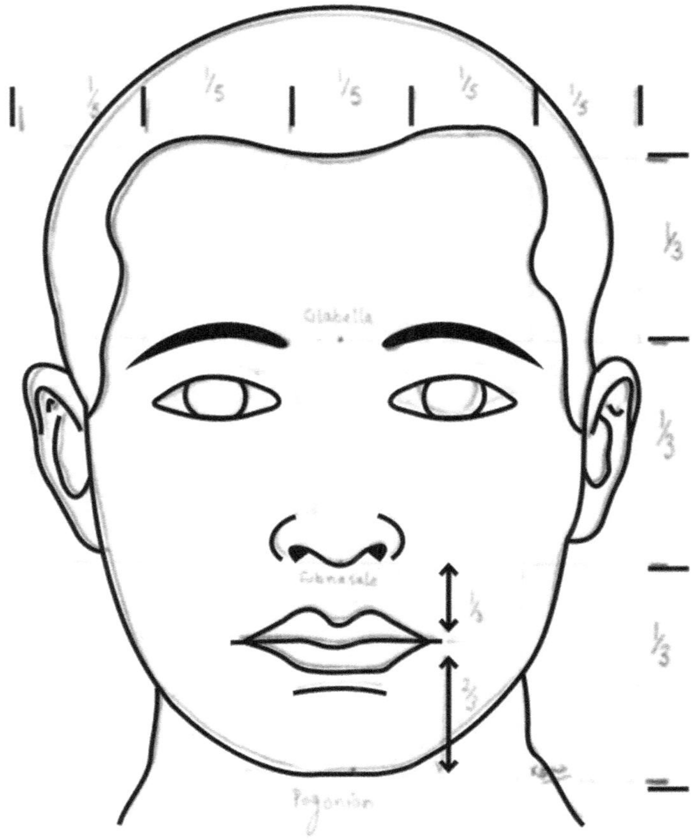

Fig. 2.5 It is showing both vertical and horizontal rule for aesthetic division of face

3. Nasal Tip—The points that need to be evaluated are tip rotation, projection (Fig. 2.6). Aesthetically, the face can divide into two equal half from the midline. In normal conditions, the width of the nasal dorsum is half of the width of intercanthal distance. The width of the nasal ala is approximately equal to the width of the eyebrow free medial border. Nasal projection is 50–60% of nasal length as per the rule of 3–4–5. It is also calculated by the division of line from the nasal tip from ala groove by an imaginary line from the upper lip and anterior part is around 50–60% in normal individual (Fig. 2.7).

Standard photographic views are [4]

1. Frontal view—It is for the assessment of facial and nasal symmetry (Figs. 2.2 and 2.4). It is useful to assess the width, symmetry and midline deviation of the bony and cartilaginous component of the nasal framework. Brow-tip aesthetic line, alar shape, lobular bulbosity, nostril size and shape are also evaluated in frontal view. Bifidality of the nasal tip is observed in this plane.
2. Right and left lateral view (profile view) (Figs. 2.6 and 2.7)—The assessment is done in relationship to the Frankfurt plane. The projection of nasal dorsum, tip, chin with nasal length and height of radix are assessed in this plane. Nasal tip rotation, break and columella show are observed in this plane. Naso-frontal, naso-labial angles, etc. are calculated in this plane.
3. Right and left lateral-Oblique view (three quarter view)—Brow-tip aesthetic line and soft tissue facets are assessed in this view.
4. Base view—It is for calculation of the shape of crura's of lower cartilage, tri-angularity, columella to lobular ratio. The shape of the nasal base is equilateral triangle ideally with

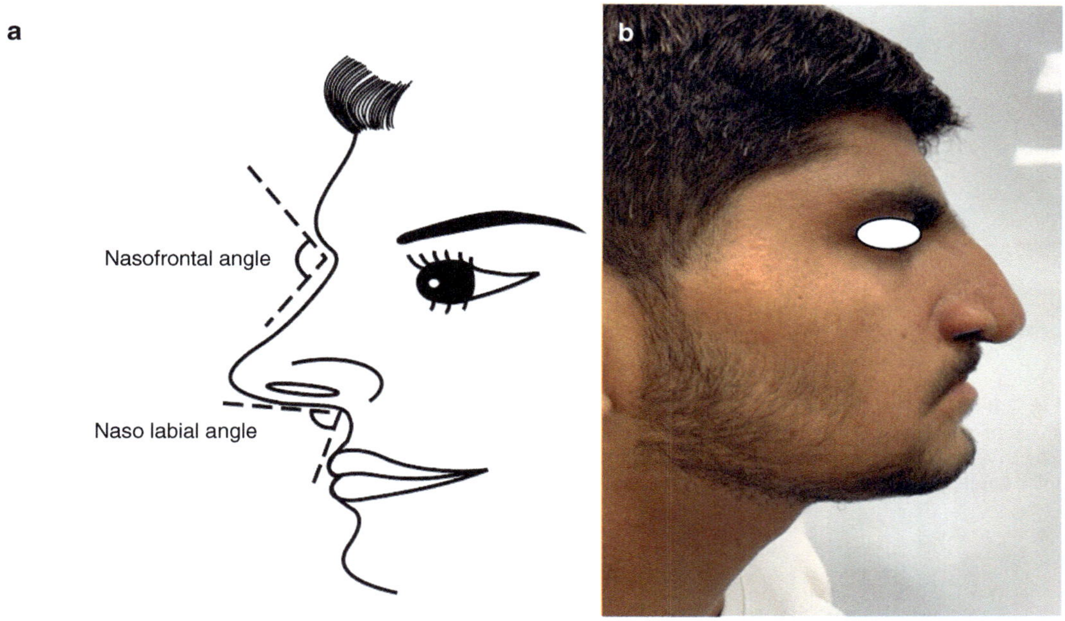

Fig. 2.6 The line diagram is representing nasolabial angle and naso-frontal angle. Naso-frontal angle is almost 180° with tip ptosis and less tip projection is visible in lateral view (Courtesy—Dr. Hitesh Verma, Associate Professor, AIIMS, New Delhi, India)

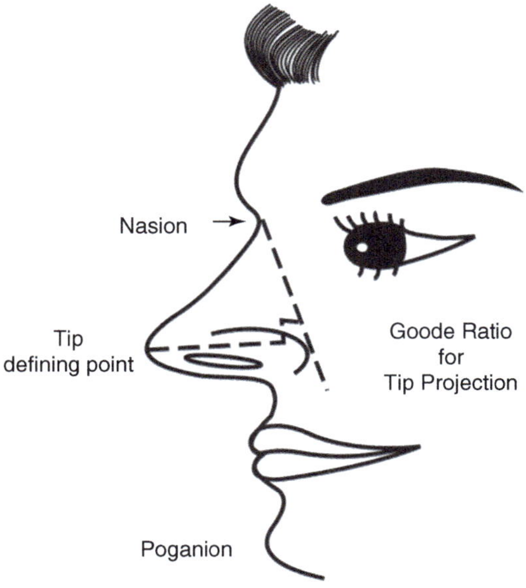

Fig. 2.7 Nasal projection is 50–60% of the length of the nose from nasion to tip defining point. Black line is the imaginary line that bisects the nasal projection line. The anterior part of line should be 50–60%

the lobular, intermediate and basal part of columella as three equal segments. Nostril is 2/3 of the height of the nose in basal view. Normal columella to lobular ratio is 2:1. Nostril shape and position, septum position, length of medial crura and basal width are also checked in this plane. Nostrils are oval shape, elongated and commonly oriented 30–45° towards the midline (Fig. 2.8).

5. Smiling view—Upper lip height, upper labial crease, nasal tip projection and nasal length are assessed in this plane. Depressor septi nasi muscle is responsible for smiling face deformity [5].
6. Skyline view (helicopter view) and Bird eye frontal view with chin up 45° are other views recommended by some author for routine practice and they are providing special details such as

Setup for Taking Photograph [6]

Digital cameras come in two categories; fixed lens (smartphone) and interchangeable lens camera (DSLR and mirrorless interchangeable

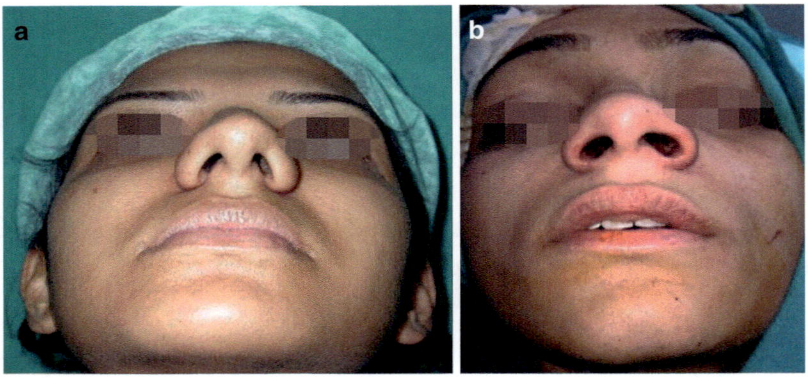

Fig. 2.8 Basal view is providing detail of nostril types, shape of crura, nostril height, etc. Figure (**a**) is showing cheek type of nostril, thick alar cartilage, narrow arch with thick basal part of columella and (**b**) is showing tube type of nostril, thin cartilage and wide arch with normal columella (Courtesy—Dr. David Victor Kumar Irugu, Associate Professor, AIIMS, New Delhi)

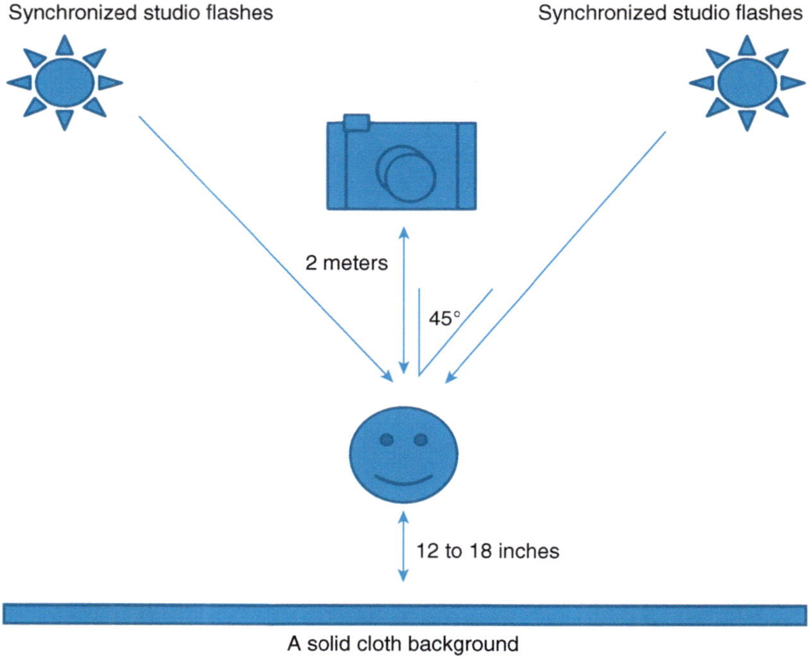

Fig. 2.9 The diagram is representing ideal setup for photography

lens). An interchangeable lens is recommended for photography because of flexibility with gaze at focal length, focus and resolution. The focal length of the camera lens should be 85–105 mm and the aperture in lens varies from f/9 to f/11. Two synchronized studio flashes are placed on either side of the camera with 45° horizontal angle between the patient-camera axis with flashlight. The makeup and jewellery should be removed with hair retracted to improve the visibility of the forehead and ear. Pre and post-operative photography should be performed in the same clothes and cloth should have a bland neck line. Solid coloured back drop preferably light blue as it is kind to all skin tones with good disparity and less glare. The patient needs to sit on the stool with a rough position of an eye within the camera (Fig. 2.9).

2.2 Part B: Open and Close Rhinoplasty and Tip Plasty

2.2.1 Introduction

Rhinoplasty is a commonly done procedure worldwide mostly for aesthetic and in some cases for functional benefit. The anatomy of the tip cartilages is complex. The nasal tip comprises the columella, lobule and ala. Lower lateral cartilage is U shaped stracture and it has two processes: the medial and lateral crura. The medial crura and overlying skin and subcutaneous tissue form the columella. The key support mechanism of the tip comprises the size, shape and strength of the lower lateral cartilages, the connection of the feet of the medial crura to the caudal edge of the septum, and the connection of the upper lateral cartilages to the lower lateral cartilages at the scroll region. Surgical strategies should keep in mind the size, shape, position and orientation of each crus including their relationships with the ipsilateral and contralateral crura of both lower lateral cartilage rings. It is important to be precise as every step has the potential for unintended as well as intended change. The most common problems are due to an under or over-projected tip. In this chapter, the methods used most widely have been described. The three basic surgical approaches are described in the literature. The approach may be selected after taking into consideration the desired outcome and patient characteristics. At the end of each surgery, the result should be a normal stable nose.

2.2.2 Approaches

Rhinoplasty is the problem-oriented practice with combination of reduction, rearrangement and amplification of tissue. Surgical treatment needs to be tailored according to deformity. Rhinoplasty surgeries are broadly classified under the external and endonasal approach. The choice of surgical approach is based on training and surgeon experience. In general, the open approach is more preferred as it provides direct visualization, allows working from both hands, provide accurate assesssment and precise rectification of deformity [7]. Practically, all deformity of the external nasal framework is managed by the open approach but more specific indications are nasal cartilages correction, difficult anatomy, post-traumatic cases, revision surgery and communicated fracture of the bony framework. In the open approach, mid-columellar stair step incision is extends on both sides along the caudal border of intermediate and lateral crus of lower lateral cartilage (marginal incision). The flap is raised in subperichondrial avascular plane and dissection is extend over the lower and upper lateral cartilage up to caudal aspect of nasal bones where dissection is extended further in the subperiosteal plane till radix. The tissue handling should be mapped according to deformity. The disadvantages are prolonged surgical time, need additional support for the cartilaginous framework, prolong postoperative edema and external scar. In the close approach, indications are limited for correction of isolated deformity of nasal tip and nasal dorsum. Infra cartilaginous, intercartilaginous and trans-cartilaginous approaches are types of incision used to expose the deformies and rest of the flap elevation is done in subperichondrial and subperiosteal plane. In the newer semiopen approach, the marginal incision is made and the rest of the procedure is done under skin. Surgical approaches to the nasal tip are of three types. Non-delivery and delivery approaches are come under close technique.

1. Non-Delivery Approaches:
   (a) Cartilage-splitting approach
   (b) Retrograde approach
      (i) Delivery approach
      (ii) External rhinoplasty

1. Non-Delivery Approach: The non-delivery approach is useful in cases where small volume reduction of the lateral crus is required and when the slight cephalic rotation of the tip is required. It is of further two types. In cartilage-splitting technique is the least traumatic of the commonly used rhinoplasty tech-

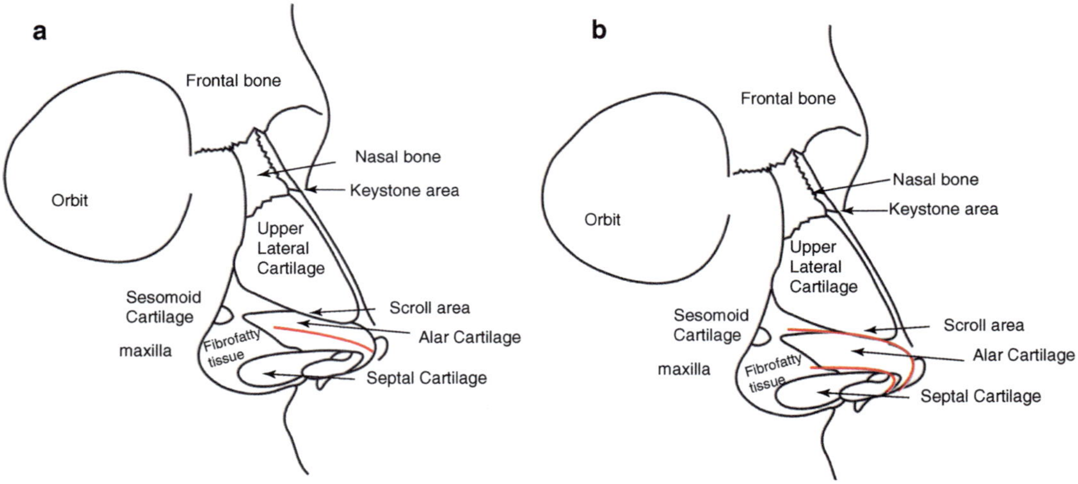

Fig. 2.10 The diagram is showing the site of the intercartilaginous incision (red line). (**b**) is showing the placement of the tip delivery incisions (Courtesy—Dr. Arvind Kairo, Associate Professor, ENT, AIIMS, New Delhi)

nique. A single incision is made at the position that overlies the cartilaginous part. Cephalic strip of cartilage with or without underlying skin can be removed. In this, an intercartilaginous incision is made followed by retrograde dissection over the lateral crus at the non-vestibular side, eversion of the lateral crus and resection of the planned cephalic portion of the cartilage (Fig. 2.10a).

2. Tip delivery is indicated when the tip is bifid, cephalically rotation and over-projected. It delivers the alar cartilages with the underlying skin and mucosa as a 'bucket handle' [7]. The incisions are made along the caudal margin and cephalic margin of the alar cartilage (Fig. 2.10b). The overlying soft tissue and skin are dissected off the alar cartilage leaving the cartilage attached to its underlying skin and mucosa.
3. External rhinoplasty is described by Gillie and popularized by Rethi [8]. Inverted V shaped incision is joined with bilateral rim incision to prepare of the columella skin flap (Fig. 2.11a). Incision should not disturb the underlying cartilage of the medial crura (Fig. 2.11b), to prevent postoperative skin necrosis and visibility of scar [7]. Skin flap is elevated and dissected till the nasal dorsum is exposed. Medial crura can be separated to expose the caudal end and dorsal area of the nasal septum.

2.2.3 Tip Defining Procedures

Under-projected nasal tip can correct by various techniques. The choice of approach can be simple removal of the cephalic strip of lower lateral cartilage, vertical division + / − strip excision of lower lateral cartilage, tip suturing and tip grafting alone or in combination [7].

1. Strip excision/division of cartilage: Tip is narrowed by trimming the cephalic part of lower lateral cartilage (Fig. 2.12). Lateral part of the lower lateral cartilage is left intact to maintain the integrity of the nasal valve. Cephalic edge of the lower lateral cartilage can be approached by a cartilage-splitting incision, tip delivery approach, or via the external rhinoplasty approach. Approximately 10 mm of lower lateral cartilage should be left in situ to avoid buckling of the cartilage.
2. Tip suturing techniques. Cephalic trimming reduces straight of the nasal value area. Tip

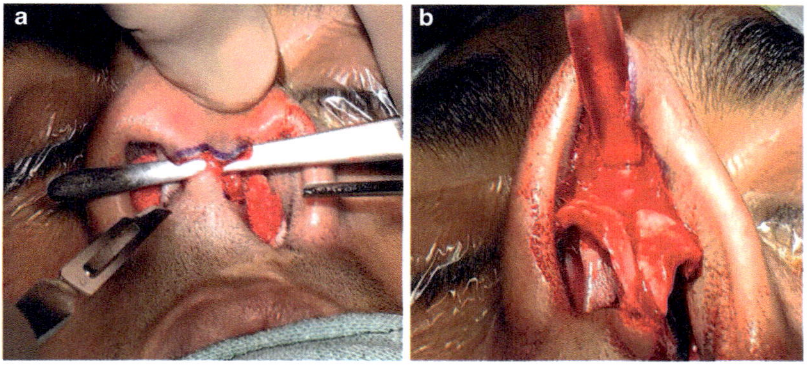

Fig. 2.11 Showing elevation of the flap by external rhinoplasty approach (Courtesy—Dr. David Victor Kumar Irugu, Associate Professor, AIIMS, New Delhi)

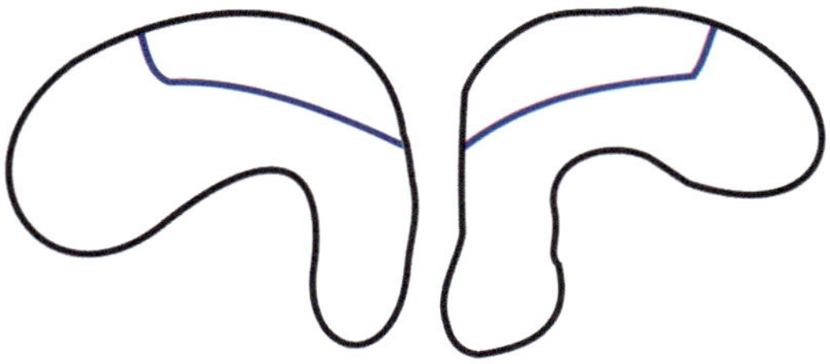

Fig. 2.12 It is showing the technique of excision of a cephalic strip of cartilage

suturing technique is free of such complications and it is reversible. Interdomal sutures are used to narrow the nasal cartilages. It is indicated when support graft is needed for tip preparation, to strengthen the medial crura and for tip projection (Fig. 2.13).

2.2.4 Management of the Overprojecting Tip

The causes of tip over-projection are alar cartilage development, nasal spine overdevelopment, caudal septal deviation, overdeveloped quadrangular cartilage, elongated columella and iatrogenic over-projection [9]. It can be done by applying complete transfixion incision. This helps in the separation of the membranous septum from the medial crural footplates. It allows the alar cartilages to be repositioned in relation to the nasal septum [7]. It can also be done by the vertical dome division technique (Goldman). Tip delivery approach followed by vertical division of the alar domes approximately 1 mm lateral to the highest point of the dome. The cartilage and its underlying mucosa are incised. The intermediate crura are rotated anteriorly and sutured with the medial crura. The classic Goldman procedure can result in irregularities of the tip, lower nasal third pinching, alar notching and a pointed 'tent pole' nasal tip which was addressed by Adamson et al. [10] They described by the placement of vertical incision medial to the high point of the dome and overlapping of the lower lateral cartilage as a method of avoiding these complications. Third technique is by interrupted strip with cartilage excision. Excising a vertical strip of cartilage from the medial [11] or lateral crura or a combination can result in better cephalic rotation of the tip. Lateral segment excision is preferred because the cartilage excision is covered by thicker sebaceous skin. Goldman tip suturing & Adamson modification are the techniques to prepare single tip in bifid nasal tip conditions [12].

2.2.5 The Under-Projected Nasal Tip

The nasal tip may appear under-projected because of disproportionately small alar cartilages or because the middle and or upper third of the nose is disproportionately large [7] Methods to increase tip projection are the Goldman tip technique, onlay graft (Fig. 2.13), lateral crural steal and shield graft. For onlay graft, conchal carti-

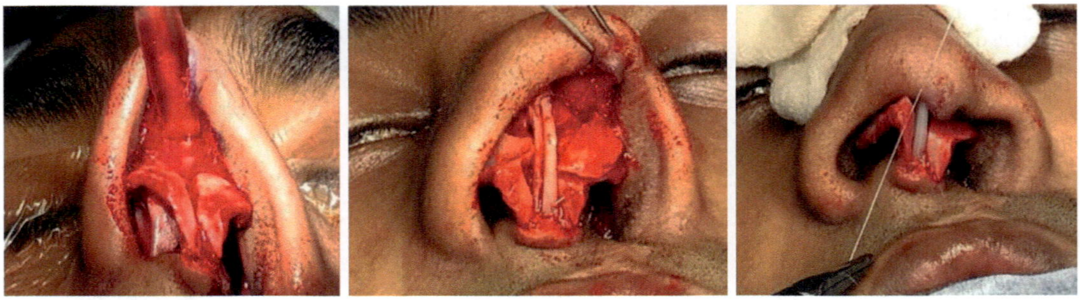

Fig. 2.13 Left ala is lower than right ala. Cartilage piece is placed over the left dome and in between both sides of medial crura. The suture is passed from the right side of right side medial ala where it was approximate with other ala before separating both ala's. Suture needs to be passed in the same fashion with other ala and supporting cartilage to prepare tip (Courtesy—Dr. David Victor Kumar Irugu, Associate Professor, AIIMS, New Delhi)

lage and septal cartilage grafts are generally used. The disadvantages of this method are that it thickens the tip of the nose. In the lateral crural steal technique, alar cartilages are dissected off the underlying vestibular skin in the intermediate crural area and the alar cartilages may be delivered. The lateral crura are then advanced to the medial crura and sutured with permanent sutures. Shield graft is useful in short columella and weak lower lateral cartilages (Fig. 2.13).

2.2.6 The Broad Nasal Tip

It is seen in thick skin people or in the abnormal shape of alar, septal cartilages. Nasal tip can be narrowed and a more triangular base be obtained by either using a Goldman tip technique or sutures to create a narrow tip.

2.2.7 Complications

Patient dissatisfaction is the most common complication of rhinoplasty [7]. This can be managed by accurate pre-operative assessment, realistic expectations and better communication. Haemorrhage and infection are other complications. Deformities relating to the nasal tip are:

(a) Pollybeak deformity: This produces loss of tip definition with supratip fullness. This may be related to scar tissue or to excessive lower lateral cartilage excision and subsequent loss tip support.
(b) Retracted ala: This is due to excessive lower lateral cartilage and/or vestibular skin excision causing retraction of the alar cartilages.
(c) Alar asymmetry is caused by unequal alar cartilage remnants.
(d) Retracted columella: This may be related to either excessive resection of the caudal edge of the septum or medial crura.
(e) Bossae: weakening and subsequent bending of the alar cartilage.

These complications are often managed with an open rhinoplasty approach for accurate diagnosis and it can be resolved by local grafts.

2.3 Part C: Nasal Dorsum Correction and Material for Rhinoplasty

The external nasal scaffold extends from the root of the nose till the nasal tip is known as the nasal dorsum. The bony nasal dorsum is formed by nasal bone and the frontal process of the maxilla and nasal part of the frontal bone. The cartilaginous part is formed by upper lateral cartilage. Deformity of nasal dorsum is described as hump (over-projected), saddle (under-projected), twisted, C and S shaped which can involve bony

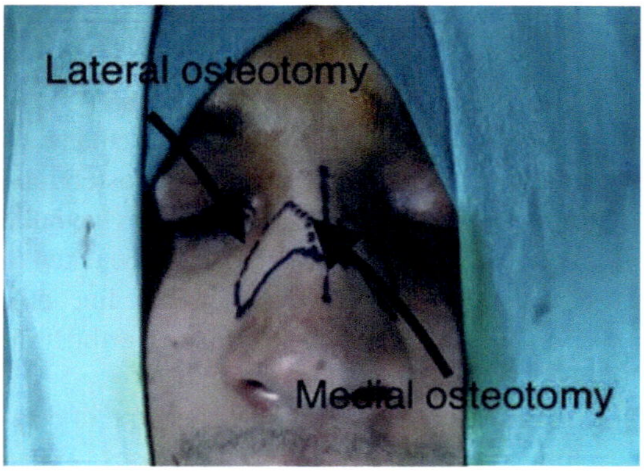

Fig. 2.14 The diagram is representing the site of medial and lateral osteotomies and how it should run to join each other

and cartilaginous part alone or in combination. The causative factors are broadly classified into congenital, traumatic and iatrogenic. Nasal dorsum deformities correction is possible with both endonasal and external approaches. The choice of approach is based on the deformity and the surgeon's preference. The first surgical step to correct the hump is the separation of upper lateral cartilage from septum after exposure. Septum proper is reduced in incremental fashion follow by bony hump correction and final modification is performed by grafting, suturing or by osteotomies alone or in combination. In saddle nose, the nasal dorsum is under-projected so grafts are needed to augment it. Various grafts and materials are used to augment saddle nose deformity. Twisted, c and s shaped nasal dorsum require osteotomies to correct deformity [12]. Following osteotomies, the nasal dorsum can be narrowed or broadened and straightened. Osteotomies are extended from the piriform aperture upwards into the nasal process of the frontal bone (Fig. 2.14). They can be done either with linear or percutaneous techniques using osteotomes. There are many types of osteotomies including lateral, medial, transverse and intermediate. Materials for the reconstruction of the nose can be autologous, homologous or allografts. In this section, we are discussing osteotomies, post-operative management, grafting materials and commonly used grafts.

1. **Lateral Osteotomy**—It is done to narrow or straighten the bony nasal dorsum. It can be done with two techniques:
   (a) Linear or single cut—It is performed intranasally. It starts from the lateral attachment of an inferior turbinate. Using an osteotome, the linear bony cut is made along nasofacial groove. Based on the site of the starting point, it is further of three types.
      (i) High-low-high technique–Taking the nasofacial groove as a reference, the osteotomy is done above the nasofacial groove (high). Incision is extending along the nasofacial groove (low) thereby leaving a small triangle of bone with the ligamental attachments, and is then merged with the medial osteotomy by curving it anteriorly (high).
      (ii) Low-low-high technique—Taking the nasofacial groove as the reference, the lateral osteotomy is started in the nasofacial groove and continued upward (low-low) to merge with the medial osteotomy by curving it anteriorly (high). The problem with this type of osteotomy is the collapse of the internal nasal valve due to the lack of preservation of the suspensory ligament attachment triangle of bone.
      (iii) Low-low-low technique—It is started in the nasofacial groove and extended upwards till the medial canthus where it is joined to the transverse osteotomy [13].

      A small triangle of bone at the piriform aperture is left intact to preserve the lateral attachments of the suspensory ligaments. The bony cut is extended along the nasofacial groove till the medial canthus where it can be joined with transverse osteotomy. Alternatively, it can be curved anteriorly from the level of inferior orbital margin to meet medial osteotomy. It is important to stay close to the maxilla while making the bony cut, otherwise it can lead to a step deformity. If it is carried higher into the thicker bone of the naso-frontal suture a rocker deformity may result.

(b) Percutaneous—it is also called perforating technique, as serial perforations are made along the route of osteotomy, through percutaneous stab incisions at nasofacial junction. Then the osteotomy is completed using digital pressure over nasal bone. This technique preserves the bridges of the periosteum, which prevent inward fall of the fractured fragment and prevent nasal collapse. This is the preferred technique in revision surgeries and difficult cases.

Complications-osteotomies are associated with the risk of inadvertent injury to the surrounding structures like the eyeball, medial canthal ligament. There can be bleeding from small arteries, but it is rare. Improper technique may lead to step deformity or rocker deformity as explained above. There may be residual scar or keloid formation in the percutaneous technique.

2. **Medial Osteotomy—**It is done to mobilize the lateral nasal wall (along with lateral osteotomy) [14]. It naturally occurs after hump removal. After medial osteotomy, upper lateral cartilage moves along with the lateral nasal wall, owing to its fixed attachment to the inner surface of the nasal wall. So care should be taken while narrowing the nasal dorsum, as it can lead to internal nasal valve collapse.

   Technique—It is done between the nasal bone and septum, from the inferior piriform aperture margin to meet transverse/lateral osteotomy superiorly at the level of the medial canthus.

   Complications—There can be injury to the upper lateral cartilages, which may lead to inverted V deformity. There may be irregular surface after hump removal. Medial osteotomy can cause internal nasal valve collapse, leading to nasal obstruction. A rare but dreaded complication might be CSF leak if the osteotomy extends too far superiorly.

3. **Transverse Osteotomy**—Small cutaneous puncture is created with a 2-mm osteotome midway between the nasal dorsum and the medial canthal region. Care should be taken to remain below the naso-frontal suture line, otherwise it may cause injury to the cribriform plate, leading to CSF leak.

4. **Intermediate Osteotomy**—This type of osteotomy is done in only select cases. When done, it should be done as the first osteotomy, as it is not possible to perform intermediate osteotomy in a free nasal bone. It can also be done by endonasal or percutaneous route. For endonasal route, intercartilaginous incision is made.

   Indications

   (a) To narrow the extremely wide nose that has a good height (bilateral osteotomy).

   (b) To correct the deviated nose with one sidewall much longer than the other.

   (c) To straighten a markedly convex nasal bone.

2.3.1 Post-Operative Management

Systemic review proposed use of intraoperative hypotensive anaesthesia, steroid, head end elevation can reduce post-operative pain and edema significantly [15]. Direct lateral nasal compression for 5 min reduces post-operative edema significantly. Other post-operative management are

(a) **Nasal packing—**It is done to stop bleeding, adhesion, septal hematoma formation (if septoplasty is concurrently done), but few articles contradict the above statement [16, 17]. It also stabilizes nasal bones from internal collapse. This should not be too tight and it can be removed after 24–48 h.

(b) **Steri-strips and external nasal splint—** Steri-strips are applied to prevent or decrease post-operative edema by its compressive effect and it also helps in psychological motivation with partially visible post-operative appearance. External nasal splint protects the loose nasal bone fragments from external pressure [18].

(c) **Cold application**—Post-operative pain, edema and ecchymosis are common after surgery. This can be minimized with the cold application as it reduces inflammation and metabolism by induced vasoconstriction. It also increases than pain threshold and reduces nerve impulse but Meta-analysis failed to show a statically significant difference.

(d) **Medications**—Pain is the main post-operative complaint and it generally lasts for a few days at a mild to a moderate level after rhinoplasty. It is more with a costal cartilage graft where it can last from weeks to a month. Muscle sparing technique and preservation of the inner laminar arch reduces the need for analgesics. Long-standing local anaesthetic should be applied at the donor site to block intercostals nerves. Post-operative antibiotics may require till the nasal pack removed.

(e) **Head end elevation**—It is to prevent/decrease post-op edema. It should be done in the initial post-operative period.

(f) **Donor site management for costal cartilage graft**—The dead space should be obliterated completely and dressing should be in place for the next 3 days to prevent post-operative hematoma formation. X-ray chest is recommended on the first post-operative day to look for pneumothorax.

(g) **Follow up**—Regular follow up should be done to ensure proper healing and post-op changes.

(h) **Photography**—Post-op photography should be done in similar background and angles for proper post-operative comparison.

2.3.2 Materials for Reconstruction in Rhinoplasty

There has been a long search for the ideal reconstruction material for rhinoplasty, but it is yet to be found. An ideal material should have some characteristics like non-immunogenic, non-carcinogenic, no foreign body reaction, not interfering with healing, must match the surrounding tissue, non-absorbable, available in adequate quantity, easy to manipulate into the desired shape, low cost. Grafts can be autologous, homologous or xenologous/semi-synthetic. It can be porous or non-porous. Porous material with pore size of 10–50 μm cannot be penetrated by macrophages, thus it is more prone to bacterial infection. If the pore size is more than macrophage penetration and tissue in growth is good, therefore less chances of infection. Materials with particle size between 20 and 60 μm have least chances of shredding of particles, which can be phagocytosed by macrophages and may lead to chronic inflammatory reactions [19].

Autografts—They can be cartilaginous or bony. Cartilage gives better matching with surrounding structure as it is soft and easy to reshape. Cartilage is very close to the ideal graft definition. It can be harvested from nasal septum, conchal or costal cartilage. Small deficit is managed by septal and conchal cartilage graft whereas large deficit is managed by costal cartilages. Right side costal cartilage graft is preferred over left to prevent injury to pericardium and post-operative misunderstanding of donor site pain from angina. The graft is generally harvested from middle (sixth–eighth) ribs and sixth costal cartilage shows more similarity with nasal dorsum in term of depth and width. Conchal and septal cartilage graft harvesting is associated with no or minimal morbidity. Pain, scar, risk of pneumothorax and relatively prolong surgery time with hospital stay are the morbidities associated with costal cartilage graft. Costal cartilage has more warping and reabsorption chances than other cartilage grafts. Warping can be minimized by complete removal of perichondrium and by delaying the insertion of graft by 30 min. Bone on other hand gives a hard un-natural feel in rhinoplasty and it can be harvest from iliac crest, ribs or split calvarium. Moreover, it has more donor site morbidity, difficult fabrication of dorsal L strut and it appear as more rigid, abnormal at the reconstruction site. Absorption rate of split calvarium is less than iliac crest bone. Post auricular fibroconnective tissue and mastoid fascia graft are used to correct minute residual deformities. Soft tissue graft is also useful to correct soft tissue loss [20, 21].

Homografts—Usually not used because of fear of transmission of slow viruses. Irradiated homologous costal cartilage is used in literature and it has no chance of virus transmission with excellent tolerance to tissue and infection. It reduces the operative time, need for auto graft but it stability of graft is questionable. In some series, it is around 70–100%. Acellular allogenic cadaveric dermis (alloderm) is used to augment tapered soft tissue encase but it has high absorption rate [20–22].

Alloplastic materials—the most accepted indication for alloplastic material is lack of sufficient autograft. It is applicable at stationary anatomical areas such as nasal dorsum as extrusion chances high at the mobile area. Scarred, thin scaffold with under-tension allograft has got high chances of extrusion.

- Gortex—Polytetrafluoroethylene (PTFE) is being marketed under the trade name of gortex. It has good tissue compatibility, the feel of soft tissue and is supplied in sheets of different thickness that can be custom cut and layered. The material can be re-sterilized if not used. There is little foreign body reaction or rejection, it is not prone to migration and the infection rate is low. It appears that Gortex is becoming the synthetic implant of choice for the nasal dorsum [8].
- Silastic—It is firm, slippery, non-porous and easily sculptural. Medical-grade silicon is called silastic. It has been used extensively in the past. It is non-immunogenic, does not react with the tissue. Its stability is based on the formation of peri-implant capsule. It is not used commonly now because of its high extrusion rate, migration, resorption of the underlying bone, changes colour of overlying skin, etc.
- Medpor is linear high-density polyethylene with interconnection pore size of 160–320 μm which makes it flexible. Pore allows in growth of connective tissue which increases the acceptability of implant at donor site. It is more user-friendly material with less extrusion rate but the cost is high.
- Hydroxyapatite material is resembled more with human bones. Its graft form coarse, highly fragile, poor moldable feature whereas granular form is more user-friendly with good take-up rate.
- Proplast and Teflon—it produces significant inflammatory reaction. It is not in use because of its high collapsibility and fragmentation rate with shearing power.
- Supramid is the polyamide mesh and it is not in use because of high chances of graft absorption.
- Polyethylene tetraphthalate mesh is easy moldable and stable graft material. It is less in use due to high infection and graft failure rates.

Commonly used terminology for grafting materials is listed below.

- Spreader graft—Autologous cartilage is placed between the nasal septum and upper lateral cartilage. Dimensions can vary from patient to patient. Commonly used dimensions are length 10–15 mm, height approx. 2 mm and width 1–2 mm. It is used commonly to increase the valve area. It can also be used as a stent for correcting mid-third C shaped deformity of cartilage, by placing it only on the concave side of septum.
- Batten graft—A small piece of cartilage is placed in the lateral nasal wall, just superior to the posterior part of lower lateral cartilage. It is used to provide strength to collapsible nasal ala.
- Shield graft—It is used to increase tip projection, done by placing a small piece of cartilage over the domes of lower lateral cartilage (Fig. 2.13).
- Caudal extension graft—It is used to increase tip support and projection.
- Turkish delight—0.5–1 mm cartilage pieces are wrapped in temporalis fascia or surgicel. It can be moulded and digitally corrected in the

first 2–3 weeks thus it reduces the chances of post-operative malposition. It has less chances of warping as graft is not compressed or battered.

References

1. Suhk J, Park J, Nguyen AH. Nasal analysis and anatomy: anthropometric proportional assessment in Asians-aesthetic balance from forehead to chin, part I. Semin Plast Surg. 2015;29(4):219–25.
2. Farkas LG, Katic MJ, Forrest CR, et al. International anthropometric study of facial morphology in various ethnic groups/races. J Craniofac Surg. 2005;16(4):615–46.
3. Pawar SS, Garcia GJM, Rhee JS. Advances in technology for functional rhinoplasty. Facial Plast Surg Clin. 2017;25(2):263–70.
4. Tardy ME Jr, dayan S, Hecht D. Preoperative rhinoplasty: evaluation and analysis. Otolaryngol Clin North Am. 2002;35(1):1–27.
5. Kalantar-Hormozi A, Beiraghi-Toosi A. Smile analysis in rhinoplasty: a randomized study for comparing resection and transposition of the depressor septi nasi muscle. Plast Reconstr Surg. 2014;133(2):261–8.
6. Swamy RS, Sykes JM, Most SP. Principles of photography in rhinoplasty for the digital photographer. Clin Plast Surg. 2010;37(2):213–21.
7. Stearns M. The nasal tip and nasolabial angle. In: Gleeson M, editor. Scott Brown's otorhinolaryngology, head and neck surgery, vol. 3. 7th ed. London: Hodder Arnold; 2008. p. 2995–3005.
8. Rethi A. Raccourcissement du nez trop long. Revue Chirurgerie Plastique. 1934;2:85.
9. Cingi C, et al. Nasal tip sutures: techniques and indications. Am J Rhinol Allergy. 2015;29(6):205–2011.
10. Adamson PA, McGraw-Wail BL, Morrow TA, Constantinides MS. Vertical dome division in open rhinoplasty. Arch Otolaryngol Head Neck Surg. 1994;120:373–80.
11. Momeni A, Gruber RP. Primary open rhinoplasty. Aesthet Surg J. 2016;36(9):983–92.
12. Bloom J, Immerman S, Constantinides M. Osteotomies in the crooked nose. Facial Plast Surg. 2011;27(05):456–66.
13. Cerkes N. The crooked nose: principles of treatment. Aesthet Surg J. 2011;31(2):241–57.
14. Lykoudis EG, Peristeri DV, Lykoudis GE, Oikonomou GA. Medial osteoectomy as a routine procedure in rhinoplasty: six-year experience with an innovative technique. Aesthet Plast Surg. 2018;42(1):256–63.
15. Adrian AO, Zachary F, Andrew RK, et al. Interventions to decrease postoperative edema and ecchymosis after rhinoplasty: a systematic review of the literature. Plastic Reconstr Surg. 2016;137(5):1448–62.
16. Repanos C, McDonald SE, Sadr AH. A survey of postoperative nasal packing among UK ENT surgeons. Eur Arch Otorhinolaryngol. 2009;266:1575–7.
17. Lee HS, Yoon HY, Kim IH, et al. The effectiveness of postoperative intervention in patients after rhinoplasty: a meta-analysis. Eur Arch Otorhinolaryngol. 2017;274:2685–94.
18. Farahvash MR, Khorasani G, Mahdiani Y, Taheri AR. The effect of steri-strip dressing on patients' satisfaction and reduction of ecchymosis in lower eyelid, malar and cheek following rhinoplasty. World J Plast Surg. 2016;5:51–7.
19. Gendeh BS, Mallina S. Graft selection in rinoplasty: indications and limitations. Med J Malaysia. 2008;63(1):35–8.
20. Cingi C, Bayar Muluk N, Winkler A, Thomas JR. Nasal tip grafts. J Craniofac Surg. 2018;29(7):1914–21.
21. Dresner HS, Hilger PA. An overview of nasal dorsal augmentation. Semin Plast Surg. 2008;22(2):65–73.
22. Murakami CS, Cook TA, Guida R. Nasal reconstruction with articulated irradiated rib cartilage. Arch Otolaryngol Head Neck Surg. 1991;117(3):327–30.

Nasal Physiology and Sinusitis

3

K. Davraj, Mayank Yadav, Preetam Chappity, Prity Sharma, Mohnish Grover, Shitanshu Sharma, Tanmaya Kataria, Kranti Bhawna, Anand Pendakur, Gurbax Singh, David Victor Kumar Irugu, Anoop Singh, and Nitin Gupta

Contents

K. Davraj
ENT, KMC, Manipal, Karnataka, India

M. Yadav
ENT, SHKM GMC, Nalhar, Nuh, Haryana, India

P. Chappity · P. Sharma
ENT, AIIMS, Bhubaneswar, Odisha, India

M. Grover · S. Sharma · T. Kataria
ENT, SMS Medical College,
Jaipur, Rajasthan, India

K. Bhawna
ENT, AIIMS, Patna, Bihar, India

A. Pendakur
Allergy Asthma ENT Clinic,
Bangalore, Karnataka, India

G. Singh
ENT, GGS Medical College and Hospital,
Faridkot, Punjab, India

D. V. K. Irugu (✉) · A. Singh
ENT, AIIMS, New Delhi, India
e-mail: irugudavid72kumar@rediffmail.com

N. Gupta
ENT, GMCH, Chandigarh, India

H. Verma, A. Thakar (eds.), *Essentials of Rhinology*, https://doi.org/10.1007/978-981-33-6284-0_3

3.1 Part A: Physiology of Nose and Paranasal Sinuses

3.1.1 Introduction

Nose and paranasal sinuses play a significant role in humidifying and filtering the inspired air, as well as contributes critically to the function of olfaction. These functions can get affected by many anatomical changes, physiological process, inflammatory conditions, and drugs. Most of the nasal cavity is lined by pseudostratified columnar ciliated epithelium, with microvilli on the surface. Mucus secretion produced by submucosal seromucinous glands and mucosal goblet cells is important for optimal functioning of the nose and paranasal sinuses. Around 0.5 to 2 L of mucus is produced every day in an individual and coordinated ciliary beat propels the mucus from each sinus in peculiar fashion to the nasal cavity and then to the pharynx.

The nasal cycle is nothing but alternate congestion and decongestion of the nasal turbinate mucosa, probably to warm and humidify the inspired air. It can be appreciated in children as young as 3 years, would be present in a majority of the adults, lasts around 2–4 h, and can persist even after cessation of nasal airflow. In physiological conditions, nasal breathing is dependent vastly on the nasal cycle. The objective assessment of nasal airway and breathing can be done by tests like acoustic rhinometry, rhinosteriometry, and rhinomanometry. The present clinical indications for these objective tests of nasal breathing include assessment of dynamic intranasal pressure changes and the site(s) of obstruction in obstructive sleep apnea, for choosing the appropriate patients for surgery, and for comparing the improvement in nasal breathing after surgery or medical therapy.

The nose is a physiological conduit through which the air is inspired and expired to the human body, whereas the paranasal sinuses are air-filled pockets in the skull, communicating with the nasal cavities. Together they are involved in humidifying and warming the inspired air, filtering the inspired air, regulation of intranasal pressure, increasing surface area for olfaction, lightening the skull weight, resonance to voice, and absorbing shock during trauma preventing injury to brain and orbit. Anatomical variations of nose and sinuses, inflammatory diseases like rhinosinusitis, systemic diseases like diabetes [1], drugs, and trauma can all influence these physiological functions. Nasal cycle is characterized by alternate nasal obstruction. It is because of changes in venous sinusoid blood volume. It lasts for 4–12 h. The autonomic nervous system controls the changes.

3.1.2 Nasal Secretions and Mucociliary Drainage

Nasal secretions are important to carry out most of the listed functions of the nose and are produced by submucosal seromucous glands and mucosal goblet cells [2].

3.1.2.1 Nasal Mucosal Lining

The distribution of glands and epithelium varies at different regions of nasal cavity, anterior vestibular part having stratified squamous lining with sebaceous glands and vibrissa, while the rest of the nasal cavity except the olfactory region having pseudostratified columnar ciliated epithelium, with microvilli on the surface [3]. Submucosal lamina propria contains the mucosal glands and the neurovascular tissues which are involved in peculiar autonomic and inflammatory responses of the nasal cavity.

3.1.2.2 Contents of Nasal Secretions

Approximately 0.5–2 L of mucus is produced every day in an individual, 95% of which is water, and rest of it contains peptides like glycoproteins, lactoferrin, lysozyme, immunoglobulins, surfactants, and antitrypsin along with some salts, and debris [3]. Nasal mucus consists of two layers, a continuous inner "sol" phase of lower viscosity surrounding the shafts of cilia; and a discontinuous outer "gel" phase of higher viscosity, which rides along the tips of the extended cilia [2, 3].

3.1.2.3 Mucociliary Drainage Pattern

Around 50–200 cilia per epithelial cell, each measuring 5–7 μm in length and 0.2–0.3 μm in diameter, clear the mucus blanket of 10–15 μm thickness [2], by beating in a coordinated and rhythmic manner [3]. The average basal ciliary beat frequency in humans is 9–15 Hz and the resultant dynamic range of mucus velocity is about 3–25 mm/min [3]. Ciliary beat to propel the mucus is coordinated and peculiarly oriented in the nasal cavity and each sinus as shown in Fig. 3.1. The mucociliary flow from the anterior sinuses is drained to posterior nasopharynx passing anteriorly and inferiorly to the eustachian tube orifice, and from the posterior sinuses to the posterior nasopharynx passing posteriorly and superiorly to the eustachian tube orifice [3].

3.1.2.4 Tests for Mucociliary Clearance

Dysfunctional mucociliary clearance is central pathology in hereditary conditions like cystic fibrosis and primary ciliary dyskinesia includ-

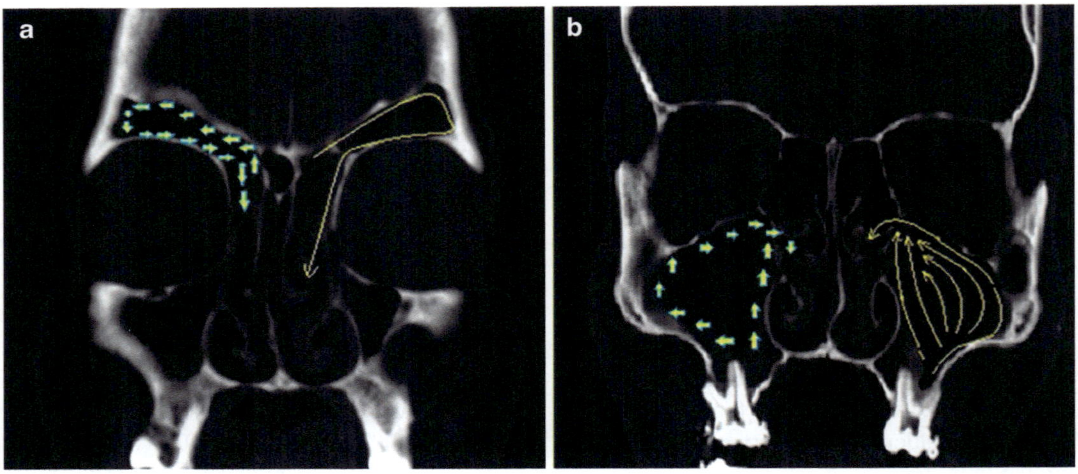

Fig. 3.1 Diagrammatic representation of sinonasal mucociliary clearance pattern. (**a**) Whorl pattern in the frontal sinus (from the medial wall through roof and lateral wall to frontal ostium in medial aspect of floor) and (**b**) Stellate pattern in maxillary sinus (from floor to maxillary ostium located in superior part of medial wall)

ing Kartagener syndrome. In addition, mucociliary clearance can get affected by commoner inflammatory diseases like chronic rhinosinusitis, by physiological stimuli like de-hydration and hormonal changes, and by pharmacological agents like anti-cholinergics and antihistamines. Saccharin test is a simple clinical test to measure mucociliary clearance, and in some cases, the movement of anteriorly placed radiolabeled dye can be detected by serial imaging.

3.1.3 Nasal Breathing

The extent and quality of nasal breathing is physiologically dependent on multiple factors including race, built, etc. but can also be influenced by local anatomical variations like septal deviation, and by the local physiological phenomenon in the nasal cavity like nasal cycle. Nasal cycle is nothing but alternate congestion and decongestion of the nasal turbinate mucosa, probably to warm and humidify the inspired air. It can be appreciated in children as young as 3 years, would be present in a majority of the adults, lasts around 2–4 h, and can persist even after cessation of nasal airflow [4].

3.1.3.1 Measurement of Nasal Breathing

Detailed history taking and thorough clinical examination of the nose including diagnostic nasal endoscopy are essential in the evaluation of nasal breathing abnormalities. These will not only be helpful in identifying the possible cause for nasal obstruction but also would enable the subjective quantification of the severity of the obstruction and thus may aid in treatment planning and prognostication in a majority of the patients. Though the objective assessment of nasal airway may be necessary often in clinical practice, the utility of these objective tests listed in Fig. 3.2. It is limited to research and trials at present.

- Present clinical indications for these objective tests of nasal breathing include
  - To know the dynamic intranasal pressures changes and the site(s) of obstruction in obstructive sleep apnea, to aid treatment planning [5].
  - For choosing the appropriate patients for surgery, and for comparing the improvement in nasal breathing after surgery or medical therapy [6, 7].
  - To demonstrate the non-restriction of the nasal airway in atrophic rhinitis or functional cases.

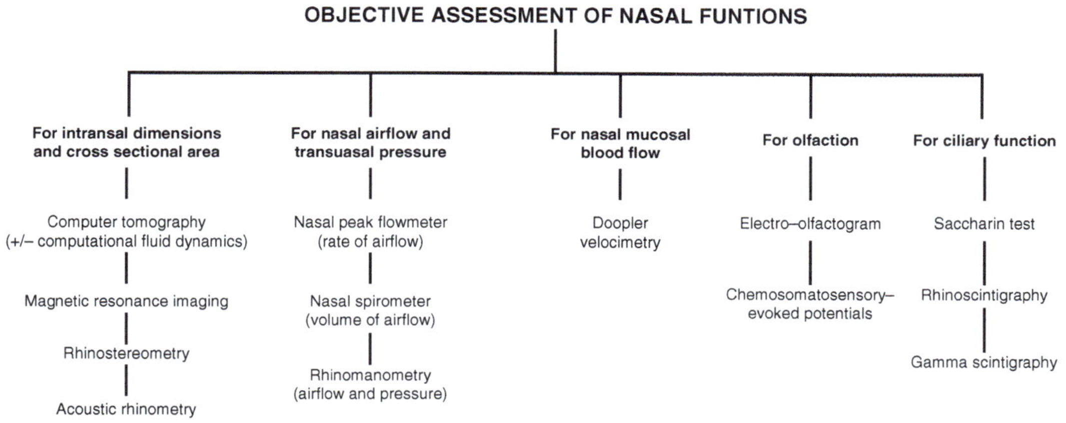

Fig. 3.2 Schematic diagram showing the objective tests for nasal functions

3.1.3.2 Important Objective Tests of Nasal Breathing

- **Test Conditions:** This needs to be done in a quiet, comfortable environment on a calm patient who has not taken any drug or tobacco or coffee before the test.
- **Acoustic Rhinometry:** Here an acoustic click is presented to each nostril separately, both before and after decongestion, and the distortions in the reflected sound wave are recorded as a computer-generated graph. Using this, the cross-sectional areas at various levels of the nose and the overall volume of each nasal cavity can be estimated separately. The first minimal cross-sectional area (CSA1) recorded corresponds to the nasal valve, and the CSA2 corresponds to the inferior turbinate [8].
- **Rhinostereometry**: For studying the changes in the nasal mucosal congestion using a microscope, mainly for the demonstration of the nasal cycle and for studying the effects of drugs on nasal blood flow.
- **Rhinomanometry:** It measures the transnasal pressure and airflow characteristics simultaneously. The transnasal pressure of one side of nasal cavity can be measured as the difference of pressure between the front of the nose and behind the nose. The posterior nasal pressure sensor can be kept at the posterior nose (pernasal/postnasal-rhinomanometry), on the opposite nostril (anterior-rhinomanometry), or at the oropharynx transorally (posterior-rhinomanometry). Air can be pumped through the nose (passive-rhinomanometry), or the patient's respiratory flow (active-rhinomanometry) can be used for measurements (Fig. 3.3).

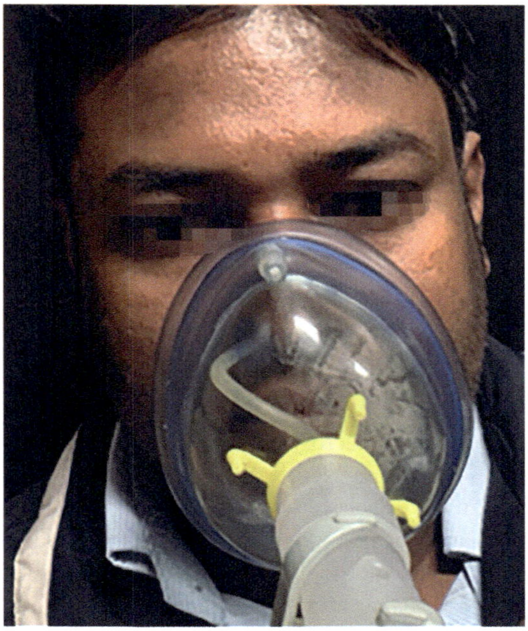

Fig. 3.3 The clinical photograph is showing anterior rhinomanometry (Courtesy—Dr. Hitesh Verma, Associate Professor, AIIMS, New Delhi, India)

3.1.3.3 References Values for Normal Adults

The nasal volume (Vol) and the minimal cross-sectional area (MCA) varies significantly between races, and the Vol and MCA of Caucasians in the non-decongested state are 0.69 cm^2 and 4.67 cm^3, respectively [9]. The normal means of total nasal resistance in the non-decongested nose is around 0.24 $Pa/cm^3/s$ in adult men about 0.24 $Pa/cm^3/s$ in adult women [10].

3.2 Part B: Olfactory Nerve and Olfactory Dysfunctions

Olfactory nerve is the special visceral afferent (SVA) nerve carrying the sense of smell or olfaction. Olfaction is an ancient, evolutionarily conserved chemosensory system. Nerves related to olfaction and taste is the only sensory nerves that lack decussation. Nerve endings are present in the superior part of olfactory cleft and adjacent nasal mucosa. The olfactory nerve enters the brain via cribriform plate and end in the olfactory bulb. Olfactory tract is formed by the efferent fiber of olfactory bulb. Olfactory tract connects primarily and secondarily with several cortical structures. Smell disorders may be caused by an impaired nasal airway or by lesions in the olfactory system, leading to reduced or distorted smell perception. Olfactory dysfunction may be the first presenting symptom of Alzheimer's or Parkinson's disease. Drugs that can cause olfactory and gustatory dysfunction are macrolides, terbinafine, fluoroquinolones. Chemical substances causing olfactory dysfunction include—acrylates, benzene, solvents, formaldehyde, cadmium, nickel dust. In head injury, occipital blows tend to produce more frequent and more severe olfactory damage than frontal blows because of coup-contra-coup injury. Olfactory epithelium has a great potential for regeneration due to its stem cell reservoir. Axel and Buck received 2004 Nobel Prize in physiology or medicine for their discoveries of odorant receptors and the organization of the olfactory system. Nasal endoscopy is the initial investigation of choice to see nasal pathology. Radiological investigation is required for intracranial lesions. Treatment policy ranges from conservative to surgical, depending on the findings. Recent advances in bio-inspired electronics have resulted in the development of potential artificial sensory systems. The first artificial olfactory system was built by Persaud and Dodd in 1982, by using a microsensor gas array based on metal-oxide structure. The current definition of "Electronic nose" was given by Gardner in 1988. Recently many artificial olfactory sensors, based on biomaterials like mammalian cells or olfactory receptors have been developed to improve the specificity of the sensors for odorants in the electronic nose and the new concept is now referred to as "Bioelectronic nose."

3.2.1 Anatomy of Olfactory Nerve

Olfactory nerve is the only cranial nerve that lacks the pre-cortical connection to the thalamus [11]. Olfactory epithelium, in the postero-superior portion of each nasal cavity, consists of somas of bipolar olfactory neurons, six to ten million in the nasal mucosa (on an area of 2.5 cm^2 in each nasal cavity [12]. These bipolar neurons are considered first order neurons in the olfactory pathway. Odoriferous particles come in contact with dendrites of these bipolar neurons which are projecting on the olfactory epithelial surface. Odorant molecules bind to G-protein coupled receptors on the dendrites of the olfactory neurons. Basal projections of these neurons ascend as unmyelinated axons which traverse through the cribriform plate in form of small nerve bundles (Fila olfactoria), there are 15–20 such bundles on each side, each forming olfactory nerves that passes through the cribriform plate surrounded by a meningeal covering (arachnoid). These Fila olfactoria penetrate the cranial cavity, pass through the subarachnoid space, immediately enter the ventral surface of olfactory bulbs, and synapse here with second order bulbar neurons. Olfactory bulb-acts as a relay station for the impulses passing between the olfactory mucosa and upper olfactory centers. It is bilateral and elliptical, ventro-dorsally oriented structure with 11–15 mm length and 4–5 mm thickness, the medial edge is convex and the lateral edge is flat. The dorsal surface is in contact with orbital and rectus gyri (inferior surface of frontal lobes), with a double layer of arachnoid separating them. The ventral surface of olfactory bulb overlies posterior 1/3 of the cribriform plate which is also the horizontal plate of the ethmoid bone. It is divided medially by crista galli, which is a vertical bony prominence in the anterior part of ethmoid. There are two grooves on each side of crista galli, which harbor olfactory tracts and are known as "olfactory ethmoidal canals." Cribriform plate has 18–22 foramina on each side through which the Fila olfactoria pass into the cranial cavity and synapse with the olfactory bulb. The microscopic laminar structure of the olfactory bulb consists of seven layers. The glomerular stratum, consisting of glomeruli of dendritic projections, is the second layer among the 7 layers of the olfactory bulb and it contains the second-order neurons which synapse with fila olfactoria. This is the first relay of olfactory sensory information. The most important second-order neurons in the olfactory pathway are Mitral cells, Tufted cells, and periglomerular cells. Each glomerulus and all the neurons synapsing in it are considered the basic functional unit of odor perception. The axonal projections of the Mitral and Tufted cells form bundles that traverse the olfactory bulb and pass dorsally, merging together to form secondary olfactory projection or olfactory tract.

Olfactory tract- it is a 28–30 mm long, thin, triangular, myelinated nervous projection with approximately 5 mm thickness anteriorly which narrows down posteriorly upto 2 mm thickness. It originates in the anterior cranial fossa and ends in the middle fossa, giving rise to olfactory trigone. During its course, the olfactory tract passes over the optic nerves, which in turn pass over the oculomotor nerves. Olfactory tract lacks Schwann cells (similar to olfactory bulb). Each olfactory tract is traverse posteriorly to end into olfactory trigone which is located above the anterior clinoid process. This olfactory trigone is basically a widening of the olfactory tract that eventually becomes triangular, it divides and gives rise to two main olfactory striata (medial and lateral) and a small central Olfactory stria, these striata eventually relay to higher brain regions. Primary olfactory cortex, anterior olfactory nucleus, olfactory tubercle, amygdaloid complex are the important central cortical structures related to olfaction (Fig. 3.4). Hippocampus, hypothalamus, thalamus, orbitofrontal cortex, cerebellum are the secondary central olfactory structures. The axons of the three olfactory striata (medial, lateral, and central) are distributed to central olfactory areas. The interactions of medial olfactory stria axons are primarily responsible for the autonomic responses associated with the sense of smell, e.g., salivation in response to odor of food or increased gastric juice

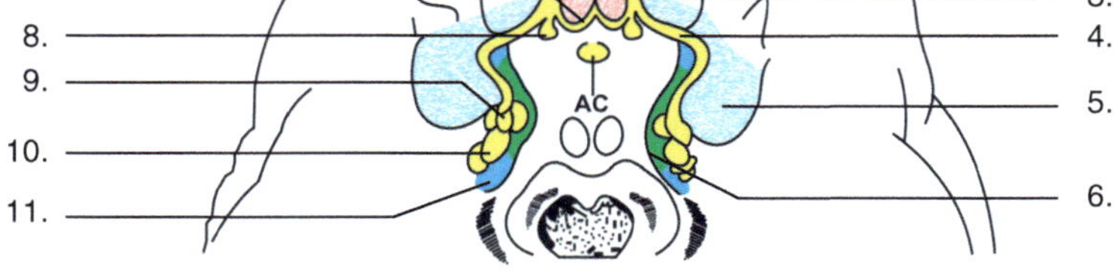

Fig. 3.4 Schematic diagram of basal view of the brain showing the ventral aspect of the frontal lobes with olfactory centers and pathways. **1**. Olfactory bulb, **2**. Olfactory tract, **3**. Anterior olfactory nucleus, **4**. Lateral olfactory stria, **5**. Insular cortex, **6**. Primary olfactory cortex, **7**. Medial olfactory stria, **8**. Olfactory tubercle, **9**. Amygdaloid complex, **10**. Hippocampal formation, **11**. Entorhinal cortex

secretion and increased intestinal peristalsis in response to the smell of food. The lateral olfactory stria has the maximum number of fibers in the olfactory tract, so it is the stria with the greatest functional transcendence. The area of the brain which is specialized in the interpretation of the olfactory sensory stimuli is the primary olfactory cortex, which is located near the uncus, in the temporal lobe and it includes—The pyriform (peri-amigdaline) and prepyriform areas.

3.2.2 Blood Supply of Olfactory Nerve

The entire course of the olfactory tract and olfactory bulb is supplied by the olfactory artery which is either a direct branch of the anterior cerebral artery or a collateral branch of the medial fronto-basal artery, which in turn is a branch of the anterior cerebral artery [13]. The blood supply of olfactory nerve also includes anterior and posterior orbital arteries also known as anterior and posterior ethmoidal arteries or accessory olfactory arteries. Other less significant arteries are Frontopolar artery, the recurrent artery of Heubner.

3.2.3 Smell Disorders

- **Hyposmia**—partial loss of smell perception.
- **Anosmia**—complete loss of smell perception.
- **Parosmia/Cacosmia/Troposmia**—the distorted perception of an existing odor, when a person perceives even pleasant odors to be foul smelling, as similar to feces, burning, rotten, or chemical odor.
- **Phantosmia**—perception of a non-existing odor (i.e., smell hallucination).
- **Hyperosmia—**increased olfactory acuity (heightened sense of smell), usually caused by a lower threshold for odor.
- Conductive smell loss—is due to impaired transport of odorant molecules to olfactory epithelia.
- Sensorineural smell loss—is due to impaired receptor function, processing, or neurotransmission.

3.2.3.1 Epidemiology

The prevalence increases with age and males are more commonly affected than females. Risk factors are increasing age, male gender, smoking, stroke, epilepsy, nasal congestion, URTIs, nasal polyps. The most common etiology for smell loss is aging. Other three major etiological factors for smell loss are—URTIs, sinonasal disease, and head trauma (Table 3.1).

3.2.4 Management of Smell Disorders

3.2.4.1 Investigations

1. **Diagnostic nasal endoscopy**—It is to exclude potential causes of conductive olfactory loss, e.g., rhinitis, nasal polyps, tumors, etc.
2. **Radiological imaging**—MRI is the investigation of choice if the nasal cavity is normal. It provides better soft tissue detail for intracranial pathology. It can also detect reduced olfactory bulb volume in congenital smell loss or parosmia.
3. **Olfactory tests**—Olfactory tests are listed below.

Table 3.1 Illustrating the etiological factor and possible causes

	Aging	URTI	Sinonasal disease	Head trauma
Presumed cause	Functional decrement in quality and quantity of olfactory receptors; ossification of cribriform plate foramina.	Viral damage of olfactory epithelium and neurons.	Nasal obstruction caused by hypertrophic mucosa and nasal polyps, cosal inflammation.	Cribriform plate injury and shearing of olfactory filaments.
Common age group	>65 years	40–60 years	20–60 years	20–50 years

(a) UPSIT (University of Pennsylvania Smell Identification Test)—This forced choice standardized test uses 40 microencapsulated odorants which are released on scratching using pencil on the standardized odor impregnated test booklets. Patients are asked to identify the odor from 4 choices provided for each odor. Hence scoring is done out of a total score of 40.
(b) Smell diskettes test—It is a questionnaire-based test with illustration.
(c) Cross-Cultural Smell Identification Test (CC-SIT)—It is 12 item cross-culture smell identification test and it is relatively quick than UPSIT. It is prepared with familiar odorant of different countries.
(d) Sniffin' sticks test—It is semi-objective test. Olfaction is assessed by calculating the mean of three subfactor threshold, identification, and discrimination.

4. **Electrophysiologic testing** of olfactory disorders usually includes the recording of olfactory event-related potentials. In response to odorant induced stimulation, the olfactory receptor neurons oscillate and the slow negative DC voltage changes recorded from the olfactory mucosa are termed Electrolfactograms (EOGs) and are regarded as compound receptor potentials of olfactory receptor neurons in the olfactory epithelium. This diagnostic tool presents the final method to confirm anosmia, but it is more used for research purposes.

3.2.4.2 Treatment Options

It depends upon the etiological factors; lifestyle modifications are breathing exercise and regular nasal douches, etc. Oral steroids may help in regaining of smell in idiopathic cases. Counseling is necessary in cases of parosmia and phantosmia. Psychiatric or neurological treatment (e.g., antidepressants or antiepileptic drugs) may be required in some patients. In cases of chronic rhinosinusitis with nasal polyposis, the highest level of evidence exists in support of use of glucocorticoids. Initial oral steroid therapy followed by topical steroid therapy seems to be more effective than topical steroid therapy alone, in decreasing polyp size and improving olfaction [14]. In nasal polyposis, surgery is reserved for cases not responding to optimal medical therapy and can improve olfaction even in some of the refractory cases. Surgical resection of olfactory neurons may lead to olfactory reinnervation from the basal stem cells, leading to recovery of smell.

3.2.5 Bioelectronic Nose

Bioelectronic nose mimics the olfactory function of the natural nose by converting chemical signals into electrical signals using novel forms of transducers. In the human nose, odorants are first recognized by olfactory receptors; nearly 400 different olfactory receptors binds with specific odor molecules. A key challenge for mimicking the olfactory system is the development of appropriate transducers to modify odor molecules into electrical signals. Advancements in nanomaterials, such as CNTs, grapheme, and conducting polymers, have enabled hybridization of olfactory receptors via nanoelectronics interface formation. The bioelectronic nose consists of primary perception elements and secondary transducers and amplifiers, inspired by biological chemoreceptors and nerve systems. So combining biological receptors with novel forms of transducers, such as microelectrode arrays (MEAs), electrochemical and optical devices, and nanomaterial-based field effect transistors (FETs) effectively convert external chemical signals into electrical signals. Optical transduction techniques, including fluorescence and calcium imaging, offer accurate and objective cue of smells with visualized binding patterns. Combined with electronic sensors, such optical transduction methods can improve the performance of the bioelectronic nose.

3.2.6 Applications of Bioelectronic Nose

1. **In medical diagnosis:** By detecting Volatile organic compounds (VOCs) released from the

body during infections, intoxication, metabolic diseases, or cancers [15].
2. **In food quality control:** It is quick and accurate method to detect microbial spoilage of food materials [16]. It is also useful to monitor the maturity of fruits so that fruits can be harvested at the best possible time and for the determination of quality and identity of cheese.
3. **In environmental monitoring:** The bioelectronic nose provides cheap, improved, and reliable method for rapid, accurate detection and quantification of environmental chemical pollutants.
4. **In smell visualization:** It is based on the bioelectronic nose which expects to enable anosmic patients to perceive smells that have not been sensed before.

3.3 Part C—Acute and Chronic Rhinosinusitis

3.3.1 Summary

Rhinosinusitis is by far the most common paranasal sinus disease encountered by rhinologists worldwide. The etiopathogenesis of acute rhinosinusitis is mostly attributed to infectious etiology, whereas chronic rhinosinusitis arises from inflammatory processes triggered by various agents. The diagnosis of this condition is given by various criteria. The European position paper on rhinosinusitis and nasal polyps (EPOS 2012) defined rhinosinusitis as a diagnosis made on clinical grounds based on the presence of characteristic symptoms, combined with objective evidence of mucosal inflammation. Evidence-based review and EPOS 2012 have recommended against routine use of antibiotics in rhinosinusitis. Steroid nasal sprays are the gold standard for the medical management of CRS. It decreases mucosal inflammation and causes partial polyp resolution. FESS (Functional endoscopic sinus surgery) is quite often required for management of CRS and very occasionally in ARS, in cases not responding to conservative management and cases with complications.

3.3.2 Introduction

Rhinosinusitis is by far the most common paranasal sinus disease. As the name suggests, it is the inflammation of the nasal and sinus mucosa. Acute rhinosinusitis (ARS) prevalence rates vary from 6 to 15% with a prevalence of recurrent ARS estimated at 0.035% [17] Chronic rhinosinusitis (CRS) represents a significant disease burden worldwide, affecting at least 11% of the population which creates substantial economic burden to healthcare systems and to the economy, by loss of productivity in the workplace [18]. Rhinosinusitis is primarily classified based on the duration of signs and symptoms (Table 3.2).

CRS is further classified into those cases with polyps and those without polyps based on endoscopic findings. A proportion of patients with polyps also fall into a unique subset, characterized by coexistent asthma and aspirin sensitivity known as Samter's triad or aspirin-exacerbated respiratory disease (AERD) [19].

3.3.3 Pathophysiology

Acute rhinosinusitis (ARS) can be viral or bacterial, with viral etiology being the most common (>95%) [20]. Predisposing factors to ARS include sinus-related anatomical factors (e.g., Haller/

Table 3.2 Rhinosinusitis is classified on the basis of duration of symptoms

Type of rhinosinusitis	Duration of inflammation
Acute	Up to 4 weeks
Chronic	>12 weeks
Sub-acute	4–12 weeks
Recurrent ARS	>4 episodes per year without evidence of CRS Each episode lasts 7–10 days
Acute on CRS	The inflammation never touch baseline

infra-orbital ethmoid cells, concha bullosa), allergy, smoking, poor mental health, Immunodeficiency, ciliary disorders, etc. The most commonly implicated viruses in ARS include rhinoviruses (50%), influenza and para-influenza viruses, adenovirus, respiratory syncytial virus, and enterovirus [21]. If bacteria do become implicated, the organisms most commonly seen are *S. pneumoniae* (27%), *H. influenzae* (44%), *M. catarrhalis* (14%) with other organisms sometimes seen including *S. pyogenes* and *S. aureus* [22]. ARS is bacterial (ABRS) if at least three of the symptoms co-exist:

1. Discolored discharge (unilateral predominance)
2. Severe local pain (unilateral predominance)
3. Fever (>38 °C)
4. Elevated ESR/CRP (Erythrocyte sedimentation rate/C—Reactive protein)
5. "Double-sickening"—Deterioration of symptoms after the initial milder phase of illness

Pathophysiological mechanisms relating to viral agents include cell invasion of the respiratory epithelium leading to inflammatory changes including mechanical changes, epithelial damage, and activation of humoral and cellular defenses. In bacterial cases, this is largely a super-infection following an initial viral insult where epithelial disruption has already occurred and there has been an associated decrease in ciliated cells and increase in goblet cells which eventually cause sinus ostial obstruction. The accumulating mucus causes an initial increase in the intra-sinus pressure followed quickly by negative pressure due to the lack of ventilation. This then sets up a vicious cycle of further congestion, mucus retention; impaired gas exchange, and pH balance and largely prevents clearance of inflammatory products and debris leading to an ideal medium for bacteria to flourish. The patients who do not respond to therapy might have the pathophysiology of biofilms, superantigens, or persistent osteitis.

Chronic Rhinosinusitis (CRS) with polyposis is characterized by an intense edematous stroma in the sinonasal epithelium, with albumin deposition, pseudocyst formation, and subepithelial/perivascular inflammatory cell infiltration. It appears to be associated with a typical T-helper 2 cell (TH2) skewed eosinophilic inflammation, with high interleukin (IL-5) and eosinophil cationic protein (ECP) concentrations in the polyps. CRS without polyposis is characterized by fibrosis, basement membrane thickening, goblet cell hyperplasia, subepithelial edema, and mononuclear cell infiltration. It exhibits a T-helper 1 cell (TH1) milieu, with increased levels of interferon-gamma (IFN-γ) in inflammed sinus mucosa and low ECP/myeloperoxidase ratios [23].

Diagnostic criteria: There are two most commonly used diagnostic criteria.

Rhinosinusitis Task Force of the American Academy of Otolaryngology–Head and Neck Surgery classification of rhinosinusitis (1997) [24] (Table 3.3).

Diagnosis requires the presence of either two major factors, or one major and two minor factors. The European position paper on rhinosinusitis and nasal polyps (EPOS 2012) defined rhinosinusitis as a diagnosis made on clinical grounds based on the presence of characteristic symptoms, combined with objective evidence of mucosal inflammation (Table 3.4) [17].

Chronic rhinosinusitis (CRS) is divided broadly into two subtypes, with nasal polyposis (CRSwNP) and CRS without polyposis (CRSsNP). Phenotype and endotype classification for CRS is also proposed in view of the number of subtypes of CRS.

3.3.4 Diagnostic Work Up

Rigid nasal endoscopy and CT scanning of the sinuses are at the present time the gold standard investigations for CRS (Fig. 3.5). Endoscopy allows the clinician to assess the nose for the presence of polyps, mucopus discharge, or middle meatal edema. The endoscope can be also used to accurately sample any mucopus for microbiological analysis [25]. CT scanning is considered mandatory for all cases requiring surgical intervention or with complications/impending complications [26]. The other tests of significance are used to enumerate the cause or exclude an differential diagnosis [27]:

Table 3.4 Clinical definition of Rhinosinusitis

Diagnostic criteria for rhinosinusitis	Symptoms should be correlated by either endoscopic and/or radiological findings
Primary symptoms (requires at least one to be present, but if both are present it is sufficient to make the diagnosis on the basis of symptoms)	Nasal blockage/obstruction/congestion Nasal discharge (anterior/posterior)
Additional symptoms (may also be present and at least one is needed if only one of the primary symptoms is present)	Facial pain/pressure Olfactory dysfunction Hyposmia/anosmia
Duration	>10 days, <3 months = acute >3 months = chronic
Endoscopy (any of these)	Nasal polyps Mucopurulent discharge (middle meatus) Edema/mucosal obstruction in middle meatus
CT scan findings (as well as or instead of endoscopic findings)	Mucosal changes within the ostiomeatal complex and/or sinuses

1. Allergy testing—skin prick testing or IgE levels (specific and total)
2. Nasal brushings for cytology
3. Nasal biopsy for the exclusion of neoplasia, to look for granulomas/vasculitis, or to examine for evidence of eosinophilia, fungal hyphae, ciliary disorders, etc.
4. Blood tests—full blood count (serum eosinophilia), ANCA (Wegener's granulomatosis), ACE (sarcoidosis)
5. Olfactory testing: Psychophysical (threshold (quantitative) and discrimination/identification (qualitative)), Olfactory event-related potentials (OERPs) (objective)
6. Physiological testing
   (a) Peak inspiratory nasal flow
   (b) Rhinomanometry
   (c) Acoustic rhinometry
   (d) Mucociliary clearance (saccharin test)
7. Ciliary function testing
   (a) Ciliary beat frequency
   (b) Ciliary beat pattern analysis
   (c) Electron microscopy

Table 3.3 Symptoms and signs of rhinosinusitis

Major symptoms/signs
Facial pain/pressure
Facial congestion/fullness
Nasal obstruction/blockage
Nasal discharge/purulence, discolored posterior drainage
Hyposmia/anosmia
Purulence on nasal examination
Fever (acute rhinosinusitis only)
Minor symptoms/signs
Headache
Fever (nonacute rhinosinusitis)
Halitosis
Fatigue
Dental pain
Cough
Ear pain/pressure/fullness

3.3.5 Radiological Staging

The common staging used for scoring of radiological findings is Lund-Mackay score [28]. This is a widely used method for documentation and comparison (Table 3.5).

For each sinus, score 0 means no opacification, score 1 means partial and 2 means complete opacification whereas for ostiomeatal complex, the score is either 0 (not obstructed) or 2 (obstructed). Each side is graded separately. A combined score of up to 24 is possible. In case of an aplastic or absent frontal sinus, a score of 0 is awarded.

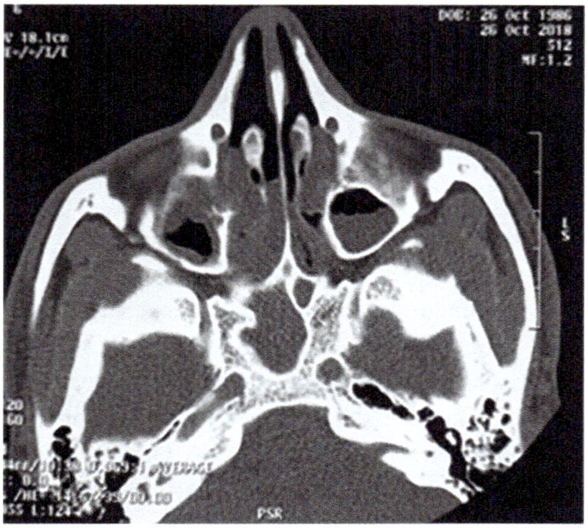

Fig. 3.5 CT scan depicting CRS involving soft tissue density in the bilateral maxillary sinus

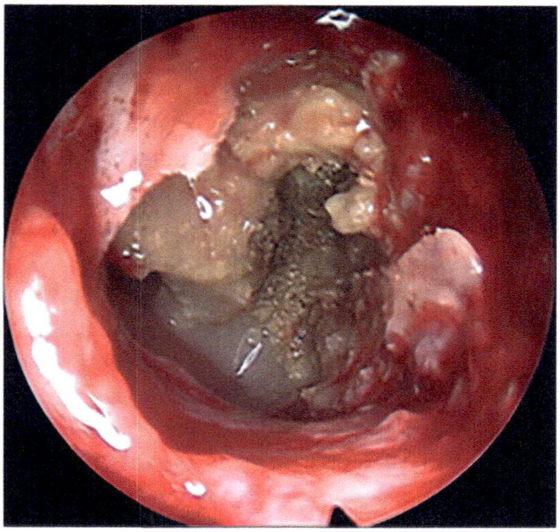

Fig. 3.6 The presence of fungal Muck with allergic mucin in the sinus differentiates CRS from allergic fungal rhinosinusitis which is an important differential diagnosis

Table 3.5 Lund-Mackay score

Score:
• 0 (no abnormality)
• 1 (partial opacification) or
• 2 (complete opacification)

3.3.6 Differential Diagnosis

Rhinosinusitis needs to be evaluated closely as many other conditions mimic rhinosinusitis. Appropriate history, endoscopy, and radiological evaluation are useful to rule out other differential diagnosis. Common diseases like fungal rhinosinusitis, benign nasal, and paranasal tumors, intermediate grade tumors like inverted papilloma, and malignancy need to be ruled out in cases not responding to treatment (Fig. 3.6).

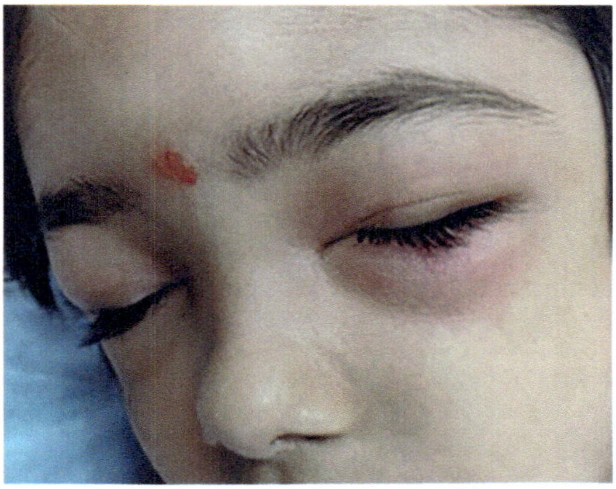

Fig. 3.7 The figure is showing left side preseptal cellulitis secondary to sinusitis (Courtesy—Dr. Hitesh Verma, Associate Professor, AIIMS, New Delhi, India)

3.3.7 Complications

Acute rhinosinusitis can cause complications due to local spread, like the erosion of lamina papyracea or through preformed foramina's (Fig. 3.7). Pott's puffy tumor or frontal subperiosteal abscess can lead to intracranial complications and thus needs early drainage and debridement. Ethmoid sinusitis can lead to orbital cellulitis and sphenoid sinusitis can lead to cavernous sinus thrombosis. Hematogenous spread can lead to brain abscess, meningitis, and toxic shock syndrome. CRS is usually associated with mucocele or pyocele formation and in case of acute exacerbation can lead to different varieties of acute complications.

3.3.8 Treatment

3.3.8.1 Antibiotics

As most cases are viral in origin, antibiotics are usually not required. Only superadded bacterial infection dictates the use of antibiotics. Due to the varied bacterial infection in ARS and CRS, the antibiotic cover is different from CRS requiring long-term antibiotics. Ideally treatment should be culture directed and re-evaluation is required for a possibility of change in antibiotics if there is no response to treatment within 72 h.

3.3.8.2 Nasal Sprays and Irrigation

Steroid nasal sprays are the gold standard for the medical management of CRS [29]. It decreases mucosal inflammation and causes partial polyp resolution. Saline and hypertonic saline nasal irrigation keeps the mucosa moist, improves naso-ciliary clearance, and prevents crust formation [30].

3.3.8.3 Oral Steroids and Anti-Histaminics

The oral steroid is immensely effective in reducing inflammation and sometimes leads to near complete resolution of polyposis (Fig. 3.8) [31]. In comparison to nasal steroid spray, it runs a higher risk of systemic side effects. As allergy can be associated, anti-histaminics and lifestyle modification plays a major role in minimizing the predisposing inflammation and recurrence of symptoms.

3.3.9 Surgery

FESS (Functional endoscopic sinus surgery) is quite often required for management of CRS and very occasionally in ARS. The role of surgery is to clear the sinus opening of any obstruction and allow the delivery of medications. Utmost care is taken to preserve the normal ciliated columnar epithelium. The surgery is usually indicated in cases not responding to long-term medical management or in cases of impending complication [32].

3.4 Part D: Frontal Sinusitis

3.4.1 Summary

The frontal sinus is one of the most complex paranasal sinuses. The frontal sinus is paired sinus and is separated by an intersinus septum that can vary in location. The frontal sinus outflow tract (FSOT) is described as an hourglass. Management of frontal

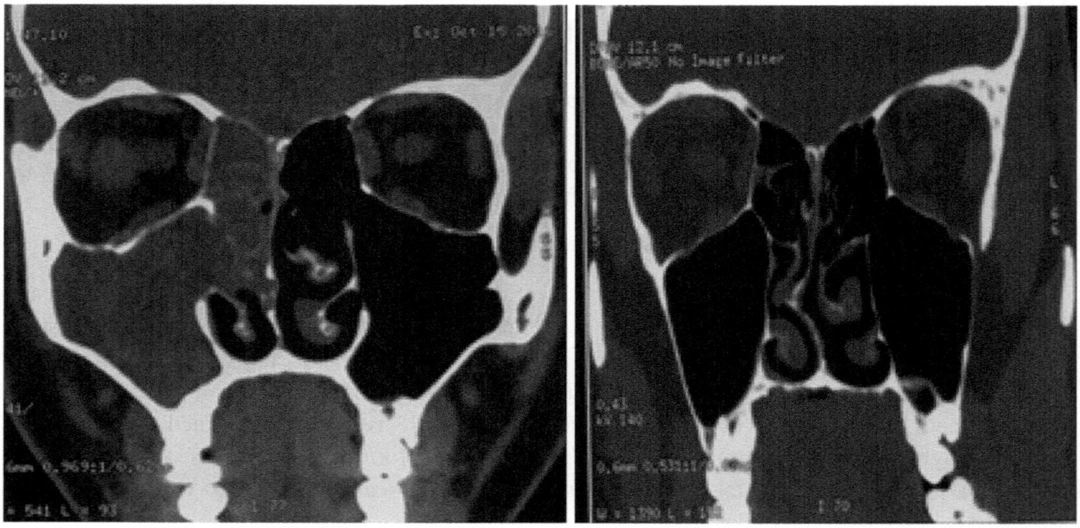

Fig. 3.8 Pansinusitis is completely resolved by oral steroid treatment (Courtesy—Dr. Hitesh Verma, Associate Professor, AIIMS, New Delhi, India)

sinus pathologies has evolved from open approaches to endoscopic approaches in the past few decades. The introduction of various classification systems like Bent and Kuhn system, Wormald classification, and the latest International frontal sinus anatomy classification system for frontal cells has helped in the surgical management of the sinus. Surgical decision making with respect to the ideal approach to the frontal sinus, can be a challenge. Hence, a thorough understanding of the available surgical techniques and the specific circumstances in which each is most effective is critical.

3.4.2 Introduction

The frontal sinus is one of the most complexes of all paranasal sinuses because of its complex drainage pathway. It is essential to clear the outflow tract in case of any pathology obstructing the drainage pathway without causing iatrogenic stenosis. Outflow tract (FSOT) is described as an hourglass. Identification of this drainage pathway helps in directing a surgeon to dissect in a way that minimizes mucosal trauma. It appears by the age of 4 years and expands in adolescence. In radiological studies, it appears by the age of 8 years. It gains its maximum size by 19 years of age. Frontal sinus is a paired asymmetric structure with intersinus septum that can vary in location. Frontal recess is a three-dimensional space (Fig. 3.9). Anteriorly, it lined by agger nasi (AN) (Fig. 3.10a), frontoethmoidal cell (FEC) and the frontal process of maxilla, frontal beak (FB), posteriorly by the upward continuation of the anterior face of the bulla (Fig. 3.10b), laterally by lamina papyracea (Fig. 3.10c) and medially by upper attachment of middle turbinate (Fig. 3.10d).

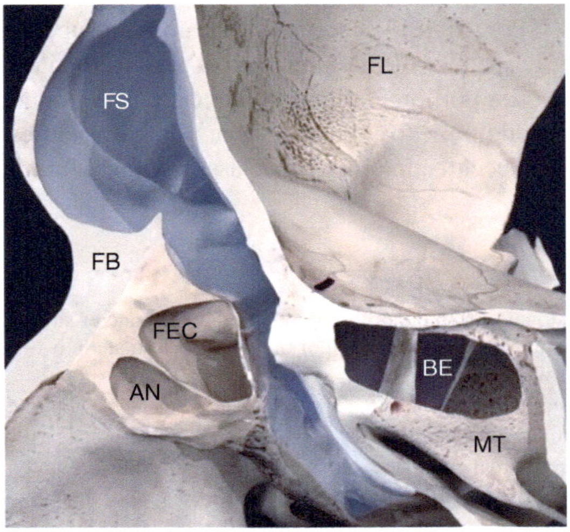

Fig. 3.9 The figure is showing the relationship of the frontal sinus and frontal recess with the surrounding structure

3.4.3 Pathophysiology

Mucociliary transport in the frontal sinus is an active inwardly directed one. Secretions climb along the intersinus septum, then pass along the roof and then along the floor drain out in FSOT. All of the secretions is not drained out of the ostium at once and some of it recirculate back into the sinus for another trip. This results in whorl like mucociliary clearance from the sinus.

3.4.4 Preoperative Workup

Non-Contrast Computed Tomography scan is the major backbone of the diagnostic workup.

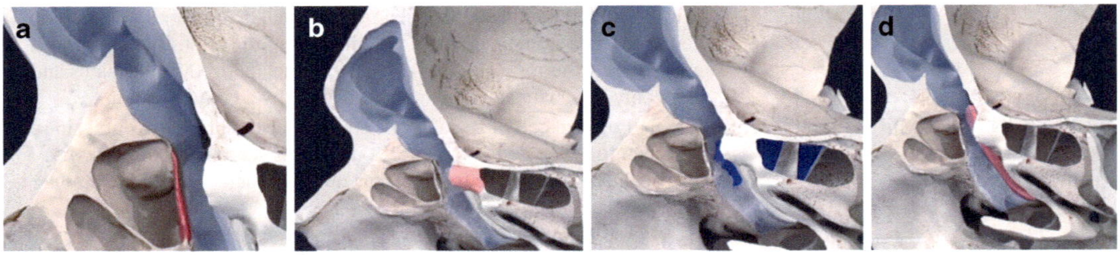

Fig. 3.10 The figure is showing the boundary of frontal recess

Parasagittal view helps in identifying the complex cells within the frontal sinus and the outflow tract. Structures to look for

1. Uncinate process—the site of its superior attachment impacts on the drainage of frontal sinus.
2. Frontal cells—they are present in 20% of patients. Bent and Kuhn divided these into four types [33]:
   (a) Type I—single cell above agger nasi
   (b) Type II—Multiple cells above agger nasi
   (c) Type III—Cell extends into frontal sinus
   (d) Type IV—Isolated frontal cell

Recently PJ Wormald proposed International Frontal Sinus Anatomy Classification [34] (Table 3.6).

Magnetic resonance imaging (MRI) is indicated in doubtful diagnosis as it provides better soft tissue detail. Tumors show enhancement in T1 sequence with contrast while fluids do not. Mucus and secretions enhance on T2 weighted scans and it is particularly useful for predicting dural involvement:

3.4.4.1 Surgical Approaches

The conservative management of acute frontal sinusitis is documented in the previous part. Factors which should be considered while dealing with frontal sinus pathology are listed in Table 3.7.

Draf classified frontal sinus surgery into four types [35]:

1. Draf I—Anterior ethmoidectomy, including the frontal recess but sparing the frontal sinus infundibulum and ostia.
2. Draf IIa—Anterior ethmoidectomy + Resection of frontal sinus floor from lamina papyracea laterally to middle turbinate medially.
3. Draf IIb—Anterior ethmoidectomy + Removal of frontal sinus floor from lamina papyracea laterally to nasal deptum.
4. Draf III (Endoscopic Modified Lothrop Procedure)—resection of the anterior superior aspect of the nasal septum as well as the inferior portion of the frontal intersinus septum in addition to bilateral type IIb procedures. Recently, International classification of frontal

Table 3.6 International frontal sinus anatomy classification

Cell type	Cell name	Definition
Anterior cells (push the drainage pathway of the frontal sinus medial, posterior, or posteromedially)	Agger nasi cell	Cell that sits either anterior to the origin of the middle turbinate or sits directly above the most anterior insertion of the middle turbinate into the lateral nasal wall.
	Supra agger cell	Anterior-lateral ethmoidal cell, located above the agger nasi cell (not pneumatizing into the frontal sinus).
	Supra agger frontal cell	Anterior-lateral ethmoidal cell that extends into the frontal sinus. A small SAFC will only extend into the floor of the frontal sinus, whereas a large SAFC may extend significantly into the frontal sinus and may even reach the roof of the frontal sinus.
Posterior cells (push the drainage pathway anteriorly)	Supra-bulla cell	Cell above the bulla ethmoidalis that does not enter the frontal sinus
	Supra-bulla frontal cell	Cell that originates in the supra-bulla region and pneumatizes along the skull base into the posterior region of the frontal sinus. The skull base forms the posterior wall of the cell.
	Supraorbital ethmoid cell	An anterior ethmoid cell that pneumatizes around, anterior to, or posterior to the anterior ethmoidal artery over the roof of the orbit. It often forms part of the posterior wall of an extensively pneumatized frontal sinus and may only be separated from the frontal sinus by a bony septation.
Medial cells (push the drainage pathway laterally)	Frontal septal cell	Medially based cell of the anterior ethmoid or the inferior frontal sinus, attached to or located in the interfrontal sinus septum, associated with the medial aspect of the frontal sinus outflow tract, pushing the drainage pathway laterally and frequently posteriorly.

Table 3.7 The factors related to patient, anatomy, and pathology of frontal sinus are listed in the consideration column. The surgical plan is listed in the surgical options column

	Considerations	Surgical options
Patient	1. Limited disease 2. Compliance issues and significant comorbidities.	Simple FESS with minimal manipulation of the frontal recess.
	Asthma and aspirin sensitivity	Comprehensive clearance of frontal recess. If recurrence see below
Anatomy	Preserved landmarks, minimum previous surgery, no complex cells	Draf type I procedure
	Poor landmarks, osteoneogenesis, multiple revision procedures, thick frontal beak, complex frontal cells	Draf type (modified endoscopic lothrop)
Pathology	Chronic frontal sinusitis with or without polyps, No previous surgery.	Draf type I procedure
	Recurrent disease, ASA with polyp, Eosinophilic mucin CRS, tumors, Lateral mucoceles. Recalcitrant.	Draf type (modified endoscopic lothrop)
	Complicated frontal sinusitis with the erosion of posterior table, anterior table osteitis, lateral extending tutors	Draf type III or an osteoplastic flap approach. Combined approach.

Table 3.8 International classification of frontal sinus surgery

No exploration	No disease
Balloon sinuplasty	May have a role in certain situations with limited disease.
Draf type I	Removing cells within the frontal recess, following FESS
Draf type IIa and b	Remove cells extending into the frontal sinus and resect bone between the lamina papyracea and middle turbinate (a) or nasal septum (b)
Draf type III, modified endoscopic lothrop (MEL), frontal sinus drillout	Resection of the floor of the frontal sinus, superior nasal septum, and intersinus septum
Osteoplastic flap + MEL Osteoplastic flap with obliteration	Above and below approach Removal of all mucosa within the sinus and obliteration with fat
Reidel's Procedure	Removal of the anterior table of the frontal sinus
Cranialization	Removal of the sinus mucosa and the posterior table.

sinus surgery is proposed on the basis of structures removed (Table 3.8) [36]. It also incorporated recent modifications in treatment policy.

The considerations for endoscopic management of frontal sinus tumors are:

1. Lesions not extending beyond a sagittal plane through the lamina papyracea are accessible endoscopically. Lesions extending beyond this may be accessible depending on the anterior-posterior dimension of the floor of the frontal sinus and the intercanthal distance.
2. Tumors arising from the medial quarter of the orbital plate of the frontal sinus may be accessible via a MEL alone or with the aid of an external trephine.
3. The junction of the anterior and posterior wall in the most lateral part of the frontal sinus may be too narrow to admit a drill. Similarly, supraorbital ethmoid cells may limit lateral access for tumor removal.
4. In general, tumors arising from the anterior wall of the frontal sinus are difficult to access endoscopically. Those arising low down may be accessible via a MEL.
5. A narrow anterior-posterior dimension of the floor of the frontal sinus (<10 mm) can limit endoscopic access and favor open or combined approaches.
6. Superior reach within the sinus may not be possible in well-pneumatized sinuses.

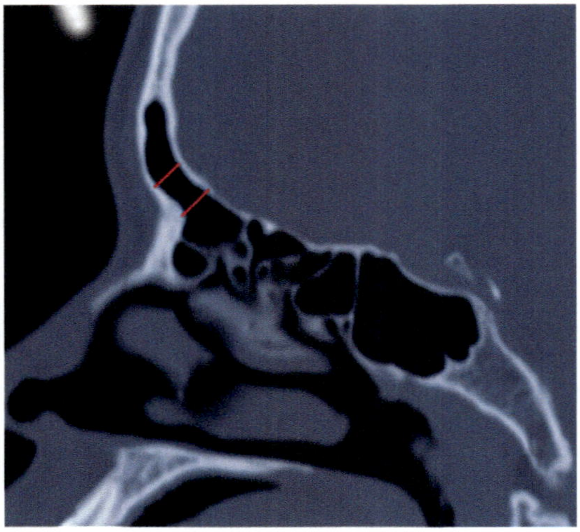

Fig. 3.11 Red lines are dividing the frontal sinus into three parts

7. Lesions originating in the lower third of the posterior wall of the frontal sinus are usually accessible via an endoscopic approach (Fig. 3.11).

3.4.4.2 Open Approaches

1. Frontal sinus trephination is performed by the creation of window in anterior wall. It starts with 1–1.5 cm incision slightly anterior or at the medial eyebrow. Periosteum over anterior wall of frontal sinus is incised and elevated. Small window made using a burr at the junction of floor and the anterior wall of the sinus. Sinus is irrigated with or without drain placement. Irrigation with color dye can aid the surgeon in detecting the sinus outflow tract endoscopically. (Mini trephination).
   Indications are:
   (a) Acute frontal sinusitis not responding to conservative management
   (b) Chronic frontal sinusitis
   (c) Depressed fracture of anterior wall of frontal sinus
   (d) Biopsy of frontal sinus lesion
   (e) As an adjuvant to endoscopic approach to localize frontal sinus especially in revision surgery
2. External frontoethmoidectomy starts with c shape incision which is placed at mid point in between nasion and medial canthus. Periosteum is incised and elevated and medial canthal ligament detached and tagged. The lacrimal sac is lifted up from the fossa. Frontoethmoidal suture line is exposed and anterior ethmoidal artery is identified and ligated. Artery forms the superior limit of dissection. Bone of lacrimal fossa and lamina papyracea is perforated as per the requirement for ethmoidectomy. Frontal sinus is accessible by removal of the floor and anterior wall of the frontal sinus.
   Indications are:
   (a) Chronic frontal sinusitis
   (b) Drainage of orbital abscess
   (c) Drainage of orbital hematoma
   (d) Orbital decompression of endocrine exophthalmos
   (e) Removal of tumor from frontal and ethmoid sinuses

   Complications
   (a) Injury to the lacrimal sac
   (b) Orbital hematomas
   (c) Closure of the nasofrontal duct by prolapsed of orbital fat, or by fibrosis and osteoneogenesis
   (d) Failure to reattach the medial canthal ligament can result in pseudohypertelorism
3. Osteoplastic Flap with and Without Obliteration
   The procedure starts with the creation of accurate template of the frontal sinus by using 6-feet Caldwell view plain radiograph. Outline of frontal sinus is marked after the creation of flap by Gull wing incision/bi-coronal incision. Periosteum is incised along the template's periphery and along the intersinus septum. Bone flap is elevated obliquely for easy reposition postoperatively. Incision is extending till the orbital rim for the easy lift of bone. Pericranium can be left attached at the lower part of bone flap for subsequent vascularity. Interfrontal sinus septa can be easily braked by osteotome or by drill. Contents of the sinus are removed. Cavity can be either obliterated with fat or is left unobliterated depending upon the indication of surgery.
   Indications

(a) Chronic frontal sinusitis
(b) Mucoceles
(c) Tumors
(d) Fractures
(e) Correction of pneumatoceles

Complications:
(a) Fracture of the bone flap, accidental intracranial entry
(b) Paresthesia and anesthesia on forehead
(c) Postoperative mucoceles

Management of frontal sinus pathologies requires a thorough understanding of the anatomy of the sinus and its outflow tract. Each case of frontal sinus pathology is unique and so requires an individualized approach for management. Though endoscopic approaches form the mainstay of frontal sinus surgery, open approaches have a role as an adjuvant to the endoscopic approach.

3.5 Part E: Complications of Sinusitis

3.5.1 Summary

Sinusitis under routine circumstances does not cause serious problems and can be often managed conservatively. Once complications arise it can take serious turn if not managed appropriately well within time. Complications can be benign/localized around the sinuses or it can be potentially serious or even fatal if it involves vital structures like orbit, cavernous sinus, and the intracranial compartment. Orbital complications are the most common and comprise around 60–75% of the total whereas local osseous complications and intracranial complications account for about 5–10% and 15–20% respectively. The proximity of orbit and brain to all the paranasal sinuses makes these structures prone to develop complications. Early stage of complications can be well managed conservatively using appropriate antibiotics but as severity increases, surgical management becomes the treatment of choice. Delayed treatment can lead to permanent sequalae and even lead to mortality.

Due to the close proximity of sinuses to the orbit and the brain, management often warrants combined efforts of ENT surgeons, Ophthalmologists, and Neurosurgeons.

3.5.2 Introduction

Complications of sinusitis can be both benign and potentially fatal. The incidence of complications has come down drastically due to the timely use of appropriate antibiotics. Generally, complications of sinusitis can be divided into three categories [37–39]

(a) Local (Osseous) (5–10%).
(b) Orbital (60–75%).
(c) Intracranial (15–20%).
(d) Other rare complications of cranial nerve palsy and optic neuropathy.

The proximity of orbit and brain to all the paranasal sinuses makes these structures prone to develop complications.

(a) **Local/Osseous/Benign Complications (5–10%)**
These complications are usually the least dangerous among all and can be managed without much morbidity to the patient (Table 3.9). They can range from
 (i) Mucocele (Fig. 3.12)
 (ii) Pott's puffy tumor (Frontal sinusitis with acute osteomyelitis)
 (iii) Facial cellulitis (Fig. 3.13)
 (iv) Facial abscess
(b) **Orbital Complications (60–75%)** [40]
Orbital complications are the most common complications of sinusitis (Table 3.10). The proximity of the eye to all the paranasal sinuses makes the orbit prone for infections and serious complications associated with sinusitis. The only soft tissue barrier is the periorbital septum. The superior and inferior ophthalmic veins are valve less and infection from the sinuses can spread to the

Table 3.9 It is showing local complication list, clinical features, and management

Complications	Clinical features	Management
Mucocele	Can present as swelling in and around the eye (ethmoid and frontal mucocele) or just some pressure symptoms or orbital symptoms (sphenoid mucocele)	Endoscopic clearance or external approach
Pott's puffy tumor	Frontal sinusitis with acute osteomyelitis. Subperiosteal pus collection in the frontal sinus leads to puffy fluctuance. • Patient presents with fever, headache, neurological findings, periorbital/frontal swelling, nasal congestion, and rhinorrhea. • May be associated with other abscess like pericranial, periorbital, epidural, subdural, and intracranial abscess if not managed adequately. • Fronto- cutaneous fistula as a late complication. • CT Scan imaging modality of choice.	Managed by combined neurosurgical and ENT team.
Facial cellulitis and abscess	These complications are local complications associated with acute sinusitis especially of the ethmoids and maxillary sinusitis.	Managed by aggressive antimicrobial therapy followed by surgery to clear the pus and open the sinuses.

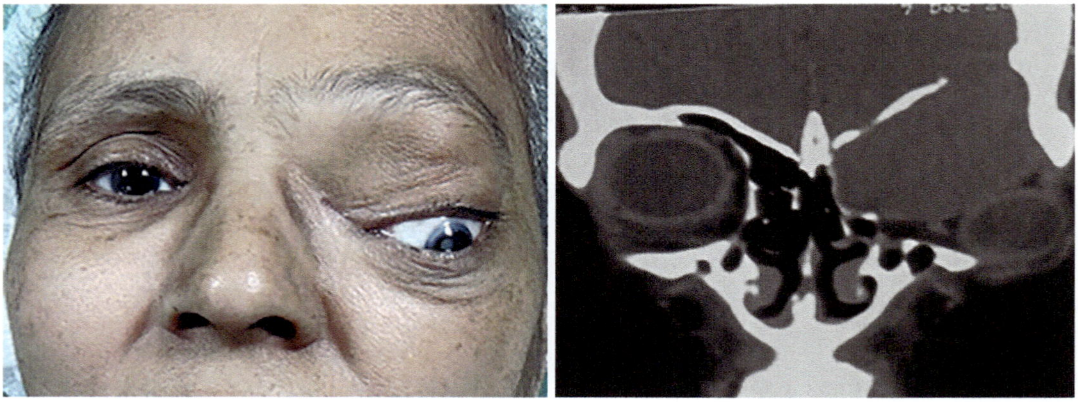

Fig. 3.12 Left side frontal mucocele. The left eyeball is pushed inferomedially and radiology is correlating with clinical photograph (Courtesy—Dr. Hitesh Verma, Associate Professor, AIIMS, New Delhi, India)

orbit very rapidly. They are given as **Chandler's criteria** [42]

(i) Preseptal cellulitis (Fig. 3.13)
(ii) Orbital cellulitis (Fig. 3.14)
(iii) Subperiosteal abscess (Fig. 3.15)
(iv) Orbital abscess
(v) Cavernous sinus thrombosis (Fig. 3.16)

(c) **Intracranial Complications (15–20%)** [43–46]

Intracranial infection due to sinusitis occurs either due to direct extension of infection or through hematogenous spread. Direct extension occurs due to either sinus wall erosion or through fracture lines or neurovascular foramina. Hematogenous spread on the other hand is

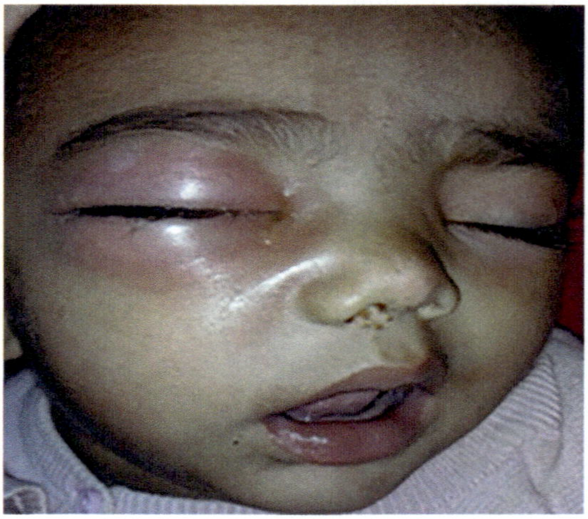

Fig. 3.13 Right side preseptal cellulitis with facial cellulitis

Table 3.10 It is showing the type of orbital complications, Symptomatology, and treatment

Orbital complications	Symptomatology	Treatment [41]
Preseptal cellulitis	• Eyelid edema and erythema • Extraocular movement intact • Normal vision • May have eyelid abscess • CT Scan: Diffuse thickness and edema of lids and conjunctiva • Least severe, most frequent	• Immediate i.v antibiotics, warm compress, and head elevation • Facilitate sinus drainage using nasal decongestants, mucolytics, and saline nasal douching.
Orbital cellulitis	• Post septal infection • Eyelid edema/erythema • Proptosis and chemosis • Impaired Extra ocular movt. • No discrete abscess • Visual acuity intact • **CT shows** low attenuation adjacent to lamina papyracea	• Immediate i.v antibiotics, warm compress, and head elevation • Facilitate sinus drainage using nasal decongestants, mucolytics, and saline nasal douching • Surgical intervention to facilitate sinus drainage if symptoms worsen in 48 h. • This could be done either endoscopic or external approach
Subperiosteal abscess	• Pus formation between periorbita and lamina papyracea • Displace orbital contents downward and laterally • Proptosis, chemosis, ophthalmoplegia • Risk for residual visual sequelae • May rupture through septum and present in eyelids • CT Scan: Rim enhancing hypodensity with mass effect adjacent to lamina papyracea	• Medical and surgical management • Look for worsening of visual acuity and EOM movements • Surgical drainage by doing external ethmoidectomy (Lynch Operation). **Remove lamina papyracea** • Endoscopic approach for medially placed abscesses • Transcaruncular approach (transconjunctival incision extend medially around lacrimal carbuncle)
Orbital abscess	• Pus formation within orbital tissues • Severe exophthalmos and chemosis • Ophthalmoplegia • Visual impairment • Risk for irreversible blindness • Can spontaneously drain through eyelid	• Drain sinuses and abscess • Incise periorbita and drain the intraconal abscess • Similar approaches as with subperiosteal • Abscess (Lynch incision, Endoscopic for medial extent)
Cavernous sinus thrombosis	• Orbital pain • Proptosis and chemosis • Ophthalmoplegia • **Symptoms in contralateral eye** • Associated with sepsis and meningismus • Radiology: Poor venous enhancement on CT. Better visualized on MRI	• Condition is very serious and warrants immediate attention • I.V Antibiotics which cross blood-brain barrier in high doses • Surgical drainage of sinuses • Mortality can be as high as 30% • Anticoagulant use to stop further propagation of clot is controversial.

through the diploic skull veins or through vessels in the ethmoid bone. Thrombophlebitis originating in the mucosal veins progressively involves the emissary veins of the skull, the dural venous sinuses, the subdural veins, and, finally, the cerebral veins. By this mode, the subdural space may be selectively infected without contamination of the intermediary structure; a subdural empyema can exist without evidence of extradural infection or osteomyelitis. Intracranial infections are (Table 3.11)

(i) Meningitis
(ii) Epidural abscess
(iii) Subdural abscess
(iv) Intracerebral abscess
(v) Cavernous sinus, venous sinus thrombosis

Intracranial involvement usually presents with common symptomatology of fever, headache, nausea, and vomiting, seizures, altered sensorium, hemiparesis, visual disturbance, and meningismus.

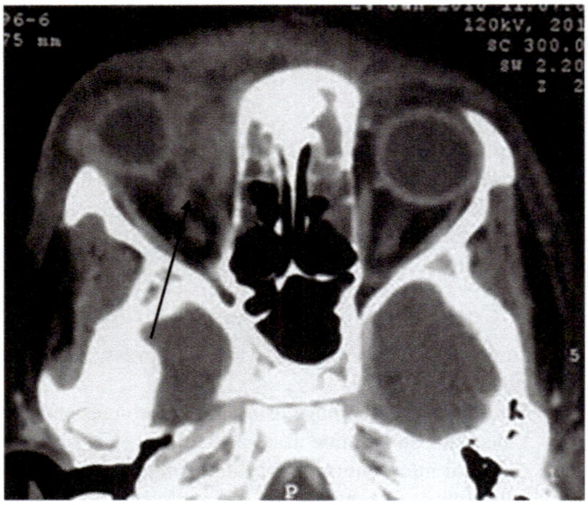

Fig. 3.14 NCCT PNS orbit is showing left side orbital cellulitis

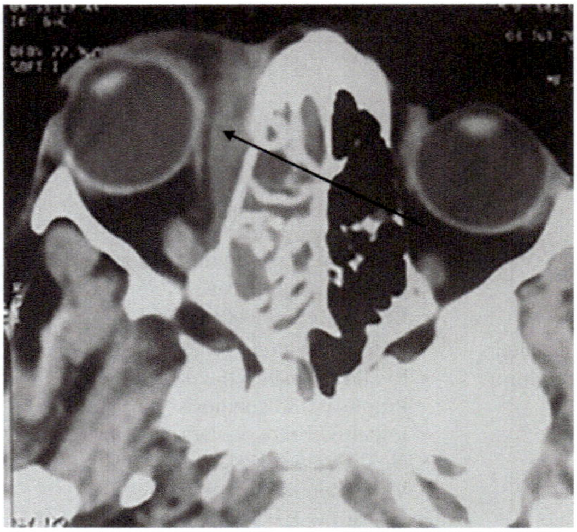

Fig. 3.15 NCCT PNS orbit is showing right side subperiosteal abscess (Courtesy—Dr. Hitesh Verma, Associate Professor, AIIMS, New Delhi, India)

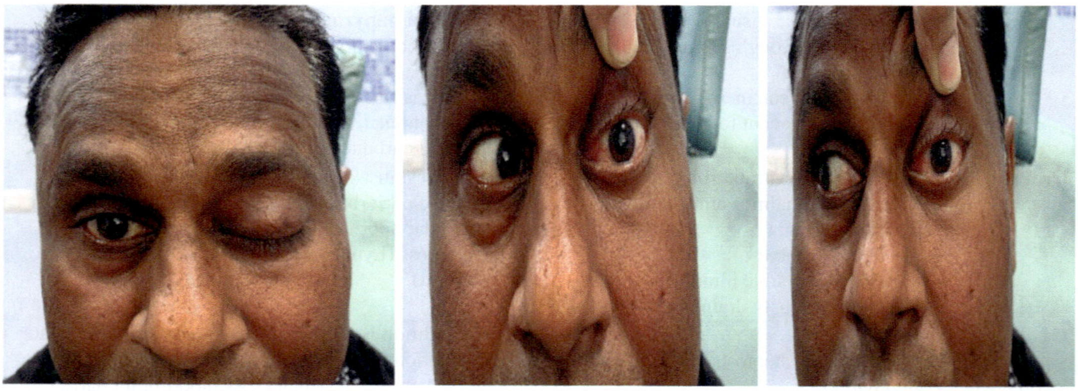

Fig. 3.16 Left cavernous sinus thrombosis (chemosis with dilated fixed pupil and restriction of extraocular movements) (Courtesy—Dr. Hitesh Verma, Associate Professor, AIIMS, New Delhi, India)

Table 3.11 It is showing the type of intracranial complications, clinical features, and management

Intracranial complications	Symptomatology	Treatment
Meningitis	• Most intracranial common complication • Headache • Meningismus • Fever • Cranial nerve palsies • Kernig's and Brudzinski sign (neck rigidity) • Usually due to involvement of sphenoid and ethmoid sinus	• Initially treated with antibiotics that penetrates blood-brain barrier • Followed by surgical drainage of the sinus
Epidural abscess	• Second most common complication • Fever, headache, nausea and vomiting, papilledema, hemiparesis, seizures • Usual sinus involved: Frontal • CT: Crescent hypodensity	• Good antibiotic coverage for long duration (may range for 4–6 weeks) • Neurosurgical intervention for drainage of abscess • Followed by ENT intervention of frontal sinus drainage (trephine, cranialization) or drainage of other involved sinuses.
Subdural Abscess	• Third most common complication. Condition of the patient deteriorates very rapidly leading to high mortality rates of residual neurological sequeal. • Headaches • Fever • Nausea, vomiting • Hemiparesis • Lethargy, coma	• **Aggressive medical therapy** • Antibiotics • Anticonvulsants • Hyperventilation, mannitol, steroids • **Drain sinuses and abscess** • Medical therapy possible if <1.5 cm • Craniotomy or stereotactic burr hole • Endoscopic or external sinus drainage
Intracerebral abscess	• Least common complication • Generally due to frontal sinus involvement followed by ethmoid and sphenoid sinus • Headache • Altered sensorium • Focal neurological deficit • Fever • Seizure, meningismus, papilledema • 60% chance of neurological sequeal and high mortality (20–30%)	• **Aggressive medical therapy** • Antibiotics • Anticonvulsants • Hyperventilation, mannitol, Steroids • Drain sinuses and abscess • Medical therapy possible if abscess <2.5 cm • **Excision or aspiration** • Diagnostic aspiration if <2.5 cm or cerebritis • Stereotactic-guided aspiration • Endoscopic or external sinus drainage
Venous Sinus thrombosis	• Retrograde thrombophlebitis from the frontal sinus may lead to thrombosis of the superior sagittal sinus. • Can be associated with other intracranial abscesses • MRI: Decreased cavernous carotid artery flow void • Mortality rate is high	• **Antibiotics, steroids, anticonvulsants** • Anticoagulation • Drain source of infection the sinuses

3.5.3 Conclusion

Complications of sinusitis have come down drastically due to timely intervention with adequate antibiotics. Complications of sinusitis can be minimal but if not addressed on time, may become potentially fatal. If these complications worsen further immediate surgical attention using endoscopic or external approach has helped reducing the mortality following these complications.

3.6 Part F: Allergic Rhinitis

3.6.1 Introduction

Allergy is a common disease the Indian incidence of which is 25–30%. In some countries, the incidence is as high as 40% of the general population, especially in young children. Though it can affects person of any age, it is generally a disease of the young. Children and adults of productive age are the common sufferers. Allergy is quite secular in affecting people of any race and of any geographical region. Women and men are both affected by allergies. Barring cardiovascular diseases and diabetes mellitus which are common ailments of older people, allergy is by far the commonest non-infective disease especially of the young. It is IgE-mediated signifying that the affected person produces IgE class of antibodies in excess to the normal range of it. The antibodies will be specific to the causative allergen. An individual with such a status is referred to be an atopic person. Allergy cuts across the entire system of human organism and can affect any part of the body but it generally affects the skin, and the mucous membrane of respiratory system and gastrointestinal system. When it affects the skin, common clinical conditions that manifest are Urticaria, Angioedema, and Atopic Dermatitis. When it affects the respiratory system, it causes Rhinitis, Conjunctivitis, Sinusitis, Serous Otitis Media, and Asthma. Nose being the main door to the respiratory system bears the brunt of allergic onslaught and so **Allergic rhinitis** is the most common manifestation of atopic allergy.

Allergic Rhinitis (AR) is the most common manifestation of atopic allergy. When the disease is persistent and when the symptoms are moderate and or severe, AR causes a considerable morbidity in the patient, especially when the patient is a young child or an adult of productive age. AR can affect all the vital functions of the nose. AR must be diagnosed clinically and specifically. Patients of AR must be treated adequately to provide relief of suffering, to prevent the development of complications, to reduce the suffering due to comorbidities and to prevent poly-sensitization.

John Bostock discovered AR when he presented an interesting case to the Medical and Chirurgical Society on 16 March 1819 "Case of a periodical affection of the eyes and chest," the first recorded description of what he later called "catarrhus aestivus" or summer catarrh, and which soon became known as hay fever [47, 48].

IgE-mediated allergy is a very common disease affecting a significant component of the general population. Children and adults in productive age are the common sufferers. Irrespective of the race and geographic distribution, the incidence of allergy is very high. Allergy cuts across the entire system of human organism and can affect any organ or any tissue but it generally affects the skin and mucous membrane of respiratory system and that of the gastrointestinal system.

Among different clinical manifestations of allergy, allergy affecting the respiratory system is the most common ailment. Nose being the main door to the respiratory system bears the brunt of allergic insult. In other words, allergy affecting the nose or AR happens to be the most common manifestation of allergy. Russel Settipane reports that 42% of Americans suffer from AR. AR has an estimated worldwide prevalence of 10–25% and is one of the most common diseases in childhood with a prevalence reaching up to 40% in some regions [49, 50]. In the year 2000, more than US$ 6 billion were spent on prescription medications for this condition [50, 51]. An estimated 14.1 million visits to a physician office are attributed to AR in the USA each year [52].

When the disease is persistent and when the symptoms are also of moderate or of severe degree, there will be a significant impact on the quality of life of the sufferer. Normal daily activities get hindered. Work and School activities are affected. Sleeplessness and tiredness result in lowering of learning and cognitive functions. All these may result in an embarrassing situation for a growing child.

AR is unfortunately undertreated and is ignored to a large extent causing the disease to cascade to neighboring tissues like conjunctiva, paranasal sinuses, middle ear, and then to the lower airways. AR is caused by many aeroallergens like tree, weed, and grass pollen; cat, dog, house dust mite (HDM), and molds. HDM is the most common indoor allergen causing perennial AR [47, 53].

Symptoms of AR appear on exposure to the causative allergens and triggers. Attempt must be made to avoid exposure to the causative allergens. However, objective evidence of raised serum specific IgE (sslgE) to an inhalant aeroallergen is essential before a patient spends time and money for extensive allergen avoidance measures. In UK general practice, diagnosis by history alone resulted in false-positive identification of allergen triggers of 32% for cat allergy, 48% for grass pollen, 75% for HDM, 54% for tree pollen, and 27% for dog when compared with formal allergy assessment including skin prick test (SPT). There is no value in extensive HDM avoidance or removal of a family pet if the sufferer is non-atopic and has no relevant allergic sensitivities [54]. Thus, objective assessment of IgE sensitivity improves accuracy in identifying allergenic triggers and accurate diagnosis [55].

Furthermore, once sslgE to an inhalant allergen is detected, the test must be interpreted correctly, and the clinician must distinguish between sensitization and allergy. At least 15% of people with a positive skin test do not develop symptoms on exposure to the relevant allergen, so the clinical history must be consistent with skin tests to confirm a clinically relevant sensitivity. For example, if a patient has year-round symptoms, severe rhinosinusitis, and nasal polyps, an isolated positive skin test to birch pollen is almost certainly irrelevant. However, they have a high negative predictive value, and therefore a patient with a negative skin prick test or no evidence of raised sslgE is likely to be genuinely non-allergic.

3.6.2 Clinical Manifestations and Differential Diagnosis

Following are the main or primary symptoms of AR:

- Sneezing
- Rhinorrhea
- Nasal Obstruction

Following are the associated symptoms of AR:

- Pruritus
- Nasal Intonation
- Slight to moderate difficulty in hearing due to inflammation spreading to the Eustachian tube and sometimes into the middle ear
- Heaviness in the Head due to sinuses getting blocked
- Lack of Concentration
- Lack of Interest in Normal Social Activity
- Mouth Breathing due to Nasal Obstruction
- Anosmia due to Inflammation affecting the Olfactory Nerve Endings

The complexity of symptoms could be a combination of several of these symptoms and can vary differently in different cases.

I. *Sneezing* in AR is the most common symptom. Sneezing can vary from one or two to as many as hundreds in a day. There are a few conditions mimicking AR. Every case of sneezing need not be of AR. Acute infective rhinitis, which is due to rhinovirus infection, would be of very recent origin. Accompanying symptoms of infection like fever, malaise, and signs of infective inflammation of the mucosa will be present. Eosinophilic non-allergic rhinitis and Nasal mastocytosis are two other conditions simulating AR but are non-atopic. The incidence of these two conditions has not been documented in India. A revision documentation of history and absence of positive correlating skin prick test will assist the diagnosis of these two conditions. Cytology of nasal secretions will reveal the preponderance of eosinophils in eosinophilic non-allergic rhinitis and of mast cells in nasal mastocytosis.
II. *Rhinorrhea* in AR can be mild to very severe and in severe cases, it can cause general weakness with lack of interest in either studies or at professional and social activities. The discharge, unless complicated by an infection, is thin and watery. Vasomotor Rhinitis (VMR) is the only other condition that mimics AR and is not uncommon in young women. In VMR, Rhinorrhea and Obstruction are commonly present, and sneezing is generally absent. Trivial stimuli like spicy food, odors, changes in temperature and humidity, sexual arousal, defecation, etc.

may act as triggers to produce the symptoms. Similar symptoms may be produced in some cases due to other systemic drugs like some antihypertensive and hormonal medication. The absence of supportive information on nasal cytology and SPT for allergy will help the diagnosis. Very rarely though, VMR may be present concomitantly with AR when it is quite a challenge for the patient and to the doctor treating the case. Cerebrospinal fluid (CSF) rhinorrhea is a rare condition that can be mistaken for the rhinorrhea of AR. History of trauma and injury to the skull must make a clinician to suspect CSF rhinorrhea. Do consider a congenital defect as a point of differential diagnosis in a very young child for CSF rhinorrhea.

III. *Nasal obstruction* is the third major complaint in AR. A Large number of patients find it difficult to cope up with this complaint when its severity is moderate or more than moderate degree. Children find it very difficult to cope up with the nasal obstruction. It is due to the swollen mucosa, which is the result of the late phase of allergic inflammation. There is a play of chemical mediators during the late phase. In addition to Histamine which is a pleiotropic mediator, cysteinyl leukotrienes, prostaglandins and Kinins are the other mediators that cause the late phase. Obstruction is usually unilateral and shifts from one side of the nose to the other every 4–6 h depending on the secretory activity of the nose. In some cases, the obstruction can become bilateral and almost complete when the sufferer will be in a miserable condition. If there is a marginally deflected septum also, the obstruction could be more on that side of the nose. Complete nasal obstruction results in the patient to become a mouth breather and if not treated early and adequately, it can affect the normal contour of a growing child's face.

Unilateral obstruction can be due to a deviated nasal septum. Very rarely a "S" shaped crooked deflection of the septum can cause bilateral obstruction. Polyps can cause unilateral and bilateral obstruction. Sometimes they are concomitantly present with AR. Ethmoid polyps are commonly associated with AR. A foreign body and a tumor are other causes of unilateral obstruction. Bilateral obstruction may be due to Rhinitis Medicamentosa, which results due to the misuse of locally applied alpha-adrenergic drugs. History of obstruction in elderly patients must make the clinician to suspect atrophic rhinitis. Examination will reveal atrophic changes of the turbinates with crusts. These days it is not uncommon to encounter atrophic rhinitis among youngsters also, especially after surgical procedures in the nose.

Pruritus in AR is a common symptom. Itching of the eyes and in inner canthi with increased tears, itching in the nose and sometimes in the ears may be present. Itching of the palate is not uncommon and can be intense. It can be so intense in some patients that they try to scratch the palatal region with a spoon attempting to obtain relief of itching.

Nasal intonation is another associated symptom commonly present when the obstruction is profound either because of allergic inflammation or when complicated by the presence of polyps.

3.6.3 Cascading Inflammation of AR Causing Complications and Comorbidities

It is quite common in many cases for AR to be concomitant with conjunctivitis. Eyes are exposed to the airborne allergens as much as the nose is. Anatomically the nose is better protected than the eyes. From another point of view, eyes have their lids to close and protect themselves which the poor nose does not possess. Though there is a difference in their structure and their physiology, they are neighbors to contend with. They are in close proximity and they are internally connected to each other through the nasolacrimal duct on either side. Tears are constantly produced in the eyes to irrigate and keep the eyes moist.

Allergic inflammation when present, cascades between the nose and the eyes conveniently to each other through the connecting nasolacrimal duct. That is how many cases of AR are cases of Allergic Rhinoconjunctivitis.

Paranasal sinuses are in close proximity to the nose. Mucous membrane in the nose and that in the paranasal sinuses is the same. In other words, there is a continuity of the same mucosa from the nose into the paranasal sinuses. Secretion from the sinuses gets drained into the nasal chambers through the ostium of each sinus. Even when the sinuses are not inflamed with allergy, inflammation of AR may and can occlude the ostium of these sinuses causing retention of fluid in the sinuses. Retention causes heaviness in the head. The heaviness or fullness in the head may result in an unpleasant status and it leads to lack of concentration in studies and at work. Cavities as they are, the sinuses normally lighten the weight of the skull being borne by the neck. Sinuses also provide resonance to the voice. When they are blocked, both of these are affected. Further, the allergic inflammation can spread to the sinuses causing sinusitis.

Inflammation of AR can spread to the middle ear through the eustachian tubes causing allergic otitis media with effusion or Glue Ear. This is especially possible when AR is inadequately treated or when it is ignored. There will be loss of hearing in speech frequency. Loss of hearing can be mild to moderate. The affected person will have a feeling of fullness in the affected ear. Tinnitus can be present. When a young child develops glue ear, it can lead to a very bad disability for the child not developing proper speech and developing improper intellectual growth. It is important to identify and diagnose this condition as early as possible. Reparative measures must be instituted quickly and aggressively.

Anosmia is possible to occur when AR is ill-treated or inadequately treated. It is clearly related to the disease duration and severity. Persistent inflammation and its effect on the umbrella of innumerable nerve endings of the olfactory nerve cause this damage. Loss of smell can be considered in children, as in adults, to be a clinical marker of disease severity [32]. This complication of AR needs a quick and detailed attention since the loss of olfaction will lead to several obstacles in a growing child's development. Loss of smell causes loss of perceiving the aroma of food which in turn results in loss of appetite and further non-secretion of saliva and other enzymes, leading to difficulty in digesting food. It may further result in nutritional deficiency which will stunt the growth of the affected child.

When allergy cascades downwards, it affects the pharynx causing pharyngitis with symptoms of the sore throat sometimes associated with slight difficulty in swallowing and a constant urge to clear the throat.

Further down when it affects the larynx, it causes laryngitis with loss of range of voice, hoarseness of voice, and loss of timbre of voice.

As it cascades further downwards, it causes comorbidity in the trachea causing tracheitis or cough variant asthma with dry cough, sometimes a very annoying difficulty to the patient especially at nights.

Bronchial asthma is the resultant condition when allergy invades the lower airways. Episodes of cough, tightness of chest, wheeze, and breathlessness which can be of varying degree are the symptoms. Significant limitation to the life of a patient happens when the disease is persistent and when the symptoms are moderate or more than moderate.

When these conditions persists, they become comorbidities. These are actually complications of AR especially when it is neglected or if AR is not treated adequately. Conjunctivitis, Sinusitis, and Asthma could be comorbidities right from the onset of AR in a few cases. Further Inquiry, Classification of the Disease and Clinical Findings on examination (Fig. 3.17):

Even before you examine a patient of suspected AR, history would be quite revealing in most of the cases. Depending on the episodes and severity of the symptoms, a patient can be classified into one of the four groups. This guidance is very helpful in making a strategy for treatment.

Anterior rhinoscopy will reveal pale, swollen mucosa with rugosity and it will be boggy

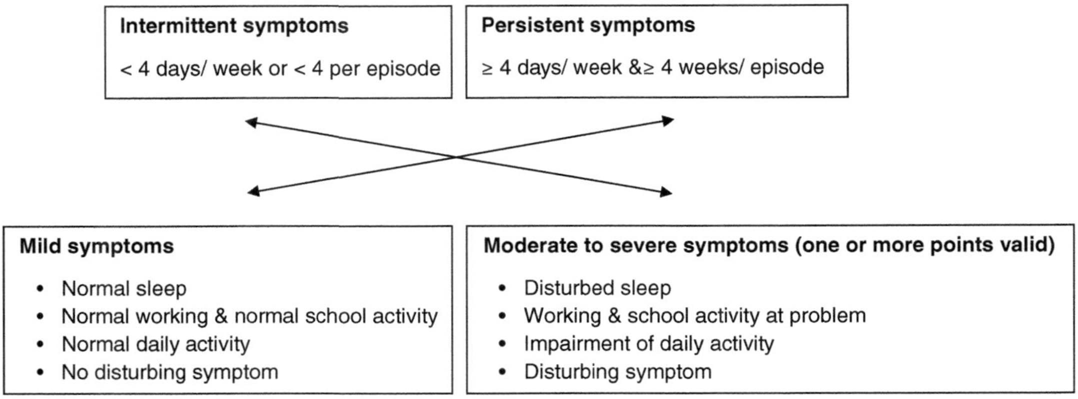

Fig. 3.17 Classification of the Disease on the basis of duration and interference in daily activities [56]

both over the septum and the turbinates. Clear transudate will be present in uncomplicated cases. The diagnostic endoscopic examination will confirm the picture of AR as also of any other comorbidity like a deflected septum and a complication like polyps, adhesions, synechiae, perforations, atrophic changes; and presence of a tumor or a foreign body. It will also provide a picture of the nasopharynx and condition of the ostia of paranasal sinuses, especially of the maxillary sinus. A telescope of 0° or a 30° and with a wide-angle profile provides adequate endoscopic examination.

When necessary, the nasal secretion can be examined for the type of cells present. To get a good columnar epithelial cell sampling, a small sterile cotton-tipped applicator can be passed under the interior turbinate and gently rubbed along the floor of the nose and is then rolled onto a clean glass slide. The procedure is done under direct vision. It may either be fixed with spray-fix for a later study or can be stained with Gram's stain or Papanicolaou stain immediately for the study. Epithelial cells, granulocytes, and mononuclear cells are looked for, and presence of bacteria is also observed. These cytograms can be of substantial help in diagnosing AR or to rule it out.

Nasal obstruction can be measured using a Rhino-manometer. It provides a measure of the nasal airway resistance present in a given case at a given time. The procedure uses a pneumotachograph to measure the flow of air through the nose.

The existence of an entity called local allergic rhinitis (LAR) with nasal production of specific IgE (sIgE) antibodies in the absence of atopy, in over 40% of non-allergic rhinitis (NAR) patients has been reported [57]. Evidence for this entity is supported by the clinical symptoms, the local production of sIgE, and a leukocyte-lymphocyte inflammatory pattern, with an increase in the nasal fluids of eosinophils, mast cells, and T lymphocytes during natural exposure to aeroallergens, as well as a positive immediate and dual response to a nasal allergen provocation test (NAPT) with local production of tryptase and eosinophil cationic protein and an increase of nasal sIgE to inhalant allergens [37]. Over recent years, increasing evidence has shown that an important number of patients previously diagnosed with NAR or idiopathic rhinitis develop a local allergy with nasal production of sIgE and a positive response to a NAPT [57]. This entity has been suggested to be entopy or LAR. These patients could also progress over time to AR [57].

3.6.4 Management of AR: Therapeutic Options (Fig. 3.18)

Unless the disease is mild, AR must not be taken for granted. It must be treated adequately. Patient must be convinced of the need to treat the inflammatory disease properly.

Allergen avoidance is easy said than done. Once the causative allergens are found and if avoidance is possible, it is the best course of

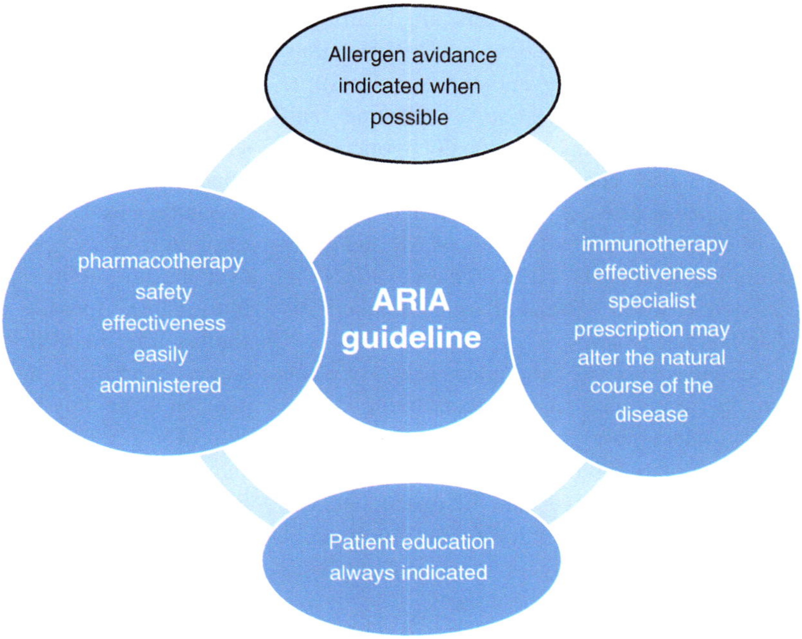

Fig. 3.18 ARIA Guidelines

Table 3.12 Effect of treatment on symptoms [58]

	Sneezing	Rhinorrhea	Obstruction	Itching	Eye symptoms
H 1-antihistamincs					
• Oral	++	++	+	+++	++
• Intranasal	++	++	+	++	0
• intra-ocular	0	0	0	0	+++
Corticosteroid					
• Intranasal	+++	+++	+++	++	++
• Oral	+++	+++	+++	+++	+++
Chromones					
• Intranasal	+	+	+	+	0
• Intra-ocular	0	0	0	0	++
Decongestants					
• Intranasal	0	0	+++	0	0
• Oral	0	0	+	0	0
Anti-cholinergics	0	++	0	0	0
Anti-leukotrienes	0	++	+	0	++

action. For pet allergens and for some food allergens, avoidance can practically be the complete solution.

A variety of molecules are available to treat and address different symptoms of AR. Depending on the severity of symptoms and morbidity, the medication must be chosen (Table 3.12).

When AR is mild, H1 blocker, an antihistamine of the new generation can address all the symptoms. First Generation antihistamines have been discarded because of the profound drowsiness they cause. New generation antihistamines provide good relief and can relieve comorbid symptoms also. Good compliance is possible because of once-a-day dosage. Several of these molecules do not cause drowsiness. There is an array of new generation molecules that have superior therapeutic exertion and a good safety profile. Such oral H1 blockers are Cetirizine, Levocetirizine, Loratadine, Desloratadine, Fexofenadine, Rupatadine, Ebastine, Olopatadine, and Bilastine. Azelastine and Olopatadine are available as locally applied antihistamines also. The onset of action is rapid and the therapeutic effect is limited to the tissue. They are of choice in very mild cases of AR and allergic conjunctivitis and as add-on therapy to INS in persistent cases of AR and allergic conjunctivitis when it is necessary.

Decongestants are sometimes necessary when there is significant nasal obstruction. Local decongestants must not be administered for more than 7–10 days for fear of rhinitis medicamentosa. Systemic decongestants like pseudoephedrine may be administered for a short duration but with caution, especially in those patients with hypertension and anxiety neurosis.

Mast cell stabilizers have a limited role. If the patient is younger than 2 years, a mast cell stabilizer like Sodium cromoglycate will be a very safe option to be applied locally in the eyes, nose, and even as an inhaler. Compliance is a challenge. If VMR is suspected as a concomitant partner of disease, addition of anti-cholinergic drops instilled intranasally may help.

Among the four main symptoms of AR sneezing, rhinorrhea and pruritus are caused by the early phase of allergic inflammation in which histamine is the main chemical mediator and that is why a H1 blocker may address these symptoms. Nasal obstruction is caused by the late phase of inflammation wherein a host of mediators play their role in causing the symptom. Only an anti-inflammatory molecule like a corticosteroid can address these symptoms. Though oral steroids are rarely required and if at all for a very short duration, intranasal steroids (INS) are the mainstay of management of such condition. They provide effective treatment for AR and are the first-line therapy for adults in moderate-to-severe cases or in individuals who are still symptomatic despite the regular use of antihistamines [53]. INS has the capability to inhibit histamine release, reduce mucus production, exert anti-edematous and vasoconstrictor activity, inhibit macrophage migration, reverse the effect of the early and late phase of inflammation, and inhibit hyper-reactivity. INS relieves all symptoms of AR, including nasal blockage, and meta-analysis shows that INS is more effective than antihistamines [53]. They act by suppressing inflammation in the nasal mucosa leading to a reduction or resolution of symptoms. There is some worry over the long-term effects of using steroids but Fluticasone furoate, Fluticasone propionate, Budesonide, and Mometasone have little systemic absorption. Mometasone which is a suspension is the only molecule recommended to be safe even for a child of 2 years and above. No significant difference in the number of symptom-free days or quality of life has been reported between the three drugs [59].

Once the disease is persistent and is not mild anymore, allergic inflammation must be addressed continuously and with adequate dose of INS. If persistent AR is inadequately treated, the cascade of inflammation does damage the anatomical structure of nasal mucosa and the turbinates. Like inadequately treated persistent asthma can cause re-modulation of lower airway smooth muscle, re-modulation of the upper respiratory area is quite possible. This is an important aspect of the management of chronic AR. If a patient is vehemently opposing INS, the Leukotriene modifier will be the next best option and it must be given regularly, for adequate period of time, and in adequate dose. Both fluticasone furoate and mometasone have been shown to reduce symptoms of allergic conjunctivitis as well as those of allergic rhinitis [60, 61]. The onset of action is variable among the steroid preparations (Table 3.13) [62]. Mometasone has the highest binding ability but flunisolide has maximum bioavailability (Figs. 3.19, 3.20, and 3.21) [63–65].

3.6.5 Leukotriene Receptor Antagonists

Leukotriene receptor antagonists (LTRA) block the effects of cysteinyl leukotrienes which are important pro-inflammatory mediators of nasal allergic reactions and whose release locally induces nasal obstruction. Although some efficacy with LTRAs has been shown in AR, the spectrum of individual responsiveness remains variable and the combination of an antihistamine and an LTRA is no more effective than an INS alone. However, it is worthwhile considering the prescription of an LTRA in patients with difficult AR and concurrent asthma, in addition to treatment with antihistamines and topical nasal steroids [53].

Systemic corticosteroids are rarely indicated in the management of AR. However, there are occasions when a short course of oral steroids may be beneficial. If the nostrils are completely blocked and if INS cannot simply enter the nasal cavities, INS sprays will not be effective of course, and therefore oral steroids may be co-prescribed along with an INS [53]. It is advisable to prescribe a good steroid molecule like Prednisolone or Methylprednisolone in adequate dose and for a reasonably good period of time like 5–7 days.

Table 3.13 Intranasal steroids—onset of action

Medication	Onset of action
Beclomethasone dipropionate	Within 3 days
Budesonide	Within 24 h
Flunisolide	4–7 days
Fluticasone furoate	Within 12 h
Triamcinolone acetonide	24 h

Even when symptoms are well under control, the inflammation of AR needs to be addressed on a continuous basis to prevent damage to the mucosa and to prevent further remodeling [28]. If a patient on INS is stable and symptom free, an attempt to reduce the daily dose may be made but the INS needs to be continued to address the "minimum persistent inflammation." Medication-sparing effect can only be achieved by allergen immunotherapy (AIT).

With INS and complementary measures, you may secure satisfactory results and the patient expectantly becomes symptom free. It means you have successfully obtained good control of the disease. All the more the allergic inflammation

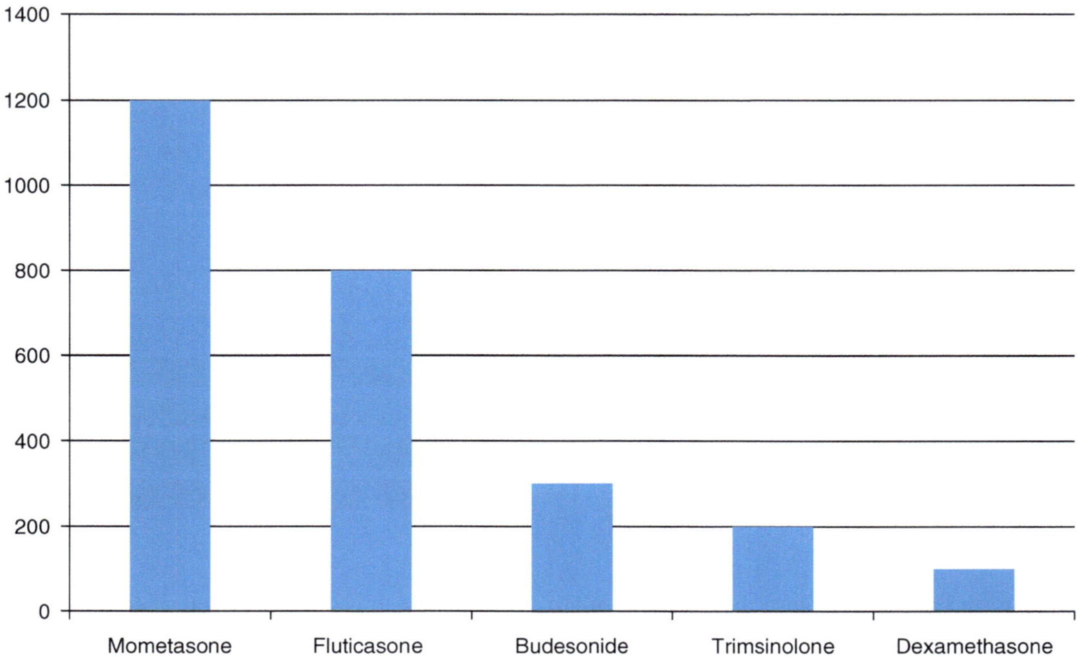

Fig. 3.19 Binding ability of steroids

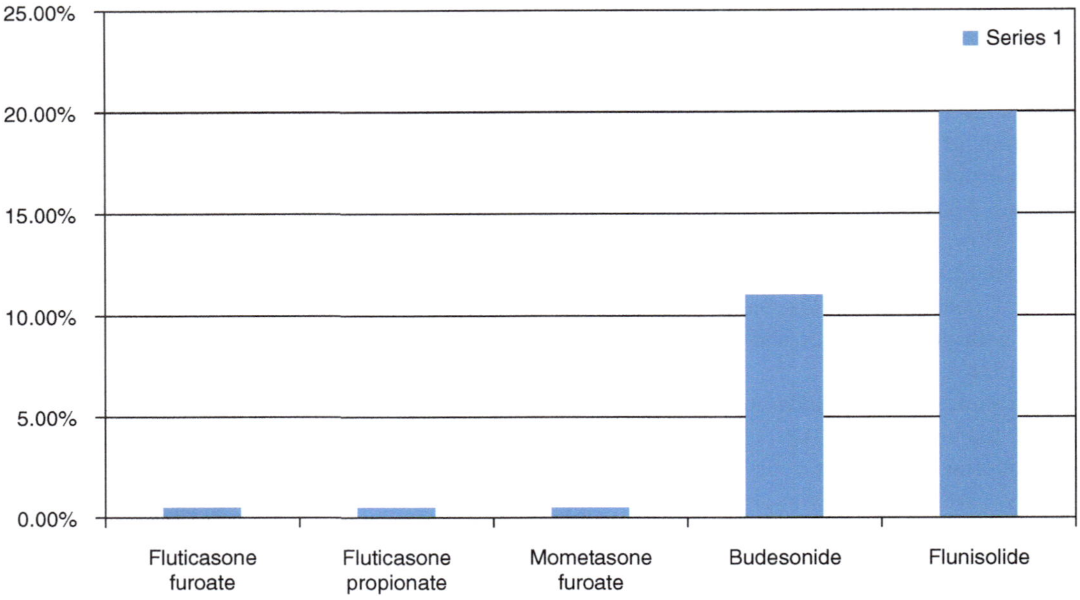

Fig. 3.20 Bioavailability of steroids

Fig. 3.21 The treatment guideline according to the severity of symptoms (ARIA Guidelines)

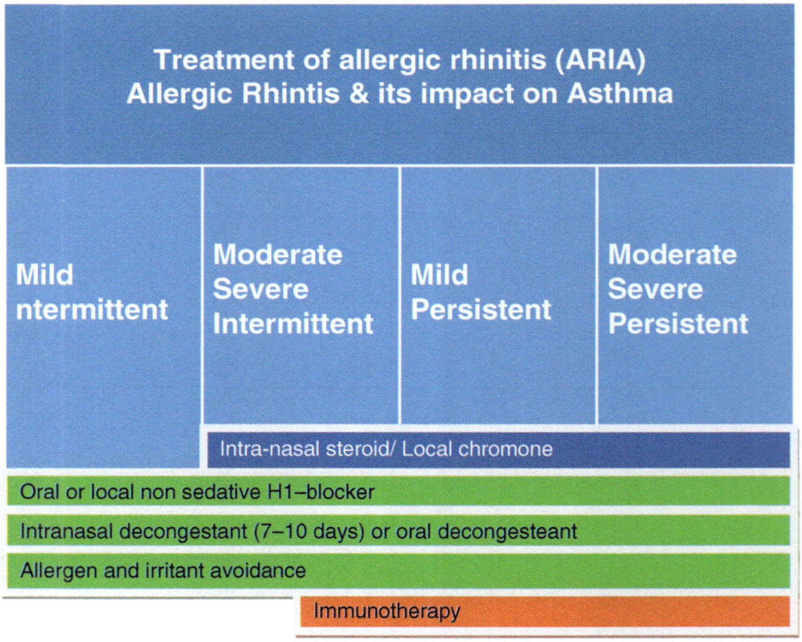

persists and prevails because the causative allergens and other triggers do persist. Even when a patient is symptom free with adequate treatment do understand that the minimum inflammation does persist. It is like a cauldron when it has been controlled. When the inflammation is raked up, it is like an inferno. That is why INS needs to be continued to address the inflammation. INS is both a reliever and a preventer. Every possible allergic attack must be prevented to further prevent re-modulation of the internal structure of the nose.

3.6.6 Difficult-to-Treat AR

When a patient is still symptomatic despite treatment with oral antihistamines and INS, the first stage is to check adherence and correct technique [53]. Clinical practice suggests that most patients who have found INS unhelpful have not persisted with treatment for an adequate period [11]. Patients should be advised that the onset of action of INS takes some time and that they should be used regularly for a minimum of 2 weeks before considering them unsuccessful [66]. Patients with seasonal AR should commence therapy 2 weeks before the pollen season as this improves efficacy [53, 67] To maximize the response to treatment, patients using INS should be given clear instructions on this aspect. They must also be advised to direct the nasal spray laterally (rather than medially towards the nasal septum) towards the lowest and anterior most part of inferior turbinate of that side and not to sniff for at least 10 min after spraying. All these measures will increase the benefit. Tipping the head back and sniffing hard decreases treatment efficacy. The spray will run down the nasopharynx and patients should be advised not to do this. To maximize effect patients may well be advised to douche with saline prior to using their nasal spray. Saline douching clears mucus and mucus plugs if any, from the nasal cavity permitting local absorption of the INS, thereby increasing its effectiveness. The use of saline douching has demonstrable benefits in symptom reduction in children and adults with seasonal rhinitis as well as in chronic rhinosinusitis [68, 69].

Depending on the severity of disease, the medication must be designed. As the patient secures benefit, step down of medication may be achieved. However, when there are episodes of flare up, step up of medication needs to be done. Once the disease is persistent, AIT must be considered especially if the patient desires a curative benefit. Proper documentation of causative allergens is necessary to institute immunotherapy. The gold standard for the specific diagnosis of allergy is SPT. Results of SPT will be the foundation for a successful AIT.

Spreading inflammatory cascade can involve several tissues and cause complications that will become permanent comorbid conditions [70]. That is why AR must be adequately treated and properly monitored. There is enough evidence to demonstrate that upper and lower airways are connected both anatomically and physiologically. In fact, they are simply upper and lower segments or components of one airway. That is why AR needs to be treated properly to prevent the onset of complications in the adjacent area and lower down in the airway, especially in the bronchi causing the onset of asthma. There is evidence of the existence of inflammation in the mucosal layers of lower airways in patients of AR without any symptoms of asthma. In cases of AR with very mild asthma, adequate dose of INS provides relief of nasal symptoms as well as those of asthma. In patients with AR, intranasal procedures to create roominess must be considered very carefully. Creating roominess by an inadvertent procedure without proper control of allergy may encourage the entry of allergens and other triggers into the lower airways causing the onset of asthma. It will become a complication, an iatrogenic surgeon-induced asthma. Surgery is never an option of management for allergy.

Some cases of AR or asthma will have comorbid symptoms in distant regions like the skin. AR or asthma can have atopic dermatitis as a comorbidity. In such a case, as you learn the details of the case, you find a strong case of allergy being the underlying disease. Treatment must include medication and other complimentary measures for both conditions. Patient must be convinced of the need for an approach to include proper inclusive medication and necessary changes in lifestyle.

Some cases of AR may have to be considered for treatment with Biological such as omalizumab. Though uncommon, rarely you encounter a case of AR where your patient is not getting stable and is not comfortable. If the patient can afford, it may be worth its while to treat such a patient with biologicals. Patient may get excellent benefits especially if there are comorbid symptoms and the relief may be for all comorbidities. You may be able to shorten the course of therapy with biologicals with the introduction of allergen immunotherapy.

Management must be holistic and integrated. Patient must be convinced of the condition being a non-infectious disease, that it needs to be addressed as one does for hypertension and or for diabetes, that the treatment with medicines provides control of disease but does not cure it, that the doctor and medication are a good part of treatment but are not the only one and, that the patient has to comply with the continuation of treatment and complementary measures for their own wellbeing. Good Rapport with the patient is necessary for a good prognosis. Periodic checkup for a good examination of the nose and to assess the treatment is mandatory. Once a patient has AR, he will continue to have it unless intervention with SPT is done to document the causative allergens and specific AIT is instituted as a curative procedure. Regular physical activity, adoption of healthy measures, and good nutrition will complement the management. Rewards to the patient and to the doctor will definitely arrive.

3.6.7 Allergen Immunotherapy (AIT)

Allergen Avoidance and Allergen Immunotherapy (AIT) are the only treatments that modify the course of an allergic disease either by preventing the development of new sensitivities or by altering the natural history of disease or disease progression [71].

AIT provides a window of opportunity for multiple benefits. Following are the benefits of AIT:

- AIT is the only available curative tool.
- AIT can alter the course of allergic disease for good.
- AIT is capable of changing the Th2 status (allergic) to Th1 status (normal).
- AIT is capable of impeding the onset of asthma in cases of allergic rhinitis.
- AIT can impede poly-sensitization.
- AIT is capable of providing medication-sparing effect.
- There is enough evidence that the benefit of AIT continues to be present for a long tenure even after concluding the therapy.
- AIT has the capacity to provide long-term protective benefit against the development of various other allergic conditions.

AIT is the administration of gradually increasing quantities of an allergen vaccine to an allergic subject, reaching a dose that is effective in ameliorating the symptoms associated with subsequent exposure to the causative allergens [71].

For an effective AIT, a proper specific diagnosis must be established. History and clinical examination are crucial but it is erroneous to make a specific diagnosis based on history alone. Causative allergens have to be determined by conducting specific allergy detection tests and correlated with the clinical manifestations.

Skin Prick Tests (SPT) can provide evidence of causative allergens and will demonstrate the presence of allergen-specific IgE (Fig. 3.22). Serum specific IgE (ssIgE) estimation can provide a quantitative evidence of the antigen-specific antibodies in the blood circulation of an allergic individual. Advantage of ssIgE estimation is that one blood sample is enough for the assay. Availability of normal skin is not a requirement. There need not be a curfew on immunosuppressive drugs when the test is conducted. The result of ssIgE may be negative but the patient may have potential allergy. A positive result is an excellent evidence of specific allergen sensitivity. SPT done with good quality allergens is the best diagnostic option. SPT offers both qualitative and quantitative measures of an allergen activity. It is fairly simple, safe, cost-effective, and reliable. SPT is hardly an invasive procedure.

Subcutaneous AIT (SCIT) or Sublingual AIT (SLIT) (Fig. 3.23) as a choice is left to the clinician and the patient considering various angles of therapy and tenure. Possibility of systemic reactions and anaphylaxis that is a major concern in

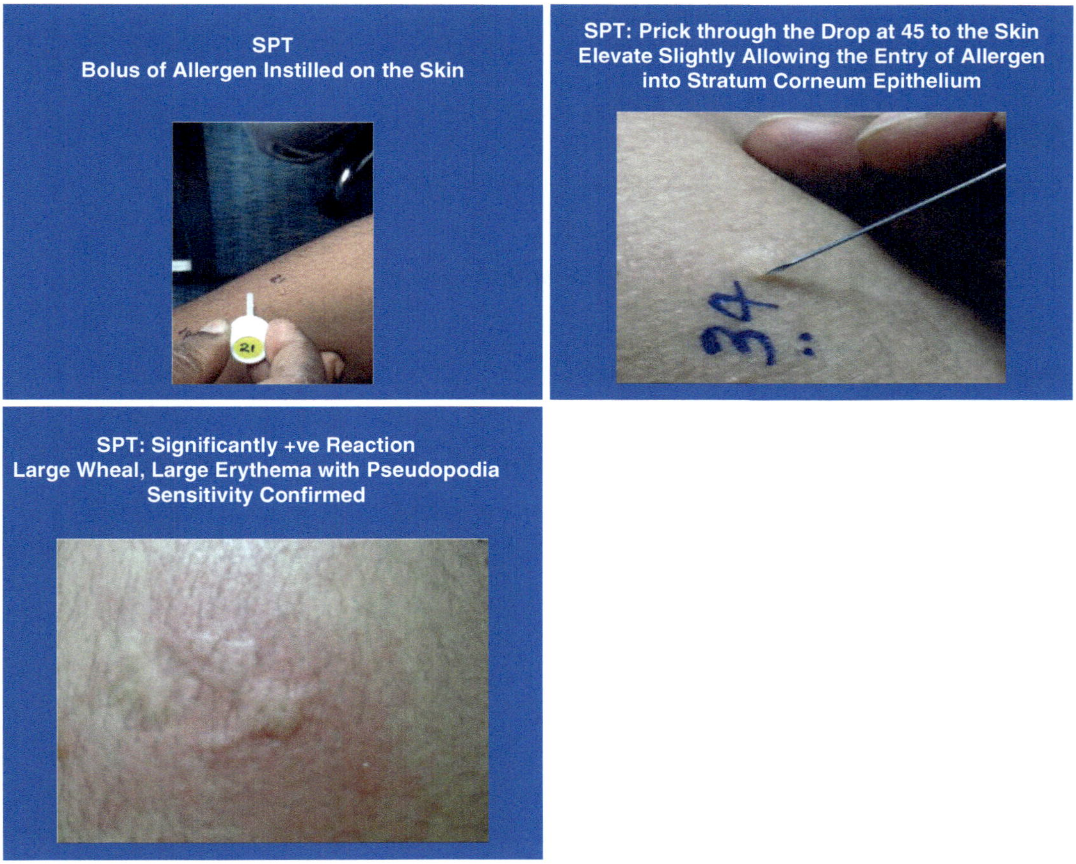

Fig. 3.22 Skin prick test

SCIT, is eliminated in SLIT. Proper diagnosis, good quality allergens, compatible and proper combination of allergens, and compliance are crucial to successful treatment by AIT.

With evidence of SLIT providing excellent therapeutic benefit to patients of AR and allergic asthma and especially with its safety profile, it has emerged and has become the option of choice for AIT. SCIT has to be administered by a medical professional. In the initial and build-up phase, injections are quite frequent. If the scheduled gap between injections is prolonged for any reason and if the following higher dose is administered, there is a risk of a systemic reaction especially if the sensitivity is high. The danger of anaphylaxis is a possibility. For AIT to become effective, the effort is necessary to reach the highest possible concentration and dose. So, compliance and safety are a major concern in SCIT. For food allergy and at present SCIT is not the accepted option. Considering all these difficulties, SLIT appears to be a safe and viable option. Much higher dose and concentration need to be achieved in SLIT for it to become success. Proper combination of allergens in the SLIT vaccine is necessary. Treatment happens in the comforts of the patient's home. It is the biggest benefit. This itself must not become a hindrance to the maintenance of treatment. SLIT works on trust. Patient and the family must be made to understand this fundamental aspect. Patient must also be made to understand that SLIT contains the same allergens to which the patient is allergic and that it is directed to shift the patient's status of allergy to normalcy, and that it does not directly relieve the symptoms like the medication does.

Sublingual Immunotherapy - SLIT

Patient: [redacted] Male 26 Years
Ref No. B03769

[redacted] Prescription No: 126348

Contents: BROUSSONETIA PAPYRIFERA POLLEN +++++ 60 %

CENCHRUS CILIARIS POLLEN ++++ 40 %

SHAKE THE BOTTLE VIGOROUSLY BEFORE ADMINISTRATION

Vials # 18 & 19: RED CAP

Concentration: 10 % Ratio – 1:10 Wt/Vol

Volume: 5.5 mL each Vial

INSTIL UNDER THE TONGUE EARLY MORNING ON EMPTY STOMACH, HOLD FOR 2 MINUTES & SWALLOW

ONCE IN 2 DAYS – 3 TIMES A WEEK WITH ONE-DAY HOLIDAY

Dose: 10 Drops each time

Dose	Date	No of Drops
1st		10
2nd		10
3rd		10
4th		10
5th		10
6th		10
7th		10
8th		10
9th		10
10th		10

Fig. 3.23 SLIT Prescription form by author's clinic

The process of AIT commences from the very first dose but it generally takes some time for its beneficial effect to reflect on the symptoms. Allergic Rhinitis, Allergic Conjunctivitis, Allergic Asthma, Sting Reactions are the classical indications for AIT. AIT may be a good option in some selected cases of drug allergy. Anaphylaxis and angioedema are conditions where AIT if possible, would be a boon to the patient and may actually be a life-saving tool. AIT has been approved as a major option of management for Atopic Dermatitis. When atopic dermatitis is so severe that it affects the social and professional life of a patient, even if the reasonable benefit can be obtained, AIT will be great. Selected cases of migraine and Meniere's disease especially with comorbid allergy conditions, would be worth the while candidates for AIT.

The beneficial effect of AIT will not be appreciable if it is administered in cases of mild allergy conditions. When the disease is persistent and when the symptoms are moderate or moderate-severe, AIT would be a great option in addition to medical management.

Successful AIT will initiate a marked enhancement of protective blocking IgG antibodies. AIT will blunt the serum concentration of specific IgE antibodies. There will be a down-regulation of inflammatory cell recruitment, activation, and mediator release. These will modify the T-Lymphocyte response to the benefit of the patient. Th2 response will get down-regulated resulting in enhanced Th1 response [72]

Poly-sensitization is a common feature in patients [73]. Poly-sensitization happens over a course of period. Poly-sensitization can be prevented by the institution of AIT early. Children are the best candidates. Re-modulation of the airways that happens due to persistent allergic inflammation is prevented with effective and early AIT. AIT also makes it cost-effective in the long run.

3.6.8 Allergens and Non-Allergic Triggers

Allergens have to be differentiated from non-allergic triggers. A clear distinction is necessary. Non-allergic triggers must never be included in prescriptions for immunotherapy. Infect they should not even be included in the tests for allergy. Many of them are inanimate subjects. They do not contain any allergen themselves. Various dusts other than house dust, smokes, fumes, perfumes, dhoop, incense, plastic, paper, cement, gravel, nylon, and polyester are such substances.

Allergens are substances that initiate and cause an allergic reaction in an individual who has developed specific IgE antibodies to those substances. They are protein in nature. They can be broadly classified into three main groups. They are Injectants or Ingestants or Inhalants.

3.6.9 SLIT as Food Allergen Immunotherapy

With SLIT, the food protein is delivered sublingually in a liquid form and then usually held for 2 min and swallowed. SLIT is thought to capitalize on the tolerogenic antigen-presenting cells in the oral mucosa [4, 5]. It is further thought that SLIT efficacy can be enhanced by exposure to the food protein in its intact form before possible epitopes are broken down through gastric digestion [74, 75].

Both in adults and children, a judicious combination of AIT, medical management, and correction of allergen-rich environment have become the hallmark of providing the complete solution to the persistent suffering of allergy patients. Wherever necessary, an effort must be made to change the existing lifestyle to suit the prevailing condition to achieve the best results. With better understanding, better techniques, quality training of specialist doctors, proper guidance by experienced allergy specialists, and better quality of allergens, AIT can only become a more powerful and sustaining tool and the option of management of allergic diseases.

3.6.10 Allergen Avoidance, Complimentary Lifestyle, and Prevention

3.6.10.1 Allergen Avoidance:

Food allergens if documented by diagnostic tests, the best course of action is to eliminate the particular food from the diet. If the allergy is severe and causes anaphylaxis or anaphylaxis type of reaction, extreme precaution is necessary. One must have very quick access to adrenaline injection. AIT is such a case may be a life-saving effort.

Pet allergy if detected, donating the pet may be the best option of the management. If this is not acceptable to the patient, AIT would be the next option.

Pollen allergy if present, during the pollen season patient must avoid being outdoors unnecessarily and especially in early mornings and later in the evenings. While going out, wearing a face mask may provide protection. Such a patient must keep the windows of their bedroom closed at night and early morning when it would be blossoming time of the plants.

Fungal spores if are the causative allergens, all places in the house must be checked for seepage and fungus infested corners and crevices. Correction measures and waterproofing of seepage areas will help. The indoor environment must be kept well ventilated and clean.

HDM and insect allergy are very common. Repeated and vigorous dust and insect controlling measures will help to a good extent both for the mites and for the insects. Minimum things must be in the bedroom especially. Corners, Crevices must be made rid of collected dust. Wardrobes and cupboards must be dust free. Curtains and carpets to be examined and if necessary, to be done away with. Maximum attention must be on the mattress and pillows. Dead or alive parts of mites and their tiny little fecal pellets are the deadly allergens. Human skin scales are the main food for the HDM. Throwing the pillow and mattress to hot sunlight and beating them up nicely will help. If the vacuum cleaner is available, it must be generously and repeatedly used on the mattress and pillows. Synthetic casings for the mattress and pillow are available. They are helpful too. Linen must be changed frequently and they must be soaked in very hot water for half hour at least before washing because dust mite allergen is heat labile. If the washing machine has heat control, linen can alternatively be washed with a minimum of 60 degrees Celsius temperature.

3.6.10.2 Complimentary Lifestyle

We are subjected to various chemicals in the food and beverages we consume. There is also a play of synthetic colors, food additives, and preservatives in most of the available out of the shelf packaged food. We must be protective of not getting exposed to these items to whatever extent we can. Many of these items though not allergens are capable of being triggers. Injurious data on long-term usage is not completely available. Preprocessed food is not health friendly. We may be subjected to harmful effects of these many known and unknown ingredients. Deficiency of Vitamin-D and Vitamin-B12 predispose us to be vulnerable to many diseases including allergy. Abundant sun energy is available. We must get ourselves exposed to sunlight for Vitamin-D. Our nutrition must contain adequate amount of protein. Sprouts, whole grains, legumes, seafood, poultry, greens, fresh seasonal and dry fruits if included into our diet, nutrition will be balanced and that itself will act as highly organic medicine to preserve good health and to protect ourselves from the disease. Some amount of physical activity regularly will make our life robust to ward off allergy. One must also try to relax for some time every day.

3.6.10.3 Prevention of Allergy:

Universal understanding and gigantic efforts are necessary to stop the usage of harmful chemicals in agriculture and horticulture. Pollution of ambient air, water, and soil must be controlled by people and governing bodies. These appear to be the major triggers all over the world. There is evidence that antibiotic administration to a pregnant woman will enhance the chance of the child to become an asthmatic. Antibiotics must be administered only when it is absolutely necessary for a pregnant woman. Breastfeeding the infant is very important to ward off many possible diseases. A person having an allergic disease must marry a person who does not have an allergy so that the possibility of their child being a non-allergic child is very high. Intranasal surgery must be avoided to a great extent in a patient of AR. Surgery is not a treatment for allergy. It can trigger the onset of asthma in a patient of AR. Platt-A Mills' hygiene hypothesis supports children growing up with pets and farm animals. Farm animals like cow release a very low-grade endotoxin. When a growing child is exposed to these farm animals, low-grade infections happen but the immune system responds positively providing an umbrella of protection. This will provide a protection to the child from developing allergy. Bactericidal and so-called Germ-check ingredients being used in toothpaste, soaps, handwash, detergents, floor cleaning solutions, and sprays could contain pesticides like Triclosan and Triclocarban. These will kill and eliminate microbiomes and will render the homes sterile. An infant or a young child growing in a sterile house has a very high possibility of developing allergy and asthma. We need clean homes, not sterile homes. It is impossible to eliminate allergy but efforts can be made to control the disease and to enforce certain benign things to prevent the onset of allergy in the coming generation.

3.7 Part G: Vasomotor Rhinitis

3.7.1 Introduction

Vasomotor rhinitis (VMR) or idiopathic rhinitis is one of the most prevalent forms of non-allergic rhinitis. It is usually seen around 30–60 years. with female predominance. Being more common in the female it is suggested that female hormones might play some role, but there is no research explaining this possibility. However as VMR may be caused by shifts in temperature and humidity, patients may experience seasonal symptoms during spring and fall. Thus, seasonal VMR can easily be confused with Seasonal Allergic Rhinitis (SAR) [76–78]. The precipitating factors are environmental conditions, such as strong smells, exposure to cold air, changes in temperature, humidity, barometric pressure, strong emotions, ingesting alcoholic beverages, and changes in hormone levels [77].

3.7.2 Pathogenesis

The exact underlying mechanisms causing VMR are not well understood. However, the most common theory explaining it, thought to be nonspecific nasal hyper-reactivity to non-immunologic stimuli on exposure. Other reasons are dysfunction of nociceptive, autonomic system alone, or both. Another concept also says the role of capsaicin-sensitive nociceptors in the nasal mucosa. Hyperactive parasympathetic innervations/hypoactive sympathetic innervations explain an autonomic imbalance towards an excess in parasympathetic innervations, some studies support that vasomotor rhinitis is more likely a result of a hypoactive sympathetic nervous system. Autonomic imbalance in favor of parasympathetic innervations results in nasal edema from vasodilatation of the nasal vasculature. Functional abnormality of sensory afferent nerves and/or C-fiber stimulation has also been suggested as possible causes of vasomotor rhinitis [79, 80].

3.7.3 Clinical Features

The predisposing factors are the changes in the environmental humidity, temperature, smoke, etc. the symptoms are persistent throughout the year. Sneezing after getting up from bed, excessive rhinorrhea, and nasal obstruction more on the dependent side are the usual symptoms. Ear and throat symptoms are absent in intrinsic rhinitis. Mucosal congestion with enlarged turbinates with smooth to modulated appearance is the standard findings on rhinoscopy (Fig. 3.24), whereas patients with predominantly excessive rhinorrhea have often distinctive appearance. Postnasal drip is another common symptom of VMR. Other less common symptoms of VMR are sneezing, nasal pruritis, and eye irritation [81].

3.7.4 Diagnosis

The diagnosis of VMR is based on the patient's history and their precipitating factors. Its diagnosis is through the exclusion of other causes. Patients usually should have normal serum IgE levels, no eosinophil in nasal smear and negative skin testing or radioallergosorbent tests (RAST) or nasal provocation test [82].

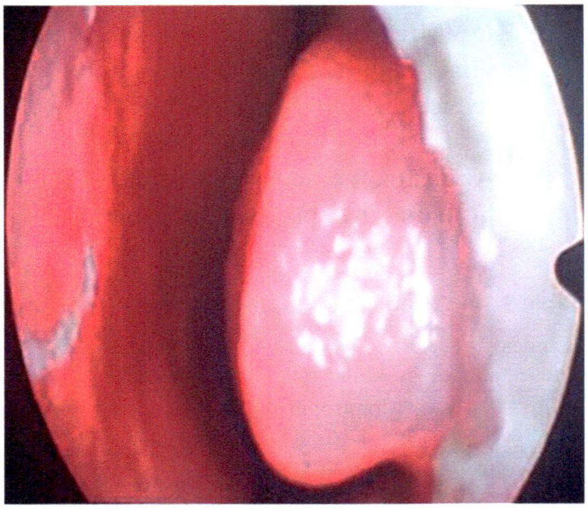

Fig. 3.24 Enlarged inferior turbinate with smooth to modulated appearance

3.7.5 Treatment

1. Avoidance: The home environment must be modified to avoid factors that initiate or exacerbate the rhinitis, like Control of humidity and temperature can lessen nasal instability or vasomotor hyperactivity.
2. Exercise: It can help reduce nasal obstruction by stimulating sympathetic nerve discharge, which produces vasoconstriction and lasts for 15–30 min.
3. Medications: First-line of treatment in vasomotor rhinitis is medical therapy in the form of topical therapy. In mild disease, one medication should be started along with the option to add a second if symptoms are not controlled by a single agent whereas in moderate disease, two agents can be started simultaneously. In severe cases, an oral medication either a decongestant or anti-cholinergic, depending on the predominating symptom can be added to the topical therapies.
   (a) Nasal Corticosteroids
   By contrast, clinical experience suggests that all nasal corticosteroids have some effectiveness in treating VMR.
   (b) Antihistamines
   It is predictable that first-generation antihistamines might reduce rhinorrhea through anti-cholinergic actions however by enlarging oral antihistamines are generally ineffective in reducing congestion in VMR. The combination of an antihistamine and a decongestant might help reduce the congestion in VMR.
   The role of intranasal antihistamines—Azelastine's efficacy in VMR is not due to histamine receptor blockade but instead, it is probably due to as an anti-inflammatory and neuro-inflammatory blocker.
   (c) Decongestants
   Both oral and topical decongestants effectively treat congestion regardless of underlying cause of VMR. However topical medications cannot be used prolong because continual use for more than 3—10 days leads to rhinitis medicamentosa.
   (d) Anti-Cholinergics
   Ipratropium bromide is a potent intranasal anti-cholinergic with utility in the treatment of rhinorrhea in VMR but it is specifically treated rhinorrhea and does little help to improve congestion.
   (e) Miscellaneous
   Topical saline spray or saline irrigation devices are help in the reduction of post-nasal drip, sneezing, and congestion.

Another therapy for VMR is topical capsaicin intranasally which helps by acting on neural fibers in the nose and thus reducing nasal hyperreactivity [83]. Algorithm for medical management is mentioned in (Table 3.14).

4. Surgical Treatment
   If Inferior turbinates are persistently hypertrophic after 3 months of medical management then it needs to be reduced to relieve nasal obstruction. Various methods of reduction are:
   (a) **Lateralization of the inferior turbinate** but it is not considered sufficient as a stand-alone procedure for the management of significant turbinate hypertrophy [84].

Table 3.14 Algorithm for the medical treatment of vasomotor rhinitis

Clinical presentation	Rhinorrhea predominant	Congestion predominant	Mixed congestion rhinorrhea
Mild	Ipratropium (IB)	topical antihistamine (TAH)	TAH or nasal corticosteroids (NCCS)
Moderate	IB+ NCCS or TAH	TAH + NCCS	TAH + NCCS
Severe	IB+ NCCS or TAH+ oral anti-cholinergic	TAH + NCCS+ oral decongestant	TAH + NCCS+ oral decongestant and anti-cholinergic

(b) **Submucosal electrocautery technique** involves the use of a single needle electrode or bipolar forceps with needle tips [85, 86]. Mucosal injury can lead to recurrent epistaxis and prolong crusting over mucosa with high risk of synechiae formation.

(c) **Submucosal radiofrequency coblation technique** differs from the electrocautery technique in that it produces significantly lower heat than that with electrocautery. Mucosal injury and epistaxis are less common than other treatment methods. The wand tip is coated in saline gel or another conductive media and activated at the head of the turbinate to produce a devascularized zone. The wand is then inserted through this zone and advanced toward the tail of the turbinate submucosally. It is then activated for a short period (e.g., 10 s), and then partly withdrawn and activated again [87].

(d) **Powered submucosal turbinate reduction** is used to reduce the amount of submucosal erectile tissue, while leaving the overlying epithelium unharmed. With the recent advent of a smaller (2.0–2.9 mm), specifically designed inferior turbinate microdebrider blade, with an incorporated tip elevator, this procedure has been made easier. The tip of the specialized microdebrider blade, or a scalpel, is then used to perform a stab incision in the head of the inferior turbinate. The microdebrider blade is then advanced (with the cutting surface facing laterally) and used to create a submucosal pocket on the infero-medial surface of the turbinate bone, using the flat tip as an elevator. Care must be taken to avoid flap perforation, while targeting the anterior and infero-medial submucosal soft tissue that contributes most significantly to nasal airflow obstruction. Submucosal resection can be carried all the way to the tail of the turbinate posteriorly.

(e) **Ultrasonic bone aspirator** to remove inferior turbinate bone is the recent advancement. This device uses ultrasonic waves to emulsify bone, with concurrent irrigation and microsuction of bone particles producing a clean surgical field; this reportedly enables removal of the inferior turbinate bone without thermal or mechanical injury to the surrounding soft tissue or mucosa.

(f) **Mucosal sacrificing techniques**

Cryosurgery to the surface of interior turbinates reduces the population of mucus glands. Scarring produced can improve the airway but the effect is short lived.

Partial turbinectomy removes a small portion (1.5–2.0 cm) of full-thickness tissue at the head of the inferior turbinate in the region of the internal nasal valve.

Laser for inferior turbinate reduction has been used for simple tissue ablation to laser mucotomy (excision of superficial mucosa), to partial or total turbinectomy with the laser used as a cutting instrument.

Total resection or "radical" turbinectomy involves the complete resection of the inferior turbinate using heavy scissors to detach it directly at its site of attachment to the lateral nasal wall. This technique can reduce the nasal resistance up to 50% but eventually fell out of favor with many surgeons owing to concerns for severe long-term complications such as atrophic rhinitis and ozaena [88].

(g) **Vidian neurectomy** It has been proposed only for non-allergic rhinitis refractory to maximal medical treatment. However, the evidence base for its benefit remains controversial. Despite its original popularity, vidian neurectomy was almost completely abandoned because of its complications and the lack of long-term effectiveness. The results showed poor long-term outcomes with the return of symptoms within a 2-year period after surgery. Malcomson in 1957 firstly suggested that the vidian nerve had a predominantly parasympathetic effect. He also suggested that it could offer relief in patients with vasomotor rhinitis (in patients with rhinorrhea predominantly) who are not responding to medical management. Sectioning of greater superficial petrosal nerve as a treatment for vasomotor rhinitis was first proposed by Zeilgelmann in 1934 which was further suggested by Murray Falconer in 1954. The different surgical techniques are described below.

(i) **Golding–Wood's transantral approach** has the disadvantage of being relatively destructive procedure and various complications like Severe bleeding from the sphenopalatine artery and its branches, Numbness of the cheek and palate, ophthalmoplegia, and even blindness can occur.
(ii) **Trans-septal vidian neurectomy** is a method in which trans-septal access is used to elevate flap over anterior and inferior wall of sphenoid body and is followed by the Identification of sphenopalatine foramen and pterygoid canal. Then Diathermy probe was passed into the pterygoid canal and vidian nerve was coagulated.
(iii) **Transpalatal vidian neurectomy** is less popular as it is associated with significant postoperative morbidity and the risk of oronasal or oroantral fistula.
(iv) **Transnasal vidian neurectomy is** primarily performed via a transseptal approach and it is a direct approach along the lateral wall of the nasal cavity. It had the advantage of providing a less invasive, more rapid, and direct method than conventional techniques but still required a rather blind dissection in the approach to the sphenopalatine foramen. Then Probe is advanced into pterygopalatine fossa via sphenopalatine foramen in posterolateral direction till the lateral end of vidian canal opening. Inadvertent trauma to the sphenopalatine artery and resultant bleeding remained a key issue.
(v) **Endoscopic vidian neurectomy (EVN)** was described by Robinson and Wormald. Improved endoscopic visualization and a better understanding of the anatomy have significantly improved the ability of the surgeon to locate and precisely resect the vidian nerve. It is well tolerated, safe, and effective in a majority of patients. It has two subtypes, i.e., type 1 or intrasphenoidal approach consists of unroofing the superior aspect of the bony vidian canal in the floor of the sphenoid sinus followed by isolating and then dividing the nerve. This approach can only be used for those well-pneumatized sphenoid sinuses in which the vidian canal is thin and isolated from the surrounding bone of the sinus floor and walls. In type 2 or transsphenoidal approach, the bone of the anterior wall of the sphenoid is removed, and this bony removal is carried out laterally to the sphenoid process of the palatine bone. The sphenoid process is resected until the vidian canal can be identified or a curved probe can be inserted and used to "hook" the vidian nerve. Once isolated, the nerve is then cut.
(vi) **Endoscopic Posterior Nasal Neurectomy (EPNN)** was emerged to avoid the postoperative complication of xerophthalmia and palatal numbness, because the posterior nasal nerve is not located as closely to the maxillary nerve as is the

vidian nerve. In this selective and distal resection of the posterior nasal nerve (the ramus emanating from pterygopalatine ganglion especially innervating nasal mucosa) was divided. Two separate techniques for EPNN have been described. The first, referred to as the transturbinate approach, is typically performed in combination with submucosal resection (SMR) of the inferior turbinate. From incision in turbinate, the mucosa of the middle meatus/lateral nasal wall is elevated and the periosteum cut and elevated until the sphenopalatine foramen (SPF) is visualized. The nerve identified as the posterior nasal nerve courses from the SPF toward the inferior turbinate is isolated and cut. Second technique uses a transnasal approach similar to that described for transnasal endoscopic sphenopalatine artery ligation and begins with a vertical incision made in the middle meatus roughly 5 mm anterior to the lateral attachment of the middle turbinate. A mucoperiosteal flap is elevated posteriorly to the crista ethmoidalis until the SPF is identified. The posterior nasal nerve is identified along with the sphenopalatine artery (SPA) which was cut [89].

Overall, the literature has shown that the endoscopic approach is associated with less morbidity than the traditional approaches.

3.8 Part H: Non-Invasive Fungal Sinusitis

3.8.1 Introduction

The non-invasive fungal rhinosinusitis spectrum includes saprophytic infection, fungal ball, allergic fungal rhinosinusitis. This spectrum of rhinosinusitis tends to affect immunocompetent individuals. Pathophysiology of the non-invasive spectrum of fungal rhinosinusitis is still speculative and enigmatic. The fungal ball affects single sinus and endoscopic removal of disease is typically curative. Allergic Fungal Rhinosinusitis is characterized by typical imaging and histopathological features and is notorious for recurrence despite of surgical removal. Fungal rhinosinusitis (FRS) is defined as the inflammation of nasal and paranasal sinus mucosa associated with fungal elements. Based on varying clinical presentation, pathophysiology, and histological appearance, FRS has been categorized into various subgroups [90, 91]. It can be acute (symptoms for 90 days), indolent condition [92]. As per the recommendations of the international society for human and animal mycology group, FRS is broadly classified into two categories based on the tissue invasion by the fungi as follows [91–93]:

1. Non-Invasive fungal sinusitis (NIFS)
   (A) Saprophytic infections
   (B) Fungal Ball (mycetoma)
   (C) Allergic fungal Sinusitis (AFS)
2. Invasive fungal sinusitis (IFS)
   (A) Acute Fulminant
   (B) Chronic invasive
   (C) Chronic granulomatous

(A) **Saprophytic Non-invasive Fungal Sinusitis (SNIFS)**
It is a recently proposed group in NIFS associated with impaired drainage of the paranasal sinuses causing colonization of the fungus. Fungal colonization of the sinonasal tract in this condition occurs following a surgical procedure or trauma leading to inflammation and ulceration/crusting of the sinonasal mucosa. The fungal deposits are restricted to the surface of the mucosa without tissue invasion. The patients are typically asymptomatic and the fungal deposits are observed as incidental findings during unrelated procedures. This form is the least described in the literature and removal of the crust is the treatment for the saprophytic infection.

(B) **Fungal Ball** [92–94]:

It is an entangled mass of fungi involving single paranasal sinus subsite usually associated with minimal mucosal inflammation. It is usually seen in immunocompetent individuals with the age range being 14–87 years with a predilection for females (~57–64% of the patients). According to the above mentioned FRS guidelines, the fungal ball is an appropriate term for this clinical entity rather than mycetoma or aspergilloma. It can present as unilateral nasal blockage or facial heaviness. The incidence of sinus involvement in the descending order is: maxillary sinus (78–84%) followed by sphenoid sinus (15–40%) and the ethmoid sinus (1–15%), however, it can involve multiple sinuses also. Pathophysiology is still unclear, however, it most likely starts with fungal spores gaining access into the paranasal sinuses spontaneously (in the geographic regions of heavy antigen exposure) or getting inoculated by surgery/trauma. The spores may then grow on obtaining a favorable environment. There are three theories mentioned in the literature regarding its development: airborne, odontogenic, and mixed.

1. *Airborne theory*: The fungal spores present in the air gain access into the sinuses through natural sinus ostia and multiply. These spores can become pathogenic on being exposed to the favorable anaerobic environment in the sinuses. The septal deviation and turbinate hypertrophy are possible contributing factors causing stasis of secretions by osteomeatal obstruction leading to the development of hypoxic environment with lowering of the pH inside the sinuses, creating a favorable atmosphere for the proliferation of fungi.
2. The *odontogenic pathway* refers to an iatrogenic affection, where the fungal colony is inoculated in the maxillary sinus owing to an oroantral communication secondary to dental extraction, periodontal lesions, or endodontic treatment.
3. The *mixed theory* combines the above two and considers both the above factors to be contributory to the disease manifestation.

Non-contrast Computer tomography of paranasal sinuses is the investigation of choice. Typically imaging shows single sinus involvement. Expansion of the involved sinus is not expected with a fungal ball, and the opacification of the involved sinus with patchy areas of high density having fine, round to linear matrix calcifications are observed. Histologically, it is characterized by the mass of fungal elements embedded in a fibrous necrotic matrix with minimal mucosal inflammatory reaction. There is no tissue invasion or granulomatous reaction in the surrounding tissue. The most commonly isolated pathogen on culture is Aspergillus species. Prior to surgery, the risk factors for the development of fungal ball, like previous sinonasal surgery, dental procedures, or any traumatic incidents, should be sought. Surgical excision with adequate sinus aeration is the treatment of choice.

(C) **Allergic Fungal Rhinosinusitis (AFRS)** [92, 94–96]:

The term was coined by Robson et al. Even though inhabitation of the sinuses by the fungal elements is common and occurs early on in life, only few individuals go on to develop AFRS. This entity is seen in immunocompetent, atopic patients; more commonly in warm and humid climates such as in the southern and southeastern the USA, India, and the Middle East. The affected sinuses contain inspissated, thick clay-like (also described as peanut butter jelly like) fungal muck with mucin varying in color from yellow, green, brown to grayish (Fig. 3.6). Microscopic examination of the eosinophilic mucin shows thick mucus from sinus mucosa admixed with dead epithelial cells, eosinophils, eosinophil degradation products like Charcot–Leyden crystals, and other inflammatory cells arranged in a layered pattern with occasional fungal hyphae.

The preferred terminology for the tenacious fungal mucin is "Eosinophilic mucin" rather than allergic mucin because of the controversies surrounding the allergic etiology of the disease. Fungal hyphae can be seen on Hematoxylin and Eosin (H&E) stain, but are best highlighted by histochemical stains such as silver stains or Periodic Acid Schiff (PAS). There is geographical variation in the fungi isolated on culture from the AFRS patients. Most commonly grown organisms are either Dematiaceous fungi (Alternaria, Bipolaris, Curvularia, Drechslera, Exserohilum, etc.) or Aspergillus sp. depending on geographical location. In India and Saudi Arabia, *Aspergillus flavus* is the commonest fungal organism cultured; while in the USA, Dematiaceous fungi can be cultured in 70–90% of cases. The pathogenesis of this disease remains unclear. It is believed to be the result of host reaction to fungal proteins instead of actual fungal infection/invasion of the tissues. Traditionally, AFRS has been considered to be a Type I hypersensitivity reaction to fungal antigens. In fact, one of the widely used diagnostic criteria for AFRS, the Bent and Kuhn criteria, includes type 1 hypersensitivity as a major criterion. However, not all patients with the pathologic diagnosis of AFRS have systemic (or even local) hypersensitivity to fungi. Bent and Kuhn [90] proposed five clinical criteria for the diagnosis of AFS: (1) nasal polyposis; (2) allergic mucin; (3) characteristic computed tomographic (CT) scan findings showing patchy hyperdense areas corresponding to fungal mucin; (4) positive fungal KOH smear; and (5) type I hypersensitivity diagnosed by history, skin test, or serology. These criteria are now referred to as major criteria.

Schubert and Goetz [96] histopathological criteria for the diagnosis of AFS:

1. Allergic mucin is present on gross and/or histopathological evaluation.
2. Either (a) Methenamine silver stain of allergic mucin is positive for fungi (without any fungal elements inside mucosa) or (b) fungal culture is positive (with or without a positive silver stain); 3) sinus mucosal H&E stain is characteristic for AFS and indistinguishable from the mucosal infiltrate in asthmatic bronchial mucosa; and.
3. Other histopathological fungal disorders are excluded.

Bent and Kuhn [97] have described major (five) and minor (six) criteria for the diagnosis of AFS in adults.

Major Criteria:

1. Type I (IgE-mediated) hypersensitivity
2. Nasal polyposis
3. Characteristic CT scan findings showing patchy hyperdensities involving sinuses
4. Allergic mucin, and
5. Positive fungal smear

Minor Criteria:

1. Concomitant Asthma
2. Unilateral disease predominance
3. Radiographic (CT scan) bone erosion
4. Positive fungal culture
5. Charcot–Leyden crystals, and
6. Serum eosinophilia

Bent and Kuhn [97] proposed diagnostic for AFRS (Table 3.15).

Currently, these are the most widely accepted and used criteria for the diagnosis of AFS. More recent studies indicate that fungal protease induced production of Th-2 cytokines attracts eosinophils, and the subsequent products of eosinophilic inflammation result in the formation of eosinophilic mucin. Non-contrast CT scan of paranasal sinus shows a heterogeneity of signals seen in involved sinus (Fig. 3.25), characterized as "starry-sky" or "serpiginous" pattern. The presence of intermittent hyperdense (corresponding to the deposition of heavy metals within eosinophilic mucin) and hypodense signals on CT scan is referred to as "double-density" sign. Treatment of this disease is not without controversies. The mainstay of treatment is the surgical removal of disease with all mucin to provide good ventilation and facilitate the delivery of topical therapy. Steroids can be used in pre and/or postoperative setting to reduce the inflammatory load and facilitate the more efficient surgical clearance of the disease with the reduction of the risk of recurrence. Utilization of antifungal therapy has been mentioned by some authors in the literature, however, the evidence for or against the same is sparse [98].

Table 3.15 Diagnostic criteria for AFRS

Stage	Endoscopic findings	Diagnostic criteria
Stage 0	No edema off mucosa and allergic mucin	Confirmed type 1 hypersensitivity by history, skin prick tests, or by serology
Stage 1	Edema of mucosa with and without allergic mucin	• Nasal polyposis • Characteristic CT finding
Stage 2	Polypoidal edema with or without allergic mucin	• Positive fungal strain or culture • Asthma
Stage 3	Polyps in the sinus with fungal debris or allergic mucin	• Fungal elements with eosinophilic mucin without tissue invasion • One-sided predominance • Bone erosion on radiology • Charcot–Leyden crystals • Eosinophilia in blood

3.9 Part I: Invasive Fungal Sinusitis

Invasive fungal sinusitis is a potentially lethal entity which if untreated can cause lot of morbidity and mortality for the patient. It is generally seen in immunocompromised patients and can involve intra-orbital or intracranial compartments. The incidence and prevalence rate is increasing progressively with more and more uses of antibiotics, chemotherapy drugs, immune-suppressive drugs, steroids, intensive care intervention, prolong life expectancy in immune deficiency patients. The risk of invasive fungal infection is more in transplanted patients. Invasive fungal sinusitis is defined by the presence of fungal hyphae within the mucosa, submucosa, bone, or blood vessels of the paranasal sinuses. Invasive sinonasal fungal infection is a silently progressive disease that, may invade the adjacent intracranial and intra-orbital compartments incurring serious morbidity. Early recognition and prompt treatment are needed in these patients. Aggressive

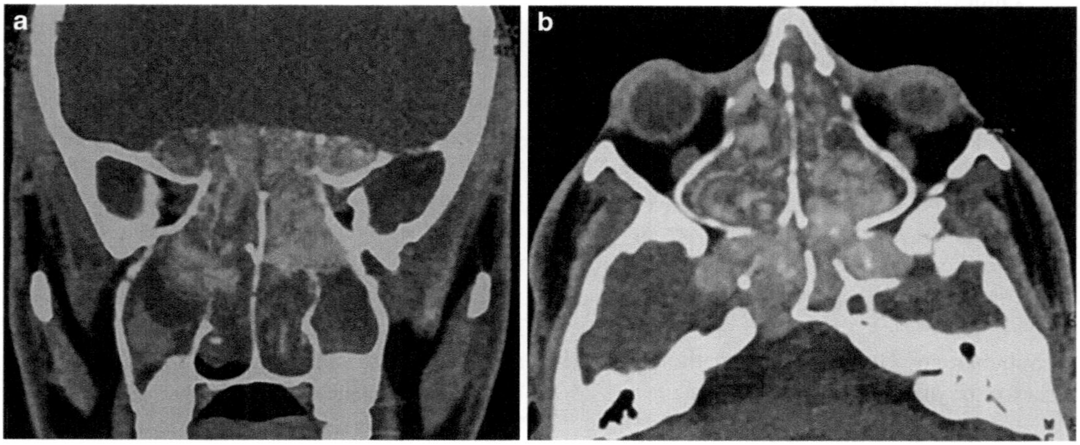

Fig. 3.25 (**a**) Axial and (**b**) coronal non-contrast CT scan of paranasal sinus of a patient with extensive allergic fungal sinusitis. Expansion of the involved sinuses occupied by the soft tissue density with patchy hyperdense areas corresponding to allergic fungal mucin can be seen. Bony thinning and remodeling leading to severe thinning and dehiscence of the roof of posterior ethmoids and the lateral wall of the sphenoid sinus can be appreciated

treatment in form of antifungal agents and extensive surgical debridement has improved the outcome in these patients. These patients need to be continuously monitored in follow-up to prevent any recurrences. It is broadly divided into two subtypes, acute invasive (fulminant) and chronic invasive. Chronic invasive can be granulomatous or non-granulomatous types.

1. **Acute Invasive Fungal Rhinosinusitis**
   It is associated with unacceptably high rates of morbidity and mortality. The exact factors underlying the pathophysiology are unclear, but the environmental load of the fungus, the specific strains, and the immune status of the host are believed to promote invasive disease. A favorable micro-aerophilic local environment is considered the trigger that initiates the proliferation and invasion of a fungal species that is usually a harmless commensal of the upper respiratory tract. Central to the pathophysiology of this disease is its angio-invasiveness. Invasive fungal rhinosinusitis is characterized by invasion of the organism into the vascular wall, with subsequent hemorrhage or ischemia [99]. The main challenges encountered in the management of this disease include the presence of the blood-brain barrier that hinders antifungal penetration intra-cerebrally, the morbidity of surgery, and the gravity of the disease's complications on the central nervous system. Vascular events are poorly tolerated in the central nervous system and one of the main causes of reported mortalities in the published literature on cerebrally invasive fungal sinusitis.
2. **Chronic Invasive Fungal Rhinosinusitis**
   Chronic invasive fungal rhinosinusitis often occurs in healthy individuals, sometime patients may have history of CRS, controlled medical comorbidities such as diabetes. Aspergillus fumigatus is the most common agent isolated [100, 101]. Chronic granulomatous invasive fungal rhinosinusitis is also known as primary paranasal granuloma and indolent fungal sinusitis.

3.9.1 Clinical Presentations

Invasive fungal infection is characterized by a mass within one or more paranasal sinuses with evidence of invasion of contiguous structures such as the base of the skull, orbit, and brain [93]. The patients have symptoms of chronic rhinosinusitis such as sinus pain, nasal discharge, headache, low-grade fever, and intermittent epistaxis. Maxillary sinus seems to be major site for the start of tissue invasion. Invasion of the fungus into the maxillary floor leads to palatal erosions. The involvement of orbital tissue, orbital apex, and cavernous sinuses are possible when the extension of infection extends beyond the ethmoid and sphenoid sinuses. The orbital apex syndrome is more commonly seen with chronic type and it can present in the form of proptosis (Fig. 3.26), orbital neuropathy, and diminished vision [101, 102]. Invasion of adjacent structures such as the cavernous sinus and anterior cranial fossa may lead to epidural abscess, parenchymal cerebritis or abscess, meningitis, cavernous sinus thrombosis, osteomyelitis, mycotic aneurism, stroke, and hematogenous dissemination [103]. Granulomatous fungal sinusitis commonly presents as proptosis or an enlarging, painless, and irregular mass in the cheek, orbit, nose, or paranasal sinuses mimicking an orbital tumor.

3.9.2 Diagnosis

Acute onset of symptoms with the rapid progression of the disease along with the uncontrolled comorbid condition especially diabetes and the presence of crusting with unhealthy nasal mucosa on nasal endoscopic examination are the features that raised the possibility of invasive fungal sinusitis. The nasal endoscopic examination reveals black-to brown crust with unhealthy, congested mucosa. Biopsy is the gold standard way to confirm the invasion of the fungus into the tissue. The presence of the fungal strains in the unhealthy nasal mucosa in fungal smear examination is very much helpful in establishing the clinical diagnosis. Mucor species are mostly seen in acute invasive fungal sinusitis whereas

Aspergillus species are mostly seen chronic invasive fungal sinusitis.

3.9.3 Imaging

CT suggests the diagnosis by showing mucosal thickening or the presence of adjoining soft tissue thickening without erosion of the bony sinus wall in acute invasive form. The absence of enhancement of nasal mucosa/turbinates raised the possibility of tissue necrosis. Hypodense lesion with osteitis and periostitis and presence of sequestrum are the other clinical features for acute invasion. In the chronic form, sinus opacification appears hyperdense due to the metallic ions concentrated by the fungus with localized erosion of the sinus wall (Fig. 3.27). It is also invaluable to assess for bony erosion into adjacent orbital and cranial cavities [104, 105]. Sometimes, tissues outside sinuses are more involved than within the sinus (Fig. 3.27b). The dense calcification is generally seen in the chronic form of invasive fungal sinusitis. CEMRI is more useful than CT for indicating the involvement of peri-sinus soft tissues such as orbit, brain parenchyma. A decrease in signal intensity on T1-weighted images and a marked decrease in signal intensity on T2-weighted images is characteristic of fungal disease, especially that is caused by aspergillus (Fig. 3.27c) [104, 105].

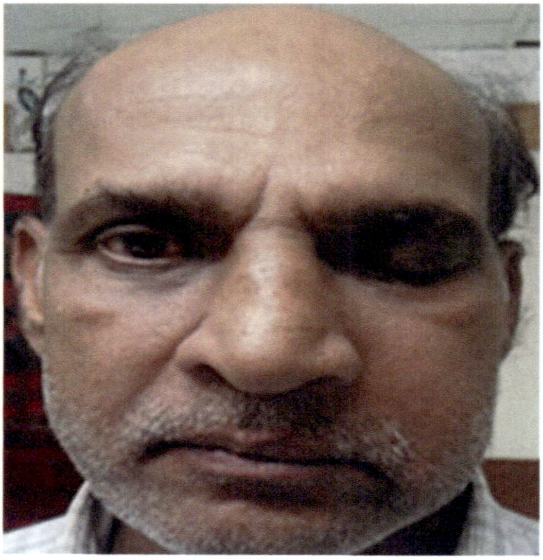

Fig. 3.26 Left orbital apex syndrome with facial nerve palsy (Courtesy—Dr. Hitesh Verma, Associate Professor, AIIMS, New Delhi, India)

3.9.4 Pathology

Histopathology shows the presence of fungal hyphae in tissue with surrounding inflammatory infiltrate with the predominance of neutrophils and associated with foci of necrosis. Invasive fungal rhinosinusitis is defined by the presence of fungal hyphae within the mucosa, submucosa, bone, or blood vessels of the paranasal sinuses. Chronic invasive fungal rhinosinusitis is characterized by the dense accumulation of hyphae

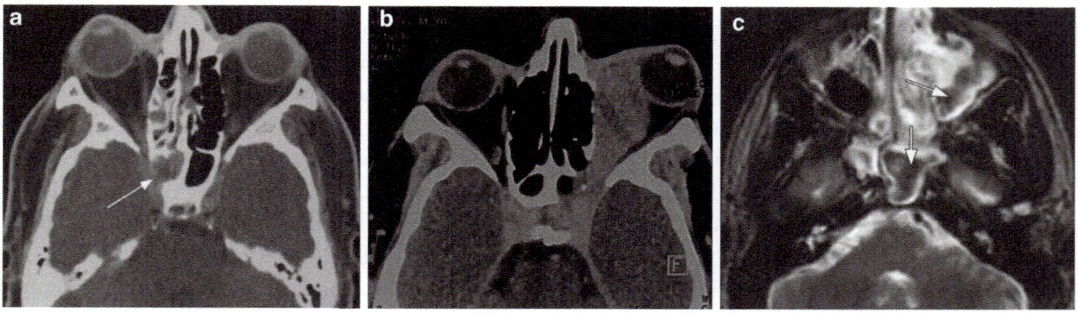

Fig. 3.27 (**a**) Axial contrast-enhanced CT scan shows right ethmoid and sphenoid sinusitis with the destruction of the lateral wall of the right sphenoid sinus (arrow). There is invasion of the right cavernous sinus with occlusion of the right internal carotid artery. (**b**) Right orbital tissue and right cavernous sinus infiltration, (**c**) (Courtesy—Dr. Hitesh Verma, Associate Professor, AIIMS, New Delhi, India), T1-weighted MR images show characteristic high signal intensity within the left maxillary, left posterior ethmoid, and sphenoid sinuses

infiltrating mucosa, blood vessels, and adjacent tissues as muscles and bones, which often exhibit necrosis and a nonspecific inflammatory infiltrate. Granulomatous invasive fungal rhinosinusitis is characterized by non-caseating granuloma with scanty fungal hyphae) within Langerhans-type giant cells, together with surrounding vasculitis and perivascular fibrosis.

3.9.5 Treatment

The standard management involves a combination of surgical debridement of necrotic tissues and long-term antifungal treatment, guided by culture results if possible, to prevent relapse. The surgical approach is determined by the CT findings. Patients with angioinvasion might benefit from a more aggressive therapeutic approach, such as higher dose of intravenous therapy, early surgical debridement, more intense assessment of response, and alternative therapy if the response is inadequate and consideration of supplementary gamma interferon therapy [106]. Amphotericin B is the initial antifungal choice for mucormycosis. Amphotericin B and Posaconazole are the drugs used to treat mucormycosis. For invasive aspergillosis—The usual adult dose of voriconazole is 6 mg/kg twice a day on day one followed by 4 mg/kg twice a day for 7 days with the option to decrease to 200 mg orally, twice a day thereafter. Therapy for those with the overt bone disease should be for at least 3–6 months and possibly for 12 months or longer. Other regime is 3–6 week course of conventional amphotericin B (1 mg/kg/day) or liposomal amphotericin B (3–5 mg/kg/day) usually secures a remission and should be followed by itraconazole or voriconazole for 6 months. Posaconazole (tablets or liquid) is an alternative to control the disease and to prevent recurrences.

3.9.6 Outcome and Follow-Up

Patients with granulomatous fungal sinusitis are believed to have a better prognosis than those with invasive fungal rhinosinusitis, although granulomatous invasive fungal rhinosinusitis tends to have a high relapse rate. Overall, morbidity and mortality appear to be lower than the acute invasive disease. Regular follow-up is indicated and should continue for about 5 years. A CT scan 1 month after surgery (Fig. 3.28) and a prolonged course of antifungal chemotherapy, with imaging repeated every 3 or 4 months and

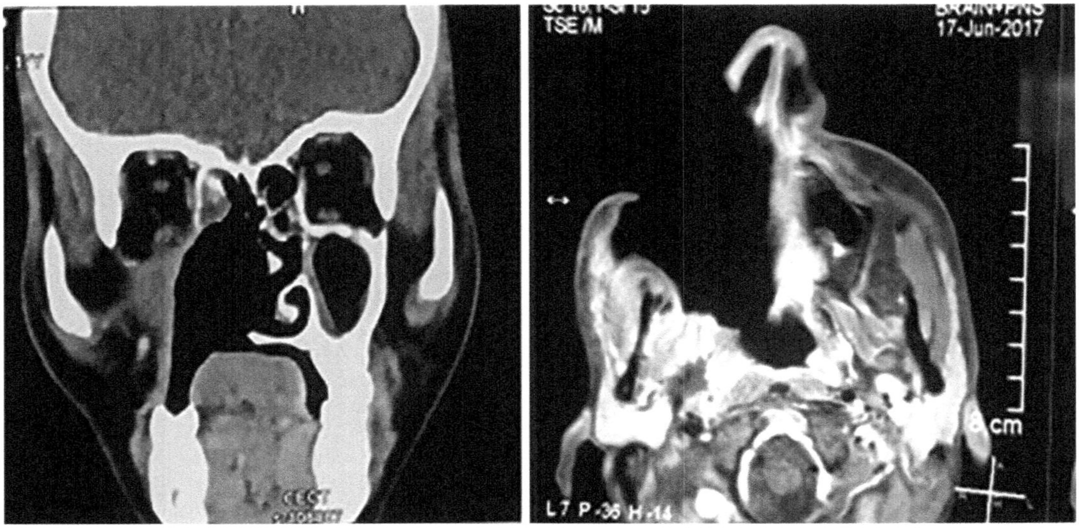

Fig. 3.28 Radiology after completion of treatment (Courtesy—Dr. Hitesh Verma, Associate Professor, AIIMS, New Delhi, India)

endoscopy every 2–3 months to evaluate recurrence should be done [107]. The post-surgical cavity can be managed after certain period of follow-up.

References

1. Gouveri E, Katotomichelakis M, Gouveris H, Danielides V, Maltezos E, Papanas N. Olfactory dysfunction in type 2 diabetes mellitus: an additional manifestation of microvascular disease? Angiology. 2014;65(10):869–76.
2. Sahin-Yilmaz A, Naclerio RM. Anatomy and physiology of the upper airway. Proc Am Thorac Soc. 2011;8(1):31–9.
3. Antunes MB, Gudis DA, Cohen NA. Epithelium, cilia, and mucus: their importance in chronic rhinosinusitis. Immunol Allergy Clin N Am. 2009;29(4):631–43.
4. Lund VJ. Nasal physiology: neurochemical receptors, nasal cycle, and ciliary action. Allergy Asthma Proc. 1996;17(4):179–84.
5. Morris LG, Burschtin O, Lebowitz RA, Jacobs JB, Lee KC. Nasal obstruction and sleep-disordered breathing: a study using acoustic rhinometry. Am J Rhinol. 2005;19(1):33–9.
6. Haavisto LE, Sipilä JI. Acoustic rhinometry, rhinomanometry and visual analogue scale before and after septal surgery: a prospective 10-year follow-up. Clin Otolaryngol. 2013;38(1):23–9.
7. Singh A, Patel N, Kenyon G, Donaldson G. Is there objective evidence that septal surgery improves nasal airflow? J Laryngol Otol. 2006;120(11):916–20.
8. Eduardo Nigro C, Faria Aguar Nigro J, Mion O, Ferreira Mello J, Louis Voegels R, Roithmann R. A systematic review to assess the anatomical correlates of the notches in acoustic rhinometry. Clin Otolaryngol. 2009;34(5):431–7.
9. Morgan NJ, MacGregor FB, Birchall MA, Lund VJ, Sittampalam Y. Racial differences in nasal fossa dimensions determined by acoustic rhinometry. Rhinology. 1995;33(4):224–8.
10. Merkle J, Kohlhas L, Zadoyan G, Mösges R, Hellmich M. Rhinomanometric reference intervals for normal total nasal airflow resistance. Rhinology. 2014;52(4):292–9.
11. Milardi D, Cacciola A, Calamuneri A, Ghilardi MF, Caminiti F, Cascio F, Andronaco V, Anastasi G, Mormina E, Arrigo A, Bruschetta D, Quartarone A. The olfactory system revealed: Non- invasive mapping by using constrained spherical deconvolution tractography in healthy humans. Front Neuroanat. 2017;11:32.
12. Hendrix P, Griessenauer CJ, Foreman P, Shoja MM, Loukas M, Tubbs RS. Arterial supply of the upper cranial nerves: a comprehensive review. Clin Anat. 2014;27:1159–66.
13. Favre JJ, Chaffanjon P, Passagia JG, Chirossel JP. Blood supply of the olfactory nerve. Meningeal relationships and surgical relevance. Surg Radiol Anat. 1995;17:133–8.
14. Vaidyanathan S, Barnes M, Williamson P, et al. Treatment of chronic rhinosinusitis with nasal polyposis with oral steroids followed by topical steroids. Ann Intern Med. 2011;154:293–302.
15. Van den Velde S, Quirynen M, van Hee P, van Steenberghe D. Halitosis associated volatiles in breath of healthy subjects. J Chromatogr B Anal Technol Biomed Life Sci. 2007;853:54–61.
16. Panigrahi S, Sankaran S, Mallik S, Gaddam B, Hanson AA. Olfactory receptor-based polypeptide sensor for acetic acid VOC detection. Mater Sci Eng C Mater Biol Appl. 2012;32:1307–13.
17. Fokkens WJ, Lund VJ, Mullol J et al. European position paper on rhinosinusitis and nasal polyps 2012. Rhinol Suppl 2012;(23):3 p preceding table of contents, 1–298.
18. Erskine SE, Verkerk MM, Notley C, et al. Chronic rhinosinusitis: patient experiences of primary and secondary care – a qualitative study. Clin Otolaryngol. 2015;41:8–14.
19. Ferguson BJ. Eosinophilic mucin rhinosinusitis: a distinct clinicopathological entity. Laryngoscope. 2000;110:799–813.
20. Bhattacharyya N. Contemporary assessment of the disease burden of sinusitis. Am J Rhinol Allergy. 2009;23(4):392–5.
21. Tatar EC, Tatar I, Ocal B, et al. Prevalence of bioflms and their response to medical treatment in chronic rhinosinusitis without polyps. Otolaryngol Head Neck Surg. 2012;146(4):669–75.
22. Seiberling KA, Conley DB, Tripathi A, et al. Superantigens and chronic rhinosinusitis: detection of staphylococcal exotoxins in nasal polyps. Laryngoscope. 2005;115(9):1580–5.
23. Conley DB, Tripathi A, Seiberling KA, et al. Superantigens and chronic rhinosinusitis: skewing of T–cell receptor V beta–distributions in polyp–derived CD4+ and CD8+ T cells. Am J Rhinol. 2006;20(5):534–9.
24. Lanza DC, Kennedy DW. Adult rhinosinusitis defined. Otolaryngol Head Neck Surg. 1997;117:S1S7.
25. Van Zele T, Claeys S, Gevaert P, et al. Differentiation of chronic sinus diseases by measurement of inflammatory mediators. Allergy. 2006;61(11):1280–9.
26. Bhattacharyya N. The economic burden and symptom manifestations of chronic rhinosinusitis. Am J Rhinol. 2003;17(1):27–32.
27. Zhang N, Van Zele T, Perez-Novo C, et al. Different types of T–effector cells orchestrate mucosal inflammation in chronic sinus disease. J Allergy Clin Immunol. 2008;122(5):961–8.
28. Lund VJ, Mackay IS. Staging in rhinosinusitis. Rhinology. 1993;31(4):183–4.
29. Zalmanovici A, Yaphe J. Intranasal steroids for acute sinusitis. Cochrane Database Syst Rev. 2009;4:CD005149.

30. Harvey R, Hannan SA, Badia L, Scadding G. Nasal saline irrigations for the symptoms of chronic rhinosinusitis. Cochrane Database Syst Rev. 2007;3:CD006394.
31. Martinez-Devesa P, Patiar S. Oral steroids for nasal polyps. Cochrane Database Syst Rev. 2011;7:CD005232.
32. Bassiouni A, Naidoo Y, Wormald PJ. When FESS fails: the inflammatory load hypothesis in refractory chronic rhinosinusitis. Laryngoscope. 2012;122:460–6.
33. Bent JP, Cuilty-Siller C, Kuhn FA. The frontal cell as a cause of frontal sinus obstruction. Am J Rhinol. 1994;8:185–91.
34. Wormald PJ, Hoseman W, Callejas C, et al. The international frontal sinus anatomy classification (IFAC) and classification of the extent of endoscopic frontal sinus surgery (EFSS). Int Forum Allergy Rhinol. 2016;6(7):677–96.
35. Draf W. Endonasal micro-endoscopic frontal sinus surgery: the fulda concept. Oper Tech Otolaryngol Head Neck Surg. 1991;2(4):234–40.
36. Saini AT, Govindaraj S. Evaluation and decision making in frontal sinus surgery. Otolaryngol Clin N Am. 2016;49(4):911–25.
37. Mamman-Prasad E, Murillo JL, Titelbaum JA. Infectious disease rounds: Pott's puffy tumour with intracranial complications. N J Med. 1992;89(7):537–9.
38. Fokkens WJ, Lund VJ, Mullol J, et al. EPOS 2012: European position paper on rhinosinusitis and nasal polyps 2012. A summary for Otorhinolaryngologists. Rhinology. 2012;50(1):1–12.
39. Epstein VA, Kern RC. Invasive fungal sinusitis and complications of rhinosinusitis. Otolaryngol Clin N Am. 2008;41(3):497–524.
40. Siedek V, Kremer A, Betz CS, Tschilsner U, Berghaus A, Leunig A. Management of orbital complications due to rhinosinusitis. Eur Arch Otorhinolaryngol. 2010;267(12):1881–6.
41. el-Silimy O. The place of endonasal endoscopy in the treatment of orbital cellulitis. Rhinology. 1995;33(2):93–6.
42. Chandler JR, Langenbrunner DJ, Stevens ER. The pathogenesis of orbital Complications in acute sinusitis. Laryngoscope. 1970;80(9):1414–28.
43. Maniglia GJ, Arnold JE, Ganz E. Intracranial abscesses secondary to nasal, sinus and orbital infections in adults and children. Arch Otolaryngol Head Neck Surg. 1989;115:1424–9.
44. Clayman GL, Adams GC, Paregh DR, Koopmann CF Jr. Intracranial complications of PNS, Sinusitis: a combined institute review. Laryngoscope. 1991;101(3):234–9.
45. Lerner DN, Choi SS, Zalzal GH, Johnson DL. Intracranial complication of sinusitis in childhood. Ann Otol Rhino Laryngol. 1995;104(4 Pt 1):288–93.
46. Johnson DL, Markle BM, Wiedermann BL, Hanahan L. Treatment of intracranial abscesses a/w sinusitis in children and adolescents. J Paedr. 1988;113(1Pt 1):15–23.
47. Schofield G, Farooque S. Recommended management and recent advances in allergic rhinitis. Drug Rev. 2014:21–8.
48. Finn R. John Bostock, hay fever, and the mechanism of allergy. Lancet. 1992;340(8833):1453–5. https://doi.org/10.1016/0140-6736(92)92634-r.
49. Björkstén B, Clayton T, Ellwood P, Stewart A, Strachan D, ISAAC Phase III Study Group. Worldwide time trends for symptoms of rhinitis and conjunctivitis: Phase III of the International Study of Asthma and Allergies in Childhood. Pediatr Allergy Immunol. 2008;19(2):110–24. https://doi.org/10.1111/j.1399-3038.2007.00601.x.
50. Stempel DA, Woolf R. The cost of treating allergic rhinitis. Curr Allergy Asthma Rep. 2002;2(3):223–30. https://doi.org/10.1007/s11882-002-0023-0.
51. McCaig LF, Nawar EW. National Hospital Ambulatory Medical Care Survey: 2004 emergency department summary. Adv Data. 2006;372:1–29.
52. Asher MI, Montefort S, Björkstén B, et al. Worldwide time trends in the prevalence of symptoms of asthma, allergic rhinoconjunctivitis, and eczema in childhood: ISAAC Phases One and Three repeat multicountry cross-sectional surveys [published correction appears in Lancet. 2007 Sep 29;370(9593):1128]. Lancet. 2006;368(9537):733–43. https://doi.org/10.1016/S0140-6736(06)69283-0.
53. Scadding GK, Durham SR, Mirakian R, et al. BSACI guidelines for the management of allergic and non-allergic rhinitis. Clin Exp Allergy. 2008;38(1):19–42. https://doi.org/10.1111/j.1365-2222.2007.02888.x.
54. Smith HE, Hogger C, Lallemant C, Crook D, Frew AJ. Is structured allergy history sufficient when assessing patients with asthma and rhinitis in general practice? J Allergy Clin Immunol. 2009;123(3):646–50. https://doi.org/10.1016/j.jaci.2008.11.005.
55. Nasser M, Fedorowicz Z, Aljufairi H, McKerrow W. Antihistamines used in addition to topical nasal steroids for intermittent and persistent allergic rhinitis in children. Cochrane Database Syst Rev. 2010;7:CD006989. https://doi.org/10.1002/14651858.CD006989.pub2.
56. Klimek L, Bachert C, Pfaar O, et al. ARIA guideline 2019: treatment of allergic rhinitis in the German health system. Allergol Select. 2019;3(1):22–50. https://doi.org/10.5414/ALX02120E.
57. Rondón C, Canto G, Blanca M. Local allergic rhinitis: a new entity, characterization and further studies. Curr Opin Allergy Clin Immunol. 2010;10(1):1–7. https://doi.org/10.1097/ACI.0b013e328334f5fb.
58. van Cauwenberge P, Bachert C, Passalacqua G, et al. Consensus statement on the treatment of allergic rhinitis. European Academy of Allergology and Clinical Immunology. Allergy. 2000;55(2):116–34. https://doi.org/10.1034/j.1398-9995.2000.00526.x.
59. Small M, Piercy J, Demoly P, Marsden H. Burden of illness and quality of life in patients being treated for seasonal allergic rhinitis: a cohort sur-

vey. Clin Transl Allergy. 2013;3(1):33. https://doi.org/10.1186/2045-7022-3-33.
60. Rodrigo GJ, Neffen H. Efficacy of fluticasone furoate nasal spray vs. placebo for the treatment of ocular and nasal symptoms of allergic rhinitis: a systematic review. Clin Exp Allergy. 2011;41(2):160–70. https://doi.org/10.1111/j.1365-2222.2010.03654.x.
61. Bielory L. Ocular symptom reduction in patients with seasonal allergic rhinitis treated with the intranasal corticosteroid mometasone furoate. Ann Allergy Asthma Immunol. 2008;100(3):272–9. https://doi.org/10.1016/S1081-1206(10)60453-X.
62. Corren J. Intranasal corticosteroids for allergic rhinitis: how do different agents compare? J Allergy Clin Immunol. 1999;104(4 Pt 1):S144–9. https://doi.org/10.1016/s0091-6749(99)70310-6.
63. Bryson HM, Faulds D. Intranasal fluticasone propionate. A review of its pharmacodynamic and pharmacokinetic properties, and therapeutic potential in allergic rhinitis. Drugs. 1992;43(5):760–75. https://doi.org/10.2165/00003495-199243050-00009.
64. Daley-Yates PT, Baker RC. Systemic bioavailability of fluticasone propionate administered as nasal drops and aqueous nasal spray formulations. Br J Clin Pharmacol. 2001;51(1):103–5. https://doi.org/10.1046/j.1365-2125.2001.01325.x.
65. Daley-Yates PT, Kunka RL, Yin Y, Andrews SM, Callejas S, Ng C. Bioavailability of fluticasone propionate and mometasone furoate aqueous nasal sprays. Eur J Clin Pharmacol. 2004;60(4):265–8. https://doi.org/10.1007/s00228-004-0763-y.
66. Bousquet J, Van Cauwenberge P, Bachert C, et al. Requirements for medications commonly used in the treatment of allergic rhinitis. European Academy of Allergy and Clinical Immunology (EAACI), Allergic Rhinitis and its Impact on Asthma (ARIA). Allergy. 2003;58(3):192–7. https://doi.org/10.1034/j.1398-9995.2003.00054.x.
67. Graft D, Aaronson D, Chervinsky P, et al. A placebo- and active-controlled randomized trial of prophylactic treatment of seasonal allergic rhinitis with mometasone furoate aqueous nasal spray. J Allergy Clin Immunol. 1996;98(4):724–31. https://doi.org/10.1016/s0091-6749(96)70119-7.
68. Garavello W, Romagnoli M, Sordo L, Gaini RM, Di Berardino C, Angrisano A. Hypersaline nasal irrigation in children with symptomatic seasonal allergic rhinitis: a randomized study. Pediatr Allergy Immunol. 2003;14(2):140–3. https://doi.org/10.1034/j.1399-3038.2003.00021.x.
69. Tomooka LT, Murphy C, Davidson TM. Clinical study and literature review of nasal irrigation. Laryngoscope. 2000;110(7):1189–93. https://doi.org/10.1097/00005537-200007000-00023.
70. Bochner BS, Hamid Q. Advances in mechanisms of allergy. J Allergy Clin Immunol. 2003;111(3 Suppl):S819–23. https://doi.org/10.1067/mai.2003.149.
71. Bousquet J, et al. WHO position paper – allergen immunotherapy: therapeutic vaccines for allergic diseases. Allergy. 1998;53(Suppl. 44):4–42.
72. Akdis CA, Akdis M. Mechanisms of allergen-specific immunotherapy. J Allergy Clin Immunol. 2011;127(1):18–29. https://doi.org/10.1016/j.jaci.2010.11.030.
73. Demoly P, Passalacqua G, Pfaar O, Sastre J, Wahn U. Management of the polyallergic patient with allergy immunotherapy: a practice-based approach. Allergy Asthma Clin Immunol. 2016;12:2. https://doi.org/10.1186/s13223-015-0109-6.
74. Akdis CA, Barlan IB, Bahceciler N, Akdis M. Immunological mechanisms of sublingual immunotherapy. Allergy. 2006;61(Suppl 81):11–4. https://doi.org/10.1111/j.1398-9995.2006.01159.x.
75. Untersmayr E, Jensen-Jarolim E. The role of protein digestibility and antacids on food allergy outcomes. J Allergy Clin Immunol. 2008;121(6):1301–10. https://doi.org/10.1016/j.jaci.2008.04.025.
76. Pattanaik D, Lieberman P. Vasomotor rhinitis. Curr Allergy Asthma Rep. 2010;10:84–91.
77. Brandt D, Bernstein JA. Questionnaire evaluation and risk factor identification for nonallergic vasomotor rhinitis. Ann Allergy Asthma Immunol. 2006;96(4):526–32.
78. Settipane RA, Charnock DR. Epidemiology of rhinitis: allergic and nonallergic. In: Baraniuk JN, Shusterman D, editors. Nonallergic Rhinitis. New York: Informa; 2007. p. 23–34.
79. Blom HM, Van Rijswijk JB, Garrelds IM, Mulder PG, Timmermans T, Gerth van Wijk R. Intranasal capsaicin is efficacious in nonallergic, noninfectious rhinitis. A placebo-controlled study. Clin Exp Allergy. 1997;27:1351–8.
80. Sarin S, Undem B, Sanico A, Togias A. The role of the nervous system in rhinitis. J Allergy Clin Immunol. 2006;118:999–1014.
81. Sin B, Togias A. Pathophysiology of allergic and nonallergic rhinitis. Proc Am Thorac Soc. 2011;8:106–14.
82. Lindberg S, Malm L. Comparison of allergic rhinitis and vasomotor rhinitis patients on the basis of a computer questionnaire. Allergy. 1993;48:602–7.
83. Scarupa MD, Kaliner MA. Nonallergic rhinitis, with a focus on vasomotor rhinitis. WAO. 2009;2:20–5.
84. Aksoy F, Yildirim YS, Veyseller B, et al. Midterm outcomes of out fracture of the inferior turbinate. Otolaryngol Head Neck Surg. 2010;143(4):579–84.
85. Elwany S, Gaimaee R, Fattah HA. Radiofrequency bipolar submucosal diathermy of the inferior turbinates. Am J Rhinol. 1999;13(2):145–9.
86. Woodhead CJ, Wickham MH, Smelt GJ, et al. Some observations on submucous diathermy. J Laryngol Otol. 1989;103(11):1047–9.
87. Cavaliere M, Mottola G, Iemma M. Comparison of the effectiveness and safety of radiofrequency turbinoplasty and traditional surgical technique in treatment of inferior turbinate hypertrophy. Otolaryngol Head Neck Surg. 2005;133(6):972–8.
88. Jourdy D. Inferior turbinate reduction. Oper Tech Otolaryngol. 2014;25:160–70.
89. Ashleigh Halderman MD, Raj Sindwani MD. Surgical management of vasomotor rhini-

tis: a systematic review. Am J Rhinol Allergy. 2015;29:128–34.
90. Sharma S. Understanding allergic fungal rhinosinusitis. Glob J Otolaryngol. 2018;13(3):GJO.MS.ID.555865.
91. Thompson GR III, Patterson TF. Fungal disease of the nose and paranasal sinuses. J Allergy Clin Immunol. 2012;129(2):321–6. https://doi.org/10.1016/j.jaci.2011.11.039.
92. Montone KT. Pathology of fungal rhinosinusitis: a review. Head Neck Pathol. 2016;10(1):40–6. https://doi.org/10.1007/s12105-016-0690-0.
93. Raz E, Win W, Hagiwara M, Lui YW, Cohen B, Fatterpekar GM. Fungal sinusitis. Neuroimaging Clin N Am. 2015;25(4):569–76. https://doi.org/10.1016/j.nic.2015.07.004.
94. Cojocari L, Sandul A. Literature review. Noninvasive fungal rhinosinusitis. Romanian J Rhinol. 2017;7(26):75–81.
95. Berlucchi M, Pedruzzi B. Allergic fungal sinusitis in children. J Aller Ther. 2012;S5:004. https://doi.org/10.4172/2155-6121.S5-004.
96. Schubert MS, Goetz DW. Evaluation and treatment of allergic fungal sinusitis. I. Demographics and diagnosis. J Allergy Clin Immunol. 1998;102(3):387–94. https://doi.org/10.1016/s0091-6749(98)70125-3.
97. Bent JP III, Kuhn FA. Diagnosis of allergic fungal sinusitis. Otolaryngol Head Neck Surg. 1994;111(5):580–8. https://doi.org/10.1177/019459989411100508.
98. Head K, Sharp S, Chong LY, Hopkins C, Philpott C. Topical and systemic antifungal therapy for chronic rhinosinusitis. Cochrane Database Syst Rev. 2018;9(9):CD012453. https://doi.org/10.1002/14651858.CD012453.pub2.
99. Panda NK, Sharma SC, Chakrabarti A, Mann SB. Paranasal sinus mycoses in north India. Mycoses. 1998;41(7–8):281–6. https://doi.org/10.1111/j.1439-0507.1998.tb00339.x.
100. Sharif MS, Ali S, Nisar H. Frequency of granulomatous invasive fungal sinusitis in patients with clinical suspicion of chronic fungal rhinosinusitis. Cureus. 2019;11(5):e4757. https://doi.org/10.7759/cureus.4757.
101. Alrajhi AA, Enani M, Mahasin Z, Al-Omran K. Chronic invasive aspergillosis of the paranasal sinuses in immunocompetent hosts from Saudi Arabia. Am J Trop Med Hyg. 2001;65(1):83–6. https://doi.org/10.4269/ajtmh.2001.65.83.
102. Soler ZM, Schlosser RJ. The role of fungi in diseases of the nose and sinuses. Am J Rhinol Allergy. 2012;26(5):351–8. https://doi.org/10.2500/ajra.2012.26.3807.
103. Hirabayashi KE, Idowu OO, Kalin-Hajdu E, et al. Invasive fungal sinusitis: risk factors for visual acuity outcomes and mortality. Ophthalmic Plast Reconstr Surg. 2019;35(6):535–42. https://doi.org/10.1097/IOP.0000000000001357.
104. Reddy CE, Gupta AK, Singh P, Mann SB. Imaging of granulomatous and chronic invasive fungal sinusitis: comparison with allergic fungal sinusitis. Otolaryngol Head Neck Surg. 2010;143(2):294–300. https://doi.org/10.1016/j.otohns.2010.02.027.
105. Siddiqui AA, Bashir SH, Ali Shah A, et al. Diagnostic MR imaging features of craniocerebral Aspergillosis of sino-nasal origin in immunocompetent patients. Acta Neurochir. 2006;148(2):155–66. https://doi.org/10.1007/s00701-005-0659-3.
106. Smith NL, Denning DW. Clinical implications of interferon-γ genetic and epigenetic variants. Immunology. 2014;143(4):499–511. https://doi.org/10.1111/imm.12362.
107. Krishnan KU, Agatha D, Selvi R. Fungal rhinosinusitis: a clinicomycological perspective. Indian J Med Microbiol. 2015;33(1):120–4. https://doi.org/10.4103/0255-0857.148407.

Granulomatous Disease and Faciomaxillary Trauma

4

Gaurav Gupta, Pooja D. Nayak, Manju Silu, Shashank Nath Singh, and Harpreet Kocher

Contents

Granulomatous diseases can affects any body. It is broadly classified into specific and non specific type. bacterial & fungal granulomatous diseases are the specific type of diseases. Granulomatosis with polyangiitis (Wegeners' granulomatosis), sarcoidosis, Churg-Strauss syndrome, NK/T cell lymphoma are the types of non specific diseases. Granuloma is the characterstic feature formed by the aggregation of macrophages. Macrophages surrounds by the layer of leukocytes. Each granulomatous disease generates

G. Gupta (✉) · P. D. Nayak · M. Silu
ENT, SP Medical College,
Bikaner, Rajasthan, India
e-mail: drgauravgupta24@gmail.com

S. N. Singh
ENT, SMS Medical College,
Jaipur, Rajasthan, India

H. Kocher
ENT, Yatharth Superspeciality Hospital,
Greater Noida, UP, India

H. Verma, A. Thakar (eds.), *Essentials of Rhinology*, https://doi.org/10.1007/978-981-33-6284-0_4

specific histopathological feature. majority of diseases are managed by specific medical managment. Atrophic rhinitis is characterized by progressive atrophy of nasal mucosa and bones within the turbinates. The symptoms are foul smell with recurrent nasal crusting, headache, epistaxis, and nasal obstruction. The endoscopic examination reveals roomy nasal cavity with brownish-green crust and atrophy of turbinates. The natural ostium of maxillary and sphenoid sinuses is visible on routine diagnostic endoscopy. The exact etiology is unknown for primary type but is usually initiates at puberty with female preponderance, indicative of endocrine inequality. Malnutrition, autoimmunity, and hereditary factor are the other important etiological factors. Prior nasal surgery, trauma, and chronic sinusitis are the common etiological factors for secondary type. A broad range of bacterial flora has been cultured in atrophic rhinitis. The primary aim of conservative treatment is regular cleaning of the nasal cavity. Nasal douches, 25% glucose in glycerine, human placental extract, etc. are tried to improve symptomatology. Surgical approaches are focused on narrowing of the nasal cavity by medialization of turbinates, by increasing the nasal septum thickness, and by narrowing of the vestibule.

The major function of the facial skeleton is providing support to sphincter muscles. Facial injuries account 10% of accidental trauma. The lines of management include the establishment of secured airway, controlled breathing, maintenance of circulation, disability assessment, and exposure of all injuries. The majority of facio-maxillary traumas are managed by semi-rigid internal fixation. The outcomes are generally assessed by fine dental occlusion, re-establishment of facial esthetics.

4.1 Part A: Granulomatous Disease of the Nose and Paranasal Sinuses

4.1.1 Introduction

Granulomatous disorders comprise a large number of diseases sharing the histological denominator of granuloma formation. Granuloma is defined as a chronic inflammatory reaction, characterized by the focal accumulation of concentric layers of cells consisting of activated macrophages called epithelioid cells and multinucleated giant cells surrounded by lymphocytes and fibroblasts. It is a type IV hypersensitivity reaction. It is a protective defense reaction by the host, where the immune system attempts to wall off substance that is foreign but is unable to eliminate. Two factors contributes to the formation of granuloma.

1. The inducer agent, which is a pathogen or foreign body, the intrinsic toxicity of which can damage the tissues.
2. The vigorous immune-inflammatory T-cell-mediated response is evoked by the pathogen/foreign body recruiting macrophages and phagocytosis secreting tissue damaging substances, during the activated stage.

Several granulomatous diseases have a predilection to involve the airways. These diseases are often characterized by a local inflammatory response in the airways, particularly in the upper nasal passages.

Etiology:

1. Infective
2. Inflammatory
3. Neoplastic

1. Infectious Granulomatous Disease:
   (A) Bacterial
   (B) Fungal
   (C) Protozoal

(A) Bacterial Granulomatous Disease:
   1. Tuberculosis—It is a form of extrapulmonary tuberculosis. Nasal tuberculosis is usually secondary either to pulmonary tuberculosis or tuberculosis of facial skin (Fig. 4.1).

      Primary disease of the nose is rare. Nasal secretions, nasal vibrissae, and the inherent resistance offered by nasal mucosa and ciliary clearance are the possible explanation for the lower occurrence of nasal tuberculosis. Tuberculosis in the head and neck region is uncommon

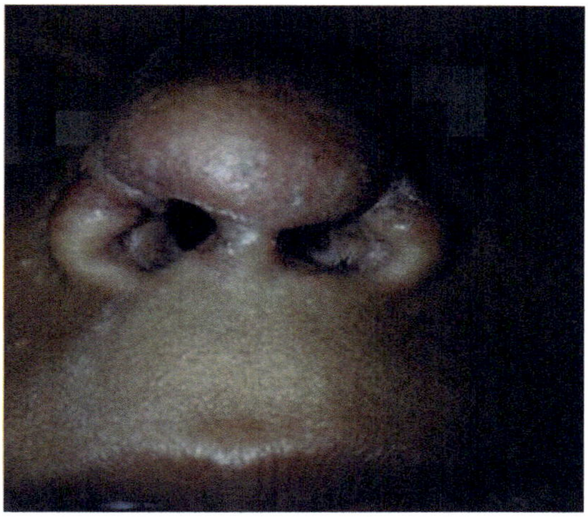

Fig. 4.1 The clinical photograph is showing nasal tuberculosis. Nasal tip and overlying skin is involved by tumor

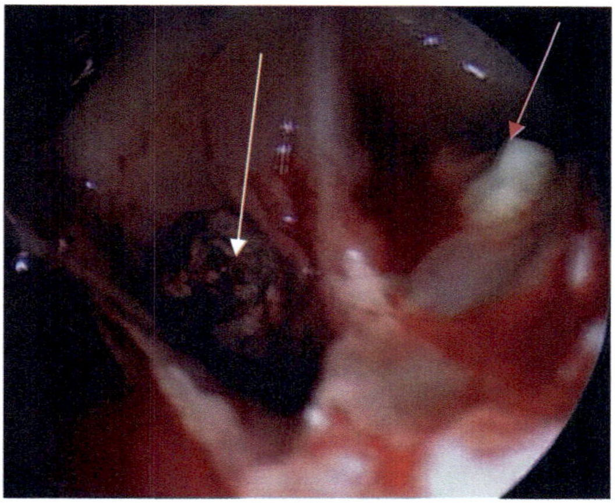

Fig. 4.2 The endoscopic photograph is showing cheesy material (red arrow) in sphenoid sinus with erosion of posterior wall with dural breach (white arrow) (Courtesy—Dr. Hitesh Verma, Associate Professor, AIIMS, New Delhi, India)

and constitutes 2–6% of all types of TB. In the last decades, extrapulmonary tuberculosis is rising due to HIV co-infection. Mycobacterium tuberculosis is the causative bacteria and it is spread by droplet formation. Nasal TB remains asymptomatic until it has progressed to the advance stage. The most common presenting symptom is nasal obstruction, discharge, epistaxis, crusting, and post-nasal discharge. On examination, nasal granuloma and ulceration can be found in cartilaginous septum, cleft of the nasal ala, or facial abscesses may be present. Sphenoid sinus, petrous apex involvement can present with retropharyngeal abscess by extension of abscess along the periosteum [1] (Fig. 4.2). Incisional or punch biopsy from the affected site is the preferred method of diagnostic sampling for ENT lesions, and tissue should be sent for: histopathology, staining for acid-fast bacilli (fluorochrome or ZN staining), culture. The treatment policy for nasal tuberculosis is administered as per national guidelines. Nasal tuberculosis is consider as bony tuberculosis & it is managed by minimum 9 month therapy.

2. Leprosy: It is a slowly progressive, chronic infectious disease caused by the bacillus Mycobacterium leprae. The nose is one of the chief organs that is affected by this disease. It is frequently deformed and disfigured and it contributes to the characteristic facies of leprotic patients. Patients can be classified into three groups, each with slightly different signs and symptoms:
   - **Paucibacillary (PB), or tuberculoid disease:** Characterized by one or a few hypo-pigmented or hyper-pigmented skin macules that exhibit loss of sensation due to infection of the peripheral nerves supplying the region. In these patients, nasal presentation is with skin lesions extending up to the nasal vestibule. The nasal mucosa is not involved.
   - **Multibacillary (MB), or lepromatous disease** is characterized by generalized or diffuse involvement of the skin, a thickening of the peripheral nerves has the potential to involve other organs, the eyes, nose, testes, and bone. The nodular form of this condition is the most advanced form of the disease. Patient can present nasal discharge and, crusting. On examination, nodular thickening of nasal mucosa in the anterior end of

the inferior turbinate is seen. Other features are Collapse of the anterior bridge of the nose with the destruction of anterior nasal spine, destruction of bony and cartilaginous portions of nasal septum.

- **Borderline, or dimorphous, Hansen's disease** is the most common form. Frequently, the initial form consisting of a few lesions, either evolves into the other forms or resolves spontaneously.

Scrapings of the nasal mucosa and skin biopsy shows the presence of acid-fast lepra bacilli which are present in the foamy appearing histiocytes called lepra cells. The treatment of leprosy is in the form of Multi Drug Therapy (MDT), which is the combination of two or three of the following drugs: Rifampicin, Dapsone, Clofazimine [2].

3. Rhinoscleroma: It is found worldwide including Central America, Chili, Central Africa, India, Indonesia, and Middle East countries. The disease usually presents in the second and third decades of life with slight female predominance. The Klebsiella rhinoscleromatis is the causative organism. It is generally found in rural areas with poor socioeconomic conditions. The exact pathogenesis of the disease is unclear. Transmission of this disease is via airborne routes. Humans are the only identified host. It is a slowly progressive disease with insidious onset and indolent course. Nasal cavity is primarily affected in 95–100% of cases. Nasopharynx, nasal sinuses, pharynx, larynx, trachea, and bronchi may also be involved. The disease progresses through three sequential and overlapping phases.
   (a) Catarrhal/Rhinitis: Patients present with non-specific rhinitis.
   (b) Granulomatous/Florid: Foul smelling purulent discharge, epistaxis, nasal obstruction, and crusting. On examination, bluish red, rubbery granulomatous lesions are seen.

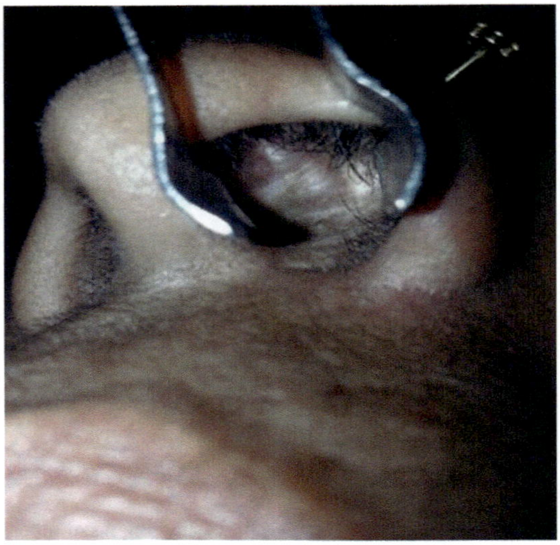

Fig. 4.3 The clinical photograph is showing complete stenosis of the left nasal cavity (Courtesy—Dr. Pirabhu S, Mch candidate, AIIMS, New Delhi, India)

   (c) Sclerotic/Cicatricial: Nasal deformities, anosmia, oral anesthesia, dysphonia, dysphagia, and stridor could happen (Fig. 4.3).

The diagnosis of Rhinoscleroma is clinched with histological confirmation. The diagnostic histological changes are seen only in the granulomatous phase. Dense infiltration by lymphocytes, plasma cells, Russell bodies, and the pathognomonic large Mikulicz cells are the histopathological features seen. Mikulicz cells are foamy macrophages with numerous cytoplasmic vacuoles containing viable and nonviable Klebsiella bacilli. They are sparse or absent in the initial catarrhal and final sclerotic stages and abundant in the proliferative phase. Extensive fibrosis and few inflammatory cells are the histological findings in the fibrotic phase. Intracytoplasmic bacilli are best demonstrated by special staining using periodic acid-Schiff (PAS), Giemsa, Gram, silver, or Warthin-Starry stains, and type III Klebsiella antigen can be detected by immunohistochemistry. Antibiotics that demonstrated efficacy includes streptomycin, doxycycline, tetracyclines, rifampicin, second and third-generation cephalosporins, sulfonamides, clofazimine, ciprofloxacin, and ofloxacin. K. rhinoscleromatis is an intracellular bacterium; it responds well to prolonged courses of rifampicin and fluoroquinolones, as these antibiotics can achieve high concentrations in macrophages. Fluoroquinolones are recommended for their excellent activity against Gram-negative bacilli, intracellular efficacy, and low toxicity profile. The current recommendation consists of a combination of ciprofloxacin and doxycycline for at least 6 months. Combination therapy is preferred due to the high relapse rates of the disease. Surgical debridement can also be considered if there is significant airway obstruction or cosmetic deformity. Other rarer complications to keep in mind include stenosis leading to respiratory obstruction (Fig. 4.3), hemorrhage, intracranial invasion, and malignancy transformation [3].

4. Syphilis: Syphilis is an infectious venereal disease caused by the spirochete *Treponema pallid.* Syphilis is acquired by direct contact, usually sexual, with active primary or secondary lesions. Infection also occurs when organisms cross the placenta to infect the fetus in a pregnant woman. *T. pallidum*'s only known natural host is human. Syphilis is a multistage disease with diverse and wide-ranging manifestations. Clinical manifestations separate the disease into stages. Primary syphilis rarely involves the nasal cavity. A single chancre at the site of inoculation develops an average of 3 weeks after exposure. It is indurate and progresses to non-purulent ulceration with regional lymphadenopathy. Secondary syphilis occurs within 3 months of initial infection and is sometimes quite subtle or disseminated mucocutaneous rash and adamant coryza. Manifestations of secondary syphilis resolve spontaneously within 3 months of appearance. Tertiary Syphilis is characterized by the formation of Gumma. Gummas are granulomatous, nodular lesions with variable central necrosis and it develops as early as 2 years after initial infection. These lesions most commonly affect the skin and bones. Nasal features are mucosal ulcerations, necrosis of nasal septum, ozoena or atrophic rhinitis, stenosis, and atresia of vestibules, Perforations of palate, and external deformities in the form of saddle nose. Lesions rarely heal spontaneously but resolve rapidly with appropriate antibiotic therapy. Congenital syphilis is divided into stages: early manifestations appearing in the first 2 years of life, late manifestations appears after 2 years, and residual stigmata. Dark ground microscopy from lesions of primary and secondary syphilis and serology are the mainstay of diagnosis. Penicillin is the drug of choice and treatment duration is based on the type of lesion [4, 5].

(B) Fungal Granulomatous Disease:

1. Rhinosporidiosis—It is caused by *Rhinosporidium seeberi.* Greater than 90% cases are reported from India, Sri Lanka, and Pakistan. It is most prevalent in southern India. The disease is mostly seen in individuals from ages 15–40. Males tend to be affected more than females by a ratio of 4:1, most likely because of greater levels of outdoor activity among males. There is no known vector for rhinosporidiosis. Nasal infection generally occurs after swimming or bathing in stagnant freshwater ponds, lakes, or rivers that contain the organism. Eye infection is believed to occur from dust or air. Mature sporangia measure approximately 100–300 microns. They are filled with large numbers of daughter cells that are called endospores. Symptoms are variable and depend on the location of the polyps. The nose and the nasopharynx are the most common

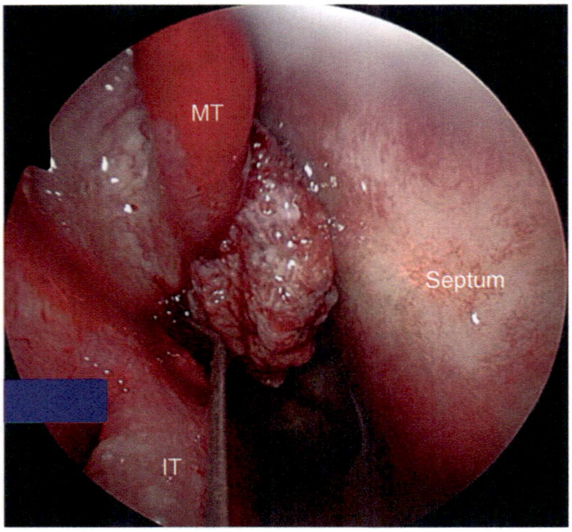

Fig. 4.4 Rhinosporidiosis of the right nasal cavity. MT(middle turbinate), IT (inferior turbinate) (Courtesy—Dr. Hitesh Verma, Associate Professor, AIIMS, New Delhi, India)

sites of infection, occurring in about 70% of cases. Patients may present with unilateral nasal obstruction and bleeding. Other symptoms may include local pruritus, coryza, sneezing, rhinorrhea, and nasal discharge. Other structures in the upper aero-digestive tract can also be affected, leading to obstruction, cough, hemoptysis, or painful swallowing.On examination red, swollen sessile, or pedunculated polyps in the nasal mucosa or the ocular conjunctivae are noted (Fig. 4.4). The presence of sporangia with endospores is diagnostic feature. The only effective treatment surgical excision of the polyps. Excision with electro-coagulation of the base of the lesion appears to be the treatment of choice in minimizing the risk of recurrence [6].

2. Histoplasmosis: It is a fungal infection caused by *Histoplasma capsulatum*. Liver, spleen, lymph nodes, bone marrow, skin, and mucosa may be involved in 1% of the cases [1]. It is typically acquired via inhalation of airborne microconidia. Most of the people with normal immune systems develop either trivial clinical histoplasmosis or are totally asymptomatic. The immunocompromised are more prone to develop disseminated disease. Histoplasma antigen detection in the urine and/or serum most sensitive method for diagnosing disseminated histoplasmosis and acute pulmonary histoplasmosis. Culture is the gold standard test but it takes up to 6 weeks to become positive. Patients with progressive disseminated histoplasmosis and those with AIDS should be treated with amphotericin B.

(C) Protozoal Granulomatous Disease:

1. Nasal leishmaniasis—In over 90% of mucosal lesions—whether primary or secondary—the nose is the only site with the disease [7]. Mucosal involvement is usually secondary to cutaneous lesions. The nasal mucosa is one of the preferred sites, especially the cartilaginous septum, vestibule, lower turbinates, and the floor of the nose. Nasal obstruction, rhinorrhea, epistaxis are the common symptoms [7]. On examination, we can find edematous anterior septal mucosa, septal nodules, septal perforation. Leishmaniotic facies ("tapir nose") when thickening and hyperemia of the nasal skin, upper lip, palate pharynx, resulting in severe deformity. Leishmaniasis is diagnosed by detecting it (or DNA) in tissue specimens. Miltefosine is the drug of choice and doses for persons whose weight is from 30 to 44 kg, 50-mg BD. For persons who weight 45 kg or above, 50-mg/TDS for 28 consecutive days. Sodium stibogluconate, ketoconazole, itraconazole, and fluconazole are other drugs used in the literature.

2. Inflammatory Granulomatous Disease:

(A) Granulomatosis with polyangiitis (Wegener granulomatosis)—It is a systemic disorder that is characterized by necrotizing vasculitis of small arteries and veins. The mean age at diagnosis is 55 years and Men and women are similarly affected. Patients may present with constitutional complaints like fever, night sweats, fatigue, loss of appetite, and weight. It is Multisystem autoimmune disease. Clinical features of WG can be divided into three categories.

- Type 1 GPA—It is characteristic by prolonged upper respiratory tract infection.
- Type 2 GPA—Pulmonary involvement is often present and is associated with a cough, hemoptysis, and cavitary lesions on chest radiography.
- Type 3 GPA is a widely disseminated form of the systemic disease and commonly consists of upper and lower airway involvement, cutaneous lesions, and progressive renal involvement.

History, examination, radiologic, and biochemical data findings help in diagnosis. The nasal cavity examination usually shows septal perforation with or without granulomatous tissue (Fig. 4.5). Patients also have abnormal erythrocyte sedimentation rate, hemoglobin, serum creatinine, and serum c-ANCA levels. These serologic findings in conjunction with nasal biopsy can provide a definitive diagnosis of WG. The c-ANCA test is highly sensitive for GPA, but a negative result does not exclude the diagnosis. The main agents used to induce remission are glucocorticoids, cyclophosphamide, and/or methotrexate [7, 8].

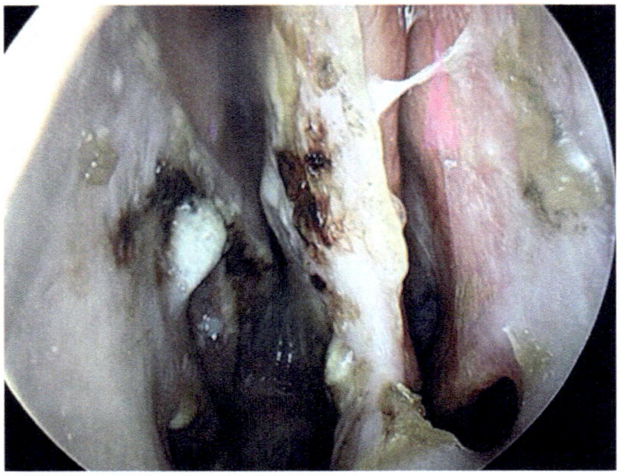

Fig. 4.5 Nasal endoscopy is showing large septal perforation with crusting and atrophy of surrounding tissue (Courtesy—Dr. Hitesh Verma, Associate Professor, AIIMS, New Delhi, India)

(B) Sarcoidosis—It frequently involves the lymphatic system, lungs, liver, spleen, and bones. It occurs most commonly between the ages of 20 and 40 years with women are slightly more often affected than men. The etiology of sarcoidosis is unknown. It is characterized by a seemingly exaggerated immune response against an unknown antigen. Sarcoidosis is manifested by the presence of multiple noncaseating granulomas in affected organ tissues. The sarcoid granuloma consists of a central area of tightly packed epithelioid cells surrounded by lymphocytes and fibroblasts. The lung is the primary organ affected by sarcoidosis. Approximately 40% of patients have extrapulmonary involvement. The involvement of the nose and paranasal sinuses by sarcoidosis is relatively infrequent with the incidence ranging between 1% and 6%. Symptoms of nasal involvement are nasal obstruction, epistaxis, dyspnea, nasal pain, epiphora, and anosmia. Nasal sarcoidosis commonly affects the mucosa of the septum and inferior turbinate. On examination, the nasal mucosa is dry and friable with crusts. Submucosal nodules with a characteristic yellow color may be noted. In more advanced disease, irregular polypoid, friable mucosa is seen and bleeds readily. More severe infiltration may lead to septal perforation or oronasal fistulae. Diagnosis is based on a combination of histologic, radiographic, immunologic, and biochemical data.

Pulmonary findings of either hilar lymphadenopathy or pulmonary fibrosis are common. Biochemical examination shows elevated serum or urinary calcium. Serum angiotensin-converting enzyme (ACE) elevations occur in 83% of patients with active sarcoidosis, which has become very useful for the diagnosis and for monitoring of relapse. The diagnosis of sarcoidosis is confirmed by the presence of noncaseating granulomas, composed of multiple epithelioid cells and Langerhans giant cells in the nasal mucosa. Negative stains for fungus and acid-fast bacilli help to support the diagnosis. Stage I sarcoidosis undergo spontaneous remission within 2 years without specific treatment. Sarcoidosis with elevated ACE values or extrapulmonary involvement usually requires treatment; this statement applies to most cases of nasal sarcoidosis. The mainstay of treatment for sarcoidosis is systemic corticosteroids. Methotrexate has been used to treat nasal sarcoidosis successfully. Nasal symptoms may be treated with nasal saline irrigations and topical nasal steroids. Secondary infections treated with culture-directed antimicrobial therapy. Surgery is advisable in medically controlled symptomatic nasal obstruction or chronic sinusitis, in selected patients [8, 9].

(C) Churg–Strauss syndrome—Eosinophilic granulomatosis with polyangiitis (EGPA) traditionally termed, Churg–Strauss syndrome is a rare systemic necrotizing vasculitis that affects small-to-medium-sized vessels. It occurs equally among men and women with mean age of 50 years. Autoimmunity is evident with the presence of hypergammaglobulinemia, increased levels of immunoglobulin E (IgE), rheumatoid factor, and Antineutrophil cytoplasm antibody (ANCA). CSS is characterized by necrotizing vasculitis of small and medium-sized vessels, Necrotizing extravascular granulomas, eosinophilia of the vessels and perivascular tissue. CSS consists of three phases:

1. A prodromal phase with allergic rhinitis and asthma
2. an eosinophilic infiltrative phase with chronic eosinophilic pneumonia (Loeffler syndrome) or gastroenteritis, and
3. A systemic, life-threatening vasculitis with granulomatous inflammation.

The patients presented with nasal crusing & polyposis, distringuished from GPA is by extensive polyposis on both side & asthma. The c-ANCA test result is also negative in CSS, although perinuclear antineutrophil cytoplasmic antibodies (p-ANCAs) is found in 70% of patients. Glucocorticoids is the treatment for CSS whereas cyclophosphamide may be helpful in life-threatening cases or in patients with poor prognostic factors. Rituximab (B-cell-depleting monoclonal antibody) has been used with favorable responses in patients with CSS refractory to conventional treatments. The anti-IgE monoclonal antibody omalizumab has demonstrated a corticosteroid-sparing effect in refractory or relapsing EGPA. Mepolizumab an interleukin-5 antagonist monoclonal antibody (IgG1 kappa) is being studied for its efficacy in CSS [8, 10].

(D) T-cell lymphoma—It is extra-nodal NK/T-cell lymphoma, nasal type (ENKL) is a rare form of non-Hodgkin's lymphoma. Disease causing destruction of the midline structures of the palate and nasal fossa, so it is also known as midline lethal granuloma. Histopathology shows the presence of polymorphic lymphoid infiltrate of mature, immature, and atypical lymphocytes, plasma cells, histiocytes, eosinophils with necrosis of cells. Immunohistochemical studies demonstrate positivity for T-cell markers like CD2, CD7, CD45RO, and CD43 and natural killer cell marker CD57.35. The causative role of EBV in the pathogenesis of T-cell lymphoma has been strongly suggested. Initial symptoms are nasal obstruction, pus, and serosanguinous nasal discharge. As the disease progresses, unilateral mucosal ulceration with extension into the palate, maxillary sinus, and upper lip is seen (Fig. 4.6). Oronasal fistula and nasal septal perforations are frequently present. The characteristic clinical feature with necrotizing atypical cell exudates on histopathology suggests the diagnosis. Therapy for localized disease is radiotherapy. Chemo-radiotherapy is the treatment for advanced lesion [11, 12]. The chemotherapy regimens are mentioned in Chap. 10.

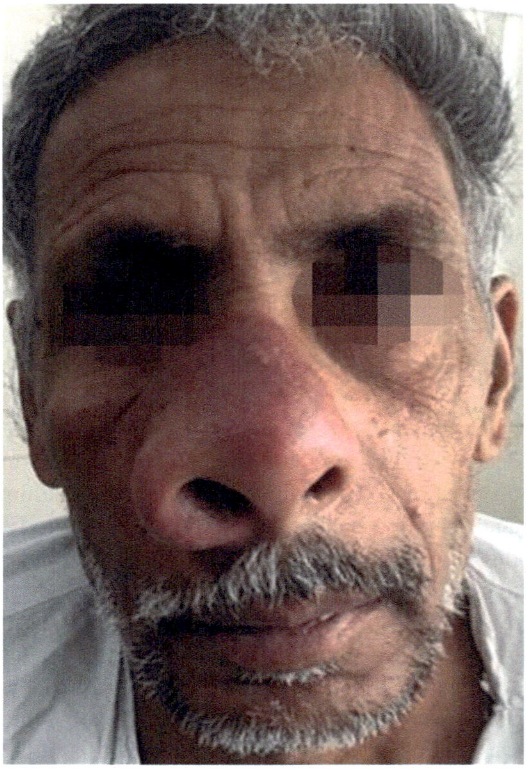

Fig. 4.6 The clinical photograph is showing reddish skin over the right half of nose with widening of ala of the right side (Courtesy—Dr. Hitesh Verma, Associate Professor, AIIMS, New Delhi, India)

4.1.2 Other Granulomatous Pathology

Inflammatory Pseudotumor (IPT)—It is benign idiopathic non-neoplastic inflammatory disease and it can involve any organ. It presents with history of the progressive, locally destructive mass lesion. Radiologically, it is infiltrative in surrounding structures so it can mimic as skull base osteomyelitis and invasive fungus sinusitis. It is isointense on T1 and hypointense on T2 MRI images. It most commonly involves orbit whereas nose and paranasal sinus involvement are relatively rare. Immunoglobulin G4 level can be raised in IPT. The final diagnosis of IPT is based on characteristic histopathology finding where tissue shows the presence of dense lymphoplasmocytic infiltration with obliterative phlebitis, storiform fibrosis. Lymphoplasmocytic infiltration is seen in IgG4 related granulomatous lesions with serum IgG level above 135 mg/dl. The most accepted treatment modality is systemic steroid, radiotherapy alone, or in combination. Surgery and immune-suppression are also mentioned as modality in few reports [13].

4.2 Part B: Atrophic Rhinitis

Atrophic rhinitis is a chronic inflammatory condition characterized by progressive atrophy of the nasal mucosa and underlying bone of the turbinates leading to the formation of thick crusts and a constant foul smell (Ozaena) in the nose. The natural ostium of the sinuses is visible in routine nasal endoscopy without effort. It can be of two types—Primary and Secondary. Histopathological examination reveals the presence of squamous epithelium instead of ciliated columnar epithelium. The choice of investigation is prescribed on the basis of history for secondary atrophic rhinitis. The selection of management is based on symptomatology and response. The first line of management is to increase mucosal clearance by nasal douches. The last management option is the closure of the nasal cavity for certain period.

Primary Atrophic rhinitis is multi-factorial in origin. Hereditary, as the disease is known to involve more than one member in the same family. In some cases, it usually involves females more than males and starts at puberty. The disease is self-limiting, tends to cease after menopause thus hormonal influence cannot be ruled out. It is more common in hot and humid climate specially in the low socioeconomic group. Nutrition has also been shown to play a vital role as deficiency of vitamin A, D, or iron or some other dietary factors have been associated with the disease and are likely causes. Autoimmune process in which viral infection or some other unspecified agents trigger antigenicity of nasal mucosa. The antibody released causes destruction of the nasal mucosa is also postulated. The most widely accepted fact is the infective process where in various organisms have been cultured from cases which are *Klebsiella ozaenae*, (Perez bacillus), diphtheroids, *P. vulgaris*, *E. coli*, Staphylococci, and Streptococci. They are all considered to be secondary invaders responsible for foul smell rather than the primary causative organism. Specific infections like syphilis, lupus, leprosy, and rhinoscleroma are the etiology for secondary atrophic rhinitis which may cause destruction of the nasal structures leading to atrophic changes. Atrophic rhinitis can also result from long-standing purulent sinusitis, radiotherapy to the nose, or excessive surgical removal of turbinates [14]. Unilateral Atrophic Rhinitis—changes in the wider side of the nasal cavity is sometimes seen in cases of marked septal deviation.

4.2.1 Pathology

The characteristic feature is squamous metaplasia of the normal ciliated columnar epithelium along with its endarteritis obliterans is seen in the mucosa, periosteum, and bone leading to atrophy of seromucinous glands, venous blood sinusoids, and nerve elements [15]. The bone of turbinates undergoes resorption causing the widening of nasal chambers. Paranasal sinuses are small due to their arrested development. Young and Taylor [16] have proposed that atrophic rhinitis is of two types, depending upon the vascular involvement into two types. Type I is major subtype (50% to 80%) and is characterized by endarteritis obliterans, periarteritis, and periarterial fibrosis of terminal arterioles as a result of chronic infection with round cell and plasma cell infiltration. Type II is minor subtype (20% to 50%) and shows capillary vasodilation with active bone resorption. Infection affects the surfactant system leading to surfactant deficit [17] through several mechanisms including, the absence of noteworthy SP-A gene up-regulation and diminution of SP-A protein reserves, also inflammatory cytokines produced in response to sepsis inhibiting the synthesis of surfactant leading to decrease the efficiency of mucociliary clearance also, surfactant deficiency impairs opsonization and phagocytosis of bacteria thus developing into a vicious cycle of colonization of nasal mucous by bacteria and causing destruction overtime.

4.2.1.1 Clinical Features

The disease is commonly seen in females and starts around puberty. Merciful anosmia is a term characterized by the foul smell from the nose but the patient herself is unaware of the smell due to marked anosmia which accompanies these degenerative changes thus making the patient a social outcast. Patient may also complain of nasal obstruction in spite of unduly wide nasal chambers. This is due to large crusts filling the nose with atrophy of nerve ending. Epistaxis may occur when the crusts are removed. Complain of decreased hearing and fullness of ear due to obstruction to eustachian tube. On examination, anterior rhinoscopy shows the nasal cavity to be full of greenish or grayish black dry crusts covering the turbinates and septum, which bleeds if removed (Fig. 4.5). On removal of crusts, nasal cavities appear roomy with atrophy of turbinates which may be reduced to mere ridges and the posterior wall of nasopharynx can be easily seen. Nasal mucosa appears pale and dermatitis of the nasal vestibule may be present. Septal perforations can be seen leading to saddle nose deformity. Atrophic changes may also be seen in the pharyngeal mucosa which appears as dry and glazed with crusts leading to atrophic pharyngitis. Sometimes the atrophic changes may extend to the laryngeal mucosa causing cough and hoarseness of voice typical of Atrophic Laryngitis. middle ear effusion, tympanic membrane retractions due to obstruction to eustachian tube causes hearing-impairment in the minority of cases [18]. Paranasal sinuses are usually small and underdeveloped with thick walls. The presence of 2 or more features beyond 6 months are in favor of atrophic rhinitis: recurrent epistaxis, episodic anosmia, nasal purulence, crusting, surgical intervention in two or more sinuses, and presence of chronic inflammatory disease [19].

4.2.1.2 Investigations

Mainly aim to establish the diagnosis by excluding secondary causes of atrophic rhinitis and other granulomatous conditions. Low hemoglobin and peripheral blood smear show microcytic hypochromic picture pointing towards iron deficiency anemia. As bacterial infection is seen, there is raised total leukocyte count (TLC) and differential leukocyte count (DLC) show lymphocytosis. Commonly, low Serum protein and plasma vitamin levels are seen due to malnutrition. Other tests done to rule out secondary causes are the erythrocyte sedimentation rate (ESR) which is raised in tuberculosis and granulomatous infection. Blood sugar is to rule out diabetes mellitus. VDRL test is to diagnose secondary to syphilis. Chest X-ray and Mantoux test/enzyme-linked immunosorbent assay (ELISA) for tuberculosis. Skin biopsy is to get the diagnosis of leprosy. Nasal biopsy is for granulomatous diseases such as lupus, leprosy, scleroma, and gumma. CT scan of paranasal sinuses shows mucoperiosteal thickening of paranasal sinuses, loss of definition of osteomeatal complex due to resorption of ethmoidal bulla and uncinate process, hypoplastic maxillary sinuses, enlargement of the nasal cavity with the erosion of the lateral nasal wall, and atrophy of inferior and middle turbinates.

4.2.2 Management Aim

Complete cure is not yet possible. Goal of treatment is to maintain nasal hygiene by removal of crusts and the associated infection, putrefying smell, and to further check crust formation. alkaline nasal douching solution is made by dissolving a teaspoonful of powder containing soda bicarbonate one part, sodium biborate one part, sodium chloride two parts in 280 ml of water. Saline acts as solvent and it washes thick mucus, crust, and debris. Nasal douches also increase mucosal humidification and ciliary function. The solution is run through one nostril and comes out from the other. It loosens the crusts and removes thick tenacious discharge. Initially, irrigations are done two to three times a day but later once every 2–3 days is sufficient. After crusts are removed, the nose is painted with 25% glucose in glycerine. This inhibits the growth of proteolytic organisms which are responsible for foul smell. In place of this antibiotic spray can also be used like Kemicetine antiozena solution contains chloromycetin, oestradiol, and vitamin D2 but antibiotics are not having much role in the treatment of atrophic rhinitis. Budesonide based nasal wash (2 ml in 1000 ml saline irrigation solution) is also recommended after saline nasal douches to improve symptomatology.

Other treatment strategies that have shown benefit are oestradiol spray which has been found to increase vascularity of nasal mucosa and regeneration of seromucinous glands for Young and Taylor Type1 not Type 2. Placental extract, when injected submucosally in the nose may provide some relief. A potassium iodide oral preparation promotes and liquefies nasal secretion [20]. Mitomycin C, platelet-rich plasma, and ozone were tried as an adjuvant treatment with nasal douches but both medications were not showed any significant benefit. Nasal endoscopic surveillance is recommended twice a year to clear crusting and to remove adhesion till symptoms persist.

4.2.3 Surgical Management

The surgeries can be broadly classified into four categories with different aims.

1. Surgeries for narrowing the nasal cavities—Nasal chambers are very wide in atrophic rhi-

nitis and air currents dry up secretions leading to crusting. Narrowing the size of the nasal airway helps to relieve the symptoms. Among the techniques followed for narrowing the nasal cavities initially Wilson injected Submucosal a mixture of 50% Teflon in glycerin paste. Then insertion of the implant under the mucoperiosteum of the floor and lateral wall of the nose and the mucoperichondrium of the septum was done and the types of implants used can be classified into two

(a) Living tissue implants
    (i) Autogenous—dermofat, bone, cartilage
    (ii) Homogenous—placenta
    (iii) Heterogenous—bioimplant
(b) Synthetic implants—acrylic, silicone, Teflon, proplast

2. Surgeries to promote regeneration of normal mucosa: Young's operation [21]—In it both the nostrils are closed completely just within the nasal vestibule by raising flaps. They are opened after 6 months or later. In these cases, mucosa may revert back to normal and crusting reduced. To avoid the discomfort of bilateral nasal obstruction, modified Young's operation was devised which aims to partially close the nostrils instead of complete closure. It is also claimed to give the same benefit as Young's (Fig. 4.7).

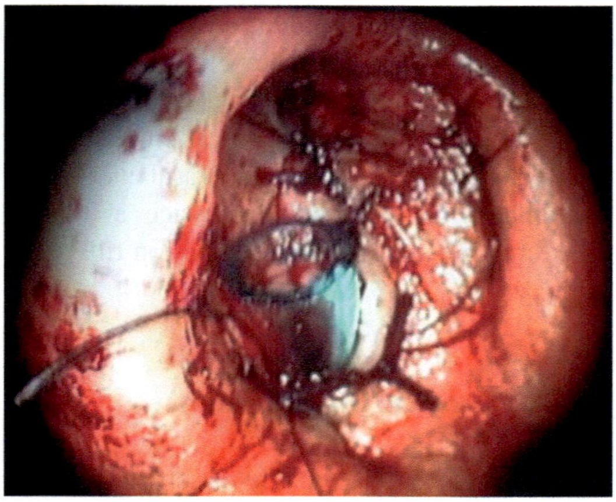

Fig. 4.7 The clinical photograph is showing modified Young's operation. The catheter is placed to prepare small size nostril (Courtesy—Dr. Hitesh Verma, Associate Professor, AIIMS, New Delhi, India)

3. Surgeries to increase lubrication of dry nasal mucosa: There are two main techniques used one is Raghav Sharan's operation [22], in which implantation of maxillary sinus mucosa is done in the nostril. And the other is Wittmack's technique, where implantation of the Stenson's duct is done (parotid duct) into the maxillary antrum.
4. Surgeries to improve the vascularity of the nasal cavities: Sympathetic tone causes vasoconstriction and emptying of the venous sinusoids via the arteriovenous anastomosis. A reduction in sympathetic tone causes venous sinusoids dilatation along with the increase in blood supply by decreasing the vasoconstriction which is being utilized in these procedures that are satellite ganglion block, cervical sympathectomy, pterygopalatine fossa block, and juxta-nasal sympathectomy.

    Number of surgical options is mentioned in literature but no control trial is performed till date for the efficacy of different procedures [20].

4.3 Part C: Maxillofacial Trauma

4.3.1 Introduction

Maxillofacial trauma presents in emergency as part of polytrauma or standalone facial trauma. The common causes include motor vehicle accidents, fall from height, or assault. Maxillofacial trauma is very commonly associated with neurological and eye trauma, along with possibility of solid viscera injury. This necessitates team approach to this entity. Like any trauma, principles of Advanced Trauma Life Support (ATLS) should be followed and attention to Airway, Breathing, Circulation, Disability, and Exposure (ABCDE) be done appropriately.

Non-comminuted maxillary fractures seldom bleed profusely. At the same time, in severe fractures nasal packing alone to control bleeding may be insufficient as splayed walls of the nasal cavity and/or palatal process of maxilla will not allow the packing to generate enough pressure to control bleeding. In such cases, airway securing followed by both oral and nasal packing can be considered (Fig. 4.8a, b).

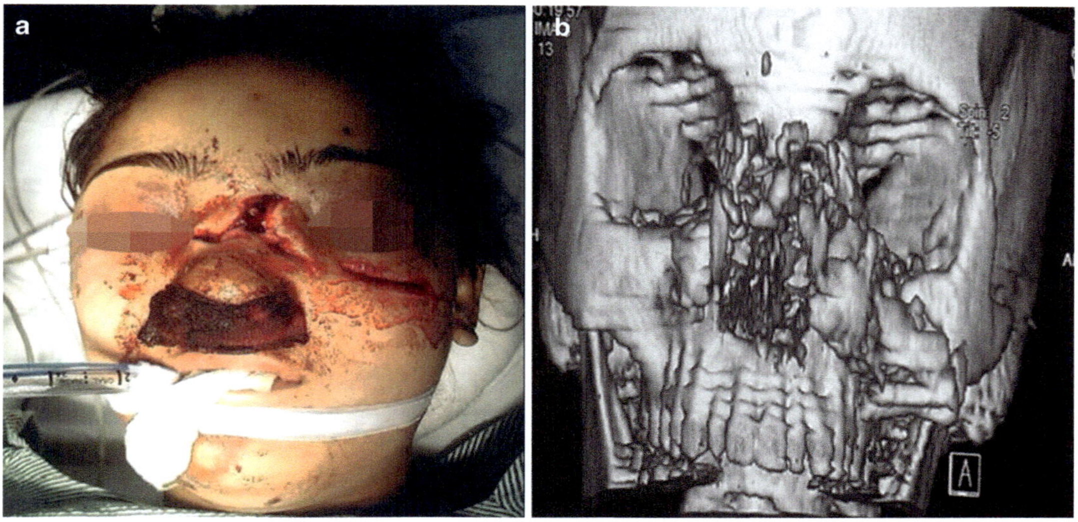

Fig. 4.8 (**a**) Patient with nasoethmoidal and bilateral maxillary fracture who needed securing of airway and oral and nasal packing to control bleeding. (**b**) 3D CT reconstruction of the same patient shows severely comminuted nasoethmoidal complex and bilateral maxillary fractures leading to splaying of lateral nasal wall. Bleeding in such a case may not be controlled by nasal packing alone

4.3.1.1 Assessment of a Maxillofacial Trauma Patient

The mechanism of injury is crucial to understanding the extent and pattern of trauma. The direction, amount of force, and object with which trauma is sustained gives an insight into the pattern of injury, hence a careful history about the circumstances how the trauma was sustained needs to be enquired. Careful attention to the scalp and facial wounds for laceration, contamination, and foreign material/debris impaction is needed. Facial skeleton should be assessed in a structured protocol to evaluate frontal bones, supra, and infraorbital margins, nasal bones, zygomatic arch and mandible. Observe for any step deformity or discontinuity. Intraoral assessment for occlusion, hematoma in the floor of mouth, missing/fractured/avulsed teeth is imperative (Fig. 4.9). Orbital assessment for telecanthus, mobility, acuity, pupillary size, and reaction should be done. Anterior rhinoscopy is done for septal fracture/hematoma. Sensation over the face along the distribution of infraorbital and mental nerves is important in preoperative period in a conscious patient. This may prevent potential postoperative medicolegal issues. Coexistent medical conditions like renal, hepatic, or cardiovascular ailments along with any coagulopathies, should be ruled out which may have a bearing on wound healing and postoperative complications.

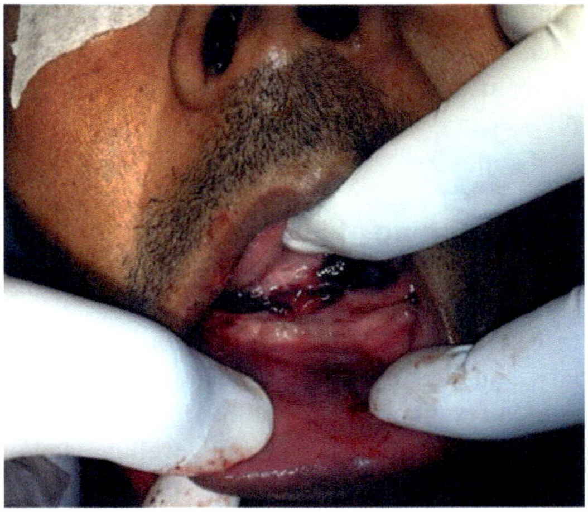

Fig. 4.9 Hematoma in floor of mouth of and edentulous patient who had fracture mandible

4.3.2 Imaging

Multidetector CT scan with three-dimensional shaded surface display is standard for evaluation

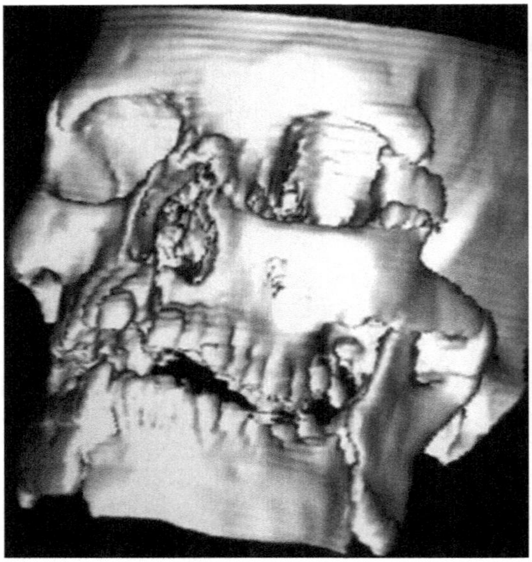

Fig. 4.10 3D shaded surface display with fractures involving left fronto-zygomatic buttress, left angle of mandible, right parasymphysis, midline maxillary, and left frontal process of the maxillary bone

(Fig. 4.10). X-ray of the skull in anteroposterior, lateral, and submentovertical view along with X-ray mandible lateral oblique view may be done if CT scan is not available.

4.3.3 Timing of Surgical Intervention

In cases of midfacial, nasal, zygomaticomaxillary complex, and frontal fractures, early operative intervention may not be feasible due to concomitant significant facial swelling and/or intracranial trauma. Hence, the surgical intervention is planned after the reduction in swelling. In patients with solid organ or hollow visceral trauma too, a definitive management of these injuries takes priority. Only after any other vital organ injury has been assessed and addressed, facial trauma care should be planned.

4.3.4 Airway Management During Surgery

For isolated mandibular, zygomaticomaxillary complex, and Le Fort 1 fractures of midface, an

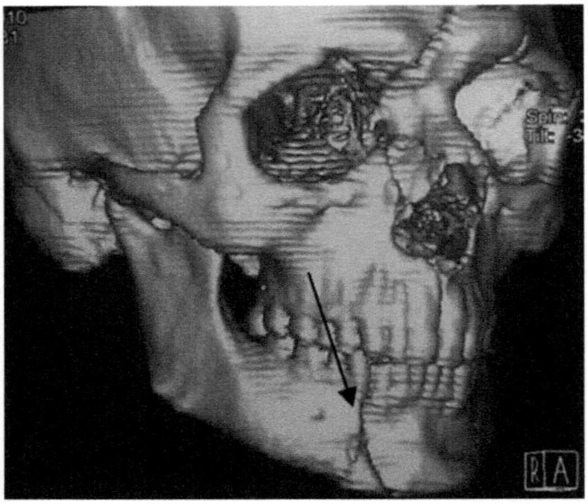

Fig. 4.11 Image shows fracture of right ramus of mandible. Also seen are midline maxillary fracture, right side Le Fort 2 maxillary fracture, and fracture of the frontal bone

nasotracheal intubation is adequate. For Le Fort 2 and Le Fort 3 fractures, a submental intubation or tracheotomy is considered.

4.3.4.1 Mandibular Fractures

Based on the location, they are divided into condylar/subcondylar, parasymphyseal (between mandibular canines)/symphyseal (between central mandibular incisors), ramus (Fig. 4.11) (posterior border of masseter to height of sigmoid notch), angle (third molar to posterior border of masseter), body (distal part of mandibular canine to distal mandibular second molar), and alveolus [23].

Condylar fractures may be intracapsular or extracapsular. Since these are often missed, a keen observation is needed during clinical examination. A small wound on the chin, malocclusion with otherwise preserved mandibular arch, diffuse parotid swelling, and parotid area crepitus are subtle pointers (Fig. 4.12a, b).

Intermaxillary fixation is done by closed (tooth-borne/bone-borne) or open techniques.

1. **Tooth-borne closed techniques**—Erich arch bars, interdental wires (Ivy loops/eyelet wires, etc.) or lingual splints.
2. **Bone-borne techniques**—skeletal suspension wires, IMF screws, external fixators, hybrid systems.

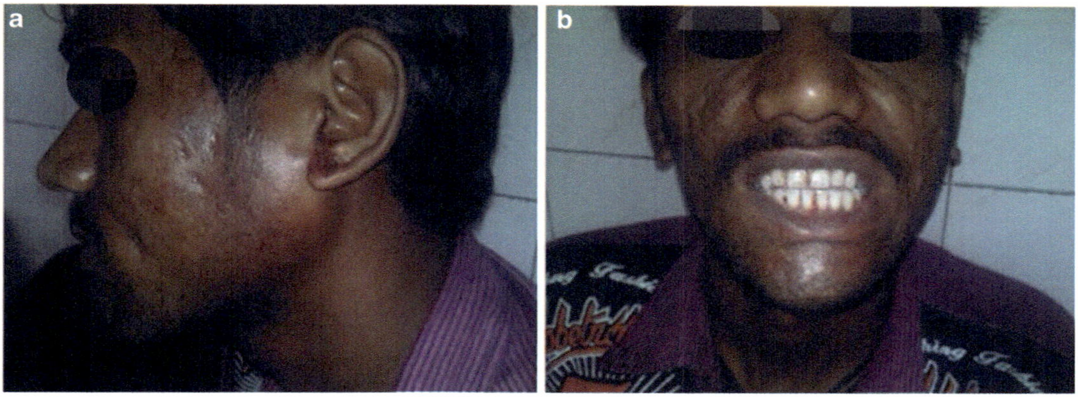

Fig. 4.12 (**a**) Left parotid swelling and ear bleeding in a patient with the left condylar fracture. The patient was otherwise well preserved with no other apparent facial injury. (**b**) Same patient showing malocclusion due to condylar fracture

Open techniques are preferable and are based on AO/ASIF guidelines. These methods include-two plate fixation, reconstruction plate, lag screws. Fracture line can be accessed by transoral/transbuccal approach (body/symphysis/parasymphysis), transcervical-submandibular approach (angle), transcervical-retromandibular approach (ramus/subcondylar), or endoscopic approach (subcondylar). Some fractures of ascending ramus and angle can be plated by transoral approach using a transbuccal device for fixation.

4.3.5 Management of Nasal Bone Fractures

Nasal fracture is classified into five subtypes on clinical basis

- Grade 0—No displacement.
- Grade 1—The deviation of nose is less than 50% of width of bridge of nose.
- Grade 2—The deviation of nose is more than 50% to almost equal of width of bridge of nose.
- Grade 3—The deviation of nose is more than width of bridge of nose.
- Grade 4—It almost reaching to the cheek.

Nasal fractures are also divided on the basis of patterns of damage.

Category 1 Fracture In this, fracture segments are generally maintained position by their inferior attachment with upper lateral cartilage. It occurs in less severe form of trauma and grade 1 fractures come under category 1 fracture. Chevallet was the first documenting person so it was also known as Chevallet fracture.

Category 2 Fracture Nasal bones, frontal process of the maxilla, and septal bones are involved in this fracture. It is seen in the more severe form of trauma. Grade 2 and above fractures come under category 2 fractures. It is also known as Jarjavay fracture (C shaped fracture).

Category 3 Fracture It involves all nasal bone with orbit, ethmoid bone, and any other facial bone. Clinically, patient may have pig-like appearance. It is also classified into two, depending upon skull base involvement. In type 2, anterior cranial base, posterior wall of frontal sinus, and optic nerve is involved.

For evaluation of nasal bone fractures, clinical assessment is most informative. Additionally, X-rays (Water's view, lateral view) and in select cases (nasoethmoidal fractures, minimally depressed fractures at rhinion/ nasion) CT may be requisitioned.

For simple fractures, closed reduction with Asch or Walsham forceps with digital manipulation is carried out (Fig. 4.13a, b). Septal straight-

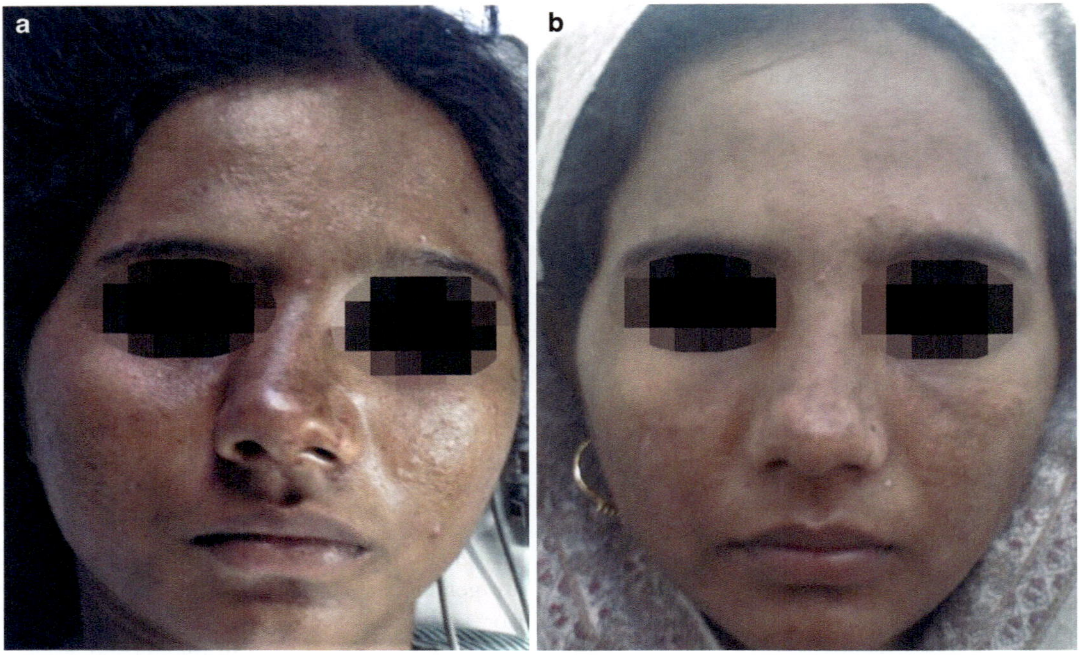

Fig. 4.13 Preoperative (6a) and postoperative (6b) image of a patient with nasal bone fracture who underwent closed reduction

ening is done if required. If significant septal cartilage and septal fracture are present, emergency septoplasty can be considered. Telescoping of fragments with significant comminution may merit external fixation using lead plates or orthopedic plates [24].

4.3.6 Zygomatic Fractures

Fractures of zygomaticomaxillary complex (ZMC) (also called trimalar, tripod, tetrapod, quadrapod) may lead to infraorbital anesthesia, trismus, diplopia, enophthalmos, palpable bony suture line abnormalities, and flattened malar prominence. Clinical evaluation includes the assessment of malar depression, mouth opening, ocular examination for mobility and diplopia, and sensation over area of V2 division. Open reduction and fixation by miniplates of ZMC fractures are carried out by using a combination of approaches: vestibular for zygomaticomaxillary buttress, subciliary/subtarsal/transconjunctival for infraorbital rim, and brow/eyebrow for lateral orbital rim [23]. Comminuted and displaced fracture of zygomatic arch are reduced and fixed by coronal approach. Non-comminuted depressed fractures of arch that are cosmetically and functionally significant can undergo closed reduction by temporal (Gilles) or vestibular (Keen) approach using periosteal or Rowe zygoma elevator.

4.3.7 Fractures of Midface

These are usually classified as Le Fort 1 (floating palate), Le Fort 2 (floating maxilla), and Le Fort 3 (craniofacial dysjunction). However, in the current scenario of high-velocity injuries, fracture lines may not follow lines of least resistance, which was the basis of this classification, and mixed fractures are more common presentation [23].

Impacted maxillae need to be disimpacted using Rowe disimpaction forceps. Definitive management is preferably by intermaxillary fixation and open reduction and internal fixation using miniplates. Fractures can be accessed by vestibular incision (Le Fort 1), a combination of vestibular and infraorbital/transconjunctival/subciliary incisions (Le Fort 2), or coronal incision (Le Fort 3).

4.3.8 Orbital Fractures

A high index of suspicion is required to diagnose orbital fractures, hence there is a need for evaluating visual acuity, visual field, and cheek area sensation in all patients of facial trauma. In children, there is also a possibility of trapdoor fractures of the orbital floor due to elasticity of bones [23], hence even in the paucity of radiological findings, it is important to have a complete visual examination. 'Blow-in' fractures, whereby the roof of the orbit may cave in due to frontal area injury, are also likely to be associated with intracranial trauma. "Blowout" fractures, generally a result of blunt trauma to orbit may be either of the medial wall (fracture into ethmoidal cells), or floor of orbit (fracture into maxillary antrum) and can result in enophthalmos or diplopia due to tethering of inferior or medial rectus muscle. These are radiologically evaluated by CT done in all three planes (Fig. 4.14). Force duction test helps in conforming the entrapped muscle.

The orbital floor defect can be approached by subciliary approach, entrapped contents freed, and defect repaired using titanium mesh, split calvarial grafts, or rib cartilage graft. There are reports of successful endoscopic repair of orbital floor fractures [25].

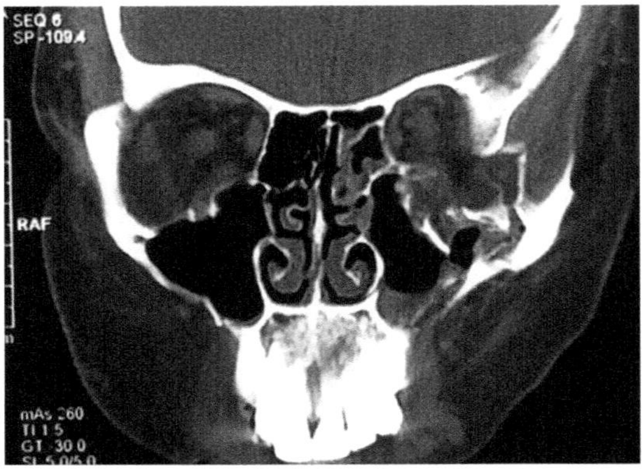

Fig. 4.14 Blowout fracture of left inferior orbital wall

4.3.9 Postoperative Care

Systemic steroids and elective postoperative ventilatory support can be considered in patients with significant facial swelling with controlled extubation in ICU/postoperative recovery.

Rigorous attention to oral hygiene and mouth opening exercises is essential to prevent infection and trismus.

References

1. Verma H, Panda S, Sikka K, Irugu DVK, Thakar A. Primary spheno-petro-clival tuberculosis. Indian J Otolaryngol Head Neck Surg. 2019;71(Suppl 3):1796–9.
2. Fischer M. Leprosy – an overview of clinical features, diagnosis, and treatment. J Dtsch Dermatol Ges. 2017;15(8):801–27.
3. Mukara BK, Munyarugamba P, Dazert S, Löhler J. Rhinoscleroma: a case series report and review of the literature. Eur Arch Otorhinolaryngol. 2014;271(7):1851–6.
4. Tsang SH, Sharma T. Syphilis. Adv Exp Med Biol. 2018;1085:219–21.
5. Fernández-López C, Morales-Angulo C. Otorhinolaryngology manifestations secondary to oral sex. Acta Otorrinolaringol Esp. 2017;68(3):169–80.
6. Almeida FA, Feitoza Lde M, Pinho JD, et al. Rhinosporidiosis: the largest case series in Brazil. Rev Soc Bras Med Trop. 2016;49(4):473–6.
7. Vega Braga FL, Machado de Carvalho G, Caixeta Guimarães A, et al. Otolaryngological manifestations of Wegener's disease. Acta Otorrinolaringol Esp. 2013;64(1):45–9.
8. Kohanski MA, Reh DD. Granulomatous diseases and chronic sinusitis, Chapter 11. Am J Rhinol Allergy. 2013;27(Suppl 1):S39–41.
9. Send T, Tuleta I, Koppen T, et al. Sarcoidosis of the paranasal sinuses. Eur Arch Otorhinolaryngol. 2019;276(7):1969–74.
10. Seccia V, Baldini C, Latorre M, et al. Focus on the involvement of the nose and paranasal sinuses in eosinophilic granulomatosis with polyangiitis (Churg-Strauss Syndrome): nasal cytology reveals infiltration of eosinophils as a very common feature. Int Arch Allergy Immunol. 2018;175(1–2):61–9.
11. Allen PB, Lechowicz MJ. Management of NK/T-cell lymphoma, nasal type. J Oncol Pract. 2019;15(10):513–20.
12. Tse E, Au-Yeung R, Kwong YL. Recent advances in the diagnosis and treatment of natural killer/T-cell lymphomas. Expert Rev Hematol. 2019;12(11):927–35.
13. Ryu G, Cho H, Lee KE, et al. Clinical significance of IgG4 in sinonasal and skull base inflam-

matory pseudotumor. Eur Arch Otorhinolaryngol. 2019;276:2465–73.
14. RA S, Kaliner MA. Nonallergic rhinitis, Chapter 14. Am J Rhinol Allergy. 2013;27(Suppl 1):S48–51.
15. Chen HS. Desquamation and squamotransformation of rhinomucosa as a prodromal sign of atrophic rhinitis. J Otorhinolaryngol Related Specialties. 1984;46(6):327–8.
16. Taylor M, Young A. Histopathological and histochemical studies in atrophic rhinitis. J Laryngol Otol. 1961;75:574–89.
17. El-Anwar MW, et al. Surfactant protein A expression in chronic rhinosinusitis and atrophic rhinitis. Int Arch Otorhinolaryngol. 2015;19(2):130–4.
18. Bist SS, Bisht M, Purohit JP. Primary atrophic rhinitis: a clinical profile, microbiological and radiological study. ISRN Otolaryngol. 2012;2012:404075.
19. Ly TH, deShazo RD, Olivier J, Stringer SP, Daley W, Stodard CM. Diagnostic criteria for atrophic rhinosinusitis. Am J Med. 2009;122(8):747–53.
20. Mishra A, Kawatra R, Gola M. Interventions for atrophic rhinitis. Cochrane Database Syst Rev. 2012;2:CD008280.
21. Young A. Closure of nostrils in Atrophic Rhinitis. J Laryngol. 1967;81:514–5.
22. Sharan R. Transplantation of the maxillary sinus mucosa in atrophic rhinitis. Indian J Otolaryngol. 1978;30:14–6.
23. Fonseca RJ. Oral and maxillofacial trauma. 3rd ed. St. Louis, MO: Elsevier; 2018.
24. Kochar HS. An innovative approach to external fixation of severe nasal bone fractures with orthopedic plates. Ear Nose Throat J. 2011;90:102–4.
25. Chen CT, Chen YR. Endoscopically assisted repair of orbital floor fractures. Plast Reconstr Surg. 2001;108:2011–8.

Diagnostic Method and Instrumentation in Rhinology

5

Gagandeep Singh, Immaculata Xess, Ankur Goyal, Ashu Seith Bhalla, Shamim Ahmed Shamim, Hitender Gautam, Zareen Lynrah, Pradip Kumar Tiwari, Ripu Daman Arora, Nikhil Singh, and Nitin M. Nagarkar

Contents

G. Singh · I. Xess · H. Gautam
Microbiology, AIIMS, New Delhi, India

A. Goyal · A. S. Bhalla
Radiology, AIIMS, New Delhi, India

S. A. Shamim
Nuclear Medicine, AIIMS, New Delhi, India

Z. Lynrah · P. K. Tiwari
ENT, NIGRIMS, Shillong, Meghalaya, India

R. D. Arora (✉) · N. Singh · N. M. Nagarkar
ENT, AIIMS, Raipur, Chhattisgarh, India
e-mail: neelripu@gmail.com

H. Verma, A. Thakar (eds.), *Essentials of Rhinology*, https://doi.org/10.1007/978-981-33-6284-0_5

Fungal rhino-sinusitis is one of the major subtypes of chronic rhino-sinusitis. It is classified into invasive and none-invasive types. Surgical clearance is the primary treatment method for non-invasive type. Non-invasive fungal sinusitis may convert into invasive type to some extent. The invasive is managed by debridement & long term antifungal therapy. The prognosis of invasive type is poor than non-invasive type. Prophylactic, incomplete & unnecessary prolong treatment raised the possibility of drug resistance. Proper identification of the causative organism, drug sensitivity against it & treatment duration reduces the risk of relapse of disease & drug resistance which intern improves the quality of life. The correct diagnosis of causative fungal organism is possible if the samples extract in correct way, timely transport to the laboratories, etc. New serological tests allow early identification of tissue invasion. Radiological interventions are commonly done for tissue diagnosis especially in hidden areas which requires extensive exposure for biopsy such as high infratemporal fossa, cranial tumour eroding middle & posterior skull base. Interventions are also indicated to control traumatic bleeding & to reduce the vascularity of vascular lesions. The procedures are performed under image guidance in head and neck region include those performed for obtaining diagnostic information or for therapeutic intent. Nuclear Medicine uses radiopharmaceuticals for diagnostic and therapeutic purposes. It plays an important role in identifying the unknown etiological factor, the staging of mass lesions of nose and paranasal sinuses pathology, to assess the treatment response. Bacteria's and viruses are involved in the majority of rhinosinusitis. Acute infection generally starts with viruses and superadded bacterial infection usually prolongs the disease duration and can complicate the outcomes. The acute type is more complicated than the chronic type. The evaluation is required generally in poor responder to the standard line of the management, complicated cases, and in chronic rhinosinusitis cases. The correct identification of the causative organism is possible by knowing the correct way of sample collection, transportation technique, etc. Endoscopes, microdebrider, radiofrequency ablation, coblator, etc. revolutionized the outcomes of surgery by improving the surgical field exposure, by providing finer details and by controlling the surgical bleeding. Navigation system allows expansion of endoscopic surgical approaches. Recent advances in the instruments allow dealing of central skull base lesions by transnasal route. The quality of life is improved significantly in comparison to traditional open trans-cranial approaches.

5.1 Part A: Diagnosis of Fungal Infections of Nose and Paranasal Sinuses

5.1.1 Introduction

Fungi are ubiquitous in the environment and we are exposed to them on a regular basis. In few individuals, fungi can cause allergic manifestations or even invasive disease in the nose and PNS, depending on underlying conditions and are collectively termed as fungal rhinosinusitis

Table 5.1 Common agents associated with fungal rhinosinusitis

Allergic fungal rhinosinusitis (AFRS)	Invasive fungal Sinusitis (IFS)
• *Aspergillus flavus* • *Aspergillus fumigatus* • *Aspergillus niger* • Other Aspergillus species • Fusarium spp. • Alternaria spp. • Cladosporium spp. • Curvularia spp. • Bipolaris spp.	• *Rhizopus oryzae* • *Rhizopus microsporus* • *Lichtheimia corymbifera* • *Apophysomyces elegans* • *Aspergillus flavus* • *Aspergillus fumigatus*

(FRS) (Table 5.1). FRS affects all age groups and socioeconomic status. FRS is neglected and often misdiagnosed in developing countries. Correct sample collection to establish an appropriate diagnosis is of paramount importance. Nasal swabs are considered inferior and biopsy specimens are the most conclusive. Once the biopsy is collected it should be transported immediately to the laboratory, immersed in normal saline in a sterile leak-proof container. Samples should always be well labeled and accompanied with complete clinical details. The samples should be processed as early as possible to avoid overgrowth of commensal flora. Samples can be stored at 4 °C if the processing is being delayed, however, if mucormycosis is being suspected the samples should not be stored at 4 °C and maintained at room temperature. Biopsy samples are processed depending on the presumptive diagnosis made by the clinician. All biopsies should be homogenized to release the fungal elements in all non-mucormycosis cases. However, if the diagnosis of mucormycosis is made, the biopsy specimen should not be homogenized as it will damage the delicate fungal elements of the Mucorales and inhibit the recovery in culture. These should instead be cut into small pieces and simply placed on the culture media. In routine, Mucorales are recovered on the culture within 3–4 days of culture and Aspergillus sp. grow within 5–7 days. Obtaining a biopsy specimen may not always be feasible. In such situations, non-culture techniques aid in establishing the diagnosis. The beta-D-glucan is a pan-fungal marker, it is positive in all cases of invasive fungal infections except mucormycosis and cryptococcosis. The galactomannan test is specific for invasive aspergillosis. Newer techniques like the lateral flow devices for detecting Aspergillus antigens and polymerase chain reaction for detecting fungal DNA in tissue specimens are under evaluation. As the nose and paranasal sinuses are in close proximity to the eye and brain, invasive type infections should be managed aggressively.

Classification of FRS: Based on histopathology, clinical features, and laboratory investigations (Fig. 5.1) [1–4].

5.1.2 Diagnosis of Invasive FRS

A high degree of suspicion should be kept for establishing a diagnosis of invasive FRS, especially in the immunocompromised patient with facial pain. The nares and oral cavity should be carefully examined for necrotic areas. Early nasal endoscopic evaluation by an otolaryngologist is essential for sampling the site. Computed tomography (CT) shows sinus involvement and may reveal bony erosions or extension of the infection. Magnetic resonance imaging (MRI) should be performed to assess intracranial and cavernous sinus involvement. Maxillary and ethmoid sinuses are the most common sites for invasive FRS. The diagnosis is dependent on histopathologic/direct demonstration of fungal elements. Isolation of the infecting fungus is necessary to guide therapy [1, 5].

5.1.3 Specimens

Tissue biopsy is the ideal sample. It should be obtained from the necrotic part of the affected site under direct visualization. Nasal scrapings have low yield, however, may be obtained in patients with bleeding diathesis. Nasal swabs should be avoided as fungal elements get trapped in fibers. Moist swabs should be obtained, if at all used, as drying of the sample will cause fungi to lose their viability. Serum samples can be sent for galactomannan antigen detection and Beta-1,3-Glucan detection and other serological markers [6, 7].

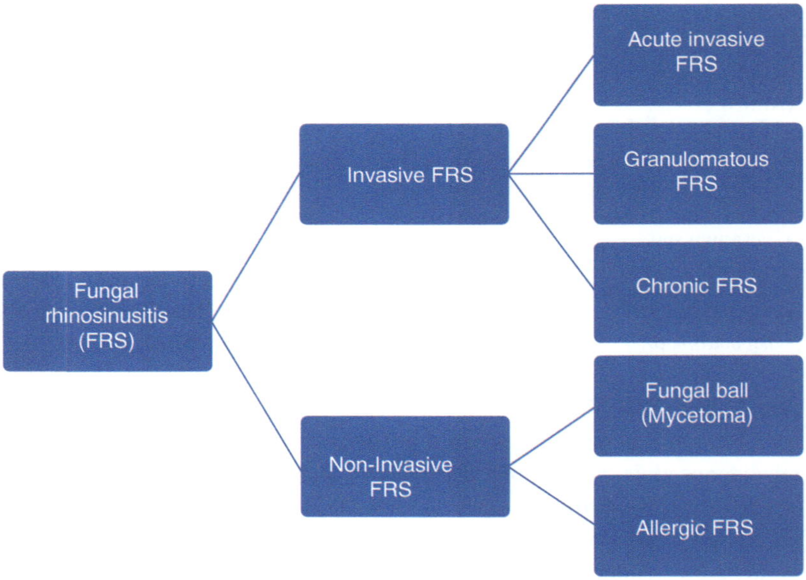

Fig. 5.1 Classification of fungal rhinosinusitis

5.1.4 Sample Transport

All tissue samples for fungal culture should be sent to the laboratory in a sterile container immersed in sterile saline. Samples should be transported immediately or within two hours of collection. Serum can be stored at 4 °C, if there is a delay in transport. However, if mucormycosis is being suspected the samples should not be stored at 4 °C and maintained at room temperature. Lower temperature causes the Mucorales to lose their viability.

5.1.5 Sample Processing

The samples should be processed as early as possible, once received in the laboratory. The tissue samples should be examined carefully for any necrotic or hemorrhagic areas. A small portion should be obtained from these areas for further processing as the fungal load is relatively higher. Depending on the presumptive diagnosis, whether aspergillosis or mucormycosis, the sample should be processed according to Fig. 5.2.

The processed samples can be examined by direct microscopy using KOH-Calcofluor White stain for fungal elements and cultured on SDA with and without antibiotics. Swabs can be plated directly on Sabouraud dextrose agar (SDA) plates. The Hyphae which are broad, aseptate, or pauci-septate, typically 8–15 μm in width with right angle branching are suggestive of mucormycosis (Fig. 5.3a). Hyphae which are septate, 4–8 μm in width with acute angle branching are suggestive of aspergillosis (Fig. 5.3b).

5.1.6 Culture and Antifungal Susceptibility Testing (AFST)

Once a culture is obtained on SDA, it can be identified based on colony characters and microscopic features on lacto-phenol cotton blue (LCB) mount. Aspergillus spp. are usually velvety to granular downy colonies where as those of mucormycetes are usually cottony, filling up the entire tube/culture plate. AFST can be performed in cases which do not respond to standard treatment. AFST is performed by the micro-broth dilution test for determining the minimum inhibitory concentrations (MICs) of antifungal drugs.

5.1.7 Serologic Tests

5.1.7.1 Beta-1,3,-Glucan (BDG)

Indicated for the presumptive diagnosis of invasive fungal disease through detection of elevated levels of BDG in serum [6]. BDG is a qualitative test & values are reported as follows:

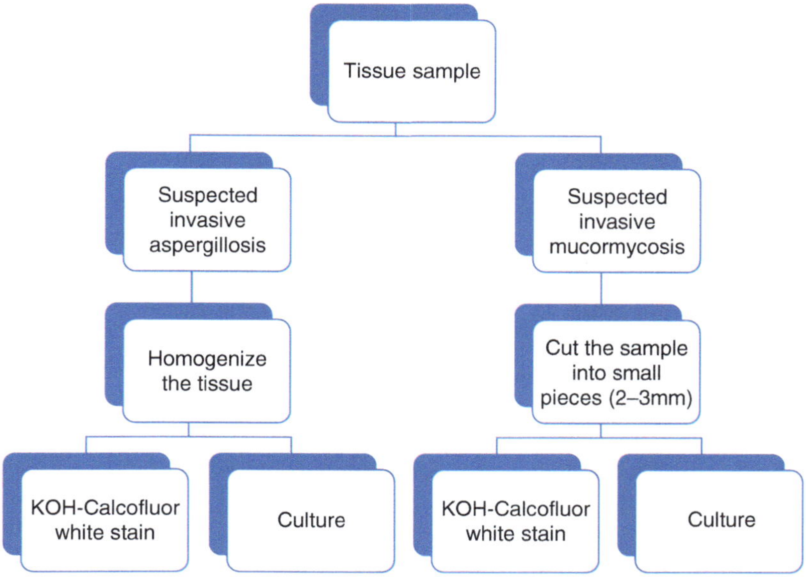

Fig. 5.2 Shows the method of processing tissue samples based on presumptive diagnosis

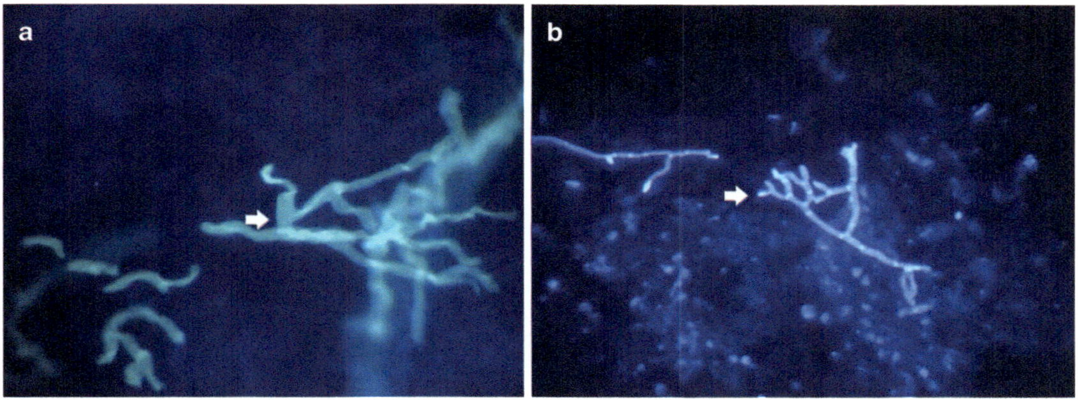

Fig. 5.3 Calcofluor white-KOH mount under 40× magnification (**a**) Broad aseptate hyphae are observed with right angle branching (arrow) and ribbon-like foldings indicating mucormycosis (**b**) Dichotomous branching at acute angle (arrow) suggestive of aspergillosis/hyalohyphomycosis

- <60 pg/mL: NEGATIVE
- ≥80 pg/mL: POSITIVE (in an at-risk patient)
- 60–79 pg/mL: EQUIVOCAL; additional sampling is necessary

A negative BDG may be seen in patients infected with

- *Cryptococcus neoformans*
- Mucorales (*Mucor, Rhizopus, etc.*)

Lower levels of BDG are found in the cell wall of *Candida parapsilosis*, which may comprise more than 30% of Candida isolates in neonatal intensive care units.

False positives may be found under the following circumstances:

(a) Bacteremic patients.
(b) Antibiotics; only amoxicillin/clavulanate and piperacillin/tazobactam (of note, antifungal therapy does not significantly affect the performance of the assay).
(c) Hemodialysis with cellulose membranes.
(d) Patients treated with iv products manufactured using cellulose filters.

(e) Surgical gauzes/sponges—transient false positives in surgical patients.

False negatives may be seen in the following circumstances:

1. Immune complex formation.

Utility of BDG:

- A **pre-emptive approach** is recommended, whereby surveillance is carried out in at-risk patients.
- **Twice weekly testing** has been recommended as a screening strategy; both in invasive aspergillosis as well as invasive candidiasis, this increases the sensitivity, specificity as well as positive predictive value (PPV) of the assay.

5.1.7.2 Galactomannan Antigen Detection

The galactomannan (GM) assay is a fairly specific and sensitive test for invasive aspergillosis. Also found in *Histoplasma capsulatum* and Fusarium spp. The aspergillus galactomannan is an immune-enzymatic sandwich microplate assay. The assay uses EBA-2 monoclonal antibodies which detect Aspergillus galactomannan. This test has been approved for diagnostic use by the U.S. Food and Drug Administration for BAL and serum specimens only. When used in conjunction with other diagnostic procedures it can be used to aid in the diagnosis of invasive aspergillosis. Galactomannan assay with serum but not BAL fluid may have prognostic value. Twice a week monitoring of neutropenic patients is often recommended. Patients with an index of ≥ 0.5 in serum and ≥ 1.0 in BAL are considered to be positive for galactomannan antigen. Specimens testing positive should be retested to confirm the positive result [7].

Cautions:

- The concomitant use of mold-active, antifungal therapy may result in reduced sensitivity.
- There are reports of positive galactomannan test results in patients receiving piperacillin/tazobactam.
- Patients with intestinal mucositis caused by chemotherapy and irradiation, which allows extra absorption of dietary galactomannan.
- False-positive Galactomannan results have been shown in patients receiving Plasmalyte for intravenous hydration or if Plasmalyte is used for BAL collection.

5.1.7.3 Aspergillus-Specific Lateral Flow Device (LFD)

Point of care test based on monoclonal antibody (mAb JF5) to detect an extracellular mannoprotein antigen that is secreted exclusively during active growth of Aspergillus species. Patient's BAL fluid samples do not need pre-treatment. Test results can be available within 10–15 min of sample receipt. LFD test results are read by the naked eye, and they have previously been shown to be reproducible between different studies and different laboratories [8].

5.1.7.4 Polymerase Chain Reaction (PCR)

Can be performed in samples that have a high degree of suspicion of fungal etiology however, direct microscopy as well as culture do not yield any results. A pan-fungal or genus-specific PCR can be performed. Extra caution should be taken while collecting samples for PCR as even little contamination with any mucosal surface may result in a false-positive PCR due to commensal fungi [9, 10].

5.2 Part B: Intervention Radiology for Rhinology

Radiology has expanded horizons not only in the diagnosis of rhinological diseases but also in the management of such patients. Radiological interventions are commonly done for tissue diagnosis as well as for bleeding control. Interventional Radiology (IR) Procedures performed under image guidance in the head and neck region include those performed for obtaining diagnostic information or for therapeutic intent (Table 5.2). Only the interventions pertaining to sinonasal lesions are discussed in this chapter. The internal carotid artery interventions are not included in this chapter. Also, the infrahyoid neck is only briefly covered.

Table 5.2 Types of IR procedures in head and neck

Diagnostic interventions	Therapeutic interventions
Image-guided FNAC and Biopsy • Infratemporal fossa	Drainage procedures • Retropharyngeal collections
Assessment of cross-circulation and vascularity on DSA	Embolization for • Epistaxis (including trauma) • Pseudoaneurysms • Preoperative embolization (JNA, Glomus tumor) • Arteriovenous malformations • Tumor erosion of arteries
Venous sampling	Jugular vein catheterization
	Sclerotherapy for venous and lymphatic malformations
	Carotid artery stenting for blowout
	Miscellaneous: • Pterygopalatine ganglion block • Radiofrequency ablation of masses • Alcohol ablation of thyroid nodules

DSA digital subtraction angiography, *JNA* Juvenile nasopharyngeal angiofibroma

Radiological interventions can be divided into *endovascular and non-vascular procedures.*

- *Non-vascular procedures* are aimed at obtaining tissue diagnosis, especially when the sinonasal masses are deep-seated or involves the infratemporal fossa (ITF).
- *Vascular interventions* are primarily done to manage oronasal bleed from arterial causes (including trauma) and preoperative embolizations to reduce intraoperative blood loss.

Majority of the radiological interventions can be done with local anesthesia and conscious sedation. General anesthesia is required for small children and when large doses of glue embolization needs to be done (since the latter cause's pain).

5.2.1 Pre-Requisites

The general *pre-requisites* include

1. Platelet count SHOULD BE ABOVE 50,000/mm^3.
2. Prothrombin time within 5 s of control or International Normalized Ratio (INR) ≤1.4.
3. Short admission, especially for vascular procedures.
4. Renal function tests, whenever intravenous contrast is to be injected.
5. Intravenous access, prior to starting the procedure.
6. Informed consent.
7. Aspirin and clopidogrel to be stopped 5 days prior and low molecular weight heparins 1 day prior to the procedure.

5.2.2 Image-Guided Sampling

Ultrasound (USG) guidance is routinely used for sampling of non-palpable lesions of the head and neck. Even for palpable lesions, ultrasound guidance may permit targeting the solid viable portions of the lesion (Fig. 5.4). Advantages of ultrasound include real-time imaging, excellent tissue contrast without radiation/intravenous contrast and thus it is commonly used for sampling of neck nodes and masses, thyroid nodules, and salivary gland lesions [11].

CT guidance is used for deep-seated lesions (for example in infratemporal fossa), bony lesions (example mandible) and for regions obscured by overlying bones or air from the aerodigestive tract. Shortest path should be employed and wherever feasible, sampling should be done along the largest dimension of the lesion. Subzygomatic (sigmoid notch/transcondylar) approach is commonly employed for targeting infratemporal lesions (Fig. 5.4).

Other approaches for suprahyoid lesions include retromandibular, paramaxillary, submastoid, transoral, and posterior [11]. While most sinonasal lesions are sampled through the nasal route, large aggressive lesions with lateral exten-

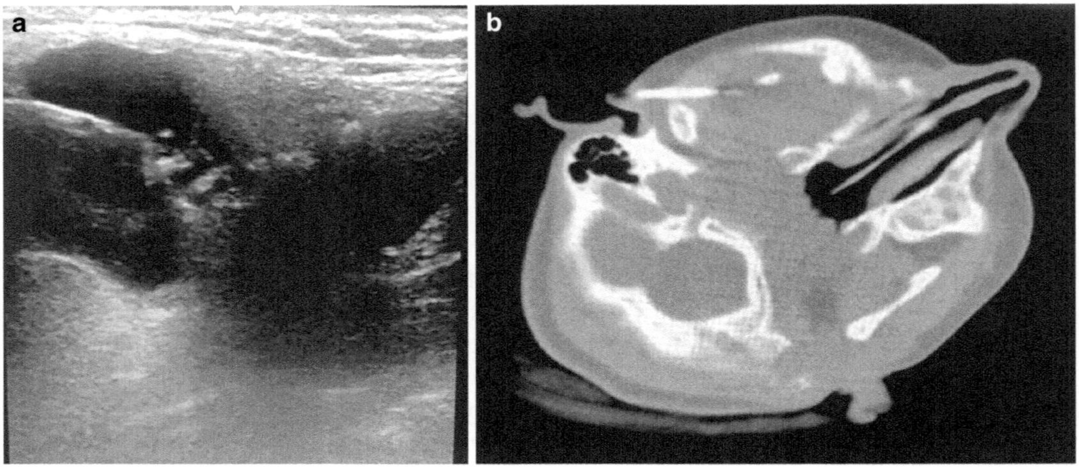

Fig. 5.4 (**a**) Ultrasound image showing sampling from necrotic nodal mass. (**b**) Axial CT image shows transcondylar approach for targeting infratemporal masses. Arrowheads denote needle

sion into ITF or beyond can be approached through CT guidance. Similarly lesions with extension into premaxillary or buccal space can be sampled under USG guidance. Addition of USG allows sampling of most solid, non-necrotic components where the yield is likely to be higher. Coaxial technique is preferred for deep-seated lesions so that access is retained for repeated passes and there is no repetitive trauma to the intervening tissues. Also, it saves time and multiple samples can be taken via the outer needle. This employs 16G outer needle and 18G inner biopsy needle. Fine needle aspiration cytology is best done with on-site pathologist and/or microbiologist to assess the adequacy of the sample [*Rapid On Site Evaluation (ROSE)* by the pathologist to check for the cellular adequacy so as to reduce recalling of the patients for a second sitting]. FNAC is done with a 21–23 gauge hypodermic/spinal needle and two-three excursions are usually sufficient. When clinico-radiological diagnosis is infection, then aspiration of the liquefied/necrotic content is useful both for identifying the pathogen as well as therapeutic purposes. However, if the neoplasm is suspected, then FNAC/biopsy from the solid component should be done. Biopsy cores are taken in case the cytology smears are inadequate or the lesion is predominantly solid. 18G cores have much better yield than 20G cores. Two-three biopsy cores are usually sufficient if the needle throw is 2 cm. Upto 5 cores may be required if length of biopsy needle hub is 1 cm.

5.2.3 DSA Assessment of Vascularity and Collateralization

Digital subtraction angiography (DSA) is done for assessment of vascularity of masses of suprahyoid neck and skull base as well as cross-circulation prior to surgery. For cross-circulation assessment, the common carotid artery ipsilateral to the side of the neoplasm is manually compressed, while contrast is injected into the contralateral internal carotid artery and DSA acquisition is done in the frontal projection (Matas maneuver) [12]. Opacification of ipsilateral brain parenchyma through patent anterior communicating artery indicates preserved cross-circulation (Fig. 5.5).

Allcock maneuver involves dominant vertebral artery injection [12] with manual carotid compression to look for posterior communicating artery patency and is done if cross-circulation is not preserved. Carotid balloon occlusion test is done by inflating an occlusion balloon in the ipsilateral internal carotid artery (cervical portion) for 20 min and evaluating ischemic tolerance. Latter

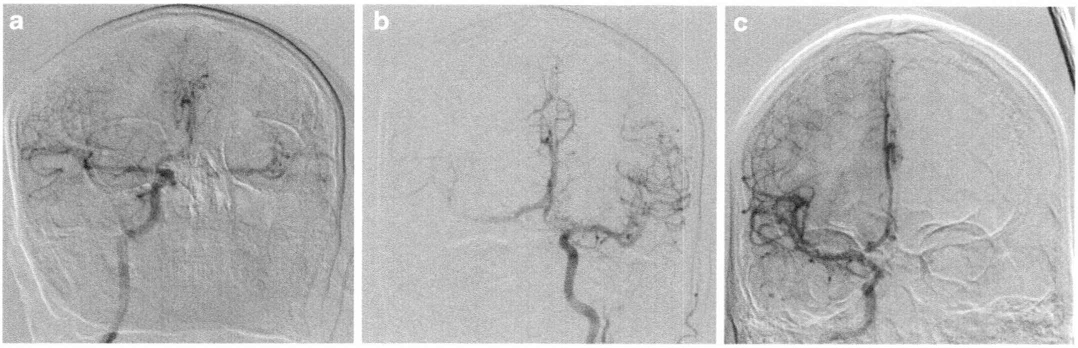

Fig. 5.5 DSA runs showing examples of cross-circulation. (**a**) DSA run through right internal carotid artery ICA (with compression of left carotid) shows preserved cross-circulation through the anterior communicating artery. (**b**) DSA run through left ICA shows preserved cross-circulation. (**c**) DSA run through right ICA shows absent cross-circulation

can be done in the most basic form by clinical neurological assessment (motor, touch sensation, language, memory, judgment tests) or more accurately by doing electroencephalography (EEG). Various imaging-based perfusion assessment studies (Single photon emission CT SPECT using Tc99m HMPAO) can also be done. The test is positive in case any neurological deficit or EEG/SPECT abnormality is detected. Though considered safe, there is mild risk of arterial dissection, thrombosis, and distal infarction (3.5%) [12]. Matas and Allcock's maneuver are safer alternatives to balloon occlusion test and can accurately predict the results of latter [12].

5.2.4 DSA Embolization in Trauma Setting

Arterial embolization procedures are commonly performed in the emergency setting for traumatic oronasal bleed not responding to packing. Selective arterial runs of bilateral internal maxillary and facial arteries are mandatory to identify the source of the bleed. DSA may show pseudoaneurysm due to traumatic injury of the artery or abnormal parenchymal blush due to bleeding from small arterioles (Fig. 5.6). Former is usually treated by selective coil embolization while the latter is managed by occluding the culprit artery using gelfoam. Sometimes the diagnostic runs may not show any abnormality on DSA, even though the patient is bleeding. Most common cause of this finding is arterial spasm secondary to trauma as well as hypovolemia. In such case, empirical embolization of bilateral internal maxillary arteries and ipsilateral facial artery is done using gelfoam. Table 5.3 outlines the commonly used embolizing agents and sclerosants.

5.2.5 DSA Embolization in Epistaxis

The first step in non-traumatic epistaxis is to identify the cause. This is done by nasal examination, endoscopy, and CT angiography. If no definite cause is apparent or there is abnormal cluster of vessels or arteriovenous malformation, then endovascular embolization is usually done. This is particularly applicable to posterior epistaxis. Depending on the finding on diagnostic runs, appropriate embolization agent is used. If no significant finding is seen and bleeding cannot be localized to one side, then empirical embolization of bilateral internal maxillary arteries is done using gelfoam/PVA particles. If bleeding can be localized to one side, then the superior labial branch (nasal septal branches) of ipsilateral facial artery is also embolized [13]. Internal maxillary artery is embolized distal to the origin of the middle meningeal artery so that sphenopalatine and descending palatine arteries are embolized [13].

Most common cause of failed embolization is bleeding from anterior and posterior ethmoidal

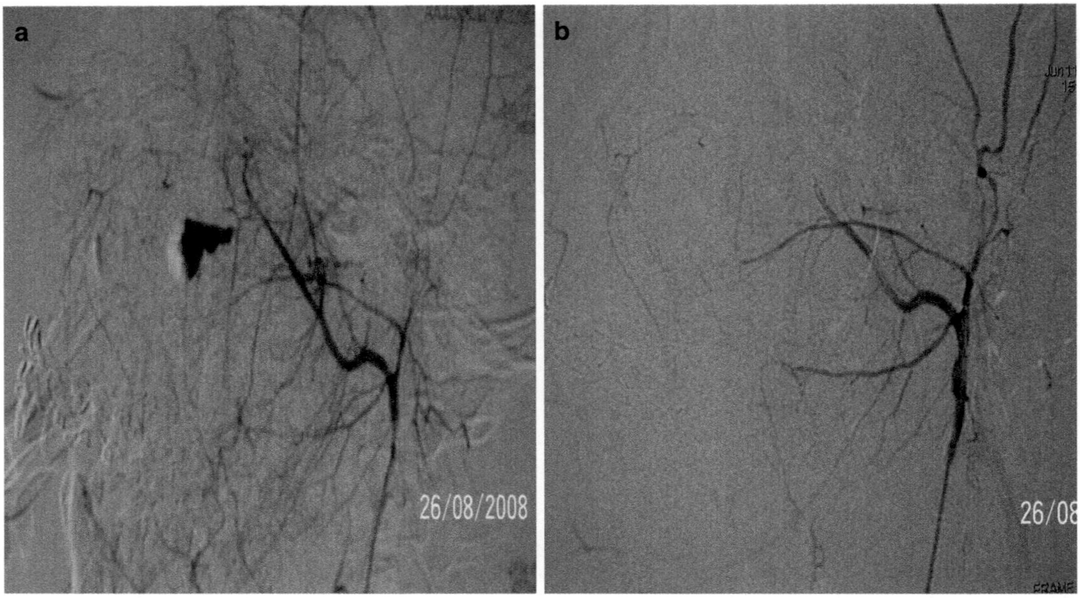

Fig. 5.6 Traumatic maxillary bleed. (**a**) Shows contrast extravasation from internal maxillary artery in the DSA run. (**b**) After gelfoam embolization, the extravasation has stopped

Table 5.3 Commonly used embolizing and sclerotherapy agents

Embolizing agents	Sclerotherapy agents
Mechanical: Coil, Microcoil, Vascular Plug, Gelfoam pledgets	3% STDS
Particulate: PVA particles, Embospheres, Gelfoam slurry	Polidocanol
Liquid: Glue	Bleomycin
Ablative: Alcohol	
Chemo-embolic agents: Chemotherapy drug with lipiodol	

STDS sodium tetradecyl sulfate

arteries (branches of ophthalmic artery); this requires surgical ligation. Reported success rates of embolization in epistaxis are 71–95% [13]. In diseases like hereditary hemorrhagic telangiectasia where multiple sessions may be needed, the main arteries must be kept patent and proximal embolization with coils should not be done.

5.2.6 DSA Embolization in Tumors

Usual indication of embolization in tumor setting is in the preoperative period to reduce the intra-operative blood loss and morbidity. This is usually done within 72 h of surgery but should not be done more than 5–7 days earlier. This is to prevent revascularization by recruitment of collaterals. Endovascular embolization is usually done. Percutaneous/endoscopic direct intralesional embolization may also be done, especially if arterial feeders are small and difficult to catheterize or if there is significant supply from the internal carotid artery. Common lesions where preoperative embolization is done include juvenile nasopharyngeal angiofibroma and glomus tumors (Figs. 5.7 and 5.8).

It may also be done for other hypervascular neoplasms like hemangiopericytoma, nerve sheath tumors, plasmacytomas, and metastases. Commonly used embolizing agent is polyvinyl alcohol (PVA) particles 300–500 μ in size. Gelfoam can also be used. Glue is used if there is excessive arteriovenous shunting or for direct embolization. Direct intratumoral glue injection can be done through percutaneous or nasal route, depending on the tumor location and extent.

All the feeding arteries (usually from external carotid artery branches) need to be embolized so that the entire tumor blush disappears. The goal is

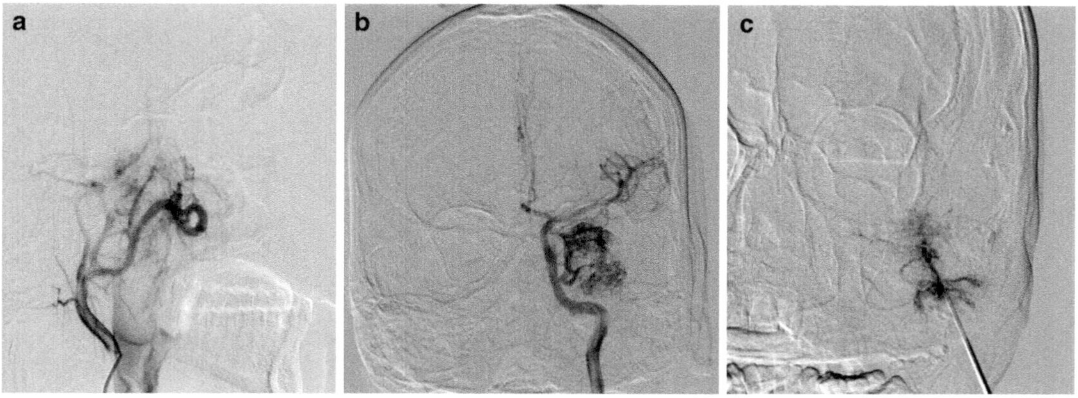

Fig. 5.7 DSA runs showing parenchymal blush of JNA. (**a**) Shows predominant supply from internal maxillary artery. (**b**) Depicts supply from internal carotid artery via vidian branch and (**c**) Demonstrates percutaneous targeting of JNA component in the infratemporal fossa

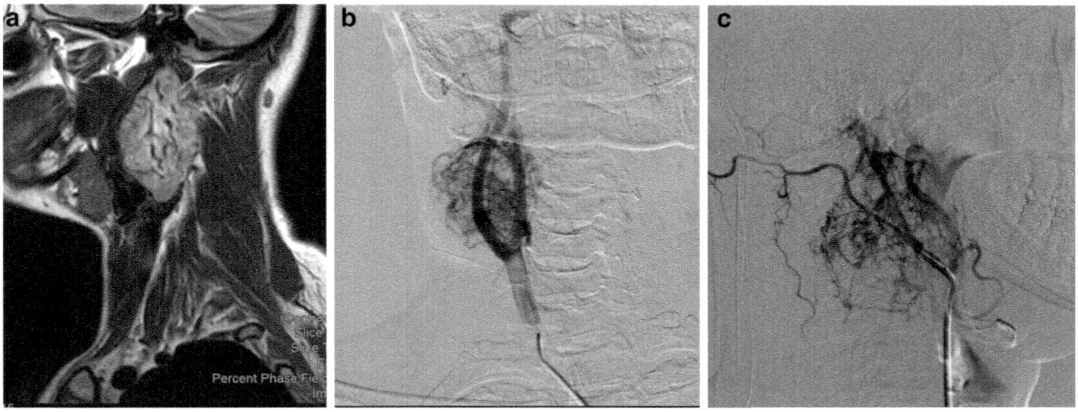

Fig. 5.8 Glomus tumor. (**a**) Sagittal T2w MRI image shows hyperintense mass with flow voids within. (**b**) DSA image RT common carotid artery runs shows splaying of ICA and ECA with intense blush. (**c**) There is predominant supply from the posterior auricular artery

to deposit the embolizing agent at arteriolar/capillary level to reduce vascularity. Feeders from the internal carotid and vertebral arteries are usually not embolized because of the risk of stroke. Few series have also tried selective chemoembolization where chemotherapy drugs are injected selectively into the feeding arteries of the tumor. This may increase the local effect of the drug on the tumor and reduce systemic toxicity. This has been mostly tried in laryngeal cancers but results have been heterogenous. Sometimes tumors may erode adjacent arteries and lead to bleeding. This is difficult to control surgically because of distorted anatomy, large tumor size, post-radiation changes, fistula, and infection [14]. CT angiography is usually done first to assess the tumor and its relationship with adjacent vessels. CT also helps to identify any pseudoaneurysm or active contrast extravasation. In such a case the corresponding artery is usually blocked with coils at the site of injury. If no site of arterial injury is identified, then tumor embolization is done to reduce bleeding.

Carotid blowout syndrome is a complication of extensive or recurrent squamous cell carcinoma of the head and neck in which there is rup-

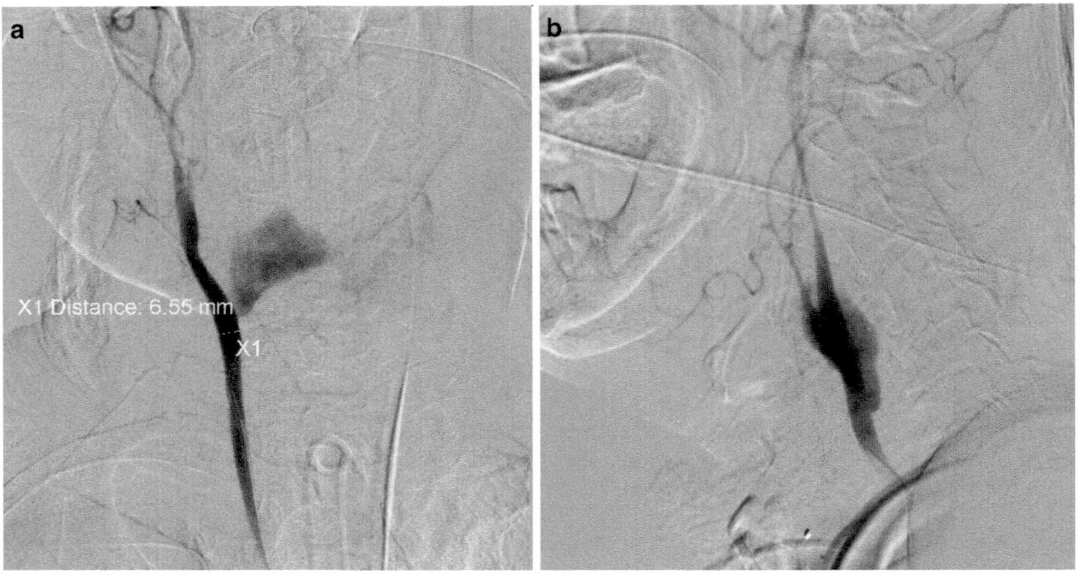

Fig. 5.9 (**a**) Frontal and (**b**) lateral DSA runs in a patient with locally invasive laryngeal cancer with carotid blowout show contrast extravasation from the distal common carotid artery

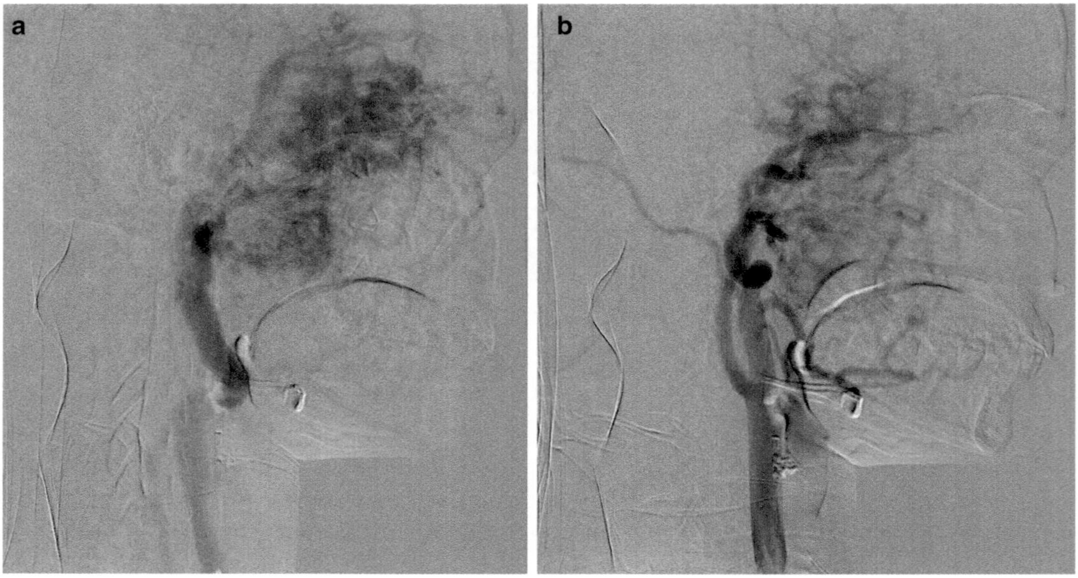

Fig. 5.10 Face AVM. (**a**) and (**b**) DSA runs in lateral projection arterial phase and late venous phase respectively show abnormal cluster of vessels getting supply from the internal maxillary artery and showing early venous shunting

ture or bleeding from the carotid artery or its branches (Fig. 5.9). This may be due to tumor eroding the vessel wall or post-radiation changes or postoperative exposure. Surgical ligation of the carotid artery is technically challenging in such a case and thus endovascular treatment is preferred. There are two options in carotid blowout. One is permanent occlusion of the carotid artery by coils or detachable balloons. However, if the balloon occlusion test is positive, then covered stent (stent graft) may be used to prevent cerebral ischemia. However, the latter does not have good long-term outcome.

5.2.7 DSA Embolization in AVMs

Arteriovenous malformations (AVMs) in the face/nose/ITF may present with pulsatile swelling and/or bleeding (epistaxis) (Fig. 5.10). Lip is often involved in such cases. Glue mixed with lipiodol is the commonly used embolizing agent. In case of large venous varices, especially when causing osteolysis of mandible, coils are used to pack the venous side of the AVM. Absolute alcohol may also be used; however, has the propensity to cause side effects due to tissue necrosis. Onyx (ethylene vinyl alcohol copolymer) can also be used especially in cases where there is direct arteriovenous fistula. For bleeding control; many times, percutaneous direct embolization is also done after endovascular control. The potential sites of dangerous anastomoses between internal and external carotid circulations need to be kept in mind in case of midline face lesions to avoid inadvertent blindness and stroke. These include nasal bridge, glabella and orbits and the anastomosis is between ophthalmic and ethmoid arteries with internal maxillary and facial artery branches. Also, such lesions usually have some drainage into the cavernous sinus as well.

5.2.8 Sclerotherapy for Sinonasal Low-Flow Malformations

Low-flow vascular malformations include venous and lymphatic malformations are commonly treated by sclerotherapy. Cystic masses in the region of glabella need to be carefully evaluated to rule out meningocele. MRI is usually recommended prior to any management to map out the entire extent of the lesion, muscle involvement, proximity to the course of nerves, orbit, and airways. Direct puncture of the lesion followed by contrast phlebography is done initially to decide the type of sclerosant, estimate its volume and look for draining veins (Fig. 5.11). The intent of sclerotherapy is the alleviation of symptoms (pain, bleeding, swelling, mass effect) and rarely curative. Sodium tetradecyl sulfate (STDS) is the commonly used sclerosant especially in case of macrocystic lesions and 3% concentration is used. Polidocanol is less effective, less painful, and incites less edema; used when the risk of side effects is more especially in case of small cystic spaces. Bleomycin is the agent of choice for microcystic lesions and incites the least inflammation, thus can be used if the lesion is close to airways. However, the cumulative dose of bleomycin should not exceed the safety limits to avoid pulmonary toxicity. Orbital extension is frequent in sinonasal lesions, thus there is potential risk of orbital inflammation post sclerotherapy. Hence risk versus benefit to be assessed based on patient

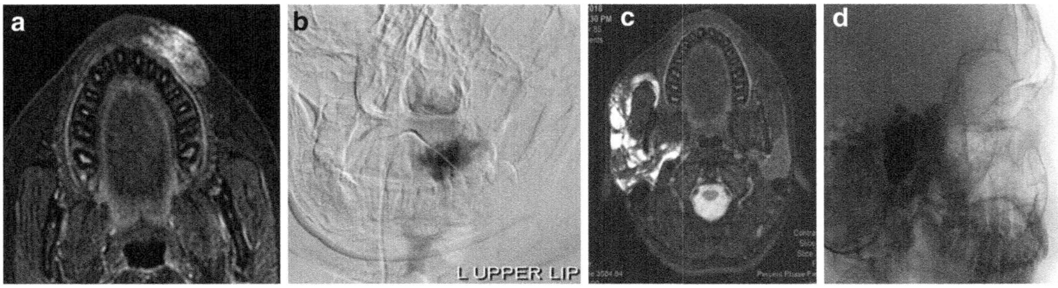

Fig. 5.11 Low-flow malformations of face. (**a**) Axial T2w MRI image shows hyperintense microcystic venous malformation in the left upper lip. (**b**) Corresponding phlebogram shows spongy pattern without any draining vein. (**c**) Axial T2w MRI image shows hyperintense lymphatic malformation involving right parotid. (**d**) Corresponding phlebogram image shows macrocystic pattern

symptoms and vision. Usual technique is foam sclerotherapy for both STDS and polidocanol to increase the surface area of contact with the endothelial wall and to slow down the clearance. The usual gap between sclerotherapy sessions is 6–8 weeks. Sclerotherapy or alcohol ablation may also be done for benign cystic lesions like colloid thyroid nodules, plunging ranula, salivary gland cysts [14].

5.2.9 Complications

Common *complications of non-vascular procedures* include pain and vasovagal reaction. There is minor risk of bleeding and infection. Injury to adjacent structures like major vessels and nerves is uncommon if a safe path has already been identified on imaging. Also, the use of thinner needles further reduces the risk. Prior radical neck surgery and radiation therapy increase the risk of vascular complications (1). Injury to nerves remains a theoretical risk in sampling procedures. Complications of sclerotherapy include pain and swelling for 5–7 days, trismus (in case of lesions in the masseteric muscles), and skin discoloration in case of superficial lesions or extravasation of sclerosant. In case of malformations around/near the nerves (example parotid lesions), there is a risk of sensory/motor loss due to post-procedural edema. These neuropathic features are usually transient. *Vascular interventions* may lead to puncture site hematomas, skin / mucosal discoloration/ulcers (due to ischemia), and rarely non-target embolization (leading to stroke or blindness) due to particle reflux and dangerous arterial anastomosis between internal and external carotid circulations [15]. Facial nerve paralysis may occur in case of embolization of the superficial temporal artery or if there is lot of post-embolization edema (alcohol/glue use). Some patients may develop post-embolization syndrome (fever, malaise, pain). There is the potential risk of raised intracranial tension post cavernous sinus thrombosis, if venous drainage is not properly mapped.

IR provides a minimally invasive treatment option with considerably less morbidity and better patient comfort [16]. With advances in the hardware of interventional radiology and increasingly available expertise, the use of IR is going to expand in ENT surgery. Both specialties need to work together for decision making to enhance patient care.

5.3 Part C: Nuclear Medicine Perspective

5.3.1 Introduction

Nuclear Medicine is a medical speciality that uses radiopharmaceuticals for diagnostic and therapeutic purposes. Recognition of nuclear medicine as a branch dates back to 1946 when Sam Seidlin became the first to report the success of radioactive iodine (^{131}I) in treating a patient with advanced thyroid cancer. Since then, there have been many discoveries and development of numerous diagnostic and therapeutic agents. The most commonly used radiotracers in diagnostic nuclear medicine are ^{99m}Tc (Technetium) labeled for planar and SPECT (Single Photon Emission Computed Tomography) imaging, and ^{18}F (Fluoride) and ^{68}Ga (Gallium) labeled for PET imaging. Nuclear Medicine plays an important role in nasal, nasopharyngeal, and paranasal sinus pathologies, by offering different types of investigations. Its use is indicated in infective pathologies and some benign and malignant pathologies.

5.3.1.1 Skull Base Osteomyelitis

Three Phase Bone Scintigraphy

Three phase bone scintigraphy is commonly used for skeletal infection imaging including skull base osteomyelitis (SBO). Three planar phases of the bone scan are: flow, pool, and delayed. Flow images demonstrate blood flow to the region of interest. Pool phase shows the soft tissue distribution of radiotracer around the region. Delayed images depict the bone uptake of radiotracer in the area. Sometimes additional SPECT/CT images are also taken. Conventional imaging for SBO is CT (Computerized tomography) is commonly performed investigation since it is relatively easy and fast method and detects demineralization and bone destruction. However, CT cannot detect the early functional changes that characterize bone infections and suffers a definite delay in detecting bony structure alterations [17]. Magnetic Resonance Imaging (MRI) is suggested to visualize intracranial spread, thrombosis, and soft tissue involvement. Both these conventional imaging techniques give anatomical details and do not allow assessment of disease activity and its response to treatment. In SBO, bone scintigraphy is indicated for the diagnosis and the extent of disease, to evaluate disease activity status, and for assessment of response to treatment. In active SBO, there will be increase in flow, pool activity, and uptake in delayed images. With SPECT/CT imaging the anatomical extent of the disease can be corroborated with functional activity. Occasionally flow and pool activity may not be significantly increased, particularly in cases of chronic osteomyelitis. In these cases, diagnosis is made on the basis of delayed and SPECT images (Fig. 5.12). The advantage of bone scan over conventional anatomical imaging is its ability to assess the functional activity of the disease. This feature can be used for response assessment, especially in immune-compromised patients in whom clinical features and laboratory parameters may not be reliable, which helps in making the decision of change or discontinuation of antibiotics. However, the disadvantage of planar bone scintigraphy is that the ongoing osteoblastic activity of the healing process may appear as false positive on scan. In such cases, WBC labeled imaging will differentiate between infection and bone remodeling. The negative predictive value of bone scintigraphy in SBO is much higher and can rule out active infection.

^{18}F FDG PET/CT

^{18}F FDG PET/CT can be used for SBO, since it is easily available and has higher resolution than planar and SPECT imaging (Fig. 5.13). As it is not a bone-specific agent, it can differentiate between bone infection and osteoblastic changes in bone healing. However, it is non-specific and can be positive in other non-infectious etiologies, like malignancy, and has higher radiation exposure to the patient than ^{99m}Tc bone scintigraphy.

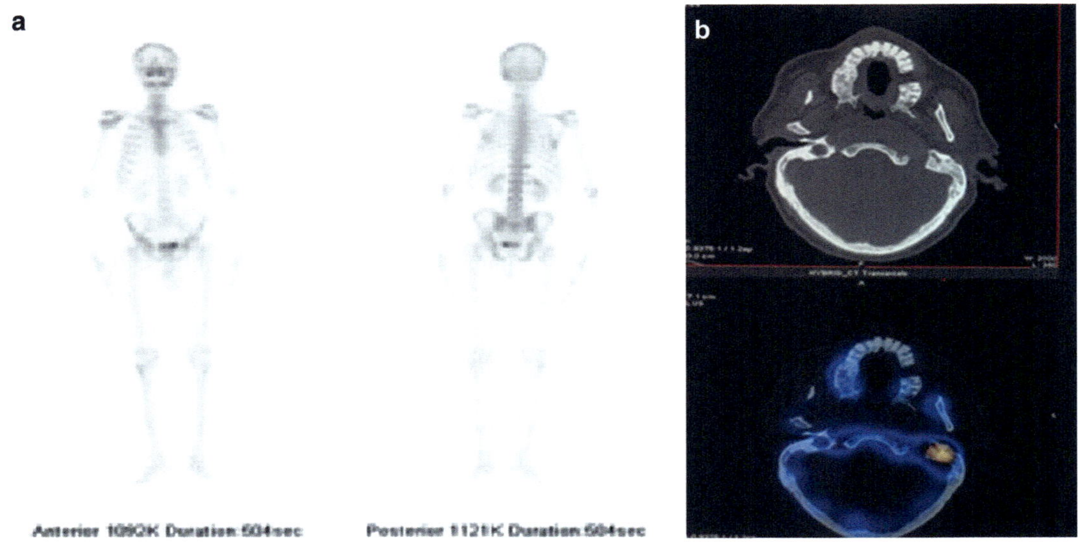

Fig. 5.12 A 40 years old diabetic patient presented with pain and discharge in the left ear for past 3 months and was referred to rule out skull base osteomyelitis. (**a**) Delayed planar images show uptake in the left mastoid region. (**b**) CT and fused SPECT-CT images reveal the focal concentration of radiotracer in left mastoid air cells which show loss of pneumatization on CT

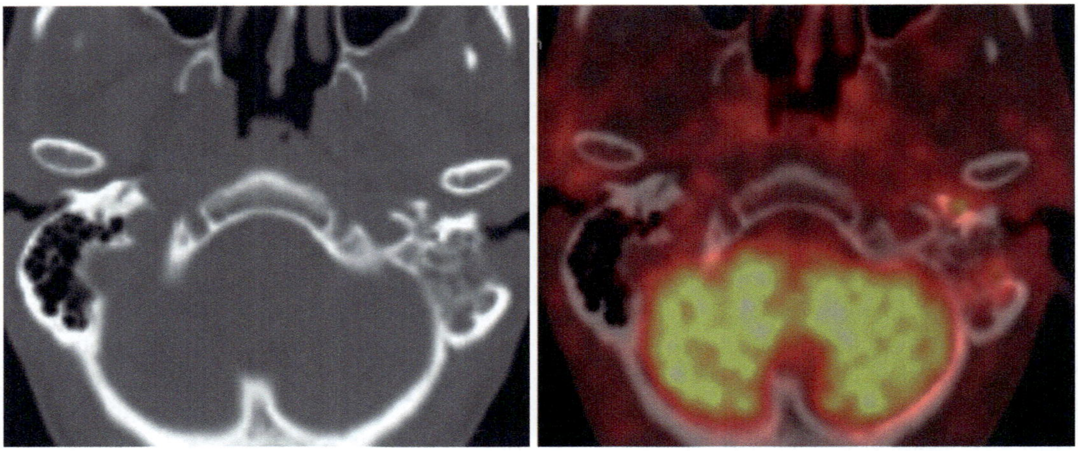

Fig. 5.13 53 years old male, with known left skull base osteomyelitis, post-left radical mastoidectomy, referred for FDG PET/CT to rule out residual disease. FDG PET/CT shows focal area of radiotracer uptake in the left styloid process and mastoid air cells, suggestive of residual disease

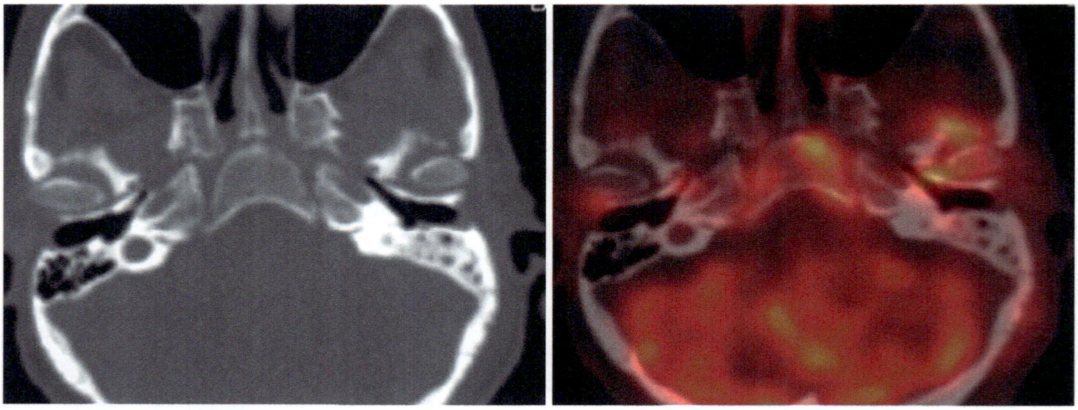

Fig. 5.14 Sixty years old female, with clinical suspicion of skull base osteomyelitis and inconclusive bone scan, underwent ^{18}F-WBC PET/CT, which revealed the involvement of left temporomandibular joint and sphenoid

WBC Labeled Imaging

White blood cells (WBC) labeling is a specific tool for infection imaging, particularly in differentiating bone infection from bone remodeling (Fig. 5.14). In this technique, autologous WBCs are labeled with radionuclide ex vivo. The commonly used SPECT based tracers are ^{99m}Tc HMPAO (hexamethylpropylene amine oxime) and ^{111}In oxine and PET-based tracer is ^{18}F labeled WBC. SPECT based tracers have less resolution as compared to PET-based tracers. Since leukocytes are directly labeled, this modality can detect ongoing infections anywhere, and can find use in fungal infections as well. The disadvantage of WBC labeled imaging is that the process is cumbersome with low yields and requires dedicated lab facility.

Tumor Imaging

(A) **Carcinoma Nasopharynx**

Conventional imaging of choice for the staging of Nasopharyngeal carcinoma (NPC) is MRI. ^{18}F-FDG PET/CT is the preferred investigation for metastatic evaluation of NPC (Fig. 5.15). MRI has high specificity, sensitivity, and accuracy for T staging of the

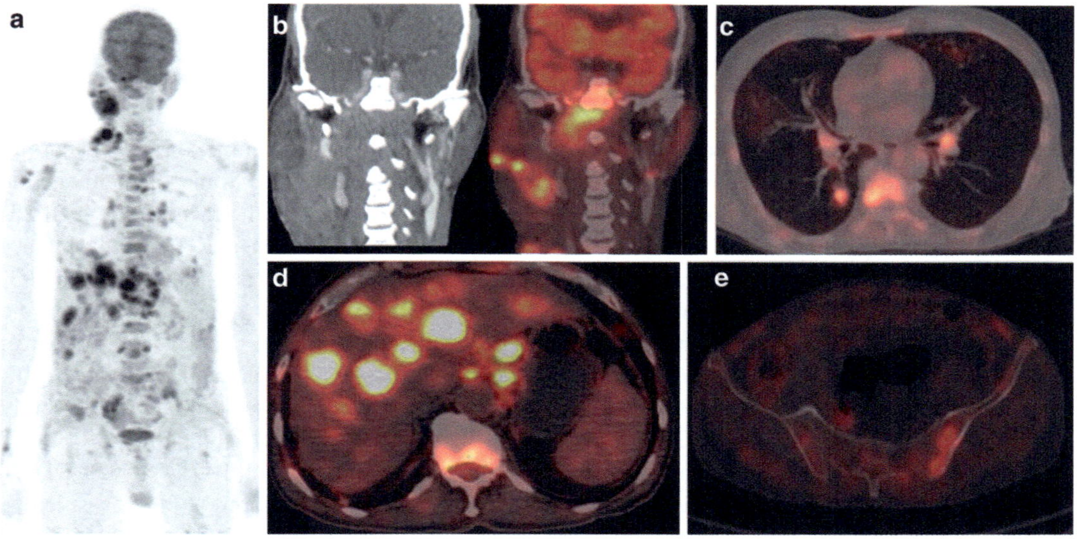

Fig. 5.15 62 year old male with biopsy proven nasopharyngeal carcinoma underwent ^{18}F-FDG PET/CT for staging. (**a**) MIP image reveals uptake in primary, cervical lymph node, lung, liver, and skeletal lesions. (**b**) Coronal section of head and neck showing intense FDG uptake in ill-defined lesion occupying the roof of nasopharynx with intracranial extension. Also seen, multiple FDG avid cervical lymph nodes. (**c**) Axial fused PET/CT images showing parenchymal lung nodule with uptake in right lung lower lobe, superior segment. (**d**) Axial fused PET/CT images showing multiple liver metastases. (**e**) Axial fused PET/CT images in bone window showing increased uptake with lytic lesion in left ilium suggestive of bone metastases

tumor. ^{18}F-FDG PET/CT has a limited role in T staging of tumor and tends to miss lesions in the skull base and cavernous sinuses due to physiologically high uptake of FDG in the brain and in early-stage tumor invasion and because of the lower resolution of PET compared with MRI [18]. Since MRI and CT depend on size criteria, it may be difficult to differentiate between small benign and malignant nodes. ^{18}F-FDG PET/CT has high accuracy in assessing N stage of tumor. ^{18}F-FDG PET/CT has a sensitivity of 97–100% and specificity of 73–97% in assessing cervical lymph nodes in patients with NPC, and MRI has a sensitivity of 84–92% and specificity of 73–97% [19]. However, PET/CT is not comparable to MRI in the detection of retropharyngeal nodes close to the primary, use of contrast enhanced CT with PET may improve this detection. According to NCCN guidelines (v1.2015) ^{18}F-FDG PET/CT is recommended for imaging of distant metastases (chest, liver, bone) for WHO class 2–3/N2–3 disease. ^{18}F-FDG PET/CT can detect residual disease in the background of postoperative and RT changes and therefore has a role to play in response assessment in these groups of patients.

(B) **Sinonasal Tumors**

Sinonasal neoplasms are rare in occurrence and comprise only 3% of all head and neck cancers. Sinonasal tumors can be of epithelial (carcinomas) or mesenchymal (sarcomas) origin. Epithelial tumors are the most common and originate from the epithelial lining, accessory salivary glands, neuroendocrine tissue, and olfactory epithelium. Mesenchymal tumors derive from the supporting tissue. Since their presentation is similar to rhinosinusitis, by the time of diagnosis they are usually much advanced. Common benign tumors in this region are papilloma and schwannoma. These benign tumors are routinely imaged with CT and MRI. However, in the presence of malignant transformation ^{18}F-FDG PET/CT has shown to have increased uptake. Therefore, PET/CT may have a role to play in cases with suspicion of co-existent malignant components.

(i) *Juvenile Nasopharyngeal Angiofibroma (JNA):*
These are benign yet locally aggressive in disease pathology. Conventionally CT and MRI are used to confirm diagnosis and disease extent. However residual disease and recurrence rate for JNA is high, ranging from 15% to 50%, which are not well detected on conventional imaging. ^{18}F-FDG PET/CT may be able to detect active residual/recurrent disease but due to physiological high FDG uptake in brain, intracranial extension and lesion close to skull base may not be well appreciated. With this consideration, ^{68}Ga-PSMA PET/CT and ^{68}Ga-DOTANOC PET/CT have been done for few patients in our department, which are showing promising results (Fig. 5.16).

(ii) *Mesenchymal Tumors:*
Mesenchymal tumor is a rare neoplasm arising from any mesenchymal tissue such as bone or soft tissue. This tumor is common in extremities, rarely occurs in sinonasal region. Some of them secrete fibroblast growth factor 23 (FGF23) which is responsible for phosphaturia and tumor-induced osteomalacia (TIO) [20]. They can present with muscle weakness, bone pain, and fractures. These tumors are small and hence difficult to diagnose. Initial whole body screening is done with ^{18}F-FDG PET/CT followed by ^{68}Ga-DOTANOC PET/CT (SSTR scintigraphy), any suspicious lesion is further evaluated with MRI and histopathology.

(iii) *Lymphoma:*
The nasal cavities and paranasal sinuses are rarely affected by primary Non-

a

b

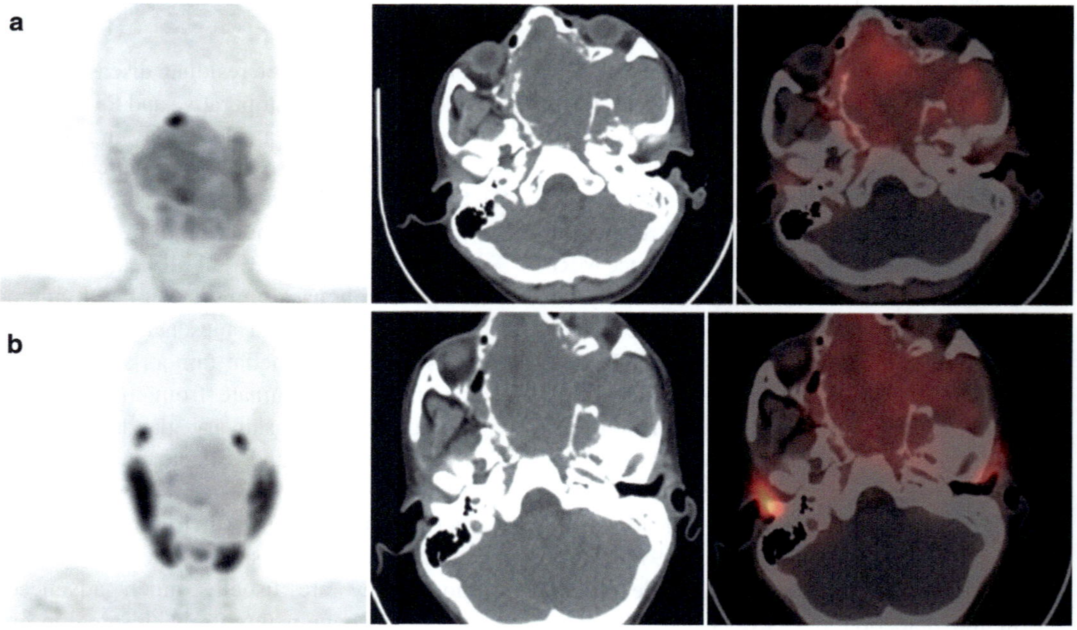

Fig. 5.16 12 year old boy with juvenile nasopharyngeal angiofibroma, underwent ^{68}Ga DOTANOC (**a**) and ^{68}Ga PSMA (**b**) PET/CT for baseline evaluation. Images reveal ill-defined lobulated mass occupying entire nasal cavity and left maxillary sinus, with erosion of sphenoid and extension into left infratemporal fossa. MIP image of DOTANOC (**a**) shows physiological uptake in pituitary gland and avid mass. Whereas MIP image of PSMA (**b**) shows physiological uptake in lacrimal and salivary glands along with the avid mass *(On going thesis- Dr. Prabhu, Dept of ENT, AIIMS, New Delhi, under guidance of Prof. Alok Thakar (ENT) & Prof Rakesh Kumar (Nuclear Medicine)*

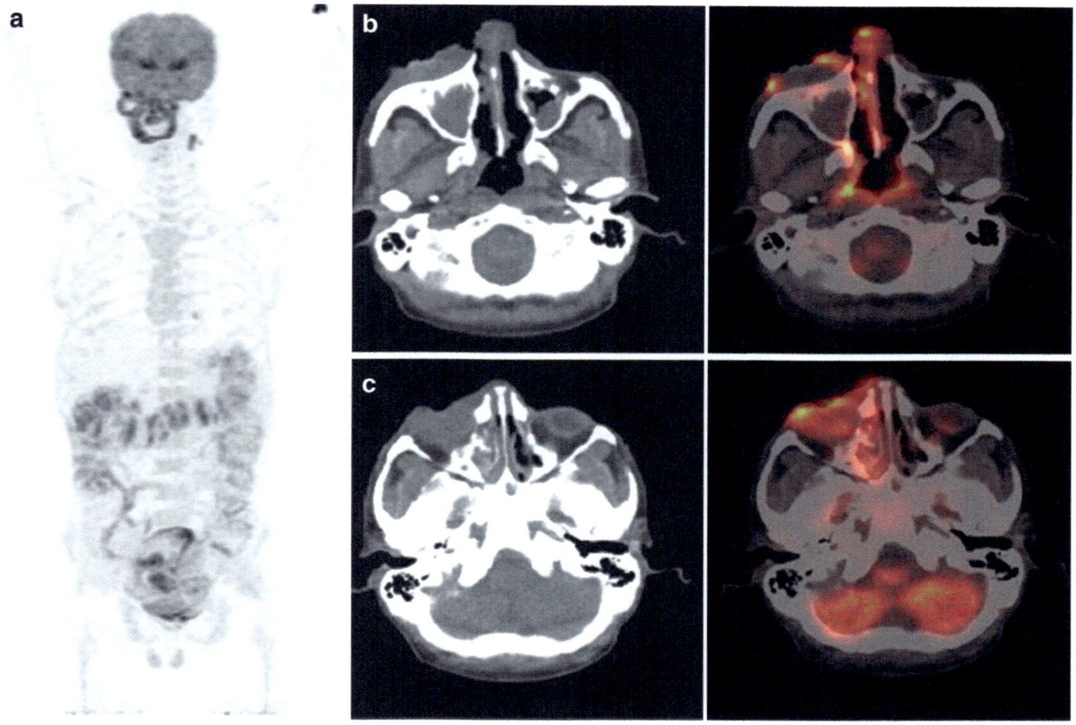

Fig. 5.17 39 year old male, with NK Tcell lymphoma of nasal cavity, underwent ^{18}F-FDG PET/CT for staging. MIP image (**a**) reveals FDG avid mass involving the nasal cavity and diffuse uptake in axial and appendicular skeleton. (**b**) Irregular soft tissue thickening of right nasal cavity and involving the nasal septum and nasopharynx, with diffuse FDG uptake. (**c**) FDG avid extension of mass into infra-orbital region of right eye and right ethmoid seen. No other lesion noted in rest of the body

Hodgkin lymphoma (NHL). Most common NHL in the head and neck region is of the Waldeyer ring, in which palatine tonsil is most common followed by nasopharynx. Primary nasopharyngeal lymphoma constitutes 8% of all head and neck lymphomas. ^{18}F-FDG PET/CT is useful for the detection of the Primary Nasopharyngeal lymphoma (PNL), its extent of disease, and response evaluation. Studies have revealed that ^{18}F-FDG PET/CT is not reliable to differentiate between PNL and NPC [21]. The nasal cavities and paranasal sinuses are rarely affected by primary NHL, these can be differentiated from squamous carcinomas of these areas on conventional imaging due to their sub-mucosal origin. ^{18}F-FDG PET/CT also has a role in the metastatic evaluation and disease activity response assessment (Fig. 5.17).

(iv) *Mucosal Melanoma:*

Mucosal malignant melanoma is a very rare tumor counting for approximately 0.8–1.3% of all melanomas. Sinonasal malignant melanoma (SNMM) accounts roughly for 4% of all head and neck melanomas and sinonasal malignancies [22]. In routine practice of head & neck radiological assessment, CT and MRI are used for initial diagnosis. These modalities have their limitation in metastatic evaluation and detection of residual/recurrent disease. ^{18}F-FDG-PET/CT imaging has higher sensitivity and specificity over conventional imaging in the staging of malignant melanoma [23]. Therefore, ^{18}F-FDG-PET/CT can be a one-stop-

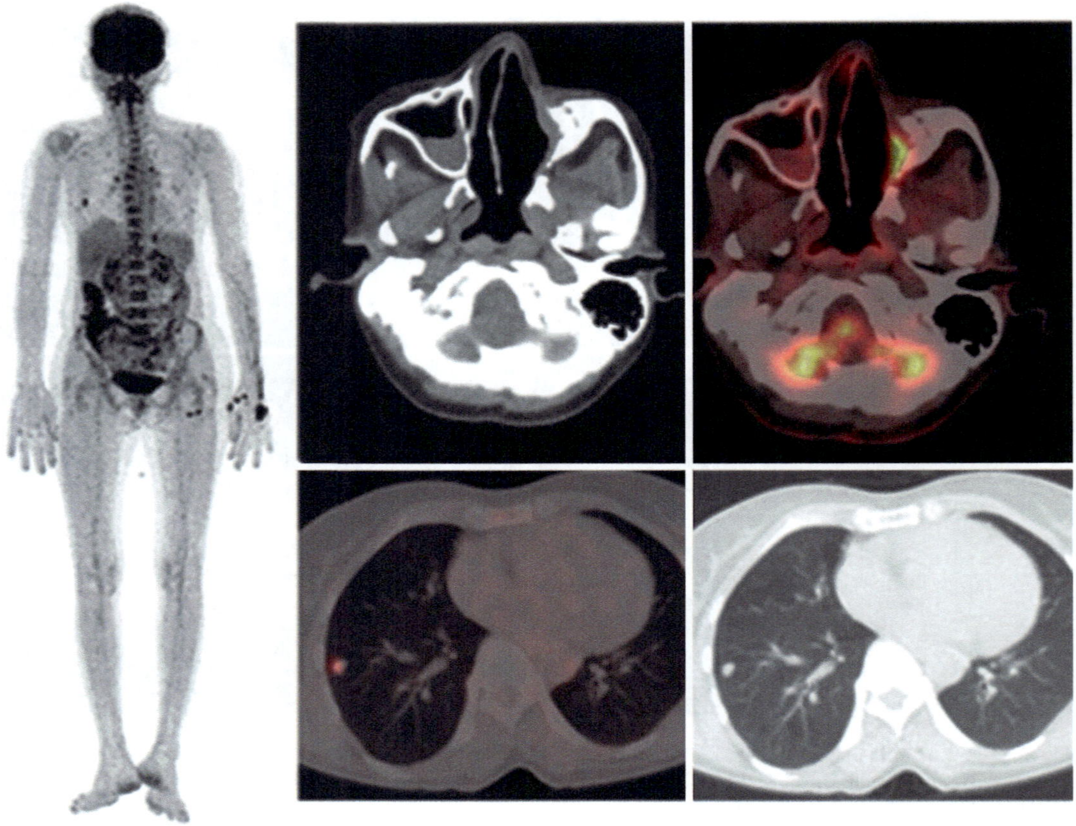

Fig. 5.18 50 years old female, with known malignant melanoma, underwent ^{18}F-FDG-PET/CT post-surgery and radiotherapy to look for disease status. (**a**) MIP image showing increased uptake in the region of nasal cavity, lungs, and axial skeleton. (**b**) Axial CT and Pet/CT fused images showing mucosal thickening in lateral wall of left nasal cavity with FDG uptake, suggestive of residual disease. (**c**) FDG avid parenchymal metastatic nodule in right lung lower lobe

shop imaging for detection of primary as well as metastatic diseases (Fig. 5.18). Studies have shown the use of ^{18}F-FDG-PET/CT in staging, restaging post-surgery, and response assessment of SNMM [24]. However, non-specific mucosal FDG uptake in local infective or inflammatory conditions may lead to misinterpretation of PET.

(v) *Olfactory Neuroblastoma:*
Olfactory neuroblastoma also known as Esthesioneuroblastoma (ENB) is a rare neuroectodermal tumor of the nasal cavity, comprising 2% of all sino-nasal neoplasms [25]. Imaging plays an important role in the diagnosis and staging of olfactory neuroblastoma. CT is essential for evaluation of the osseous involvement of the cribriform plate, fovea ethmoidalis, and lamina papyracea. MRI assesses the soft tissue extent and dural involvement of the disease. Like other neuroectodermal tumors, ENB shows MIBG (Meta-iodo benzyl guanidine), a nor-epinephrine analog, concentration. ^{123}I labeled MIBG for diagnostic planar and SPECT and ^{131}I labeled MIBG for therapeutic indications are already in use for extra-nasal neuroblastoma. MIBG scintigraphy has been found to be useful in differentiating olfactory neuroblastomas from other nasal tumors [26]. ^{18}F-FDG-PET/CT is used for staging, restaging, and follow up of ENB [27]. Some studies have shown

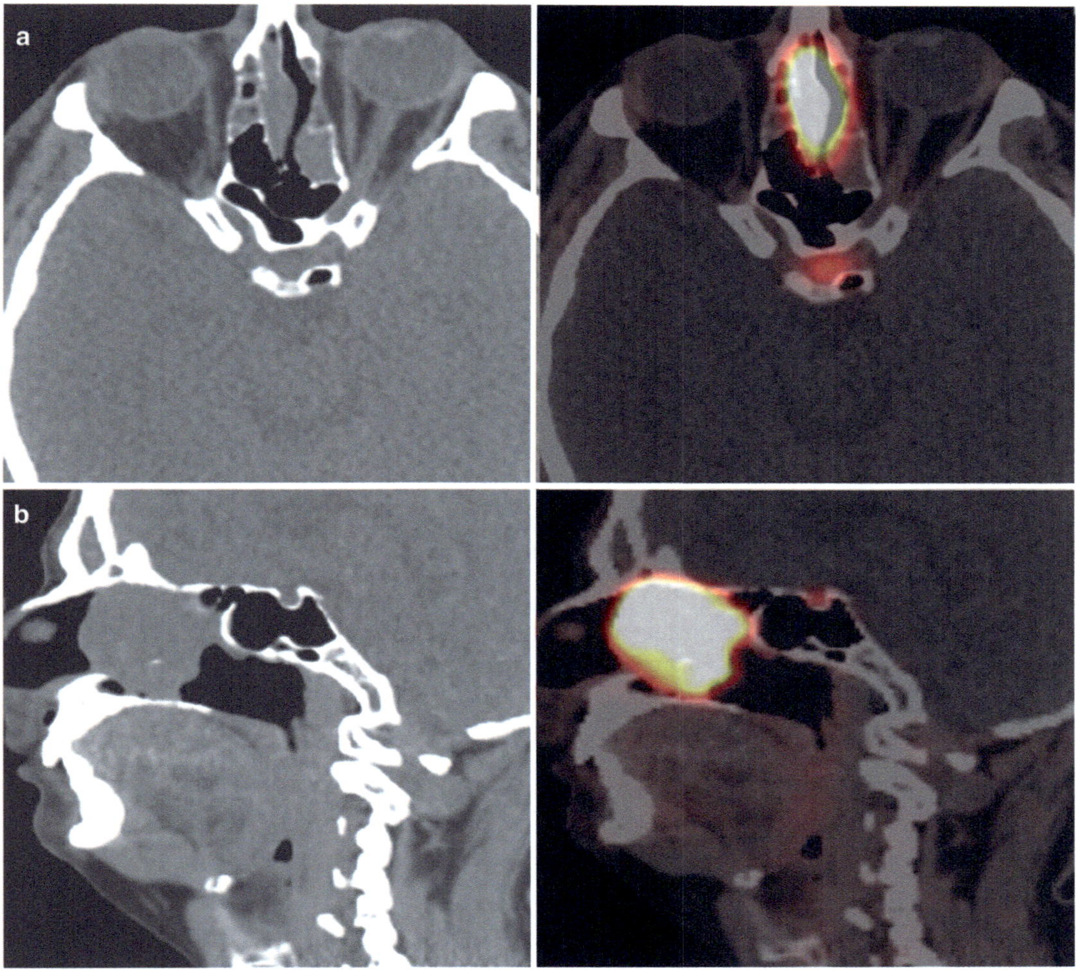

Fig. 5.19 33 years old male, with suspected nasal neuroendocrine carcinoma, post three cycles of docetaxel, underwent ^{68}Ga DOTANOC PET/CT. (**a**) Axial CT and PET/CT fused images showing sift tissue mass in right nasal cavity with intense tracer uptake. (**b**) Sagittal CT and PET/CT fused images showing mass occupying the right nasal cavity. Biopsy revealed olfactory neuroblastoma

the superior diagnostic role of Choline-based PET (^{18}F or ^{11}C labeled) over FDG PET, however, more data is required to establish this [28]. High expression of Somatostatin Receptors (SSTR), particularly SSTR-1 and 2, has been documented in tumor cells of neuroblastoma [29]. Extending from this knowledge Savelli et al. have reported SSTR scintigraphy and peptide receptor radionuclide therapy (PRRT) in a case of ENB, they have reported good uptake of ^{68}Ga DOTANOC in tumor and response to ^{90}Y DOTATATE (Fig. 5.19) [30].

(vi) *Occult Primary:*
Carcinomas of unknown primary (CUP) account for 5–10% of head and neck cancers [31]. Oropharynx is one of the most common sites of origin of head and neck occult primaries, accounting for nearly 90% of CUPs, the nasopharynx and hypopharynx are relatively less common 'hot spots' for occult primary tumors [32]. When conventional imaging, i.e.,

CT and MRI, fail to localize occult primary, PET/CT becomes the next investigation of choice. FDG PET/CT scan has an overall staging accuracy of 69–78%, a positive predictive value of 56–83%, a negative predictive value of 75–86%, a sensitivity of 63–100%, and a specificity of 90–94% in CUP [33]. Apart from the localization of primary, PET also assists in identifying more feasible sites for biopsy. However, FDG PET/CT also has its drawbacks, the presence of infective/inflammatory pathology in nasal cavity and paranasal sinuses may give rise to false positives.

(C) **Sentinel Lymph Node Scintigraphy**
Sentinel lymph node biopsy is based on the identification of the predictable pattern of lymphatic drainage to a primary tumor, and its role as an effective filter for tumor cells [34]. Histopathological confirmation of the involvement of sentinel lymph node helps in limiting unnecessary neck dissections. There are various techniques for the identification of the sentinel lymph nodes, commonly used are the dye method and radiotracer method. In the radiotracer method, the radiolabeled colloid suspension is injected at the primary site, and planar and SPECT/CT images are acquired at 15, 30, and 60 min from injection. SPECT/CT provides anatomical confirmation of lymph node level of the sentinel lymph node. During surgery, the exact location of the nodes may be confirmed using a hand-held gamma detector probe. These identified lymph nodes are then biopsied to look for the spread of malignancy, and assist in decisions regarding neck dissection. Few sentinel lymph node scintigraphy studies have been done for sino-nasal malignancies, showing an increment in the identification of involved nodes of up to 14% [35].

(D) **Therapeutic Potential**
Tumors expressing somatostatin receptors (SSTR) like NET of the nose and paranasal sinuses, may be considered for peptide receptor radionuclide therapy (PRRT) targeting these receptors, such as ^{177}Lu (lutetium), ^{90}Y (yttrium), or ^{225}Ac (actinium) labeled DOTATE. Olfactory neuroblastoma like other neuroblastomas is amenable to ^{131}I-MIBG therapy. JNA has been shown to express both SSTRs and PSMA, therefore, theoretically can receive PRRT or PSMA labeled ^{177}Lu or ^{225}Ac therapy.

5.4 Part D: Bacteriology and Virology

5.4.1 Introduction

Antonie Philips van Leeuwenhoek was the first scientist who observed bacteria. Bacteria are single cell organism seen by light microscopy which unlike viruses is able to multiply by binary fission as well as survive outside other cells. After birth, the nasopharynx of a new born does not remain a sterile site for more than 48 h. With rapid acquisition of colonizing bacteria initially from the maternal genital tract and later followed by organism which are either ingested or received from carrier skin. The normal indigenous flora consists of gram-positive and gram-negative, aerobic and anaerobic bacteria including the oral streptococci, Bacteroides species, Corynebacterium species, and Neisseria species.

5.4.1.1 Bacteriology of Nose and PNS

Common cold (Rhinitis) is defined as an inflammation of the nasal mucous membrane or lining. Bacterial agents are responsible for 10–15% of cases of rhinitis which include *Chlamydia pneumoniae, Mycoplasma pneumoniae,* and Group A streptococci [36]. Maxillary sinus is the most commonly involved sinus. The subsequent order of frequency of sinus involvement is the ethmoid, frontal, and sphenoid sinuses) [37]. *Streptococcus pneumoniae* and *Haemophilus influenzae* are the most common etiological agents among community-acquired cases (50–60%). *Moraxella catarrhalis* is responsible for around 20% of cases in children. Methicillin-resistant *Staphylococcus aureus* (MRSA) concern is emerging. Among anaerobes, *Prevotella* spp. *Fusobacterium* spp., are found [38]. Among chronic sinusitis, common pathogens are *S. pneumoniae, H. influenzae, and M. catarrhalis. Other pathogens that are* less frequently seen are anaerobic streptococci, Prevotella spp., and *Fusobacterium* spp. *M. catarrhalis* is one of the possible agent in chronic sinusitis in children [36].

Nosocomial sinusitis is a relatively common occurring complication, mainly in critical care. Risk factors are nasal intubation, nasal-enteric tube. Bacterial species that are prevalent in environment of hospital are the common etiological agents for nosocomial cases including, *Staphylococcus. aureus, Pseudomonas* spp., *Klebsiella pneumonia,* etc. Such infections are commonly polymicrobial and multidrug resistant. During the last three decades, extrapulmonary tuberculosis (EPTB) has gained special attention because of the human immunodeficiency virus (HIV) pandemic. *Mycobacterium tuberculosis* most frequently reaches the lung and rarely involves paranasal sinuses and nasopharynx. It reaches the nose and facial bones through blood stream or lymphatics. Antral lavage examination for AFB and culture for *Mycobacterium tuberculosis* can facilitate early diagnosis, there by avoiding surgical intervention.

Steps and Site of Specimen Collection [39]

1. Rhinitis: The sample is collected from anterior nares. If pus is found on anterior rhinoscopy, dry swab is applied over it to collect sample. If no pus is found, the swab is moistened first and then the anterior nares are swabbed. Swab specimen should be taken from at least 1 cm inside the nares. The transport medium for the swab is mainly for staphylococcal carriers. To culture the lesion, the sample is to be collected from the advancing margin of the lesion. For nasopharyngeal swab, flexible swab stick is inserted per nasal, it is passed through the nasal cavity till it impinges on the nasopharynx, and then rotate for 5–10 s. Swab can be moistened with Stuart's or Amie's medium. (This moistening is only for bacterial etiology suspected). Thin wire or flexible swab is dipped into transport medium. Transport to laboratory immediately.
2. Sinusitis is the clinical diagnosis. Maxillary sinusitis is the most common type of sinusitis, and specimen is collected by aspiration and subjected to culture and susceptibility testing [36, 40]. Therapy can be modified according to the etiological agent and treatment response. As nasal cavity is colonized heavily with respiratory flora, contamination of sample collected from paranasal sinuses is quite common. To help in differentiating true infection from contamination, quantitative methods can be helpful. Colony count of at least 10^4 colony-forming units per milliliter (CFUs/mL) of aspirated material is suggestive of infection.
3. General instructions for specimen transport: The specimen should reach the laboratory as soon as possible. Ideally specimen must reach the laboratory within <2 h. If specimen is taken in odd hours, it can be store at 4 °C (This only applies to Virus etiology as mentioned with Coronavirus). For suspected Bacterial etiology, we can keep the specimen at room temperature maximum for 24 h. It should not be refrigerated, Sinus drainage is unacceptable for smear or culture because of contamination with naturally occuring flora.

Nasal smear is also useful to evaluate eosinophils. It may help in diagnosing the suspected cases of allergic rhinitis. Even in uncomplicated cold, polymorpho-nuclear leukocytes predominance in nasal secretions can be seen and does not always a marker for bacterial superinfection. Routine microbiological investigations like bacterial cultures or antigen detection are required when specific bacterial etiological agent like group A streptococcus, nasal diphtheria, or *Bordetella pertussis* is suspected.

5.4.2 Staining Procedures

- Gram Stain: It divides the bacteria into Gram-positive and Gram-negative bacteria.
- Ziehl–Neelsen Technique: It divides the bacteria into acid fast and non-acid fast. *Mycobacterium tuberculosis* being acid fast,

is presumptively diagnosed with this technique.

- Albert Stain: It is performed for *Corynebacterium diphtheriae*, will appear as green bacilli with purple-blue metachromatic granules and in typical arrangement.

5.4.3 Culture Media Are Required to Isolate the Bacteria from the Clinical Specimens

1. Primary Plating Medias are blood agar, MacConkey agar, chocolate (Heated blood agar) agar. It is for isolation of aerobic bacteria (Figs. 5.20, 5.21, and 5.22).
2. Lowenstein-Jensen (LJ) medium: It is used for isolation of *Mycobacterium tuberculosis.*

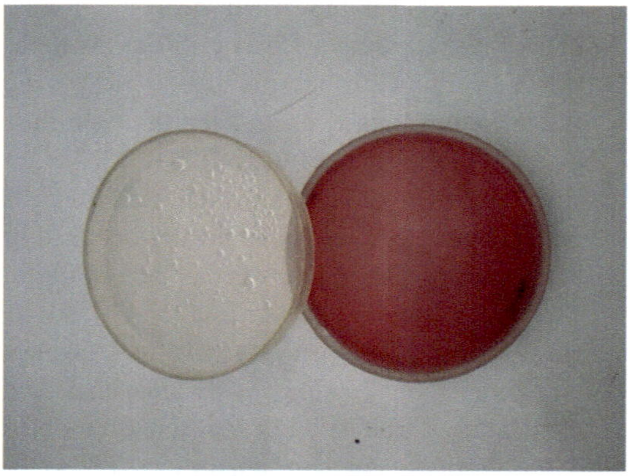

Fig. 5.20 MacConkey Agar

3. Loeffler's serum slope and Potassium tellurite agar (PTA): It is used for isolation of *Corynebacterium diphtheriae.*
4. Blood agar and Pike's medium (Blood agar containing crystal violet and sodium azide): For *Streptococcus spp.*
5. Robertson's cooked meat medium (RCM), PRAS (pre-reduced anaerobic sterilized) transport medium, Stuart's transport medium for anaerobes.

Growth from the medium can be identified by conventional biochemical tests, automated identification system, or MALDI-ToF {Matrix-assisted laser desorption/ionization (MALDI), and the mass analyzer is time-of-flight (TOF) analyzer}.

5.4.3.1 Storage of Media

Bacterial cultures are generally stored on agar plates or in stab cultures in the refrigerator at 4 °C. Long-term storage methods should be considered for maximum bacterial viability like:

1. Freezing samples
2. Freeze-drying (Lyophilization)

5.4.4 Nucleic Acid Amplification Techniques (NAAT)

It is increase the yield of sample. The various NAATs used are Polymerase chain reaction

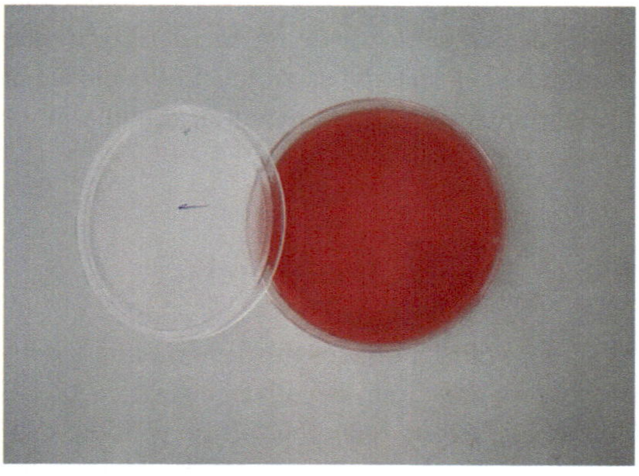

Fig. 5.21 Blood Agar

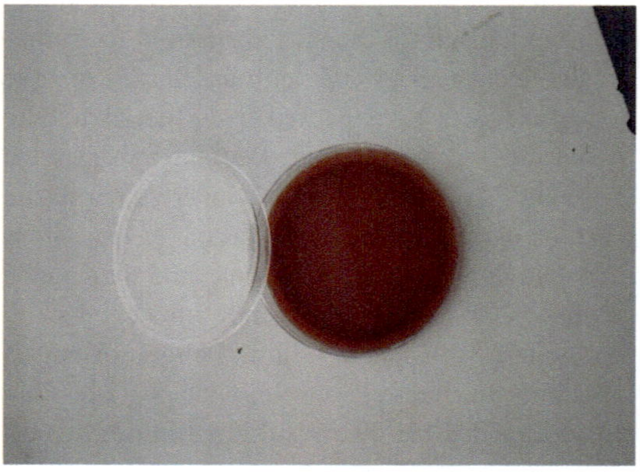

Fig. 5.22 Chocolate Agar

(PCR), Real-time polymerase chain reaction, Ligase chain reaction (LCR), Transcription-mediated amplification (TMA), Nucleic acid sequence-based amplification (NASBA), and Strand displacement amplification (SDA) [41].

The PCR technique involves three basic steps to amplify the number.

1. DNA extraction from the organism
2. Amplification of extracted DNA
3. Gel electrophoresis of the amplified product

5.4.5 Antibiotic Sensitivity, Resistance, and Prevention

Testing for antibiotic sensitivity is often done by the Kirby-Bauer method or automated antibiotic susceptibility system. Small disc containing antibiotics are placed onto a plate upon which bacteria are growing. If the bacteria are sensitive to the antibiotic, a clear ring, or zone of inhibition, is seen around the disc indicating poor growth. Antibiotic resistance occurs when bacteria change in some way that reduces or eliminates the effectiveness of drugs, chemicals, or other agents designed to cure or prevent infections. The bacteria survive and continue to multiply causing more harm. Bacteria can do this through several mechanisms. To preserve the potency of existing antibiotics, overall antibiotic use must be decreased. Physicians, pharmacists, and the general public must avoid the careless use of these valuable drugs. Antibiotics must be prescribed only for bacterial infections and in the proper dose for the correct amount of time.

5.4.6 Viruses in ENT

Viruses are the smallest unicellular organisms, are obligate intracellular. Viruses are the most primitive microorganisms infecting man. Viral infections are responsible for rhinitis in 20–25% of cases. In rhino-pathologies of viral origin, the microscopic picture is characterized by fairly aspecific cellular changes gathered under the term "ciliocytophthoria," which comprises degenerative alterations of the ciliary ultrastructure (shortening and focal or even general loss of the cilia), the cytoplasm (contraction of the cytoplasm, or even shortening of the upper portion of the cell body), the nucleus (chromatin margination with a ground-glass appearance and intranuclear inclusions). The range of viruses that commonly infects the respiratory tract is notoriously wide (rhinovirus, coronavirus, respiratory syncytial virus [RSV], adenovirus, parainfluenza virus, coxsackievirus, cytomegalovirus). However, no specific cytomorphologic alteration has been found till date that could represent a turning point in epidemiology, despite viral infections accounting for the bulk of human infectious diseases, or in prognosis and therapy. Some have strongly linked with the carcinogenesis of several tumor types, particularly Burkitt's lymphoma and nasopharyngeal carcinoma (NPC) with Epstein-Barr virus (EBV).

5.4.7 Laboratory Diagnosis of Viral Diseases

Laboratory Diagnosis of Common Cold [37]: The culture, antigen detection, PCR, or serologic methods are the commonly employed diagnostic methods for viral pathogens that cause the common cold. As such, routine diagnostic methods neither required nor of any help in cases with common cold. It is only helpful when therapy with an antiviral agent is required for specific etiological agent. As such, viruses have been infrequently isolated from patients with acute sinusitis. Timing of sinus aspiration may be responsible for this. Sinus aspiration is usually done in persistent sinusitis when case has been symptomatic for at least 7–10 days [42]. Normally, by this time, viral infection may be diminishing. Respiratory viruses have been recovered from approximately 10% of sinus aspirates. Approximately 30–40% of sinus aspirates in cases with acute sinusitis are not positive for any bacteria. It is presumed that many of these infections are, in fact, viral. Nasopharyngeal and oropharyngeal swab is also collected to evaluate virus. Swab should be Dacron or polyester flocked swab. For transport of samples for viral detection, Viral transport medium (VTM) containing antifungal and antibiotic supplements to be used. Avoid repeated freezing and thawing of specimen. Transport the sample to laboratory at 4 °C. If specimen is required to be stored, store at 4 °C less than equal to 5 days while at −70 °C for >5 days.

5.4.7.1 Detection Methods for Viruses

Direct Demonstration of Virus is done by electron microscopy, immune-electron microscopy, Fluorescent microscopy, Light microscopy. ELISA, direct immunofluorescence (IF), Immunochromatography (ICT) test, flow through assays are the methods for detection of viral antigens. Hemagglutination Inhibition assay (HAI), neutralization test, and complement fixation test (CFT) are the conventional techniques for detection of the specific antibodies. Enzyme-linked immunosorbent assay (ELISA) is a technique used to detect antibodies to infectious agents in a sample. Antibodies are made in response to infection and so an antibody ELISA can indicate whether or not an animal has been in contact with a certain virus. Molecular methods include RT-PCR is for RNA and DNA detection. The isolation of virus is done by animal inoculation method, embryonated egg inoculation method, and by tissue cultures such as organ culture, explant culture, cell line culture [43].

5.5 Part E: Advanced Instruments in Rhinology

The normal anatomy of the nose and paranasal sinuses is highly variable and complicated. Certain parts were very difficult to access with existing cold instruments so clearance of disease from these areas was difficult. With the advent of the concept of functional endoscopic sinus surgery, preservation of uninvolved mucosa is very important so outcome of surgery is better. It improves the quality of life to great extent. With the advancement in instrumentation in the field of rhinology, the knowledge of normal anatomy and its variation is improved, handling of diseased and normal healthy mucosa is improved, access to difficult area is also improved so the disease clearance is better than with cold instruments which in term reduce the chances of recurrence and residual disease. Sinonasal region is surrounded by vital structures such as brain and orbit. Inadvertent injury to these vital structures can create devastating complications. Powered instrument also reduces the rate of complications and fear to handle disease close to these vital structures, which in turn reduces the morbidity, mortality, and financial burden on community. Endoscopes, debrider, coblator, navigation system, ultrasonic aspirator, radiofrequency ablation, etc. are advances in the last two decades.

1. Endoscopes—It is prepared by using fiber optics and powerful lens systems to provide lighting and visualization of the relatively inaccessible areas through conventional instruments. The portion of the endoscope inserted into the body can be rigid or flexible. Hopkins rod lens system was developed to provide endoscopes of different length, diameter, and angle to provide visualization in certain areas. The rigid endoscopes commonly used are 2.7, 3, and 4 mm in diameter. 2.7 mm is for pediatric and 4 mm is for adult nasal procedures. Visualization is better with the increase in diameter of endoscopes as more light can transmit to the surgical field. The working length of nasal endoscopes is 18 cm. Nasal endoscopes are available in various degrees such as 0, 15, 30, 45, 70, and 90° (Fig. 5.23) [44]. 0° and 30° endoscopes are the most commonly used endoscopes. With the increase in degrees, we can see more hidden part of nose and paranasal sinuses. Seventy degree endoscope is useful for visualization of frontal sinus and maxillary sinus floor. All the endoscopes are now autoclavable. 0° nasal endoscope comes with green color coding. Fifteen and thirteen degrees endoscopes comes with white and red color coding. Color coding for 45°, 70°, 90° endoscopes are blue, yellow, and black respectively.

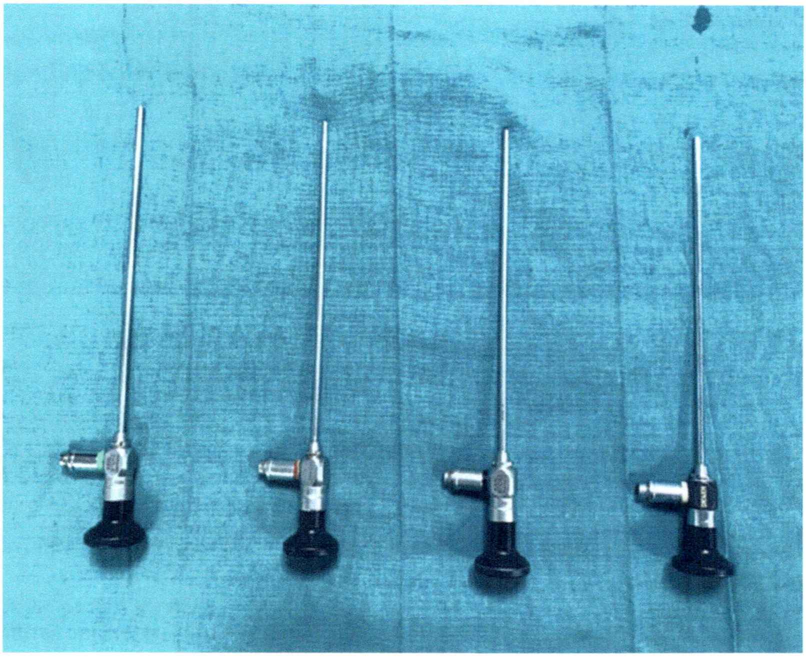

Fig. 5.23 Nasal endoscopes

Video endoscopes are mechanically similar to fiber-endoscopes. They have charged couple device (CCD) 'chip' and supporting electronics mounted at the tip, to and fro wiring replacing the optical bundle and further electronics and switches occupying the site of the ocular lens on the upper part of the control head [45]. A CCD chip is an array of 33,000–100,000 individual photo pixel receiving photons reflected back from the mucosal surface and producing electrons in proportion to the light received. The advantages are improved image quality, improved monitor view, removing the necessity to grasp the instrument close to the surgeon eye has hygienic advantages and it also improved instrument design and handling techniques. The only limiting factor is no direct viewing. Endoscopic observation can further increase by the light source and digital camera.

Light Source further augment visualization by increasing light output. With the advent of the xenon light source (peak wavelengths in the 800–1000 nm range), visualization has markedly improved. Xenon sources have been observed to be 3 times greater than that of standard halogen sources, with white rather than yellow-tinted light quality. In comparison to halogen light, xenon is more robust and efficient, with greater life, less heat creation. The drawback of xenon bulbs is the cost to install and replace, it takes a few seconds to attain full glow and give off more glare.

Digital cameras use chips that process color information. Modern 3-chip cameras have spate chips to process each of the three primary colors, red, blue, and green. This markedly enhances video quality [46].

2. Microdebrider—Microdebrider is a powered instrument. It is an extremely helpful surgical tool in modern endoscopic sinus surgery [47]. Handpiece, interchangeable blades, and machines are the components of microdebrider. The handpiece is connected with suction and irrigation source which is cylindrical or piston drip in design (Fig. 5.24). The blades have cylindrical back part for easy connection with handpiece. It contains two hollow shafts. The outer shaft allows suction and irrigation through and around the blades whereas the inner shaft rotates or oscillates with in outer

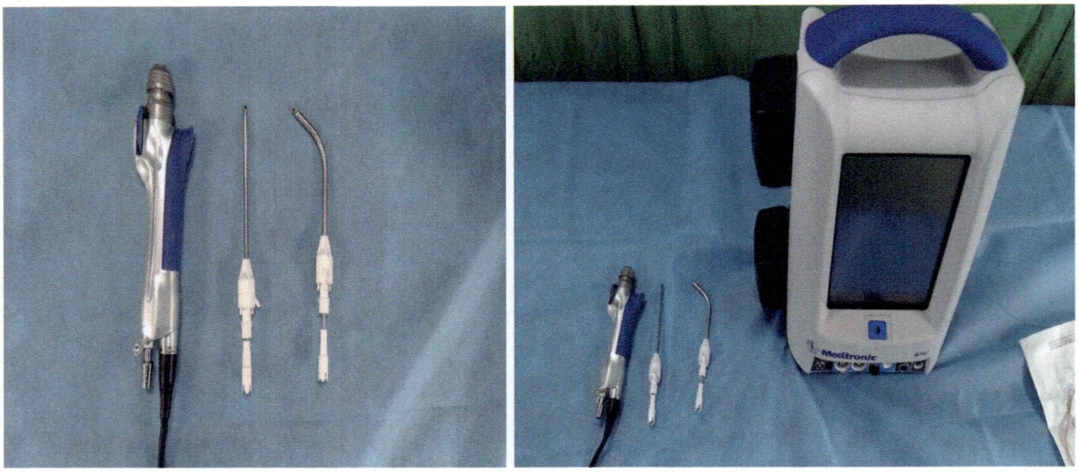

Fig. 5.24 Microdebrider hand piece, blades, and machine (Courtesy—Dr. Hitesh Verma, Associate Professor, AIIMS, New Delhi, India)

shaft. For surgical ease, blades are available in wide range in term of size and angles. Straight edge blades allow clear tissue cut without injury to surrounding mucosa whereas serrated edge blades allow rapid tissue removal. Frontal sinus and the deeper part of maxillary sinus can be accessed by more angled blades. Recent modification in design increases the application of microdebrider such as inferior turbinate reduction, correction of septal spur [48]. The mode and speed can be control by footplate of microdebrider.

Microdebrider acts by indrawn of soft tissue by the suction portal. This tissue is sheared off by the revolving blade between the inner and outer cannulas. Irrigation is classically incorporated into the device, applied by another set of tubing, and pumped into the blade to assist the movement of debrided tissue. The irrigation helps to prevent blockage of the device by the debrided tissue. The slower the revolving speed of the blade, the big is the tissue nibble. At higher speed rates, the instrument becomes less effective for debridement of tissue but it is more effective for drilling of bone. Oscillation mode is used for tissue debridement and it is around 5000 rotations per minute. Other mode is rotation, it is used for drilling and it is around 15,000 rotations per minute. The sheared bits of debrided tissue are sucked by the suction effect. Microdebrider also improves surgical field by its suction and irrigation mechanism. The Advantages are the preservation of surrounding healthy mucosa, it allows precise tissue removal and decreases surgical time [49]. It is commonly used for the removal of polyp and tumor tissue of nose and paranasal sinuses. Current technology advances have added cauterization of bleeders by delivering bipolar cautery effect via the end of the blade. These blades themselves are surrounded by layers of insulation causing a sandwiching of the inner and outer electrodes [50].

3. Coblator—Coblator term is originated from "Controlled ablation". It is a kind of bipolar radiofrequency ablation that works at relatively low temperatures (typically 60–70 C) by unsettling molecular bonds and allowing tissues to melt [51, 52]. Soft tissue melting makes use of bipolar radiofrequency energy. This energy is made to flow through a conductive medium like normal saline. When current from radiofrequency probe passes through saline medium it breaks saline into sodium and chloride ions. These highly energized ions form a plasma field strong enough to break organic molecular bonds within soft tissue causing its dissolution. The excellent conduc-

tivity of saline is used in this technology. This conductivity is responsible for high energy plasma generation. Low temperature limits the thermal damage to surrounding tissues with a depth of penetration 2–4 mm. The stages of plasma generation are (Fig. 5.25).

(a) First stage is characterized by the transition from bubble to film boiling. This decreases heat emission and causes increase in surface temperature.
(b) Second stage is vapor film pulsation. Tissue ablation occurs during this stage.
(c) Third stage—Reduction of amplitude of current across the electrodes.
(d) Fourth stage: Dissipation of electron energy at the metal electrode surface.
(e) Fifth stage (stage of thermal dissipation of energy): This stage is essentially due to the combination of plasma ions, active atoms, and molecules. Plasma contains H and OH ions. These ions makes plasma destructive. Hydroxy radicals causes protein degradation. When coblation is being used to perform surgery the interface between the plasma and dissected tissue acts as a gate for charged particles.

Radiofrequency generator, foot pedal, irrigation system, and wand are the components of coblator (Fig. 5.26). Radiofrequency (RF) generator generates RF signals. It is managed by the microprocessor. This generator is competent in adjusting the settings as per the type

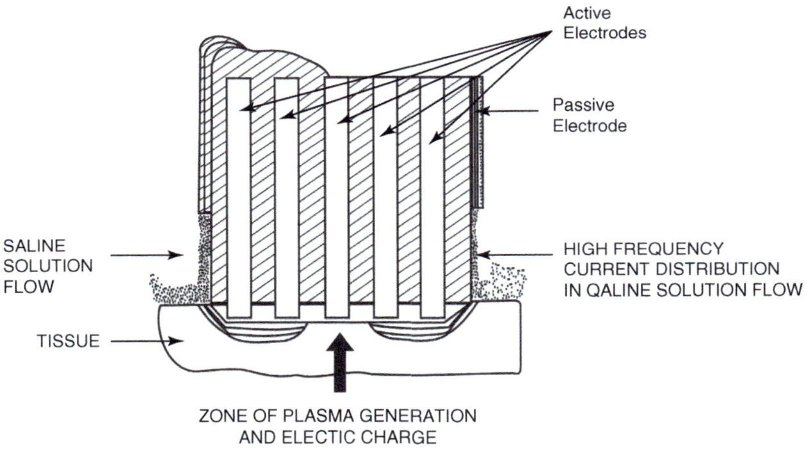

Fig. 5.25 Diagrammatic representation of mechanism in coblation wand. (Coblation wand has two electrodes, i.e., Base electrode and active electrode. These electrodes are separated by ceramic. Saline flows between these two electrodes. Current generated flows between these two electrodes via the saline medium. Saline gets broken down into ions thereby forming active plasma which ablates tissue

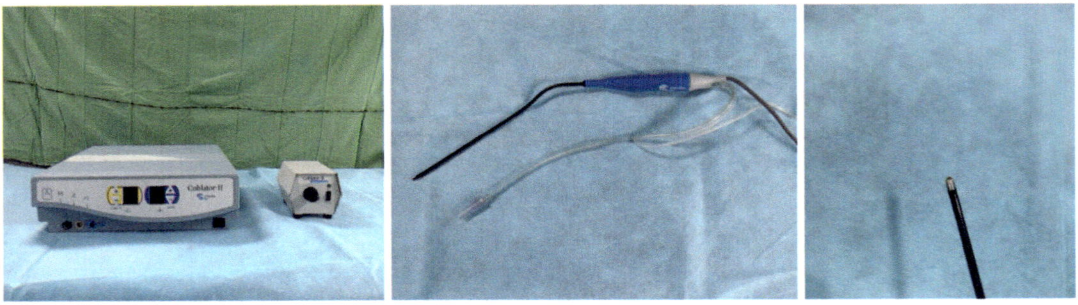

Fig. 5.26 Radio frequency generator, irrigation system and wand (Courtesy—Dr. Hitesh Verma, Associate Professor, AIIMS, New Delhi, India)

of wand inserted. It automatically senses the type of the wand and adjusts settings accordingly. For coblation, the plasma setting is 7 and for cauterization, non-plasma setting is 3. Foot pedal control has two color-coded pedals. The yellow one is for coblation and the blue one is for RF cautery. This device also emits different sounds when these pedals are pressed indicating to the surgeon which mode is getting activated. There are different types of wands available to perform coblation procedure optimally [53–55].

The efficiency of ablation can be improved by its intermittent application, copious irrigation, and by using cold saline. Cold saline can be prepared by placing the saline pack in a refrigerator overnight.

It is primarily useful in adenotonsillectomy, removal of vascular lesion of sinonasal region. The a**dvantages** are less bleeding, limited surrounding tissue damage.

4. *Surgical Navigation System*

   It is also known as image-guided surgery (IGS) and has emerged as a critical tool during the era of endoscopic surgery. Structures in the skull base are either embedded or closely adherent to the bone, making this region ideal for IGS. Steps of image guidance machine for rhinology and skull base surgery are

   (a) Preoperative 0.5–1 mm cuts in all plans of radiology of nose and paranasal sinuses are acquired in CD and it needs to be uploaded in IGS machine.
   (b) The head mount universal tracker is attached to the patient.
   (c) Registration: It relates the patient in OT to pre-op acquired image data sets and is used to establish the relation between two coordinate systems. It is done by using anatomical landmarks that are visible on patient and image data, e.g., Tragus, outer canthus, inner canthus, nasion. The position of the tip of probe is identified by tracking device and coordinates are fed back to navigation software. With the use of fiducial markers the registration process is complete (Fig. 5.27) [56, 57].
   (d) Tracking—It is the mechanism of following the position of patient/instruments within the operative field. It provides dynamic positional information. Tracking system must be precise, consistently accurate, fast enough to provide >25 readings/s, insensitive to changes in air temperature, unaffected by metal objects. Tracking systems are based on either magnetic field or based on infra-red light sensors [58].

The Mechanism is that every point in the patient's sinuses/surface landmarks has *x*, *y*, *z* coordinate (Real coordinates). The patient's CT scan image will also have a corresponding *x*, *y*, *z* coordinates (Virtual coordinates). IGS works by matching and correlating the real and virtual coordinates. It produces 3D localization information for navigation during sur-

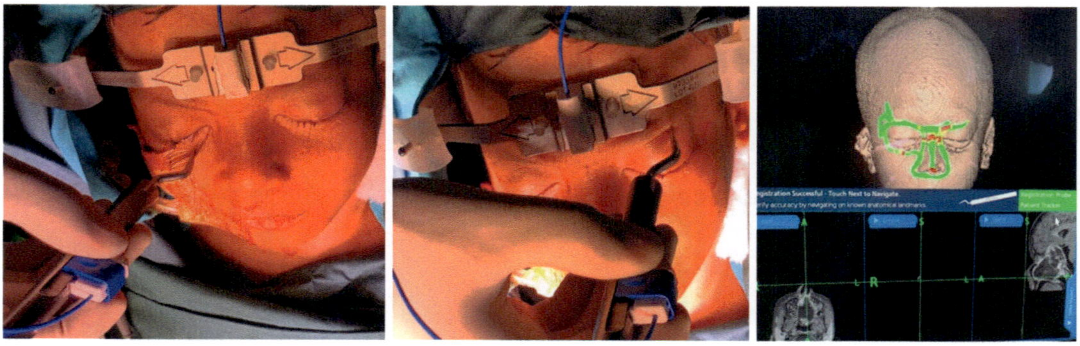

Fig. 5.27 Registration and tracking for navigation system (Courtesy—Dr. Hitesh Verma, Associate Professor, AIIMS, New Delhi, India)

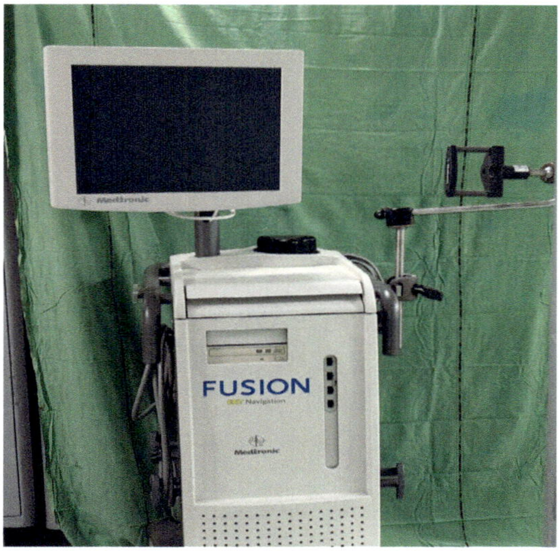

Fig. 5.28 Navigation system (Courtesy—Dr. Hitesh Verma, Associate Professor, AIIMS, New Delhi, India)

gery. The components of navigation system are head-mounted universal tracker, Overhead optical tracking camera, Optical LEDs placed on the universal tracker, navigation pointer and other navigation devices, Monitor and Software: simultaneous view of axial, coronal, and sagittal sections (Fig. 5.28) and the frontal sinus outflow pathway with an orange line. This surgical plan may be imported into the navigation system.

Clinical applications of IGS are in
(a) FESS, esp. revision sinus surgeries because no recognizable anatomical landmarks [59].
(b) Extensive mass lesion of nose and PNS with distorted anatomy.
(c) Extended endoscopic surgery for skull base such as pituitary surgery, nasal tumor with intracranial extension [60].
(d) Excision or drainage of petrous apex and internal auditory meatus tumors by transphenoid approach.

5. *Ultrasonic Aspirator*—It is called by Cavitron ultrasonic surgical aspirator (CUSA). The machine is worked by the mechanism of creation of cavitation. It is a process of creation of the vapor form of liquid when the machine is subjected to diminish pressure at sustained ambient temperature so that boiling of liquid occurs due to pressure reduction. Cavitation is formed on the minus side of a pressure cycle, when the tip of probe is retracting with sufficient frequency and amplitude, resulting in the formation of shock waves. Cells expands and burst by increasing pressure. It is more confined to the tissues with high water proportion such as fat, mass lesion. Blood vessels, nerves, and other healthy tissue mostly unaffected by the process. Gas and fluid are aspirated by negative pressure device. It works by generating the ultrasonic waves up to the range of 23 KHx [61]. The steps for the CUSA application are (Fig. 5.29).
(a) Irrigation fluid came out from handpiece with a speed of 3–40 ml/min. Aspiration of gas and liquid occurs at the tip with a maximum pressure of 500 mmHg.
(b) When the vibrating tip comes in contact with tissue, it breaks cells.
(c) Twenty-four kilo hertz generating handpiece is useful to break tough, fibrous, and calcified tumors while the small 35 kHz handpiece is useful during procedures requiring precision, tactile feedback, and delicate control.
(d) A wide variety of tips enables customization of the handpiece for each procedure, depending on the consistency, location, and depth of the targeted tissue.

Suction and Irrigation mechanism of CUSA draws tissue toward the vibrating tip and creates a tip/tissue pairing effect. It keeps the operating site clear [62, 63]. It can be useful in all kind of surgeries in the field of rhinology and skull base such as inferior turbinoplasty, septoplasty, DCR, FESS, etc. The advantages are safety, reduction in operating time, quality improvement, and facilitation of selective surgeries.

6. *Radiofrequency Ablation*—It acts by ablation with minimally invasive and usually appropriate for inoperable patients with other comorbidities. It requires a less hospital stay or can be performed on an outpatient basis. It preserves more normal healthy tissue [64–66]. RF ablation has been used for the treatment of

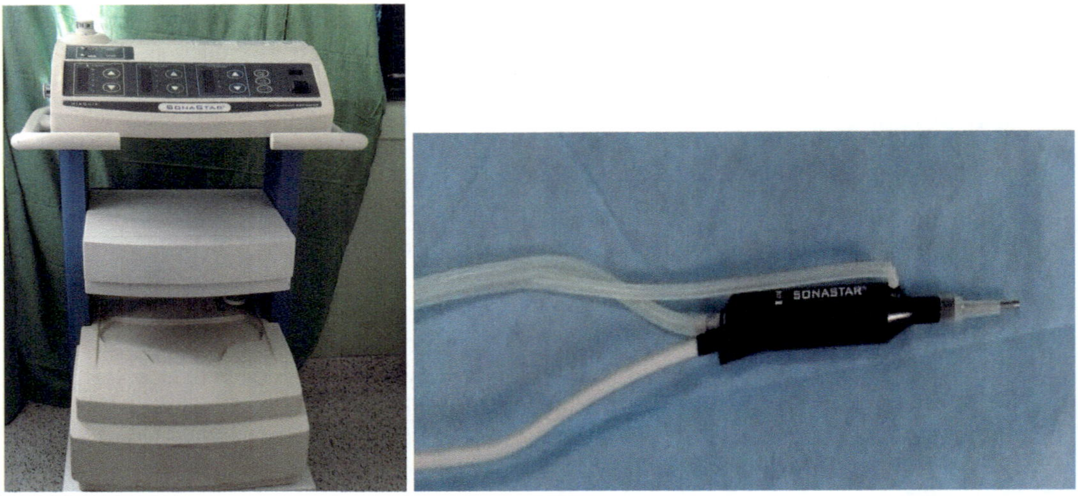

Fig. 5.29 Ultrasonic aspirator (Courtesy—Dr. Hitesh Verma, Associate Professor, AIIMS, New Delhi, India)

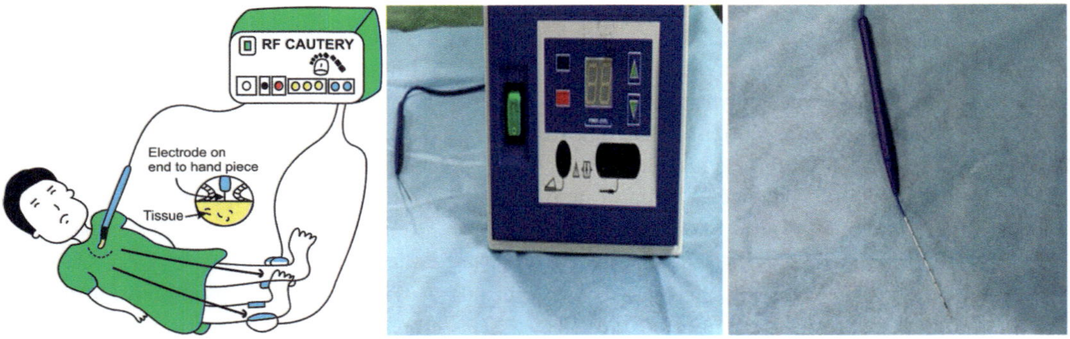

Fig. 5.30 RF ablation circuit and machine (Courtesy for figure **b** and **c** Dr. Hitesh Verma, Associate Professor, AIIMS, New Delhi, India)

various neoplasms, including metastasis from a variety of primary tumors [67, 68]. The act by deposition of power into tumors induces thermal injury resulting in a tumoricidal effect. RF ablation involves the flow of electrical alternating current through tissues whereby ionic shakeup and resistive heating of the tissues occurs. In order to set up this current, the RF ablation system requires a closed-loop circuit comprised of an electrical generator, a needle electrode, a patient (a resistor), and large dispersive electrodes (or "grounding pads") (Fig. 5.30).

The nature of the thermal hurt depends on the tissue temperature and the duration of heating. Successful ablation can only be achieved by optimizing heat production and minimizing heat loss. Successful RF ablation can be reduced when tissues are heated to greater than 100 °C and/or when charring of tissues occurs. An important element of effective ablation is the extent of the ablation zone. In order to assure eradication of microscopic tumoral extensions, the ablation zone needs to include areas beyond the tumor margin. This is called the ablation margin, and safe ablation margins varies depending on the organ being ablated and should preferably be approximately 1 cm. Principles of RF ablation is based on

(a) Joule heating—rapid alternating current (~460–480 kHz) passing through a resistive medium is converted into thermal energy
(b) RF ablation: electrode → tissue → ground pads
(c) AC current → ionic agitation → friction causes tissue heating

RF acts by tissue heating (protein denaturation), tissue boiling (water vaporization and tissue disruption) which leads to breakdown of cell membranes, vascular thrombosis, red cell fragmentation, and cell death. It is primarily used for inferior turbinate reduction. Superficial ulceration of mucosa, crusting, and adhesion are the complications of RF in rhinology.

7. *Hydrodebrider*—The mucosal biofilm formation is the major cause of failure in FESS [69]. It protects bacteria from immune-system and antibiotic penetration [70, 71]. It leads to the generation of strong antimicrobial resistance to usual medical and surgical treatments. Hydrodebrider allows controlled delivery of a shear force to the mucosal surface of the sinonasal cavity and has claimed as a useful adjunct in the disruption of the biofilm structure. It is thought to be worked by providing a controlled shear energy that helps mechanically in dislocation of mucosal biofilm [72]. It consists of an endoscopic suction irrigator with 270° articulation designed to apply irrigation under pressure during sinus surgery. The handpiece delivers a rotating spray of pressurized saline at 5 ml/s, enabling access to all of the sinuses but for frontal sinus, the handpiece includes a streamlined 2.2 mm diameter tip and fixed 80° articulation for accessing the frontal sinus. It works by providing simultaneous suctioning and irrigation. It is important to allow recirculation and avoid pooling of solution. The multidirectional irrigation (five radial and one axial holes) allows the fluid to reach hidden recesses. It is useful to lavage of sinuses and to remove fungal muck in non-invasive fungal sinusitis.

References

1. Chakrabarti A, Denning DW, Ferguson BJ, Ponikau J, Buzina W, Kita H, Marple B, Panda N, Vlaminck S, Kauffmann-Lacroix C, Das A, Singh P, Taj-Aldeen SJ, Kantarcioglu AS, Handa KK, Gupta A, Thungabathra M, Shivaprakash MR, Bal A, Fothergill A, Radotra BD. Fungal rhinosinusitis: a categorization and definitional schema addressing current controversies. Laryngoscope. 2009;119(9):1809–18.
2. Callejas CA, Douglas RG. Fungal rhinosinusitis: what every allergist should know. Clin Exp Allergy. 2013;43(8):835–49.
3. Grosjean P, Weber R. Fungus balls of the paranasal sinuses: a review. Eur Arch Otorhinolaryngol. 2007;264(5):461–70.
4. Chakrabarti A, Rudramurthy SM, Panda N, Das A, Singh A. Epidemiology of chronic fungal rhinosinusitis in rural India. Mycoses. 2015;58(5):294–302.
5. Patterson TF, Thompson GR, Denning DW, et al. Practice guidelines for the diagnosis and management of aspergillosis: 2016 update by the infectious diseases society of America. Clin Infect Dis. 2016;63(4):e1–e60.
6. Cho HJ, Hong SD, Kim HY, Chung SK, Dhong HJ. Clinical implications of serum galactomannan measurement in patients with acute invasive fungal rhinosinusitis. Rhinology. 2016;54(4):336–41.
7. Theel ES, Doern CD. β-D-glucan testing is important for diagnosis of invasive fungal infections. J Clin Microbiol. 2013;51(11):3478–83.
8. Heldt S, Hoenigl M. Lateral flow assays for the diagnosis of invasive aspergillosis: current status. Curr Fungal Infect Rep. 2017;11(2):45–51.
9. Valero C, de la Cruz-Villar L, Zaragoza Ó, Buitrago MJ. New panfungal real-time PCR assay for diagnosis of invasive fungal infections. J Clin Microbiol. 2016;54(12):2910–8.
10. Arvanitis M, Anagnostou T, Fuchs BB, Caliendo AM, Mylonakis E. Molecular and nonmolecular diagnostic methods for invasive fungal infections. Clin Microbiol Rev. 2014;27(3):490–526.
11. Gupta S, Henningsen JA, Wallace MJ, Madoff DC, Morello FA, Ahrar K, et al. Percutaneous biopsy of head and neck lesions with CT guidance: various approaches and relevant anatomic and technical considerations. Radiogr Rev Publ Radiol Soc N Am Inc. 2007;27(2):371–90.

12. Kikuchi K, Yoshiura T, Hiwatashi A, Togao O, Yamashita K, Honda H. Balloon test occlusion of internal carotid artery: Angiographic findings predictive of results. World J Radiol. 2014;6(8):619–24.
13. Krajina A, Chrobok V. Radiological diagnosis and management of epistaxis. Cardiovasc Intervent Radiol. 2014;37(1):26–36.
14. Gandhi D, Gemmete JJ, Ansari SA, Gujar SK, Mukherji SK. Interventional neuroradiology of the head and neck. AJNR Am J Neuroradiol. 2008;29(10):1806–15.
15. Broomfield S, Bruce I, Birzgalis A, Herwadkar A. The expanding role of interventional radiology in head and neck surgery. J R Soc Med. 2009;102(6):228–34.
16. Kulkarni SS, Shetty NS, Dharia TP, Polnaya AM. Pictorial essay: Vascular interventions in extra cranial head and neck. Indian J Radiol Imaging. 2012;22(4):350–7.
17. Fayad LM, Carrino JA, Fishman EK. Musculoskeletal infection: role of CT in the emergency department. Radiographics. 2007;27:1723–1736 (Stacy GS, Kapur A (2011) Mimics of bone and soft tissue neoplasms. Radiol Clin N Am 49:1261–1286.
18. Mohandas A, Marcus C, Kang H, Truong M-T, Subramaniam RM. FDG PET/CT in the management of nasopharyngeal carcinoma. Am J Roentgenol. 2014;203(2):146–57.
19. Kao CH, Hsieh JF, Tsai SC, et al. Comparison of 18-fluoro-2-deoxyglucose positron emission tomography and computed tomography in detection of cervical lymph node metastases of nasopharyngeal carcinoma. Ann Otol Rhinol Laryngol. 2000;109:1130–4.
20. Chong WH, Molinolo AA, Chen CC, Collins MT. Tumor-induced osteomalacia. Endocr Relat Cancer. 2011;18(3):R53–77. https://doi.org/10.1530/ERC-11-0006.
21. Cho K-S, Kang D-W, Kim H-J, Lee J-K, Roh H-J. Differential diagnosis of primary nasopharyngeal lymphoma and nasopharyngeal carcinoma focusing on CT, MRI, and PET/CT. Otolaryngol Head Neck Surg. 2012;146(4):574–8. https://doi.org/10.1177/0194599811143471
22. Thompson L, Wieneke J, Miettinen M. Sinonasal tract and nasopharyngeal melanomas: a clinicopathologic study of 115 cases with a proposed staging system. Am J Surg Pathol. 2003;27:594–611.
23. Swetter S, Carroll L, Johnson D, Segall G. Positron emission tomography is superior to computed tomography for metastatic detection in melanoma patients. Ann Surg Oncol. 2002;9:646–53.
24. Goerres GW, Stoeckli SJ, von Schulthess GK, Steinert HC. FDG PET for mucosal malignant melanoma of the head and neck. Laryngoscope. 2002;112(2):381–5.
25. Howell MC, Branstetter BF, Snyderman CH. Patterns of regional spread for esthesioneuroblastoma. AJNR Am J Neuroradiol. 2011;32:929–33. https://doi.org/10.3174/ajnr.A2401.
26. Sasajima T, Kinouchi H, Tomura N, Watara J, Mizoi K. High uptake of ^{123}I-metaiodobenzylguanidine related to olfactory neuroblastoma revealed by single-photon emission CT. Am J Neuroradiol. 2000;21(4):717–20.
27. Dublin AB, Bobinski M. Imaging characteristics of olfactory neuroblastoma (Esthesioneuroblastoma). J Neurol Surg B Skull Base. 2015;77(1):1–5.
28. Wu H-b, Wang Q-s, Zhong J-m, Zhou W-l, Li H-s, Qiao-yu W. Preliminary study on the evaluation of olfactory neuroblastoma using PET/CT. Clin Nucl Med. 2011;36:894–8.
29. Watanabe N, Nakanishi Y, Kinukawa N, et al. Expressions of somatostatin receptor subtypes (SSTR-1, 2, 3, 4 and 5) in neuroblastic tumors; special reference to clinicopathological correlations with international neuroblastoma pathology classification and outcomes. Acta Histochem Cytochem. 2014;47(5):219–29.
30. Savelli G, Bartolomei M, Bignardi M. Somatostatin receptors imaging and therapy in a patient affected by esthesioneuroblastoma with meningeal metastases. A classic example of theranostic approach. J Neurooncol. 2016;127:617–9. https://doi.org/10.1007/s11060-016-2067-3.
31. Pavlidis N, Briasoulis E, Hainsworth J, Greco FA. Diagnostic and therapeutic management of cancer of an unknown primary. Eur J Cancer. 2003;39(14):1990–2005.
32. Cianchetti M, Mancuso AA, Amdur RJ, Werning JW, Kirwan J, Morris CG, Mendenhall W. Diagnostic evaluation of squamous cell carcinoma metastatic to cervical lymph nodes from an unknown head and neck primary site. Laryngoscope. 2009;119(12):2348–54.
33. Calabrese L, Jereczek-Fossa BA, Jassem J, et al. Diagnosis and management of neck metastases from an unknown primary. Acta Otorhinolaryngol Ital. 2005;25(1):2–12.
34. Ross GL, Soutar DS. Sentinel node biopsy in head and neck cancer: preliminary results of a multicenter trial. Ann Surg Oncol. 2004;11:690–6.
35. Ene P, Popescu RC, Voiculescu S, et al. Sentinel lymph node — work hypothesis in sinonasal carcinoma treatment. Maedica (Buchar). 2011;6(4):308–12.
36. Scott B. In: Tille PM, editor. Bailey & Scott's diagnostic microbiology. 13th ed: Elsevier Mosby; 2014.
37. Bennett JE, Dolin R, Blaser MJ, editors. Mandell: Mandell, Douglas and Bennett's principles and practice of infectious diseases. 8th ed: Elsevier; 2015.
38. Kasper DL, Fauci AS, Hauser SL, Longo DL, Jameson JL, Loscalzo J (eds) Harrison: Harrison's principles of internal medicine, 19th ed. McGraw Hill; 2015.
39. Garcia LS, Isenberg HD, editors. Isenberg: clinical microbiology procedural handbook. 2nd edition update. ASM Press; 2007.
40. Lee VS, Davis GE. Culture-directed topical antibiotic treatment for chronic rhinosinusitis. Am J Rhinol Allergy. 2016;30(6):414–7. https://doi.org/10.2500/ajra.2016.30.4380.
41. Rom D, Bassiouni A, Eykman E, et al. The association between disease severity and microbiome in chronic

rhinosinusitis. Laryngoscope. 2019;129(6):1265–73. https://doi.org/10.1002/lary.27726.
42. Aring AM, Chan MM. Current concepts in adult acute rhinosinusitis. Am Fam Physician. 2016;94(2):97–105.
43. Liu P, Lu L, Xu M, et al. A novel multiplex PCR for virus detection by melting curve analysis. J Virol Methods. 2018;262:56–60. https://doi.org/10.1016/j.jviromet.2018.09.010.
44. Chandra RK, Conley DB, Kern RC. Evolution of the endoscope and endoscopic sinus surgery. Otolaryngol Clin N Am. 2009;42(5):747–52.
45. Marsh BR. Historic development of broncho-esophagology. Otolaryngol Head Neck Surg. 1996;114(6):689–716.
46. Wootton C. Digital image formats, Chapter 6. In: A practical guide to video and audio compression: from sprockets and rasters to macro blocks. Burlington, MA: Focal Press; 2005. p. 115–46.
47. Sindwani R, Manz R. Technological innovations in tissue removal during rhinologic surgery. Am J Rhino Allergy. 2012;26(1):65–9.
48. Beswick DM, Rodriguez KD, Olds CE, et al. Quantification of maxillary sinus accessibility via a middle meatal antrostomy. Am J Rhinol Allergy. 2015;29(5):394–6.
49. Selivanova O, Kuehnemund M, Mann WJ, Amedee RG. Comparison of conventional instruments and mechanical debriders for surgery of patients with chronic sinusitis. Am J Rhinol. 2003;17(4):197–202.
50. Kumar N, Sindwani R. Bipolar microdebrider may reduce intraoperative blood loss and operative time during nasal polyp surgery. Ear Nose Throat J. 2012;91(8):336–44.
51. Grobler A, Carney AS. Radiofrequency coblation tonsillectomy. Br J Hosp Med (Lond). 2006;67(6):309–12.
52. Coblation product brochure. https://www.smith--nephew.com/global/assets/pdf/products/surgical/sportsmedicine/08427f%20multi-electrode %20technology%20brochure.pdf. Accessed July 30, 2016.
53. Sergeev VN, Belov SV. Coblation technology: a new method for high frequency electrosurgery. Biomed Eng. 2003;37(1):22–5.
54. Belov SV. Use of high-frequency cold plasma ablation technology for electrosurgery with minimized invasiveness. Biomed Eng. 2004;38(2):80–5.
55. Qi B, Ren C, Wang D, Li SZ, Wang K, Zhang Y. Uniform glow like plasma source assisted by preionization of spark in ambient air at atmospheric pressure. Appl Phys Lett. 2006;89:131503.
56. Albritton FD, Kingdom TI, DelGaudio JM. Malleable registration mask: application of a novel registration method in image guided sinus surgery. Am J Rhinol. 2001;15:219–24.
57. Raabe A, Krishnan R, Wolff R, Hermann E, Zimmermann M, Seifert V. Laser surface scanning for patient registration in intracranial image-guided surgery. Neurosurgery. 2002;50:797–801. discussion 802–3
58. Azuma R, Bishop G. Improving static and dynamic registration in an optical see-through hmd. In: Proceedings of the 21st annual conference on computer graphics and interactive techniques. New York: ACM Press; 1994. p. 197–204.
59. Metson R. Image-guided sinus surgery: lessons learned from the first 1000 cases. Otolaryngol Head Neck Surg. 2003;128:8–13.
60. Neumann AM Jr, Pasquale-Niebles K, Bhuta T, Sillers MJ. Image-guided transnasal endoscopic surgery of the paranasal sinuses and anterior skull base. Am J Rhinol. 1999;13:449–54.
61. Chan KK, Watmough DJ, Hope DT, Moir K. A new motor-driven surgical probe and its in vitro comparison with the Cavitron Ultrasonic Surgical Aspirator. Ultrasound Med Biol. 1986;12:279–83.
62. Deppe G, Malviya VK, Malone JM Jr. Use of Cavitron Ultrasonic Surgical Aspirator (CUSA) for palliative resection of recurrent gynecologic malignancies involving the vagina. Eur J Gynaecol Oncol. 1989;10:1–2.
63. Chopp RT, Shah BB, Addonizio JC. Use of ultrasonic surgical aspirator in renal surgery. Urology. 1983;22:157–9.
64. Gillams AR. The use of radiofrequency in cancer. Br J Cancer. 2005;92:1825–9.
65. Gillams A. Tumor ablation: current role in the kidney, lung and bone. Cancer Imaging. 2009;9:68–70.
66. Bilchik AJ, Rose DM, Allegra DP, Bostick PJ, Hsueh E, Morton DL. Radiofrequency ablation: a minimally invasive technique with multiple applications. Cancer J Sci Am. 1999;5:356–61.
67. Lencioni R, Crocetti L, Cioni R, et al. Response to radiofrequency ablation of pulmonary tumours: a prospective, intention-to-treat, multicentre clinical trial (the RAPTURE study). Lancet Oncol. 2008;9:621–8.
68. Dupuy DE, Mayo-Smith WW, Abbott GF, DiPetrillo T. Clinical applications of radiofrequency tumor ablation in the thorax. Radiographics. 2002;22:259–69.
69. Potera C. Forging a link between biofilms and disease. Science. 1999;283:1837–9.
70. Cavaliere R, Ball JL, Turnbull L, Whitchurch CB. The biofilm matrix destabilizers, EDTA and DNaseI, enhance the susceptibility of nontypeable Hemophilus influenzae biofilms to treatment with ampicillin and ciprofloxacin. Microbiology. 2014;3:557–67.
71. Berlanga M, Gomez-Perez L, Guerrero R. Biofilm formation and antibiotic susceptibility in dispersed cells versus planktonic cells from clinical, industry and environmental origins. Antonie Van Leeuwenhoek. 2017;110:1691–704.
72. Valentine R, Jervis-Bardy J, Psaltis A, Tan LW, Wormald PJ. Efficacy of using a hydrodebrider and of citric acid/zwitterionic surfactant on a Staphylococcus aureus bacterial biofilm in the sheep model of rhinosinusitis. Am J Rhinol Allergy. 2011;25:323–6.

Tumours of Nose and Paranasal Sinuses

6

Gyan Nayak, Hitesh Verma, Rakesh Kumar, Rupa Mehta, Nikhil Singh, Kuldeep Thakur, Kapil Sikka, Anchal Kakkar, and Deepali Jain

Contents

G. Nayak
ENT, PGIMER, Chandigarh, India

H. Verma (✉) · R. Kumar · K. Thakur · K. Sikka
ENT, AIIMS, New Delhi, India
e-mail: drhitesh10@gmail.com

R. Mehta · N. Singh
ENT, AIIMS, Raipur, Chhattisgarh, India

A. Kakkar · D. Jain
Pathology, AIIMS, New Delhi, India

H. Verma, A. Thakar (eds.), *Essentials of Rhinology*, https://doi.org/10.1007/978-981-33-6284-0_6

6.1 Part A: Benign Lesions of Nose and Paranasal Sinuses

6.1.1 Introduction

The benign tumours of the nose and paranasal sinus represents a vast and varied group of lesions. These tumours are often diagnosed late due to their rarity of the condition and similar presentation to chronic rhinosinusitis. These lesions are usually indolent and diagnosis can be delayed. It is prudent to consider the diagnosis of benign tumours of the nose and paranasal sinuses in the setting of unilateral nasal symptoms with bleeding. With the advent of endoscopes, instrumentation, and navigation system, it is possible to detect in the early stage and initiate safe treatment thus, reducing morbidity.

6.1.2 Clinical Presentation

The clinical presentation in the majority of the condition mimics the symptoms of chronic rhinosinusitis like nasal obstruction, nasal discharge, postnasal drip, hyposmia, or anosmia. Nasal bleeding can be seen in vascular tumours and inverted papilloma. Facial deformity, telecanthus can be seen in fibrosseous lesions of maxillofacial bones. Although visual symptoms are rare but visual blurring and diplopia can be presenting complaints due to the pressure effect on the orbital contents. WHO classified Sinonasal tumours according to their tissues of origin viz. epithelial, mesenchymal, hematolymphoid, neural, germ cell tumours, and other tumour-like conditions like reparative granuloma [1].

6.1.3 Benign Tumours of Epithelial Origin Sinonasal Papilloma

6.1.3.1 Inverted Papilloma (Shneiderian Papilloma, Inverting Type)

WHO has classified sinonasal papilloma into three histopathological subgroups: exophytic papilloma, inverted papilloma (IP), and oncocytic papilloma [1]. Inverted papilloma is the most common tumour among these subgroups.

IP is also known as Ringertz tumour or Schneiderian papilloma, and arises from the lateral nasal wall and is a locally aggressive tumour with the tendency to recur after its excision. These tumours were first described by Ward in 1884 and later characterised by Ringertz in 1935. Inverted papillomas constitute 0.5–4% of sinonasal tumours and the chances of turning into malignancy reaches up to 5% [2]. Males are more commonly affected with M:F ratio of 3.4:1 and commonly presents in the 6th–7th decade of life. The various risk factors associated with inverted papilloma are nickel, organic solvents, welding fumes, etc. [3, 4] A close association between the human papillomavirus (HPV) and inverted papilloma has also been suggested but the evidence is inadequate to validate its role in its etiopathogenesis [5].

Histologically, the classical hallmark appearance is digitiform proliferation of squamous epithelium into the underlying stroma with an intact basement membrane. There is well-differentiated columnar or ciliated respiratory epithelium with variable degrees of squamous differentiation [6].

HPV and Inverted Papilloma The role of HPV and inverted papilloma has been studied to find out its correlation in its etiopathogenesis. Kashima et al. suggested on the basis of polymerase chain reaction detection of HPV DNA in specimens to be etiologically related to sinonasal papillomas, inverted papillomas, and squamous cell carcinomas [5]. McLachlin et al., in a study of 22 patients, found HPV DNA to be present in inverted papilloma as well as its association with squamous cell carcinoma (SCC), which suggested its role in the etiopathogenesis and malignant transformation [7]. Retrospective studies have concluded that HPV infection might represent the initiation in the oncogenesis of inverted papilloma [8, 9].

In contradiction to the above studies, many studies have shown conflicting evidence. Kraft et al. detected HPV-11 in only 1 out of 29 inverted papillomas. There was no evidence of HPV where inverted papilloma is associated with SCC [10]. A study of 66 patients did show HPV isolation; however, subsequent analysis revealed that the presence of HPV DNA was neither a statistically significant predictor of the recurrence of inverted papilloma nor was it a statistically significant risk factor for associated SCCs [11]. These conflicting findings suggest that HPV may represent mere incidental colonisation rather than a causative agent.

6.1.4 Clinical Presentation

The common symptoms include nasal obstruction and epistaxis. Larger tumour size may present with facial swelling and visual symptoms. The diagnostic nasal endoscopy reveals vascular, friable multilobulated mass filling the nasal cavity, arising from the lateral nasal wall near the osteomeatal complex (Fig. 6.1). Tumour mass can extend into the maxillary and ethmoid sinus. Krause has classified the tumour depending on its extension (Table 6.1) [12]. Contrast-enhanced computed tomography shows remodelling and focal erosion and may show focal hyperostosis at the attachment site (site of origin). A convoluted, "cerebriform," pattern is characteristic of inverted papilloma on T2/STIR and post-gadolinium T1-weighted MR images (Fig. 6.2) [13].

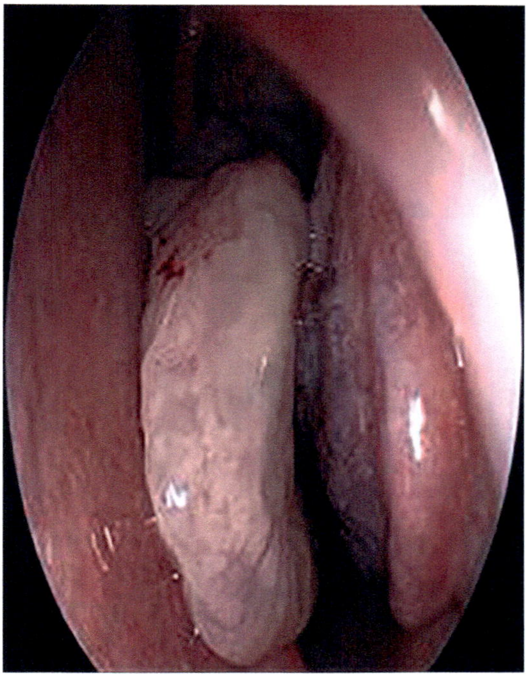

Fig. 6.1 The inverted papilloma arising from the left osteomeatal complex

Table 6.1 Krouse's classification of inverted papilloma

Stage	Tumour extension
1	Disease limited to the nasal cavity
2	Disease extends to ethmoid sinus and medial and superior wall of maxillary sinus
3	Tumour involves lateral and inferior aspects of the maxillary sinus or extension into the frontal or sphenoid sinus
4	Extranasal extension or malignancy

Medial maxillectomy has been the standard of care for inverted papillomas for many decades. Lateral rhinotomy or sublabial approach is still being used to access the tumour in resource-limited settings. Currently, endoscopic Denker is the preferred approach for medial maxillectomy [14–16]. Endoscopic Denker approach involves

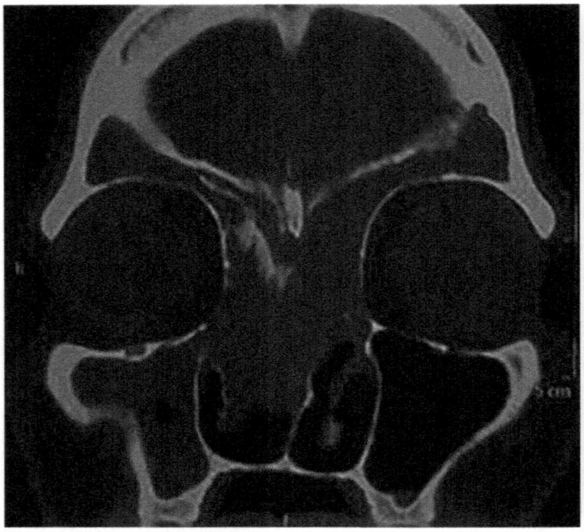
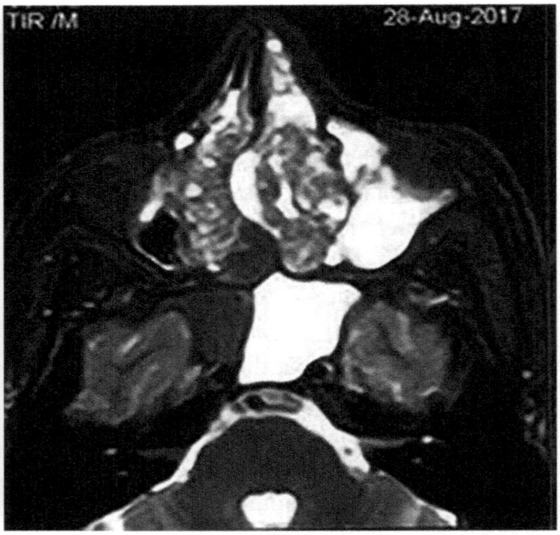

Fig. 6.2 NCCT PNS orbit (coronal cut) is showing homogenous mass filling both side frontal, ethmoid sinuses with focal hyperostosis (black arrow) in the region of the right frontal outflow tract. The right maxillary sinus is also filled up by secretions as the ostium is not wide and air–fluid level is visible within the sinus. MRI Nose and PNS (axial cut) are showing characteristic "cerebriform" pattern (black arrow) in nasal cavity and ethmoid sinuses. (Courtesy—Dr. Hitesh Verma, Associate Professor, AIIMS, New Delhi, India)

drilling of the thick bone of the lateral wall of the pyriform aperture from the anteromedial part of the maxillary sinus. This significantly improves the surgical accessibility to the posterolateral wall and infratemporal fossa. The commonly reported complications are bleeding, infraorbital hypoesthesia, epiphora, orbital fat exposure, alar collapse, etc.

Radiation therapy as adjuvant therapy is used for local recurrences at some centres, but this remains controversial [17]. However, regular follow-up and subsequent surgical management remains the treatment option for the vast majority of recurrent cases.

6.1.5 Schneiderian Papilloma (Oncocytic Type)

These types of papilloma are a variant of Schneiderian papilloma where the columnar cell lining have oncocytic features. The high content of cytochrome C oxidase and mitochondria establishes this oncocytic appearance. Other synonyms are cylindrical cell papilloma, columnar cell papilloma [1]. In contrast to inverted papilloma, there is equal distribution among the sexes and HPV has not been isolated from these variants.

6.1.6 Schneiderian Papilloma (Exophytic Type)

These are the papillomas arising from the Schneiderian membrane with rich papillary fronds and fibrovascular cores covered by layers of epithelium [1]. Other synonyms are transitional cell papilloma, fungiform papilloma, septal papilloma. These tumours are more commonly seen in men (2–10 times) between 20–50 years of age. In contrast to inverted papilloma, these variants are localised more on the lower anterior nasal septum with no significant lateralisation. They are infrequent on the lateral nasal wall. Malignant change in exophytic papilloma is rare.

6.1.7 Salivary Gland Adenoma

Only 25% of glandular tumours are benign in the nose and paranasal sinus tract. The common veining tumours are pleomorphic adenoma, myoepithelioma, and oncocytoma. Pleomorphic adenoma presents with non-specific signs and symptoms like nasal obstruction, discharge, and occasional bleeding. These are more common between 20 and 50 years of age. Most of the cases arise from the submucosa of the bony and cartilaginous part of the nasal septum. Treatment is surgical with wide local excision.

6.1.8 Benign Tumours of Bony and Cartilaginous Origin

6.1.8.1 Osteoma

Osteomas are benign, slow-growing osteoblastic lesions and the most common type of benign sinonasal tumours [18]. They are incidental findings on computed tomography of patients with sinus symptoms. These tumours are mostly asymptomatic and occasionally present with symptoms of headache, nasal discharge, epiphora, forehead swelling, ocular pain, etc. The most common location of osteoma is in the frontal sinus followed by ethmoid, maxillary, and more rarely the sphenoid sinus (Fig. 6.3). However, rarely, the turbinates can be involved causing obstruction to frontal recess, nasolacrimal duct and can also lead to mucocele formation. Osteomas have slight male preponderance and are usually diagnosed between the second and fifth decades.

These tumours are histologically divided into three categories as shown in Table 6.2 [19]. Osteomas can also be associated with Gardner syndrome, a form of familial adenomatous polyposis with epidermoid cysts, lipomas, and desmoid tumours [20]. High-resolution computed tomography of paranasal sinus and orbit assesses the site of attachment and gauges the extent of the lesion. Differential diagnosis of nasal osteoma includes other fibroosseous lesions like fibrous dysplasia and ossifying fibroma.

Table 6.2 Histological types of osteoma

Types of osteoma	Histology
Ivory osteoma	Lobulated, made of compact dense bone containing a minimal amount of fibrous tissue
Mature osteoma	Spongy, mature bone with conspicuous fibrous tissue
Mixed osteoma	Findings of both ivory and mature osteoma

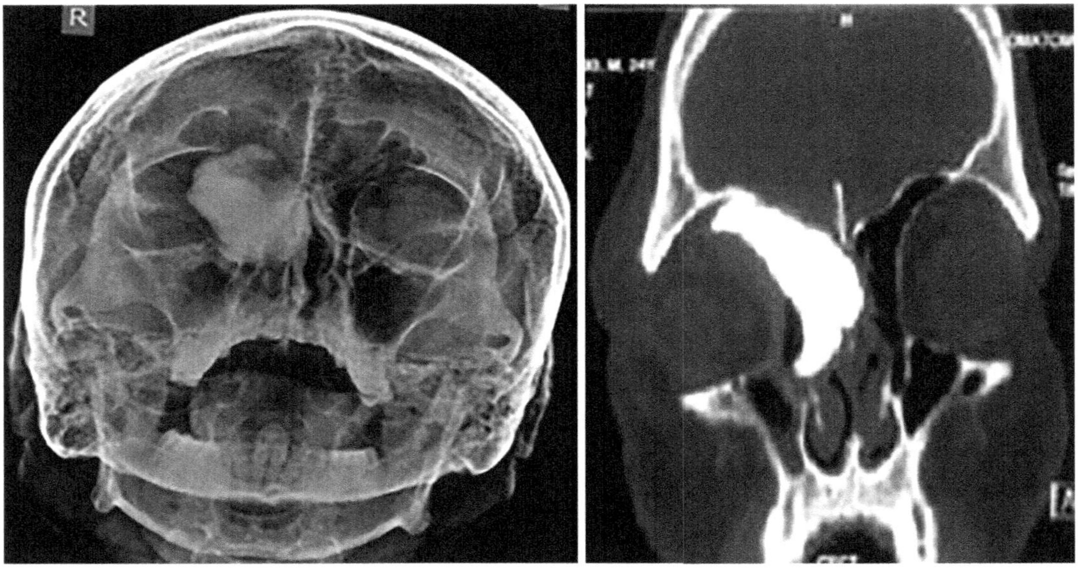

Fig. 6.3 Water's view is showing radio-opaque mass in the region of the right ethmoid and frontal sinus floor. NCCT PNS orbit (Coronal cut) is showing ivory osteoma of the right anterior ethmoid region. (Courtesy—Dr. Hitesh Verma, Associate Professor, AIIMS, New Delhi, India)

Treatment of osteoma depends upon the signs and symptoms. These tumours are slow-growing in nature and there is a general consensus in favour of a wait-and-watch policy provided there are no symptoms and the lesion does not encroach critical structures like optic nerve, orbit, frontal mucocele, facial deformity. Local resection by endoscopic or external approach is the treatment of choice.

6.1.8.2 Chondroma

Chondromas are extremely rare and any cartilaginous tumour more than 2 cm in this site should be considered potentially malignant unless proven otherwise.

6.1.9 Fibroosseus Lesion

Fibroosseous lesions comprise a diverse group of conditions of cranio facial skeleton which includes developmental lesions, reactive or dysplastic lesions, and neoplasms. These lesions are characterised by the replacement of normal bone by variable fibroblastic connective tissue matrix [21]. The WHO and Eversole classification of fibroosseous lesions is shown in Table 6.3 and Table 6.4, respectively [1, 22].

6.1.9.1 Fibrous Dysplasia

Fibrous dysplasia (FD) is a benign dysplastic skeletal lesion where the normal bone is replaced by disorganised and immature bony and fibrous tissue. FD may affect a single bone (monostotic) or more than one bones (polyostotic). Monostotic FD is more common in the craniofacial skeleton with the maxilla affected more commonly than the mandible. Polyostotic FD may be associated

Table 6.3 WHO classification of fibroosseous lesions

Fibroosseous conditions	Subtypes
Ossifying fibroma	
Fibrous dysplasia	
Osseous dysplasia	(a) Periodical osseous dysplasia, focal osseous dysplasia, florid osseous dysplasia, familial gigantiform cementoma
Central giant cell granuloma	
Cherubism	
Aneurysmal bone cyst	
Solitary bone cyst	

Table 6.4 Eversole classification of fibroosseous lesions

Fibrosooesus pathology	Disease	Subtypes
1. Bone dysplasia	a. Fibrous dysplasia	i. Monostotic
		Ii. Polyostotic
		Iii. Polyostotic with endocrinopathy (McCune–Albright syndrome)
	b. Osteitis deformans/Paget's disease	
	c. Pagetoid heritable bone dysplasia of childhood	
	d. Segmental odontomaxillary dysplasia	
2. Cemento-osseous dysplasia	a. Focal cemento-osseous dysplasia	
	b. Florid cemento-osseous dysplasia	
3. Nflammatory/reactive process	a. Focal sclerosing osteomyelitis	
	b. Diffuse sclerosing osteomyelitis	
	c. Proliferative periostitis	
4. Metabolic disease	Hyperparathyroidism	
5. Neoplastic conditions	a. Ossifying fibroma	
	b. Juvenile ossifying fibroma	i. Trabecular
		ii. Psammomatoid
	c. Gigantiform cemetoma	

with endocrine abnormality and skin pigmentation and this variant is known as McCune–Albright syndrome [23].

FD occurs in the first two decades of life with equal preponderance in males and females. The most common symptoms are painless swelling and asymmetry of the facial skeleton. Involvement of nose, paranasal sinuses, and foramina of the skull base, orbit can cause symptoms such as nasal obstruction, headache, proptosis, visual abnormality, hyposmia/anosmia. Diagnosis of this condition requires clinical, radiological, and histological assessment. Key radiological features on CT scan show radiolucent/radiopaque depending upon the degree of calcification leading to a typical "ground glass" appearance (Fig. 6.4). This mottling appearance blends with the surrounding normal bones with ill-defined margins [24].

Histological feature depends upon the grade of ossification and calcification within the immature matrix and the trabeculae assumes classic "Chinese figure script" pattern [22, 23]. These lesions tend to become quiescent after puberty. Only cosmetic deformity can be corrected by surgical contouring of the affected site. However, continuous growth in later life with visual symptoms will require surgical decompression of the optic nerve [25, 26].

6.1.9.2 Ossifying Fibroma

Ossifying fibroma are true benign tumours among all the fibroosseous lesions. Ossifying fibroma of craniofacial skeleton divided into following types:

- Ossifying fibroma of Odontogenic origin (Cemento-ossifying fibroma)
- Juvenile Ossifying fibroma (JOF)
  - (a) Trabecular Juvenile Ossifying fibroma (TrJOF)
  - (b) Psammomatoid Juvenile Ossifying fibroma (PsJOF)
- Gigantiform cementoma

Ossifying fibromas are generally unifocal lesions except the gigantiform cementoma which are typically multifocal in presentation [22, 23]. Radiologically OF are well-defined unilocular mass and due to the expansile nature, the cortex is thinned out (Fig. 6.5). The radiolucency on computed tomography scan can vary and depends upon the degree of calcification. Treatment is usually surgical excision by enucleation or curettage. The recurrence rate is low in most of the cases.

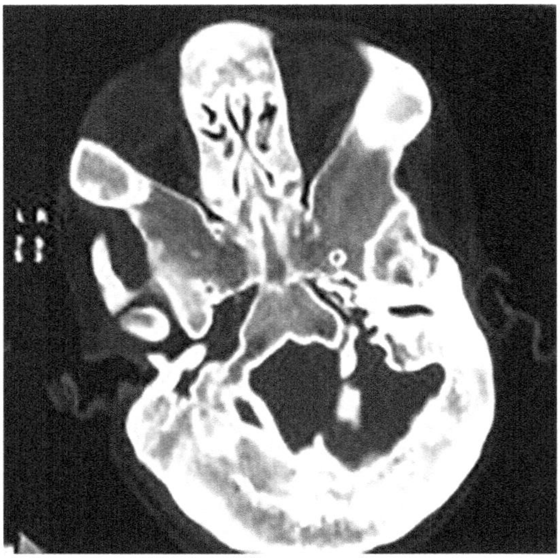

Fig. 6.4 NCCT Head is showing fibrous dysplasia involving all skull base bones. (Courtesy—Dr. Hitesh Verma, Associate Professor, AIIMS, New Delhi, India)

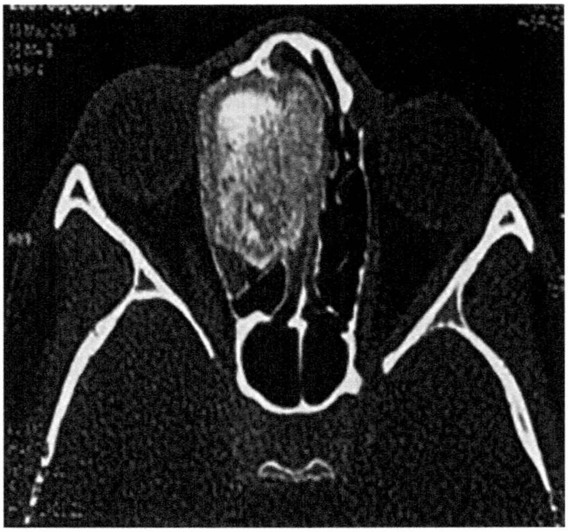

Fig. 6.5 Unilocular expansile mass lesion in right anterior ethmoid region. It is pushing lamina papyracea and eyeball laterally

6.1.10 Benign Vascular Tumours

6.1.10.1 Lobular Capillary Haemangioma (Pyogenic Granuloma)

Sinonasal haemangioma accounts for up to 25% of non-epithelial neoplasms in this region. Lobular capillary haemangioma are benign vascular lesions and are also known as haemangiomatous granuloma, granuloma gravidarum, granulation tissue-type haemangioma, etc. The term "pyogenic granuloma" is a misnomer as neither there is any infective aetiology nor any granuloma formation [27].

A lobular capillary haemangioma is a circumscribed lesion comprising lobules of capillaries lined by endothelial cells and supported by prominent pericytes. The lobules are separated by fibro-myxoid stroma with few mitotic figures but never atypical [28]. Most commonly affects women in their second to third decade of life. This can be explained by the high incidence of pregnancy during this time period. These tumours may occur during the first trimester of pregnancy, but the incidence increases until the seventh month of pregnancy. They occur in approximately 2% of all pregnant females with the most common presentation being a rapidly growing nasal mass with recurrent epistaxis. The most frequently affected site is the septum followed by the turbinate and the sinuses [29].

Management of these lesions depends upon the timing and severity of presentation. Most of them resolve spontaneously after the end of pregnancy. Surgical intervention is considered in patients with multiple episodes of epistaxis or whose lesions fail to resolve after pregnancy. Endoscopic surgical resection and cauterisation is the standard of care with a high success rate [30, 31].

6.1.11 Other Rare Lesions

1- Neurogenic tumours

Neurofibroma and schwannoma are the neurogenic benign tumour of the nose and paranasal sinuses. Neurogenic tumours are a relatively rare entity of this region. Maxillary sinus is the most common site of origin. Symptomatology is the same with other benign lesions and surgical excision is the treatment of choice.

2- Dermoid

Dermoid cyst is the commonest midline congenital mass lesion of the nasal dorsum. It is formed due to incomplete obliteration of neuroectoderm of frontonasal region. It can present in the form of cyst, sinus, and fistula with or without intracranial extension (Fig. 6.6). Both CT and MRI are required to assess tract extent and for treatment plan (Fig. 6.7). The presence of bifid crista raised the possibility of intracranial extension of the tract. MRI of the skull base region is required in such suspected cases to map the tract extent. External rhinoplasty, vertical midline, lateral rhinotomy, horizontal trans-nasal, and endoscopic approaches are used to excise the nasal part of the tract. The choice of approach depends on the external opening of the tract. Neurosurgical team is required to excise the intracranial part [32].

6.2 Part B: Angiofibroma, Its Medical and Surgical Management

Angiofibroma is first described by Hippocrates in the fifth century. Other names are, e.g., juvenile nasopharyngeal angiofibroma, nasopharyngeal fibroma, juvenile angiofibroma. It accounts for 0.05% of all head and neck tumours. It is more prevalent in familial adenomatous polyposis (FAP) group patients. It is a benign, locally aggressive unencapsulated vascular tumour. It has both vascular and fibrous elements. Various authors proposed different theories for its origin. The most recent and accepted theory is that it is a vascular malformation and maybe it arises from persistent tissue of the first branchial artery. The nasopharynx is the most common site of involvement. It takes origin from sphenopalatine foreman and extends medially in the nasal cavity, laterally into pterygopalatine fossa, and superiorly into the cranial cavity. The symptomatology can vary from unilateral nasal obstruction to life-threatening epistaxis. It appears grossly as

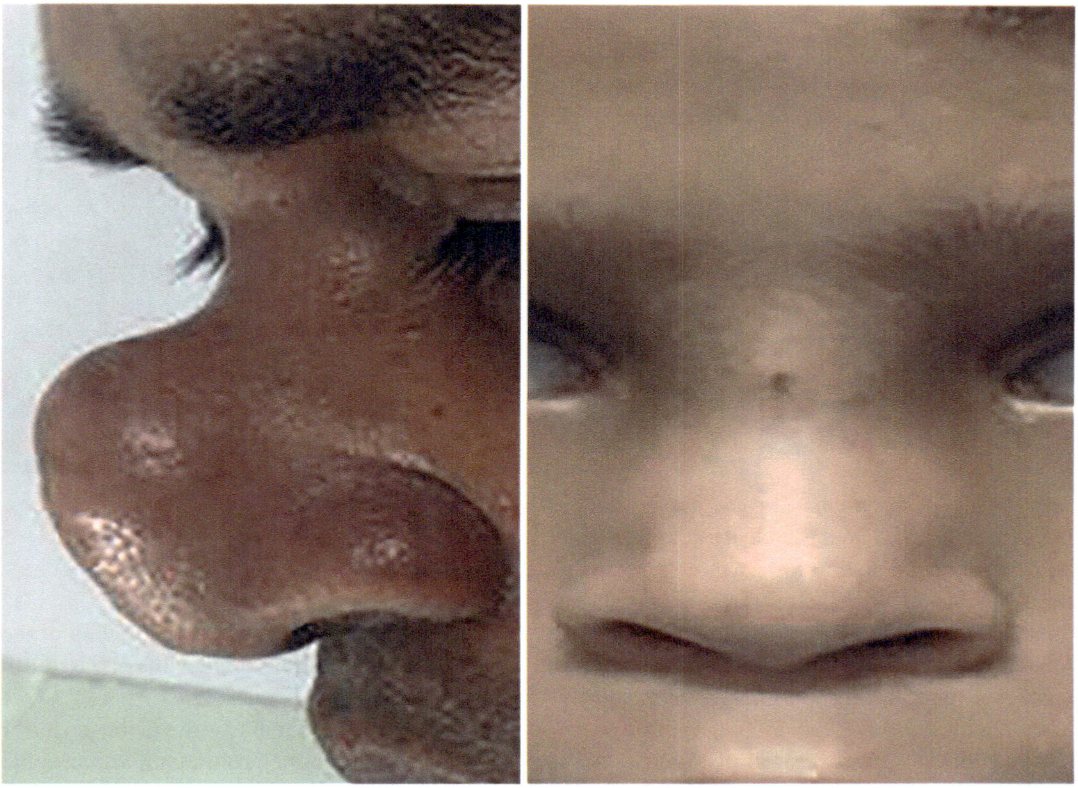

Fig. 6.6 Clinical photographs are showing cystic, fistulous external presentation. (Courtesy—Dr. Hitesh Verma, Associate Professor, AIIMS, New Delhi, India)

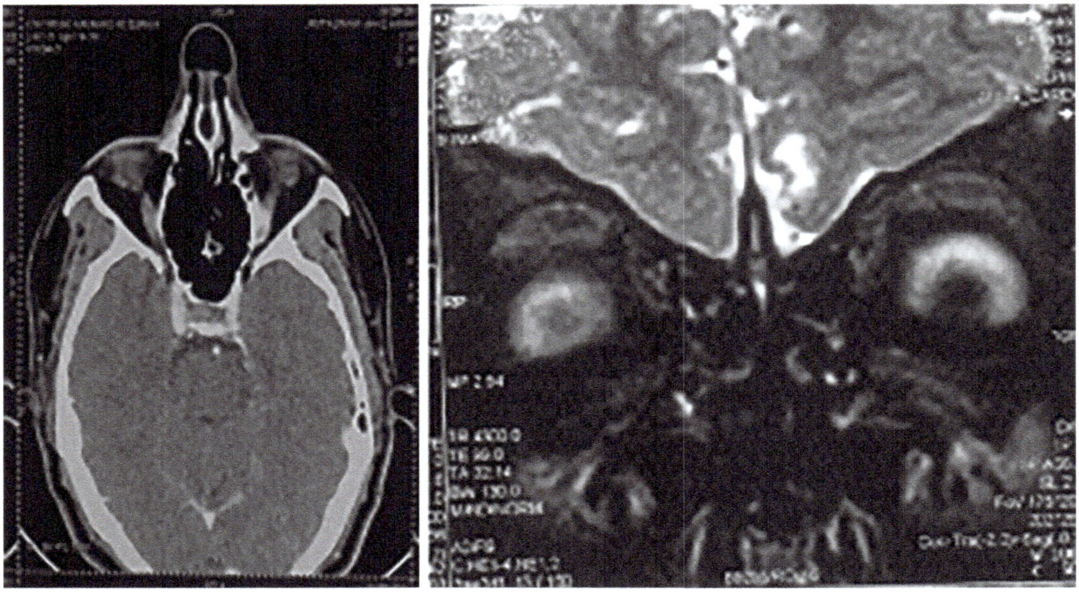

Fig. 6.7 NCCT PNS is showing bifid crista galli and corresponding MRI is not showing intracranial extension of tract. (Courtesy—Dr. Hitesh Verma, Associate Professor, AIIMS, New Delhi, India)

pinkish-grey colour lobular mass. Microscopically, blood vessels are immature with poorly developed surrounding muscular layers. Mutation and expression of β catenin, p-53, C-KIT, C-MYC, VEGF receptor, and BMI-1 are found in the tissue of angiofibroma. The most accepted treatment modality is surgical which can be endoscopic or external. The choice of approach is based on tumour extent and surgeon experience. Radiotherapy and hormonal therapy are the other treatment modalities.

6.2.1 Extensions

Sphenopalatine foreman (SPF) is present in the lateral nasal wall. The nasal cavity communicates with the pterygopalatine fossa via a sphenopalatine foreman. The foreman is covered by palatine bone inferiorly and sphenoid bone superiorly. Sphenopalatine artery and nerve to the lateral nasal wall and nasopalatine nerve enter into the nasal cavity via the foreman. Angiofibroma gets origin from the superior aspect of foreman and it tends to spread submucosally in close by less-resistant anatomical sites. It follows the standard pathway of spread because of its fixed site of origin and characteristic tumour behaviour. It can extend medially into the nasal cavity, paranasal sinuses, nasopharynx, and oropharynx. It can invade within the cancellous bone of the basisphenoid region. The lateral extension involves the pterygopalatine fossa (PPF), where It can push the posterior wall of the maxilla anteriorly which is known as the Holmen–Miller sign. It further extends laterally and it involves the infratemporal fossa (ITF), temporal fossa, and cheek (Fig. 6.8). It can extend behind the pterygoid plates (PP) [33].

Superiorly, it enters into the intracranial cavity mostly via inferior orbital fissure, orbit, superior orbital fissure (Fig. 6.9) [34]. The intracranial extension is found in 10–20% of cases but dural infiltration is very rare. Other pathways are:

1. Nasal cavity®ethmoid roof®erosion of fovea ethmoidalis or cribriform plate®intracranial.
2. Nasal cavity®erosion of skull base at planum and sphenoid sinus roof® or lateral wall and intracranial.

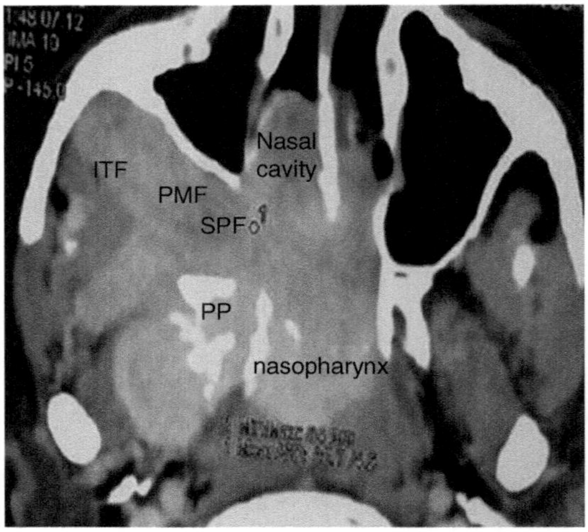

Fig. 6.8 CECT PNS orbit is showing characteristic extensions of JNA

3. From ITF it may erode the greater wing of the sphenoid and middle cranial fossa (lateral to cavernous sinus).
4. It can enter the cranial cavity via the posterior wall of PPF. Foramen rotundum, vidian canal are the natural communication site with the cranium.
5. Rarely Infratemporal fossa® temporal fossa®intracranial by the erosion of squamous part of the temporal bone.

Demographic Features [35] It is seen in the first two decades of life. It is found exclusively in males and it may be explained by the presence of high androgen, oestrogen receptors. Nasal obstruction (70–90%) and recurrent epistaxis (40–60%) are the most common ways of presentation. Facial pain, persistent rhinosinusitis, and headache are the other symptoms. Conductive hearing loss and ear fullness occur after the blockage of eustachian tube opening in the nasopharynx. Proptosis and facial asymmetry appears in the advanced stage. Clinical examination shows the presence of mucoid discharge in the nasal cavity, anterior displacement of the soft palate, and widening of space behind the last upper molar. Nasal endoscopy reveals a single large pinkish-red lobular mass filling choana and posterior part of the nasal cavity. It pushes the posterior part of the middle turbinate anteriorly.

Investigations

Contrast CT of the nose and paranasal sinuses is the first basic investigation (Fig. 6.8). Angiofibroma is highly intense after contrast administration because of rich vascularity. Angiofibroma spreads in a characteristic way, so CT also helps in confirming the diagnosis. Radiology helps in locating the site of origin and it also helps in mapping the extension of tumour which indeed helps in deciding the treatment policy [36, 37]. Erosion of anterior most of vidian canal favours the theory that it arises from medial most of PPF [38]. CT angiography is helpful by providing feeder detail preoperatively (Fig. 6.10). Digital subtraction angiography (DSA) is an invasive method and it also helps in the mapping of feeding vessels. DSA-based

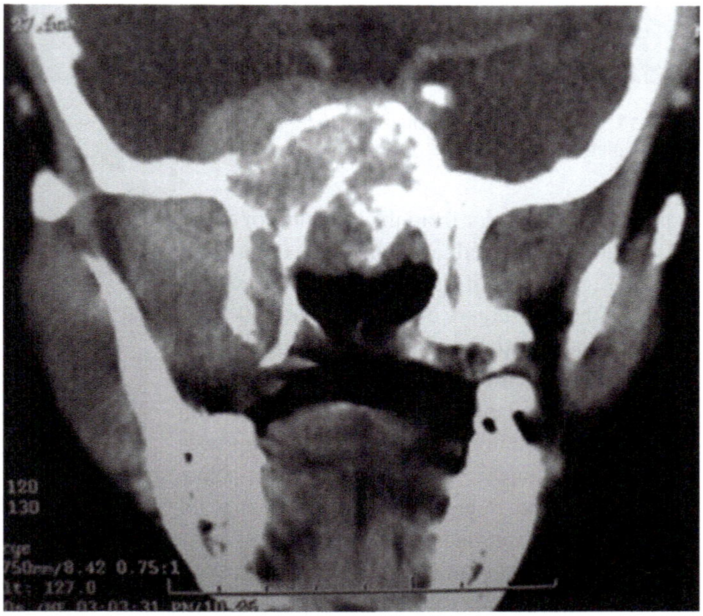

Fig. 6.9 Contrast enhancing mass is involving of both cavernous sinuses, sphenoid sinus, retropterygoid space and right ITF

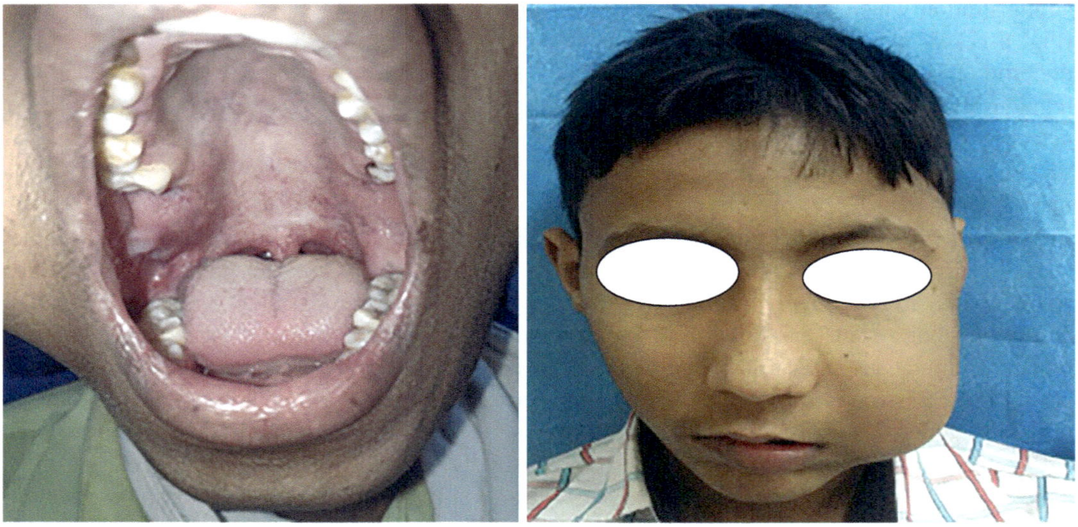

Fig. 6.10 The clinical photograph is showing the widening of space behind the last right molar with a bulged and displaced soft palate. Two different swellings are appreciated by extension of JNA in the temporal fossa and cheek region

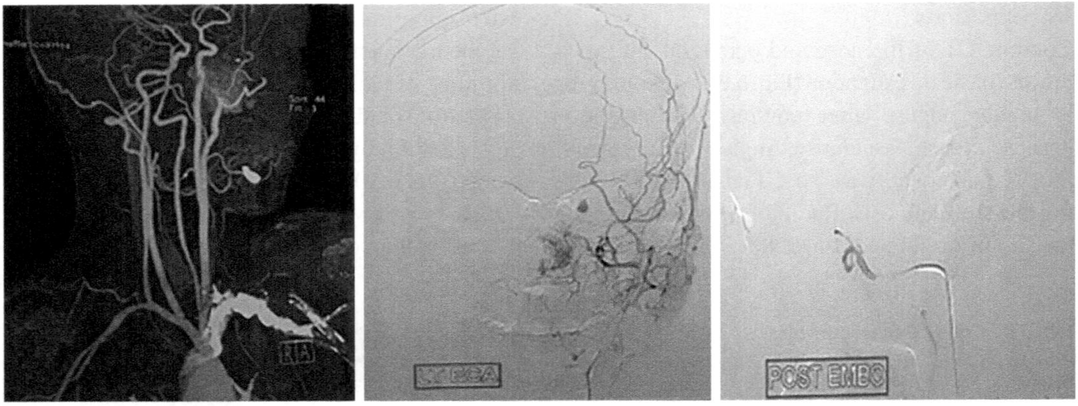

Fig. 6.11 CT angiography is showing feeder and tumour blush. Loss of tumour vascularity post embolisation is visible in DSA pictures

embolisation of feeder from the branches of external carotid artery reduces bleeding intraoperatively (Fig. 6.11). It is most effective within 24–48 hrs before surgery and it can reduce 60–70% of blood loss. Initial studies create doubt on the effectiveness of embolisation on tumour excision by secondary inflammation but advancement in technology and embolisation materials improves the surgical outcome. Selective and super-selective embolisation reduces accidental slippage of material into the internal carotid system.

On MRI [37], angiofibroma is hypointense on T1 and intermediate to hyperintense on T2. Tumour shows hyperintensity after contrast administration which appears as bags of worms (Fig. 6.12). MRI is reserve for a condition like doubtful diagnosis, invasion into cranial fossa, relationship with cavernous sinus and dura, to detect a residual tumour in the postoperative period, to assess the response of medical management. The temporary control of the carotid system in the neck or balloon occlusion of the internal carotid artery may be required to deal with tumour receiving major blood supply from ICA.

Recent studies show the presence of prostate-specific membranous antigen in angiofibroma tissue. PMSA PET scan is indicated for the detection of residual tumour in the postoperative period where MRI raised residual possibility (Fig. 6.13) [39].

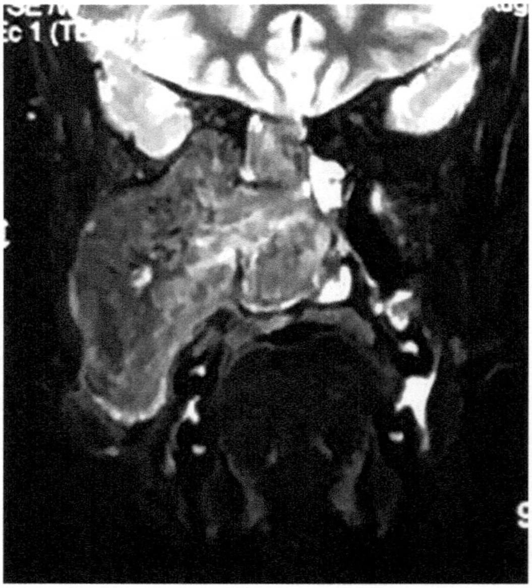

Fig. 6.12 Bag of worm appearance in MRI T2 image

Feeding vessels The branches of the internal maxillary artery are the most common feeder. Sphenopalatine is the most common feeding branch of the maxillary artery. Palatine arteries and ascending pharyngeal artery are the other common arteries. As the tumour grows, it can get vascularity from other vessels of the ipsilateral side or contralateral side (36%). Internal carotid artery feeder generates when mass extends into the orbital, cranium and with gross skull base involvement but vidian artery can supply tumour in early stage because of its proximity with the site of origin. Tumour receives feeder from the ophthalmic artery and sometimes direct branch from the internal carotid artery. The vertebral and basilar artery can also provide feeders [40].

6.2.1.1 Staging System

Sessions proposed the first staging system. Chandler, Fisch, Radkowski, Pittsburgh, Andrew, Onerci staging systems are the other staging system proposed at different points of time [35]. Radkowski staging system is the most popular staging system.

- Stage 1a—JNA is limited to the nasal cavity and/or nasopharynx (Fig. 6.14a).
- Stage 1b—extension into one or more paranasal sinuses.
- Stage IIa—minimal extension into PPF (Fig. 6.14b).

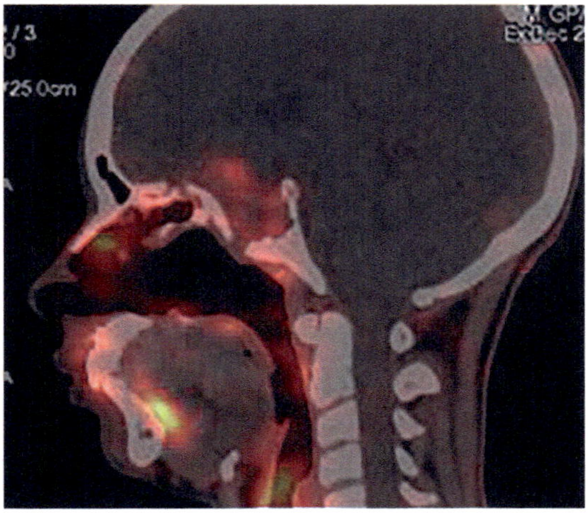

Fig. 6.13 PMSA PET scan showing dye uptake in sphenoid sinus and close by intracranial part. *(Ongoing thesis—Dr. Prabhu, Dept of ENT, AIIMS, New Delhi, under the guidance of Prof. Alok Thakar (ENT) and Prof Rakesh Kumar (Nuclear Medicine))*

- Stage IIb—JNA occupies PPF completely with or without erosion of orbital bones.
- Stage IIc—extension into ITF with or without cheek or posterior to the pterygoid plate (Fig. 6.14c).
- Stage IIIa—skull base bone erosion with minimal intracranial extension.
- Stage IIIb—gross intracranial extension ± cavernous sinus (Fig. 6.9).

Syndermann's staging system [41] is based on residual tumour blush post embolisation (Fig. 6.11). Residual tumour blush is because of blood supply from the internal carotid artery.

- Stage 1—Tumour is confined medial to midpoint of PPF, nasal cavity, and no vascularity after embolisation.
- Stage 2—Tumour extention into paranasal sinuses and lateral part of PPF without any residual vascularity.
- Stage 3—Extracranial tumour beyond stage 2 (ITF, orbit, skull base erosion) without residual vascularity.
- Stage 4—Stage 3 tumour with residual vascularity.
- Stage 5—Intracranial extension. M (medial) and L (lateral) are used for medial and lateral to the cavernous sinus.

Diagnosis The typical demographic profile of a patient with a characteristic radiological spread pattern is sufficient enough to make a diagnosis. The biopsy is not indicated because it can lead to excessive bleeding.

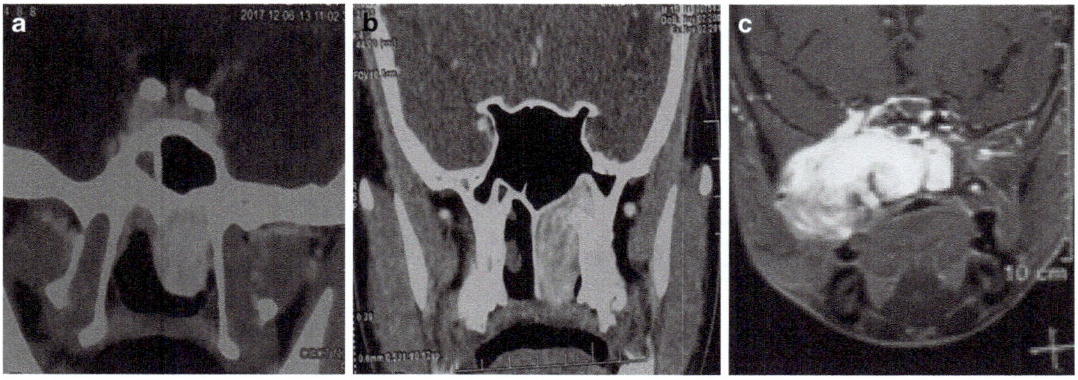

Fig. 6.14 Different stages of JNA. (**a**) stage Ia, (**b**) stage IIa, (**c**) stage IIc

6.2.1.2 Histopathology

It is circumscribed, non-capsulated mucosa covered lobular mass lesion. Colour depends on the vascular component of the tumour (pinkish-white to red). Microscopically, it is formed by fibrocellular stoma with spindle cells and haphazardly arranged dense collagen matrix with the irregular vascular pattern. The vessels are dilated and lacks true muscle layer [42].

Differential Diagnosis Angiomatous polyp, infected antrochoanal polyp, benign (hemangioma, paraganglioma) or malignant tumour (hemangiopericytoma) are differential tumours for angiofibroma. The demographic features, clinical features, and pattern of spread helps in differentiating these tumours from JNA [35, 43].

6.2.1.3 Treatment

Surgical treatment is the gold standard treatment. The choice of approach can vary between centres based on the surgeon's experience and hospital setup. The majority of centres are shifted from open surgical methods (lateral rhinotomy, Weber–Fergusson, transpalatal, sublabial, midfacial degloving, Le Fort 1 approach) to endoscopic method because of improving anatomical knowledge, advancement in technology, and expertise [44]. Endoscopic Denker's, septal window, anterior maxillotomy, and small posterior sublabial incision allow easy dealing of ITF extension of JNA by endoscopic approach (Fig. 6.15). Posterior septectomy increases space within the nasal cavity. Literature supports the use of endoscopic excision till stage IIIa of the Radkowski staging system [44]. Tumour removal in toto or piecemeal showed a similar recurrence pattern if the extension of tumour is well assessed intraoperatively.

Open anterior (lateral rhinotomy, Weber Ferguson or maxillary swing) and lateral approach (subtemoral approach with or without craniotomy) is indicated for large volume tumour with gross skullbase involvement and when tumour is lateral to ICA, significant residual vascularity after embolization (equal to more than 50%) (Figs. 6.16 and 6.17).

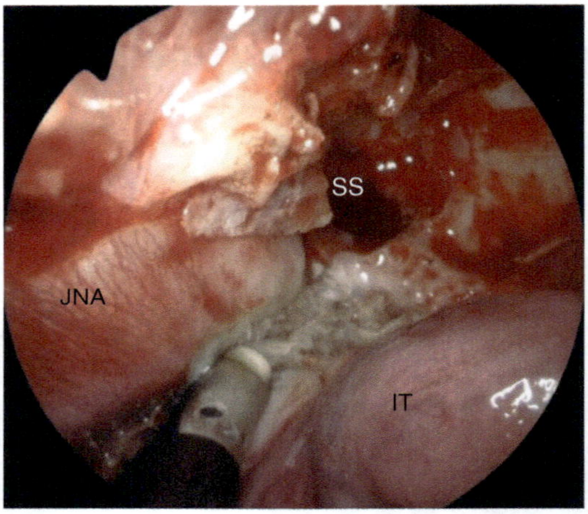

Fig. 6.15 Endoscopic picture is showing a bloodless field with coblator while separating JNA from the surrounding

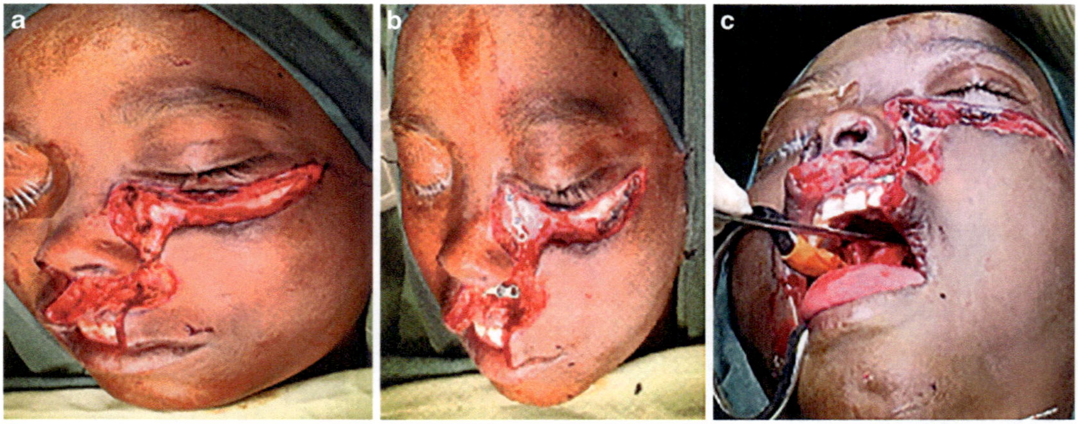

Fig. 6.16 Maxillary swing approach. (**a**) Weber–Fergusson's incision is made, (**b**) plating for postoperative approximation, (**c**) raising of palatal flap

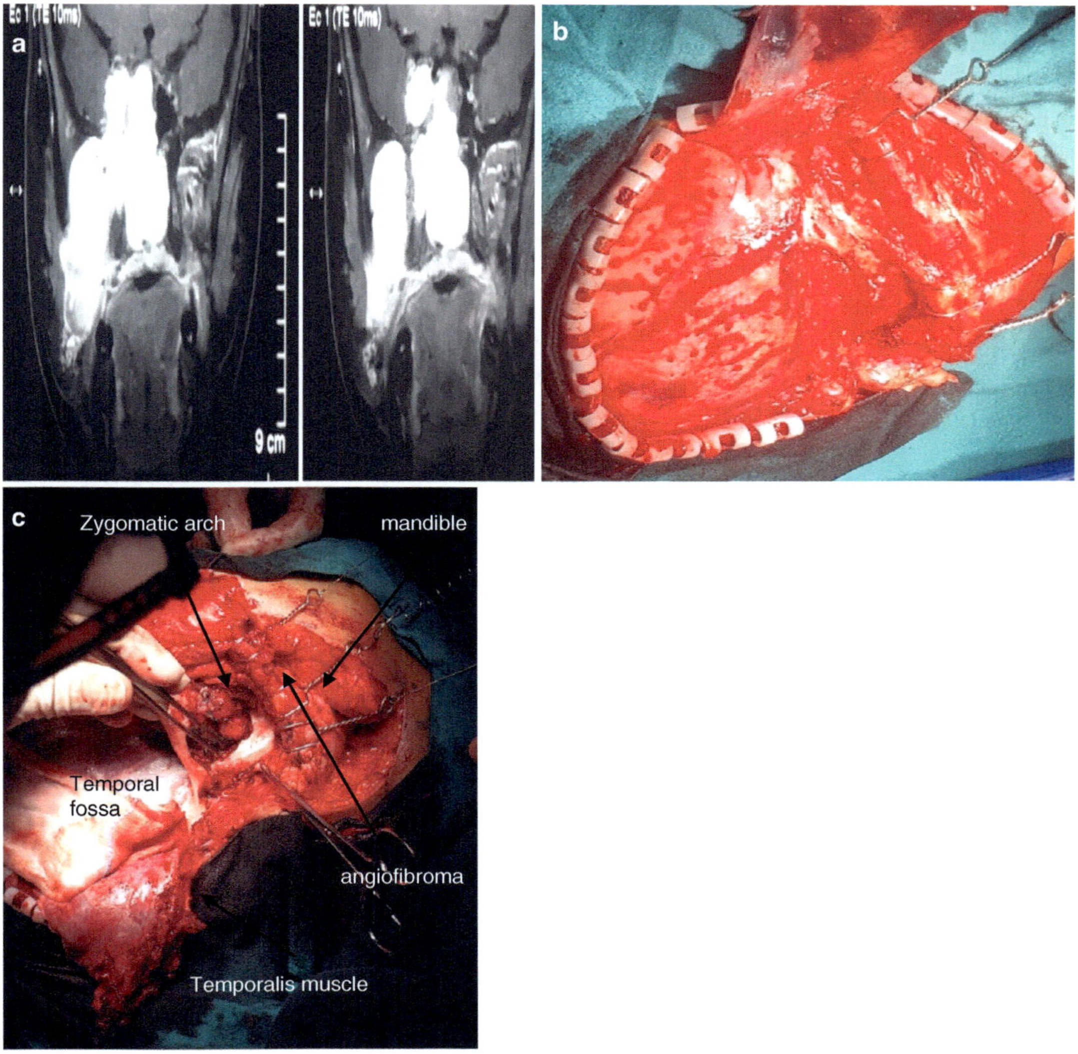

Fig. 6.17 Preauricular subtemporal approach for right side. (**a**) JNA 3b, (**b**) flap elevation, (**c**) exposure of tumour

Excision of residual tumour lies in close proximity with ICA, dura, optic nerve and cavernous sinus is challenging as tumour handling can lead to significant morbidity [45]. Hypotensive anaesthesia, reverse Trendelenburg position, proper decongestion, preoperative embolisation, and coblation of peritumoral tissues are the measures to reduce the amount of intraoperative bleeding significantly (Fig. 6.15). Large-volume tumour, an extension of tumour into vidian canal and infiltration into the cancellous bone of skull base, inexperienced surgeon, and early age of onset are the major factors for tumour residual.

Medical Management Immunohistochemistry shows the presence of oestrogen α, oestrogen β, androgen, and vascular endothelial growth factor (VEGF) receptors in tumour tissue. It is an oestrogen suppressive tumour and testosterone responsive tumour. Diethylstilbestrol was initially used for shrinkage but it has a long list of adverse effects. Flutamide therapy is a non-

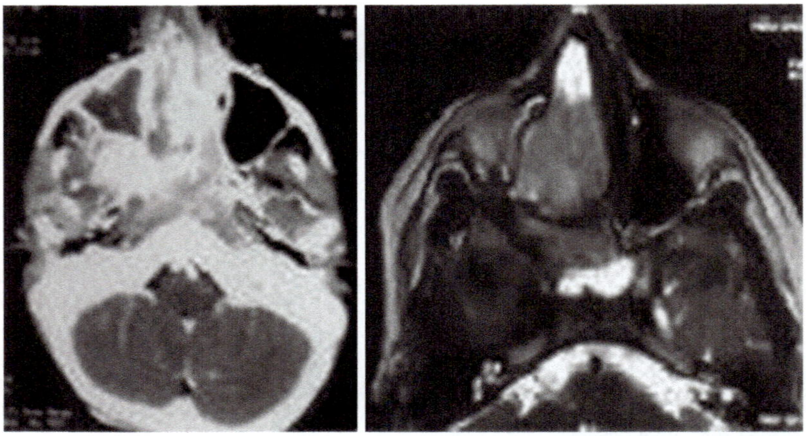

Fig. 6.18 Radiology is showing a reduction of the stage from pretreatment II C to II A of the Radkowski stage

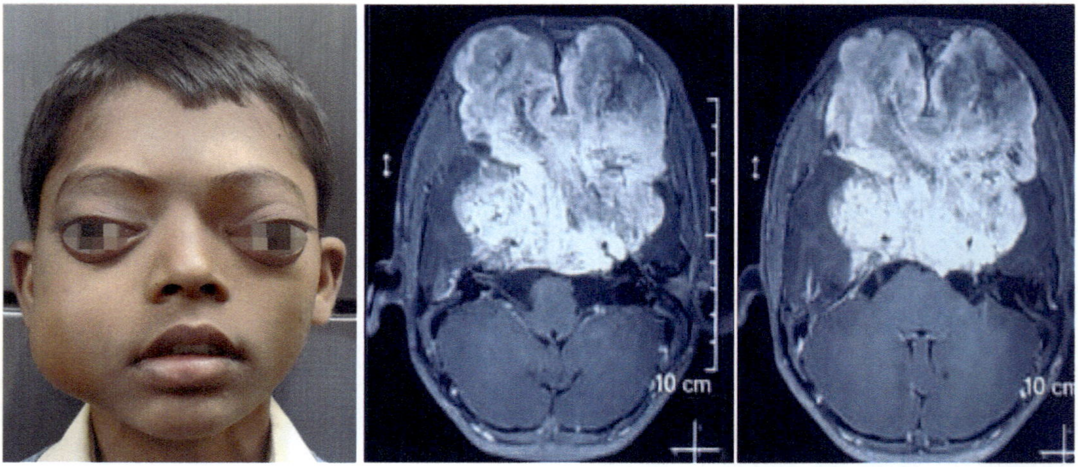

Fig. 6.19 Clinical photograph is showing bilateral proptosis, with fullness in the right cheek. CECT is showing hyperintense mass with 360-degree involvement of the bilateral carotid artery

steroidal, anti-androgenic drug without feminising side effects and limited reversible adverse effects. The dose is 10 mg/kg/day for 6 weeks. The response rate ranged from 7 to 44% and it was found more in post-puberty patients (Fig. 6.18). It is also effective in reducing episode number and amount of blood loss in the preoperative period [46, 47].

Radiotherapy is indicated for unresectable tumours (Fig. 6.19), in patients with persistent residual lesion even after multiple surgeries and when residual lies close to the vital structure where surgery is very much challenging. The dose ranges from 30 to 55 Gy with tumour control rate ranging from 70 to 90%. The side effects are cataract, panhypopituitarism, growth retardation, temporal lobe necrosis, and secondary malignancy. Recent techniques such as IMRT can reduce the risk of complication rate, but limited literature is available [48, 49].

Surveillance The advised radiological investigation is MRI and it can be performed after pack removal or at 3 months postoperative period after [46]. The surrounding inflammation interferes in the diagnosis of residual lesion. PMSA PET scan is indicated when MRI is doubtful. When no lesion is found in 5 years' follow-up period, then

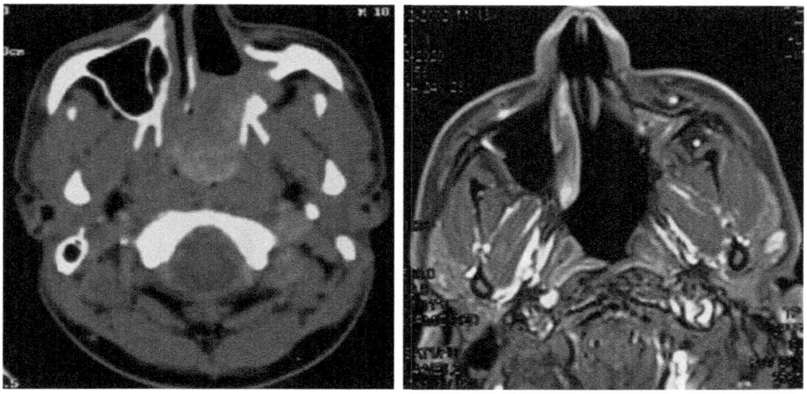

Fig. 6.20 Preoperative CECT and postoperative surveillance (3-months interval) MRI scan for residual detection

the patient can be labelled as disease-free (Fig. 6.20).

6.3 Part C: Cancer of Nose and Paranasal Sinuses

Cancers of the nose and PNS are very rare, and account for 0.2–0.8% of all neoplasms. Overall, they form <3% of all head and neck cancers. The symptoms of nose and PNS tumours are similar to those of common disorders such as chronic rhinosinusitis and thus cause a delay in diagnosis. The commonest age of presentation is in the fifth and sixth decade of life with a male predilection (Male:Female:: 2:1) [50]. The most commonly involved sinus is the maxillary (70%) > ethmoid (20%) > frontal and sphenoid sinuses. A wide variety of histologies may be encountered although Squamous Cell Carcinoma (SCC) is the most common malignant tumour. The TNM staging system is slightly complex and different for different regions of the nose and paranasal sinuses. A correct documentation of staging is required for treatment planning, prognostication, and information transfer.

6.3.1 Aetiology

Several carcinogenic compounds have been identified with inhalation of these carcinogens being responsible for ~40% of reported sinonasal malignancies. Exposure to industrial fumes, nickel refining processes, alkaline battery manufacture industry, leather tanning, soldering, welding has been reported to cause cancer of paranasal sinuses.

Squamous cell carcinoma has been associated with softwood dust, nickel, mustard gas, asbestos industry workers. African mahogany appears to be the most carcinogenic of all agents. Adenocarcinoma, especially the interstitial variant, is mostly associated with hardwood dust in the furniture industry, clothes and leather industry. Biologically active compounds in wood dust impair mucociliary clearance and predispose to carcinogenesis [51].

Human Papilloma Virus (HPV) infection has an increased risk of malignant transformation of inverted papilloma. However, no significant association between cigarette smoking and alcohol in sinonasal cancers has been noted.

6.3.2 Patterns of Tumour Spread

The most common route of spread is by local invasion. Orbit and cranium are seperate from nose and paranasal sinuses by thin bone. The paranasal sinuses other than the maxillary sinus are in close proximity to orbit and cranial cavity which makes them more vulnerable even at low volume of tumour. Natural foreman allows early spread of tumour.

Local Invasion Periosteum, perichondrium, and dura appear to act as a momentary fence and oppose tumour growth to some degree [52, 53]. The bone of the anterior maxilla, medial wall and floor of orbital, roof of the frontal sinus and olfactory cleft are very thin and readily destroyed by tumour. The clinical presentation is based on the area of involvement. Maxillary sinus tumours generally present with medial spread or anterior/inferior wall breach. Inferior orbital fissure and thin orbital floor allows early orbital involvement but periorbita is the relatively tough lining that limits orbital tissue involvement to certain extent. Posterior breach involves infratemporal fossa, pteryomaxillary space and pterygoid plates which is relatively rare [54]. Öhngren described a line running from the medial canthus of the orbit to the angle of the mandible. Superiorly based tumours are more aggressive and poorly differentiated, whereas inferiorly based tumours are more amenable to treatment with a better prognosis. Orbit is involved by the lateral and inferior spread of ethmoid and frontal sinus tumours. Anterior cranial fossa is involved by the superior spread of tumours. Cavernous sinus is involved by lateral spread, nasopharynx by inferior spread, nasal cavity and ethmoid sinuses by anterior spread of sphenoid sinus tumours.

- *Regional spread*: Nodal disease is a marker of locally advanced disease and lymphatic spread to regional nodes is seen in around 25–35% of patients. Submandibular and jugulodigastric nodes are the most commonly involved lymph nodes by anteriorly placed tumours, when tumour breaches anterior bony wall, whereas, posteriorly placed tumours involve retropharyngeal lymph nodes. Anterior spread has a better prognosis than posterior spread.
- *Distant metastases*: It is unusual at the time of presentation and develops in less than 20% of patients with adenocarcinomas, whereas, for SCC, it is around 10% [55]. The most common sites for metastases are bone, brain, liver, lung, and skin (Fig. 6.21).

6.3.3 Clinical Features

The clinical presentation is depending on the site of involvement. Nasal symptoms are the most common. The usual manifestations are unilateral nasal obstruction, persistent sinusitis, recurrent epistaxis, foul-smelling nasal discharge, facial pain, etc. Epiphora is due to blockage of the nasolacrimal duct (Fig. 6.22).

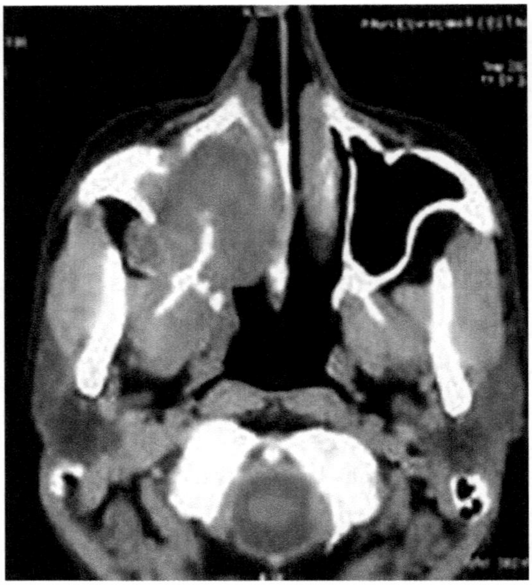

Fig. 6.21 Tumour of left maxillary sinus involving ITF, pterygoid plates, pterygoid muscles, and nasal cavity

Oral symptoms are seen in 25–30% of patients. These symptoms manifest in the form of loose teeth, pain in maxillary teeth, and palatal fullness (Fig. 6.23). Muscles of mastication, nerves are involved by tumour extension into infratemporal fossa or by pterygoid muscle infiltration and patients are present with symptoms of trismus.

Numbness of the cheek is the sign of inferior orbital nerve infiltration. Distortion of nose and face is a late feature (Fig. 6.22). Pattern of eyeball displacement is helpful in pinpointing the involved sinus. Auditory manifestations are in the form of hearing loss, secondary to serous otitis media due to nasopharyngeal extension. Cranial nerve II, III, IV, V1, V2, and VI nerves are seen after orbital apex and cavernous sinus involvement. Cranial nerve involvement is a manifestation of advanced disease; it indicates poor prognosis.

Diagnosis Clinical staging requires detailed local examination with neck evaluation for cervical lymphadenopathy, cranial nerve function, and ophthalmological evaluation. Nasal endoscopy is done with a diagnostic purpose to see the characteristic of mass and with a therapeutic purpose to obtain tissue for biopsy (Fig. 6.24). Contrast CT scan of nose and paranasal sinuses 3–5 mm axial, coronal, and sagittal images are required to document staging of the tumour. Coronal images are obtained for involvement of the orbital floor and skull base and axial images are obtained for extension through the posterior wall of the maxillary sinus into the pterygopalatine fossa and infratemporal fossa (Fig. 6.25). It also helps to evaluate the tumour involvement of the retro-orbital and orbital apex region. Sometimes, reconstructed images are required to pinpoint bony erosion. However, the limitations of CT scan are in the evaluation of periorbita, dural involvement to see whether the tumour has invaded or is just abutting these structures. It is

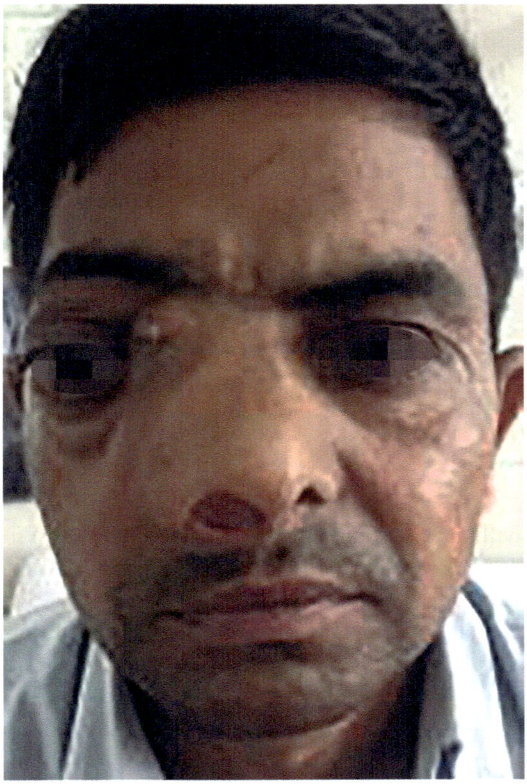

Fig. 6.22 Nasal mass (Right) with fullness of right nasal cavity ulceration of skin in medial canthus and lateral/inferior displacement of right eyeball (clinical stage is T4). (Courtesy—Dr. Hitesh Verma, Associate Professor, AIIMS, New Delhi, India)

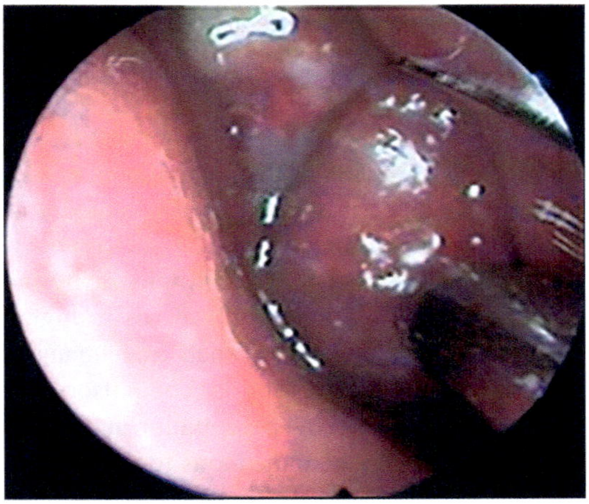

Fig. 6.24 Nasal endoscopy is revealing a mass in the left nasal cavity (clinical stage T2)

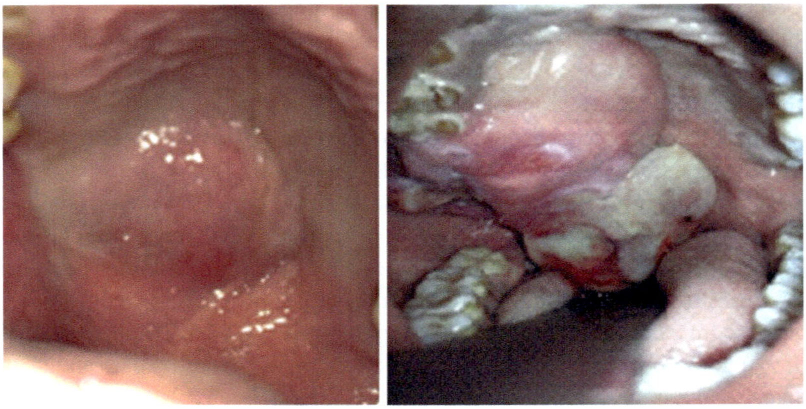

Fig. 6.23 Palatal bulge and ulceration with loosening of teeth by inferior spread of maxillary sinus tumour

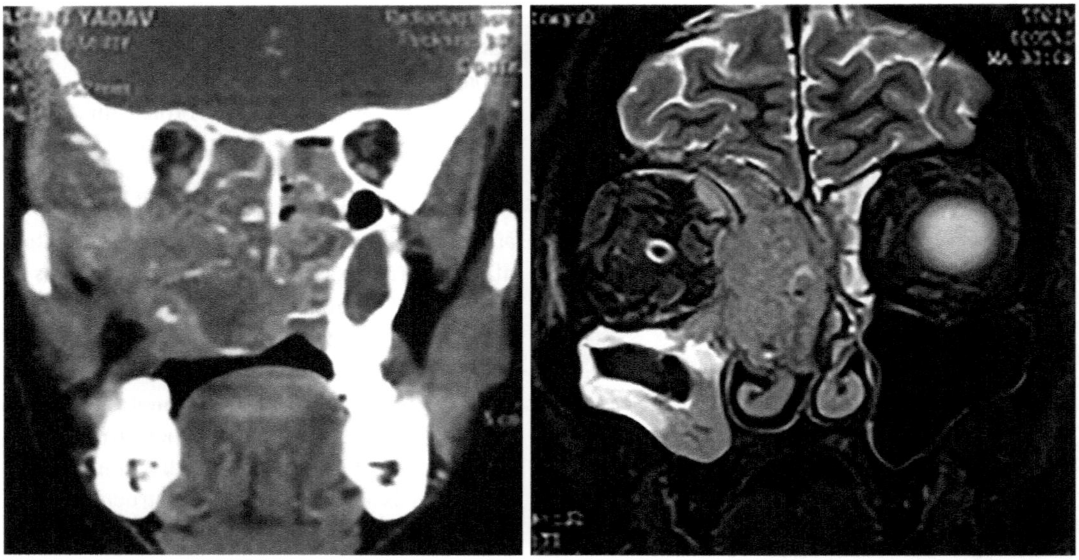

Fig. 6.25 CECT Nose and PNS showing the extent of a sinonasal tumour (T4a stage). MRI is showing right periorbital infiltration with retained section in right maxillary sinus (T4a stage)

difficult to differentiate tumour from soft tissues and secretions owing to their similar densities. MRI is prescribed in such cases as it provides us better soft tissue details and it differentiates tumour from secretion [54, 56]. Angiography and embolisation have limited indications in highly vascular malignant lesions, such as hemangiopericytoma. Histopathology is compulsory for tissue diagnosis. Unusual presentation and abnormal recurrence are the indications for PET scan.

6.3.4 Histopathology

Squamous cell carcinoma (SCC) is the leading histopathological diagnosis. Adenocarcinoma and adenoid cystic carcinoma accounts for around 10% of nose and PNS tumours. The tumours have a male preponderance and are seen mostly in sixth to seventh decades of life. Sinonasal tumour mostly arise from the lateral nasal wall whereas tumours arise from paranasal sinuses. SCC is well-differentiated in a majority of cases (85%). Esthesioneuroblastoma originates from basal cells of the olfactory epithelium. It accounts for less than 5% of sinonasal malignancies and it has bimodal age distribution (peak at 20 and 50 of age). It has female preponderance with the potential of inducing paraneoplastic syndrome by releasing peptides. Sinonasal undifferentiated carcinoma, melanoma, and hemangiopericytomas are other common differential diagnoses for sinonasal tumours [57, 58].

Staging it is devised for carcinomas of the maxillary sinus, ethmoid sinus, and the nasal cavity and is not applicable to mesodermal tumours, olfactory neuroblastoma (OAN) for which other grading systems have been devised. TNM Classification (AJCC 2018) is proposed for nose and paranasal sinuses lesions [59].

6.3.5 Stage with Description

6.3.5.1 T Staging

Maxillary Sinus

- **T1** Tumour confined to the maxillary antrum mucosa without bone erosion.
- **T2** Tumour produces bone erosion or destruction, except the posterior wall of the antrum, and it also includes tumour extension into the hard palate and/or middle meatus.
- **T3** Tumour infiltrates in whichever of the subsequent: maxillary sinus posterior wall, sub-

cutaneous tissues over maxillary sinus, ethmoid sinus, medial wall and floor of orbit, pterygomaxillary space.
- **T4a** Tumour infiltrates in whichever of the subsequent: anterior orbit stuffing, pterygoid plates, cheek skin, cribriform plate, infratemporal fossa, sphenoid or frontal sinuses (Fig. 6.25).
- **T4b** Tumour infiltrates in whichever of the subsequent: apex of orbit, dura, brain, cranial nerves except maxillary division of trigeminal nerve, nasopharynx, or clivus.

Ethmoid Sinus

- **T1** Tumour confined to the ethmoid sinuses with or without bony erosion.
- **T2** Tumour extends into the nasal cavity.
- **T3** Tumour extends into anterior orbit and/or maxillary sinus.
- **T4a** Tumour infiltrates in whichever of the subsequent: anterior orbital stuffing, skin over nose or cheek, negligible anterior intracranial extension, pterygoid plates, sphenoid or frontal sinuses.
- **T4b** Tumour infiltrates in whichever of the subsequent: orbit apex of orbit, dura, brain, cranial nerves except maxillary division of trigeminal nerve, nasopharynx, or clivus.

Nasal Cavity

- **T1** Tumour involves only one subunit of the subsequent: septum, floor, lateral wall, and vestibule of the nasal cavity.
- **T2** Tumour involves two subunits or ethmoid.
- **T3** Tumour infiltrates into the orbit anteriorly and/or maxillary sinus.
- **T4a** Tumour invades any of the following: anterior orbital stuffing, skin over nose or cheek, negligible anterior intracranial extension, pterygoid plates, sphenoid or frontal sinuses.
- **T4b** Tumour infiltrates in whichever of the subsequent: apex of orbit, dura, brain, middle cranial fossa, cranial nerves except maxillary division of trigeminal nerve, nasopharynx or clivus.

N Staging

- **NX** Local lymph nodes cannot be assessed.
- **N0** No local lymph node metastasis.
- **N1** Metastasis in a solitary ipsilateral lymph node, 3 cm or less in maximum measurement exclusive of extranodal extension.
- **N2**
- **N2a**—Metastasis in a solitary ipsilateral lymph node, more than 3 cm but not more than 6 cm in maximum measurement exclusive of extranodal extension.
- **N2b**—Metastasis in several ipsilateral lymph nodes, none more than 6 cm in maximum measurement exclusive of extranodal extension.
- **N2c**—Metastasis in bilateral or contralateral lymph nodes, none more than 6 cm in greatest dimension, without extranodal extension.
- **N3a** Metastasis in a lymph node more than 6 cm in greatest dimension without extranodal extension.
- **N3b** Metastases in a solitary or several lymph nodes with clinical extranodal extension.

The staging template is mentioned in Table 6.5.

The staging system for olfactory neuroblastoma is first proposed by Kadish and then it was modified by Morita [60]:

Stage 1: Tumour confined to nasal cavity

Stage 2: Tumour confined to the nasal cavity and paranasal sinuses

Stage 3: Extension of tumour away from nose and paranasal sinuses (intra-orbit or intracranial)

Stage 4: Any previous stage with cervical lymph node or distal metastasis

Table 6.5 Staging template

Stage			
O	Tis	N0	M0
I	T1	N0	M0
II	T2	N0	M0
III	T1/2	N1	M0
	T3	N0/1	M0
IVa	T1/2/3	N2	M0
	T4a	N0/1/2	M0
IVb	T4b	Any N	M0
	Any T	N3	M0
IVc	Any T	Any N	M1

Dulgurov proposed a new staging system for esthesioneuroblastoma [61]:

- T1 is confined to the nose and PNS without superior ethmoid cells and sphenoid sinus involvement.
- T2 is T1 + sphenoid sinus with or without erosion of cribriform plate.
- T3 is any stage with intraorbital and intracranial extension without dural infiltration.
- T4 is brain parenchyma involvement.

The presence of regional and distal metastasis is marked as N1 and M1. Dural involvement is noticed in 25% and lymph node metastasis in 5% of cases. Hyems et al. proposed a histopathological grading system on the basis of tumour cell architecture, degree of differentiation, nuclear pleomorphism, mitotic index, tumour necrosis, and nature of the matrix. They graded histology into four subtypes where type 1 is least aggressive and type 4 is most aggressive [62].

Surgical and other management for sinonasal malignancies is mentioned in Chaps. 7 and 10.

6.4 Part D: Nasopharyngeal Carcinoma

6.4.1 Summary

Nasopharyngeal carcinoma (NPC) is the most common neoplasm arising in the nasopharynx which shows remarkable geographical difference in incidence across the world. NPC is uncommon in the United State but is endemic in many areas in the world, particularly southeastern China and Hong Kong where the incidence is as high as 20–30 cases per 100,000 population. The main factors believed to be associated with the development of NPC are EBV, genetic, and environmental; however, we are still unable to assimilate these information to translate knowledge into prevention, early detection, and improved survival outcome. The most common clinical presentation is palpable cervical lymphadenopathy (50%) followed by blood-stained nasal discharge (41%), deafness (30%), and cranial nerve palsy in about 10% of cases. Nasopharyngosocopic examination reveals growth and provides a suitable area for biopsy under direct visualisation. The use of immunohistochemical markers will help to differentiate NPC from other malignancies in the nasopharynx.

Computed tomography has been the cornerstone of radiological staging for many years; however, magnetic resonance imaging has been used increasingly because of its superior definition in detecting soft tissue changes and intracranial involvement. Bone scan and positron emission tomography are other reliable investigations to look for distant metastasis.

In recent years, treatment of NPC had undergone several paradigm shifts resulting in improved prognosis. Advances in the planning and delivery of radiation treatment and the addition of chemotherapy have been demonstrated to improve disease control rates in locally advanced NPC. In general, patients with stage 1 are treated by radiation therapy alone, whereas, stage II, III, and IV are treated by concurrent radiotherapy and chemotherapy. Surgery should be considered as a first-line treatment of residual or recurrence disease at the primary site (rT1 and limited rT2). Technical advances have enabled surgeons to perform endoscopic or robotic surgeries as salvage, reducing the morbidity from traditional open resections. Patients with NPC cases are followed up and assessed with office-based rigid and/or fibro-optic nasal endoscopy. Positron emission tomography–computed tomography, CT, or MRI scan should be carried out at 3 months from completion of treatment to assess response.

6.4.2 Anatomy of Nasopharynx

It is also known as postnasal space, located in the centre of the head behind the nasal cavity and above the oropharynx. It is a region where thorough clinical examination as well as adequate exposure for surgical resection is difficult. Anatomically, the roof is formed by the body of sphenoid bone, sphenoid further slants downwards in front of arch of atlas and body of axis to form the posterior wall. The floor is formed by the upper surface of the soft palate. The lateral wall is formed by the eustachian tube opening in the upper part and superior constrictor muscle in the lower part. Fossa of Rosenmuller, also called lateral pharyngeal recess, is an important structure lying in the lateral wall, which is bounded anteriorly by torus tubarius and levator palatine muscle, posteriorly by the posterior wall of the nasopharynx and retropharyngeal space, laterally by parapharyngeal space, and inferiorly by the upper edge of superior constrictor muscle (Fig. 6.26a, b). Its superior boundary is the skull base with important openings including foramen spinosum, foramen ovale, and carotid canal. The internal carotid artery is separated from the apex of the lateral recess by only a thin layer of fibroconnective tissue.

Blood supply of the nasopharynx is from branches of the internal maxillary artery, ascending pharyngeal artery and venous drainage is to the pterygoid plexus. Sensory supply is from branches of the maxillary nerve and lymphatic supply drains into the retropharyngeal and cervical lymph nodes.

Tumours of Nasopharynx A broad range of neoplasms arise in the nasopharynx from epithelial to mesenchymal, lymphoid, and neuroectodermal cells (Table 6.6) [63].

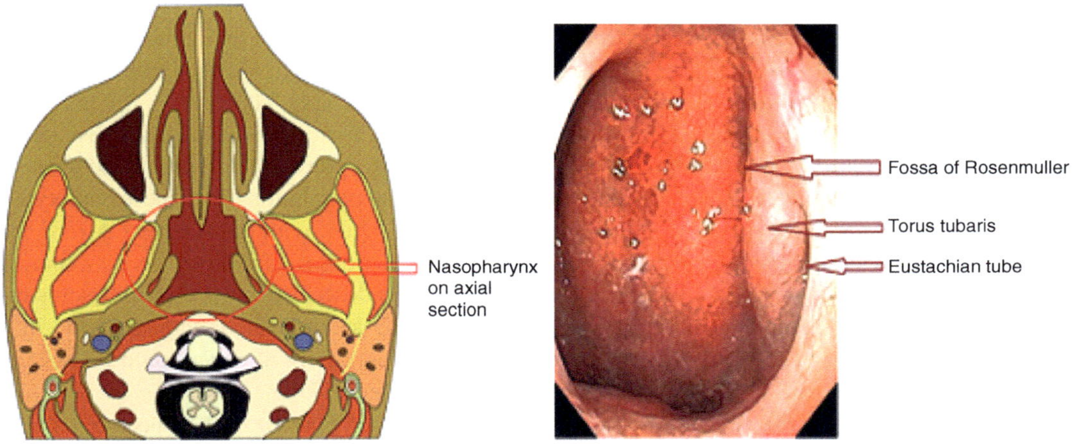

Fig. 6.26. Axial view of nasopharynx and the endoscopic view of nasopharynx from left choana

Table 6.6 (Pathology fourth edition WHO classification)

Carcinomas	Nasopharyngeal carcinoma	Non-keratinising SCC	8072/3	Soft tissue tumours	Nasopharyngeal angiofibroma	9160/0
		Keratinising SCC	8071/3	Haemato-lymphoid tumours	Diffuse B cell lymphoma	9680/3
		Basaloid SCC	8083/3		Extra-osseous plasmacytoma	9734/3
	Nasopharyngeal papillary adenocarcinoma		8260/3		Extramedullary myeloid sarcoma	9930/3
Salivary gland tumours	Adenoid cystic carcinoma		8200/3	Notochordal tumours	Chordoma	9370/3
	Salivary gland anlage tumours					
Benign and borderline lesions	Hairy polyp					
	Ectopic pituitary adenoma		8272/0			
	Craniopharyngioma		9350/1			

6.4.3 Benign Tumours

It Includes salivary gland tumours, hyperplastic lymphoid tissue, adenoid hypertrophy, nasopharyngeal cyst, papilloma, juvenile angiofibroma, and choanal polyps.

Malignant Tumours Include lymphomas, salivary gland tumours, and NPC.

6.4.4 Nasopharyngeal Carcinoma

Nasopharyngeal carcinoma (NPC) has unique epidemiology, pathogenesis, and evolving treatment modalities which have undergone several paradigm shifts over the last 30 years. Recent advances in the treatment planning and delivery of radiation therapy and the better understanding of the delivery of chemotherapeutic agents over the decades have contributed to the improvement in prognosis. Globally NPC is a rare cancer with 80,000 new cases reported per year and accounts for 0.7% of all cancers [64]. Compared with other cancer types, NPC is uncommon with a very unique pattern of geographical distribution. In non-endemic areas like North America and Europe, the incidence rate is low (<1 case per 100,000 population) whereas in high-risk areas such as Hong Kong and Southern China, the annual age-standardised incidence rate among male is as high as 20–30 cases per 100,000 population and 8–15 cases per 100,000 population [65, 66]. A most common site is the fossa of Rosenmüller followed by the superior posterior wall of the nasopharynx.

Aetiology The main factors believed to be associated with NPC include Epstein–Barr Virus (EBV), genetic and environmental factors.

- *Epstein–Barr Virus:* Epstein–Barr Virus is a herpesvirus with a central DNA core and an enveloped capsid. Infection with EBV occurs in early childhood and tends to be asymptomatic. In acute and convalescent phase of infection, the immunoglobulins (IgG and IgM) to antigens (nuclear core early antigen [EA] or the viral capsid antigen [VCA]) rises. Hence, in the majority of any population, IgG VCA and EA will be raised; however, in NPC, the IgA VCA and EA raises [67]. EBV antigens are also present on NPC cells and express lytic antigens (latent membrane proteins 1, 2, 3) and nuclear antigens (Epstein–Barr nuclear antigens 1–6). In NPC, EBNA-1 is always expressed and LMP-1 is consistently expressed in significant levels. EBNA-1 is responsible for maintaining viral episome in the tumour cells, whereas LMP-1 has been shown to induce cellular growth by inducing epithelial hyperplasia and altered keratin gene expression [68, 69]. In addition, expression of LMP-1 and EBNA-1 is not seen in normal nasopharyngeal epithelium cells.
- *Genetic factor:* The association of human leukocyte antigen (HLA) alleles with NPC is well established; HLA A2, Bw46, B17, Bw58, DR3, and DR9 have been consistently found more prevalent in NPC in contrast to the general population [70]. These haplotypes are associated with an increased risk for NPC. Deletions in chromosomes 3, 9, and 11 have been described in NPC. Family clusters with NPC are not uncommon as NPC in a first-degree family member could be as high as eight times [71].
- *Environment factors:* It has been seen that diets high in preservatives containing nitrosamines such as salted fish, eggs, and vegetables are associated with NPC. Other environmental factors associated with NPC include chemical fumes and wood dusts [72].

Clinical Features The most common presentation in NPC is palpable cervical lymphadenopathy (50%) mainly high level V and level II. Others may present with nasal symptoms (30%), otological symptoms (20%), cranial nerve palsy 20% (III, IV, V, VIth nerves), or distant metastasis 3% (spine is the commonest site of distant metastasis). Unilateral secretory otitis media presenting as deafness (30%) in adults is a warning sign and is believed to be secondary to eustachian tube dysfunction.

Around 1% of NPC cases may have dermatomyositis as a paraneoplastic syndrome which can develop concurrently with NPC, late after diagnosis, or months before the NPC is clinically apparent [73].

Assessment Patients should be assessed with rigid and fibro-optic nasal endoscopy which reveals exophytic mass that may occupy the whole postnasal space (Fig. 6.27). Ulcerated growth may be present and in about 10% of NPC patients, the lesion is submucosal.

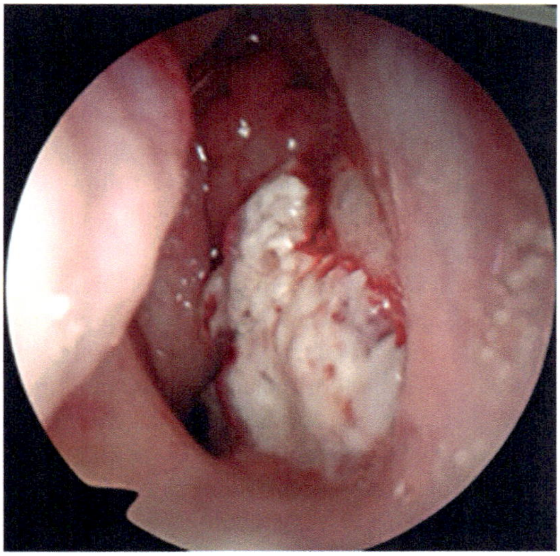

Fig. 6.27 Endoscopic view of nasopharyngeal tumour: A tumour can be seen obliterating the right nasal choana

Multislice computed tomographic scan of head, neck, and chest is an essential investigation particularly useful in delineating clival and skull base erosion. Magnetic resonance imaging provides superior definition in detecting soft tissue changes and intracranial involvement (Fig. 6.28a, b).

Diagnosis The gold standard in the diagnosis of NPC is the histopathological confirmation. The immunohistochemical markers such as cytokeratin, epithelial cell markers, and Epstein–Barr encoded ribonucleic acid (EBER) will help in differentiating NPC from other malignancies.

Cytology Fine-needle aspiration with immunohistochemical staining for EBER from enlarged neck lymph node can often differentiate between metastasis from undifferentiated carcinoma and squamous cell carcinoma.

Other Staging Investigations Other staging investigations include chest radiograph, CT scan of lungs and liver, liver ultrasound, and bone scan. Among these, bone scan has the highest pick-up rate, which is consistent with the skeleton being the most common distant site of metastasis. Positron emission tomography (PET-CT) is another imaging tool; however, literature is scant

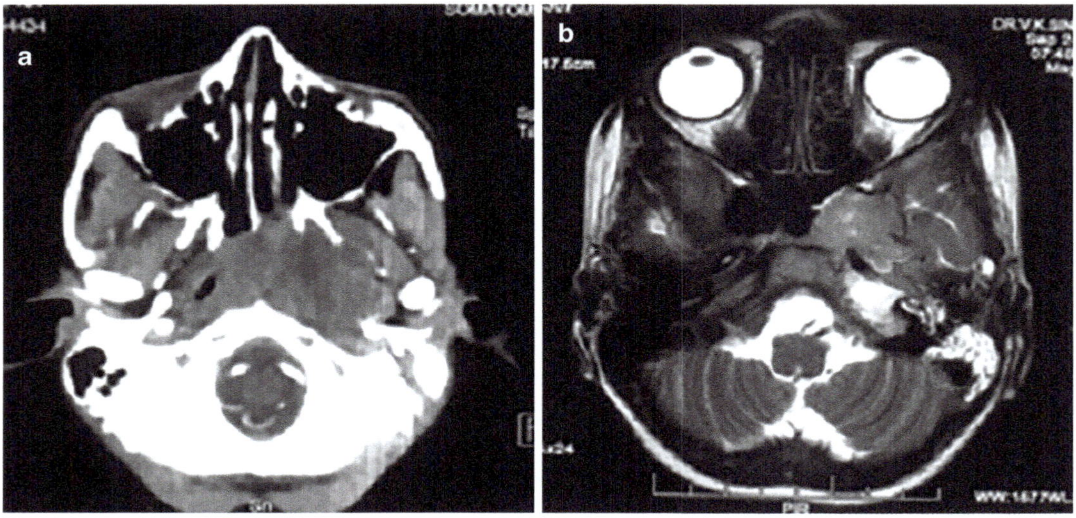

Fig. 6.28 (**a**) Contrast-enhanced computed tomography (axial section) of left nasopharyngeal carcinoma. (**b**) T2w axial section, left nasopharyngeal carcinoma

on the efficacy and cost-effectiveness of using PET-CT as a sole staging tool to assess the primary and regional metastasis. A recent meta-analysis has confirmed the reliable performance of PET-CT in the evaluation of distant metastasis, with a pooled sensitivity of 83% and specificity of 97% [74].

EBV DNA copies may be measured by polymerase chain reaction techniques which correlate with the stage of disease and are useful as an indicator of treatment response. Immunoserology (VCA-IgA, EA-IgA, EBVNA1-IgA) and EBV DNA can be used as screening methods.

Pathology: WHO histological classification: Three types:

- Type I—Keratinising squamous cell carcinoma
- Type IIa—Differentiated non-keratinising carcinoma
- Type IIb—undifferentiated non-keratinising carcinoma
- Type III—Basaloid squamous cell carcinoma

In endemic areas, the non-keratinising subtype constitutes most cases (>95%) and is invariably associated with EBV infection. On histopathology, abundant lymphoid cells are seen intermixed with malignant epithelial cells.

Staging of Nasopharyngeal Cancers The eighth edition of AJCC Classification and staging [59] is given in Table 6.7.

- Differential diagnoses include lymphoma, extramedullary plasmacytoma, melanoma, rhabdomyosarcoma, and adenoid cystic carcinoma.

Treatment: Non-keratinising NPC is a radiosensitive tumour and radiotherapy is the mainstay of treatment, whereas surgery is reserved for salvage of radiation failure.

- Intensity-modulated radiation therapy techniques are the standard of care, and integrating CT or MRI images into the 3D planning system provides accurate spatial information on the normal organ and tumour target which enables more flexible adjustment of the beam direction.
- Radiotherapy (RT) is the mainstay for the radical treatment of NPC (stage I).
- Concurrent chemoradiotherapy followed by adjuvant cisplatin and fluorouracil or neoadjuvant chemotherapy followed by concurrent chemoradiotherapy offers significant improvement in overall survival in stage III and IV diseases [75, 76].

NCCN Guideline [77]

- T1, N0, M0: Definitive radiotherapy to nasopharynx and elective RT to neck.
- T1, N1–3; T2–4, N0–3: Clinical trials (preferred) or Concurrent chemo/RT followed by adjuvant chemotherapy or induction chemotherapy followed by chemo/RT or concurrent chemo/RT not followed by chemotherapy.
- Any T, any N, M1: Clinical trials (preferred) or Platinum-based combination chemotherapy followed by RT or concurrent systemic therapy/RT as clinically indicated or observation or concurrent chemo/RT or RT or surgery in select patients with oligometastatic disease.
- Cetuximab or nimotuzumab, monoclonal antibodies in combination with induction chemotherapy has shown better overall survival and 3-years' disease-free survival in patients with locally advanced NPC treated with intensity-modulated radiotherapy [78].

Treatment of Local Recurrence Brachytherapy, high-dose external reirradiation, or surgery has comparable results in terms of treatment outcome in patients with early local recurrence, but their toxicity profile is quite different. Nasopharyngectomy is mainly reserved for lesions that do not involve skull base or internal carotid artery (rT1 and limited rT2) whereas external beam reirradiation is an alternative to surgery for rT2 disease and is often the only option for more advanced disease (advanced rT2, rT3–4). Brachytherapy is only suitable for small recurrences confined to the central nasopharynx. Few radioresistant tumours like adenoid cystic carcinoma should be treated with upfront surgery followed by radiotherapy.

Table 6.7 Staging: eighth edition of AJCC Classification and staging

T category		T criteria	
Tx		Primary tumour cannot be assessed.	
T0		No tumour recognised, but EBV-positive cervical lymph node(s).	
T1		Tumour limited to nasopharynx, or involvement of oropharynx and/or nasal cavity without parapharyngeal space infiltration.	
T2		Tumour with involvement to parapharyngeal space and/or neighbouring soft tissue involvement (medial pterygoid, lateral pterygoid, prevertebral muscles).	
T3		Tumour with infiltration of bony structures at the skull base, cervical vertebra, pterygoid structures, and/or paranasal sinuses.	
T4		Tumours with intracranial extension, involvement of cranial nerves, hypopharynx, orbit, parotid gland, and/or extensive soft tissue infiltration beyond the lateral surface of the lateral pterygoid muscle.	
N category		**N criteria**	
Nx		Regional lymph nodes cannot be assessed.	
N0		No regional lymph node metastasis.	
N1		Unilateral metastasis in cervical lymph node(s) and/unilateral or bilateral metastasis in retropharyngeal lymph node(s), 6 cm or smaller in greatest dimensions, above the caudal border of cricoid cartilage.	
N2		Bilateral metastasis in cervical lymph node(s) 6 cm or smaller in greatest dimension, above the caudal border of the cricoid cartilage.	
N3		Unilateral or bilateral metastasis in cervical lymph node(s), larger than 6 cm in greatest dimension, and/or extension below the caudal border of cricoid cartilage.	
M category		**M criteria**	
M0		No distant metastasis	
M1		Distant metastasis	
When T is ...	And N is...	And M is...	Then the stage group is...
Tis	N0	M0	Stage 0
T1	N0	M0	Stage I
T1,N0	N1	M0	Stage II
T2	N0	M0	Stage II
T2	N1	M0	Stage II
T1,T0	N2	M0	Stage III
T2	N2	M0	Stage III
T3	N0	M0	Stage III
T3	N1	M0	Stage III
T3	N2	M0	Stage III
T4	N0	M0	Stage IVA
T4	N1	M0	Stage IVA
T4	N2	M0	Stage IVA
Any T	N3	M0	Stage IVA
Any T	Any N	M1	Stage IVB

Surgery in form of nasopharyngectomy should be considered as a first-line treatment of residual or recurrence disease at the primary site (rT1 and limited rT2).

Surgical Approaches to Nasopharynx
Anterior approaches:

1. Trans-palatine approaches

Indications:

- Benign and malignant tumours of the posterior nasopharyngeal wall (2 cm or less in size)
- Access to tumour extending to clivus and craniocervical junction

Contraindications:
- Nasopharyngeal tumours size >2 cm
- Significant intracranial extension
- Tumours extending to parapharyngeal space, infratemporal fossa, cavernous sinus, and peritubal space

2. Transmandibular–transcervical approach:
   Indications:
   - Nasopharyngeal tumours extending into the anterior infratemporal fossa

   Contraindications:
   - Dural invasion >2 cm2 and intracranial involvement
   - Invasion of parasellar and posterior infratemporal region
3. Lateral approaches: infratemporal fossa type C:
   Indications:
   - Tumour that extends into the temporal bone with the involvement of the epipharynx
   - Contraindications:
   - Advanced disease extending to sella, contralateral middle fossa, anterior skull base
4. Anterolateral approach: Maxillary swing technique (Fig. 6.16)
   Indications:
   - Nasopharyngeal tumours with limited extension into the anterior infratemporal region

   Contraindications:
   - Lesions involving petrous ICA and petrous apex
   - Lesions extending into parasellar and/or posterior infratemporal region
5. Combined approaches: Subtemporal–preauricular infratemporal fossa approaches (Fig. 6.17)
   Indications:
   - Large tumours (T4) involving infratemporal space extending into the nasopharynx, cavernous sinus, and middle cranial fossa

   Contraindications:
   - Bilateral ICA involvement
   - Bilateral involvement of optic chiasma
   - Lesion extending into posterior cranial fossa
6. Facial translocation:
   Indications:
   - Extensive tumours (T4) of anterior and middle skull base extending into orbit, paranasal sinus, and posterior cranial fossa with intracranial involvement
   - Contraindications:
   - Bilateral involvement of ICA
   - Bilateral involvement of optic chiasma
   - Lesion extending into posterior cranial fossa

Robotic Nasopharyngectomy Transoral robotic nasopharyngectomy has many advantages which include good visualisation of the lateral aspect of nasopharynx and avoidance of cutting palatal muscles including tensor veil palatine which can cause velopharyngeal insufficiency. This new technique is a feasible operation for salvage of recurrent nasopharyngeal carcinoma mainly rT1 and limited rT2 NPC. Early results have shown a high control rate, low morbidity, and comparable operating time to open surgeries. It is indicated in [79]:

1. Smaller tumours in posterior wall/roof of nasopharynx.
2. Fossa of Rosenmuller without lateral extension.
3. Tumour should be more than 1 cm from ICA and the course of ICA should not be medial to the medial pterygoid plate.

Contraindications:

1. Tumour located less than 1 cm from ICA
2. Tumour extending lateral to lateral pterygoid plate
3. Tumour with invasion of pterygopalatine fossa or maxillary sinus

A major disadvantage is the lack of tactile sensation which makes the surgeon unaware that the tip of the instrument has reached the bony clivus or the inability to palpate ICA which is in the lateral aspect of the area of dissection.

Endoscopic Nasopharyngectomy A minimally invasive, safe, and efficacious option for selected primary and locally radiorecurrent tumours with comparable survival to open approaches. This technique approaches the nasopharynx through the natural orifices with added high magnification and avoids the inherent morbidities associated with open procedures. However, long-term evaluation with longer follow-up data is required. Three types of nasopharyngeal endoscopic resection (NER) are:

1. Type I NER: Involves resection of posterior wall of nasopharynx
2. Type II NER: Involves resection of tumours extending superiorly to the sphenoid sinus
3. Type 3 NER: Is trans-pterygoid approach to posterolateral nasopharynx with removal of eustachian tube and pterygoid plates

Initial results are promising with local control comparable to conventional open surgical techniques, with most series having a 2-years' local control of over 80% [80, 81].

Treatment of Regional Recurrence Reirradiation for nodal failure is associated with poor results and high complications. Neck dissection remains the treatment of choice for residual or metastatic neck disease whenever possible. Prognosis often remains poor in neck residue patients. Surgical salvage of nodal recurrence has a 5-years' local control of 66% and 5-years' overall survival of 37% [82].

Distant Recurrence The traditional first-line chemotherapeutic regimen for metastatic NPC is a combination of cisplatin and 5-fluorouracil and the median overall survival is around 12 months.

Brachytherapy This modality can be used either as a primary treatment modality or in the management of recurrent cancers. For patients with T1–2 NPC, it can be used either as two-dimensional high-dose-rate brachytherapy or three-dimensional image high-dose-rate brachytherapy with acceptable complications. For recurrent NPC, image-guided ^{125}I is an effective treatment modality with better survival and minimal damage [83].

Immunotherapy Expression of EBV antigens is important as these antigens are being targeted in immunotherapy such as viral-specific adoptive cell therapy. These strategies may emerge as the main modality of treatment and can offer a durable remission in advanced nasopharyngeal carcinoma [84].

Photodynamic Therapy (PDT) FDA-approved therapy involves a combination of light-activated photosensitiser, visible light, and molecular oxygen to selectively destroy tissue. Antitumour effect is derived by three mechanisms: the destruction of tumour-associated vasculature, direct cytotoxic effect, and induction of inflammatory reaction against tumour cells. Photofrin, first-generation FDA-approved photosensitiser, is administered via intravenous injections with 24–48 hours incubation with light of wavelength 630 nm. Its longer clearance time is a drawback of photofrin-mediated PDT. A number of second-generation photosensitisers (5-Aminolevulinic acid, hexyl-ALA, and Meta-tetra (hydroxyphenyl) chlorine) were discovered and have potential advantages over first-generation drugs including better tumour selectivity, faster clearance, and higher chemical purity. Light sources commonly used for PDT include laser diode, laser, filtered broadband light, and light-emitting diodes. It can be used in residual and recurrent cases and initial studies have shown improvement in recurrent tumours of less than 10 mm in depth [85].

Follow-Up With the introduction of a concurrent chemoradiation regimen, recurrence has dropped to less than 10%. Most failures occur within 2 years of treatment. Patients with NPC cases are followed up and assessed with office-based rigid and/or fibro-optic nasal endoscopy. Positron emission tomography–computed tomography, CT, or MRI scan should be carried out at 3 months from completion of treatment to assess response.

Outcome In general, patients with non-viral-associated nasopharyngeal carcinoma (i.e. HPV-negative, EBV-negative tumours) had worse outcomes than patients with viral-associated tumours. The average 5 years survival rates with treatment are [86]:

- Stage I: 100%
- Stage II: 90%
- Stage III: 67%
- Stage IV A: 67%
- Stage IV B: 69%
- Stage IV C:18%

Adenoid Cystic Carcinoma Adenoid cystic carcinoma (ACC) arising from minor salivary glands in this region is relatively rare and has a progressive clinical course. These lesions are characterised by local infiltration and neural invasion and can extend from the nasopharynx into the orbital cavity, along the cranial nerve canal and anterior skull base. Most often, they tend to be locally aggressive and have high tendency of recurrence. Magnetic resonance imaging is the investigation of interest as it detects perineurial invasion and has a superior definition in detecting soft tissue changes. It is widely used for monitoring the response of treatment. Complete surgical resection is an important goal in the treatment; however, close resection margins in an anatomically complex area, adjuvant therapy becomes an integral part of treatment [87]. Endoscopic surgery is becoming a promising approach for early-stage disease.

ACC grows slowly, recurs frequently, and metastasises to distant organs, particularly lungs, and therefore, its long-term prognosis is poor. The solid component of tumour on histology, advanced tumour stage, and the perineurial invasion appears to be associated with an unfavourable prognosis.

Nasopharyngeal Papillary Adenocarcinoma Primary nasopharyngeal papillary adenocarcinoma is an extremely rare tumour which is reported to occupy 0.48% of all types of NPC [88]. These tumours have features resembling papillary carcinoma thyroid with nuclear positive expression of thyroid transcription factor-1 (TTF-1) and therefore can be confused with metastatic papillary thyroid carcinoma histologically but these lesions are thyroglobulin-negative.

These tumours commonly arise from surface epithelium in the posterior and superior aspect of the nasopharynx. Histologically, tumour cells have a papillary architecture with mild nuclear atypia and invasive growth pattern. On immunohistochemistry, these tumours are TTF-1 V, CK-7, CK-19, and CEA positive. Complete surgical excision is the treatment. Adjuvant radiation therapy is advised in case of incomplete excision [89].

Chordoma Chordoma is a low-grade malignant tumour arising from notochord remnants showing epithelial–mesenchymal differentiation. They mostly arise from clivus in the head and neck region in 25–35% of cases. These lesions are slow-growing and invade local structures, and malignant transformation occurs in third to fourth decade of life. Metastasis is rare and if occurs, metastasise to lungs, bones, skin, and lymph nodes. They can have varied presentations, depending on their location. Cranial tumours may present with chronic intractable headache, cranial neuropathy, inferior extension results in nasal or nasopharyngeal mass, nasal obstruction, nasal bleeding, and cerebrospinal rhinorrhoea. Histologically shows lobular growth pattern separated by connective tissue septae (typical multivacuolated physaliferous cells). Immunohistochemistry shows positivity for cytokeratin, vimentin, and S-100 [90]. Staging is done by radiological investigations (CECT/CEMRI) and is a prerequisite for appropriate management. Treatment options include surgery (gross total resection) +/− radiotherapy or radiotherapy. Endonasal endoscopic skull base approach has allowed a high rate of gross as well as microscopic clearance of disease [91]. Due to the locally invasive nature of the lesion, complete excision may not be possible leading to a high recurrence rate. Five and 10 years overall survival rates are 50% and 20%. Tumour necrosis and volume of tumour more than 70 ml are independent poor prognostic factors.

6.5 Part E: Pathology of Lesions of the Nose and Paranasal Sinuses

Lesions of the nose and paranasal sinuses include inflammatory lesions as well as benign and malignant neoplasms. With increasing ease of availability of high-throughput molecular diagnostic platforms, newer genetically defined entities are being identified, leading to escalating complexity of classification systems. This chapter covers the salient diagnostic features and genetic alterations in the frequently encountered lesions of this region.

6.5.1 Sinonasal Neoplasms

The nasal cavity and paranasal sinuses play host to a wide spectrum of benign and malignant neoplasms. These neoplasms may be exclusive to this region, may occur here more frequently than at other head and neck sites, or may occur elsewhere in the body but are important in the sinonasal tract due to differential diagnostic considerations. They include benign and malignant tumours of epithelial, mesenchymal, neuroectodermal, and hematolymphoid origin, as shown in Table 6.8 [92, 93].

6.5.2 Carcinomas

Carcinomas are tumours of epithelial origin. Sinonasal carcinomas represent fewer than 5% of all head and neck tumours. They may arise from the respiratory epithelium of the sinonasal region, or from the subepithelial mucoserous glands. They are diagnosed primarily based on morphology and immunohistochemistry. However, improvements in molecular techniques in recent years have led to a more specific categorisation of sinonasal carcinomas, with many poorly differentiated tumours being redefined into more specific categories based on molecular genetic features.

Table 6.8 Classification of sinonasal tumours

Epithelial		Mesenchymal			Others
Malignant	Benign	Malignant	Borderline	Benign	
Squamous cell carcinoma and variants	Sinonasal papillomas	Biphenotypic sinonasal sarcoma	Glomangiopericytoma	Leiomyoma	Neuroectodermal *Olfactory neuroblastoma* *Ewing sarcoma* *Mucosal melanoma*
SMARCB1-deficient sinonasal carcinoma	Respiratory epithelial lesions *Respiratory epithelial adenomatoid hamartoma* *Seromucinous hamartoma*	Undifferentiated pleomorphic sarcoma	Solitary fibrous tumour	Hemangioma	Lymphomas *Extranodal NK/T cell lymphoma* *Plasmacytoma* *Plasmablastic lymphoma*
NUT carcinoma	Salivary gland tumours *Pleomorphic adenoma*	Malignant peripheral nerve sheath tumour	Fibromatosis	Schwannoma	Sinonasal teratocarcinosarcoma
Neuroendocrine carcinomas		Fibrosarcoma	Epithelioid hemangioendothelioma	Neurofibroma	Ectopic pituitary adenoma
Adenocarcinoma		Rhabdomyosarcoma			Meningioma
Sinonasal undifferentiated carcinoma (SNUC)		Synovial sarcoma			
		Leiomyosarcoma			
		Angiosarcoma			

6.5.2.1 Squamous Cell Carcinoma (SCC)

SCC is a carcinoma with squamous differentiation, arising from the sinonasal surface epithelium. SCCs occur de novo, or, less frequently, by malignant transformation of sinonasal papillomas. They are classified as keratinising and non-keratinising types. The keratinising type of SCC is associated with smoking and resembles keratinising SCC at other head and neck sites. It displays nests and cords of atypical squamous cells with evidence of maturation, i.e. keratinisation, in a desmoplastic stroma. Keratinising SCCs are graded as well into moderately or poorly differentiated tumours based on the extent of keratinisation (Fig. 6.29a). Non-keratinising SCC has been found to be associated with transcriptionally active high-risk HPV. It is morphologically characterised by ribbon-like and nested architecture, and pushing borders (Fig. 6.29b). Tumour cells appear basaloid, with scant cytoplasm and ovoid nuclei (Fig. 6.29c). These tumours are not graded as keratinising SCC are HPV-related tumours demonstrate diffuse p16 staining, and are HPV positive by in DNA and mRNA situ hybridisation techniques. Rare morphological subtypes of SCC occasionally encountered in the sinonasal tract include spindle cell (sarcomatoid) SCC, lymphoepithelial carcinoma, papillary SCC, basaloid SCC, and verrucous carcinoma. SCCs are immunopositive for cytokeratins including CK5/6, epithelial membrane antigen (EMA), and squamous markers p63 and p40. Staining with these markers is extremely helpful in establishing the diagnosis of spindle cell SCC [94].

6.5.2.2 SMARCB1-Deficient Sinonasal Carcinoma

SMARCB1-deficient sinonasal carcinomas are recently identified aggressive neoplasms characterised by biallelic inactivating alterations (deletions, intragenic mutations) in the *SMARCB1* tumour suppressor gene on 22q11.2, which can be demonstrated by loss of immunoexpression of INI1, the protein product of this gene. Prior to their identification, they were mostly diagnosed as non-keratinising SCC or sinonasal undifferentiated carcinoma (SNUC). These tumours show a variable admixture of basaloid (Fig. 6.30a), plasmacytoid (Fig. 6.30b), and rhabdoid cells with abundant eccentric eosinophilic inclusion-like cytoplasm (Fig. 6.30c). In addition, they may also show oncocytic cells in a glandular pattern, mimicking adenocarcinomas. Inverted papilloma-like growth, pagetoid spread along respiratory epithelium, and clefting artefact around tumour islands are other features that may be present. Necrosis, frequent mitoses, and intracytoplasmic clear vacuoles are present in the tumour cells. On immunohistochemistry, they show loss of INI1 immunostaining (Fig. 6.30d), are diffusely cytokeratin-positive, and show variable staining with p63, p40, CK5/6, and neuroendocrine markers [95, 96].

6.5.2.3 NUT Carcinoma

NUT carcinoma is a novel, poorly differentiated, aggressive carcinoma characterised by *NUTM1* gene rearrangements with various fusion partners, most frequently *BRD4*. NUT carcinomas

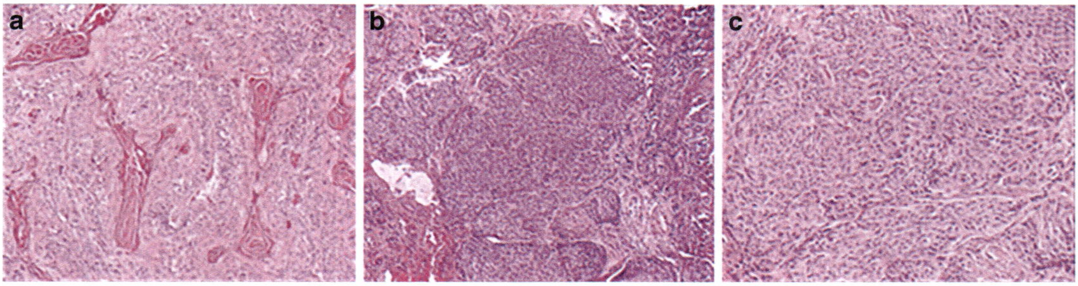

Fig. 6.29 Keratinising squamous cell carcinoma showing irregular nests of cells with abundant pink cytoplasm and keratin pearls (**a**); non-keratinising squamous cell carcinoma showing large rounded nests with smooth borders (**b**) containing tumour cells with scant cytoplasm (**c**)

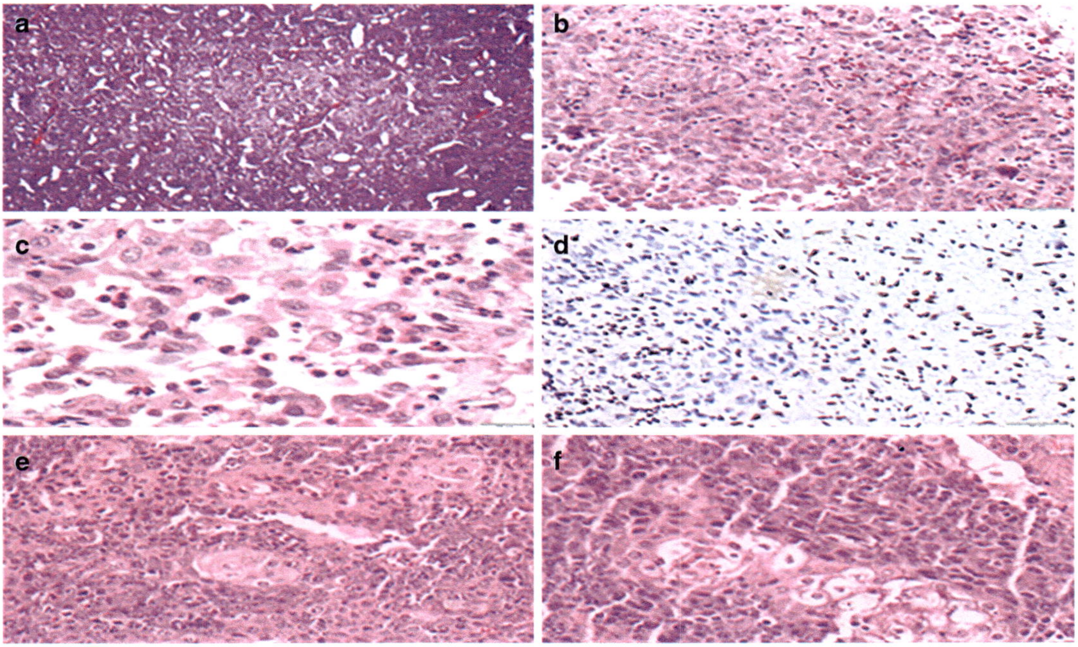

Fig. 6.30 *SMARCB1*-deficient sinonasal carcinoma with "blue" basaloid cells showing empty vacuoles (**a**), "pink" plasmacytoid (**b**) and rhabdoid (**c**) cells, and loss of INI1 staining (**d**); NUT carcinoma showing undifferentiated basaloid cells (**e**) with foci of abrupt squamous differentiation (**f**)

have been described at midline locations in the head and neck including the sinonasal region and parotid gland, and in the mediastinum and lung. These tumours are composed of sheets and nests of undifferentiated basaloid cells (Fig. 6.30e), with foci of abrupt squamous differentiation including clear cells and squamous eddies (Fig. 6.30f). The tumour cells may display spindling and peripheral palisading. Interspersed inflammatory cells may be present. The tumour cells show diffuse immunopositivity with cytokeratin, p63, p40, and NUT protein [97].

6.5.2.4 Adenocarcinoma

Sinonasal adenocarcinomas are glandular neoplasms that arise from glandular cells in the respiratory mucosa. Non-salivary-type sinonasal adenocarcinomas are classified as intestinal and non-intestinal types.

Intestinal-type adenocarcinomas (ITACs) are sinonasal glandular neoplasms that resemble gastrointestinal adenocarcinomas, hence the name. They develop through intestinal metaplasia of the lining epithelium of the sinonasal region. They present as exophytic masses that extensively invade surrounding tissue. They show a variety of histological patterns, including papillary (Fig. 6.31a), tubular, solid, and mucinous. Mixed patterns are frequent. Mucinous, goblet, and signet-ring cells containing intracytoplasmic mucin are present; intraluminal and extracellular mucin may also be seen. The tumour cells are cuboidal to columnar with pseudostratified nuclei (Fig. 6.31b) showing variable crowding and loss of polarity which increase with increasing grade from low through intermediate to high. The tumour cells are immunopositive for CK20, CDX2 (Fig. 6.31c), villin, and MUC2, similar to colonic adenocarcinomas; variable staining for CK7, EMA, and CEA is also seen. Focal positivity for neuroendocrine markers is frequent. Mutations have been identified in *KRAS*, *HRAS*, *TP53* genes, like in colonic adenocarcinomas. Solid, mucinous, and signet ring patterns have been found to be associated with poor prognosis in these tumours [98].

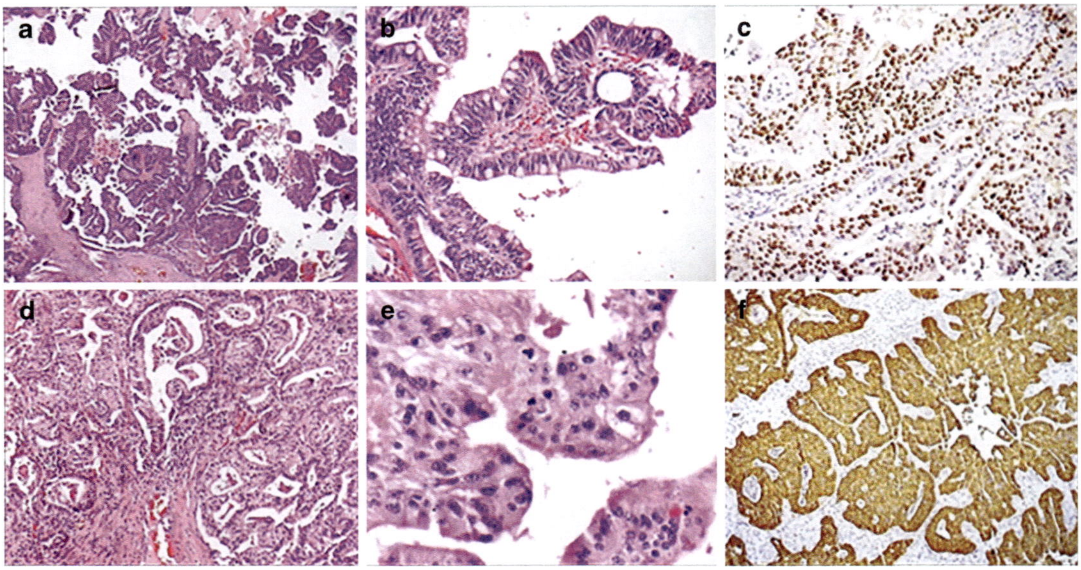

Fig. 6.31 Intestinal-type adenocarcinoma with papillary structures (**a**) lined by tall columnar cells with stratification of nuclei (**b**) immunopositive for CDX2 (**c**); non-intestinal-type adenocarcinoma with tubuloglandular pattern (**d**), cuboidal cells (**e**) and CK7 positivity (**f**)

Non-intestinal-type adenocarcinomas (NITACs) are sinonasal adenocarcinomas that do not show the features of salivary gland neoplasms and do not have an intestinal phenotype. They show papillary, tubuloglandular (Fig. 6.31d), solid architecture with a single layer of cuboidal to columnar cells lacking cilia (Fig. 6.31e), with mild to moderate (in low grade) or severe (in high grade) nuclear pleomorphism. Low-grade tumours have well-formed back-to-back glands; high-grade tumours have predominantly solid pattern with sheet-like growth of tumour cells. Scant intracytoplasmic or intraluminal mucin may be present. Tumour cells are immunopositive for CK7 (Fig. 6.31f) and are negative for CK20, CDX2, and villin. INI1 expression is retained, unlike in SMARCB1-deficient sinonasal carcinomas with glandular architectural patterns [99].

6.5.2.5 Neuroendocrine Carcinomas (NECs)

Neuroendocrine carcinomas (NECs) in the sinonasal tract are relatively rare, with the majority being poorly differentiated NECs, which are high-grade carcinomas with evidence of neuroendocrine differentiation. NECs are graded as well, moderately or poorly differentiated NEC based on mitotic count and presence of necrosis. Poorly differentiated NEC includes small cell NEC and large cell NEC, of which the former outnumbers the latter. Small cell NEC (Fig. 6.32a) is composed of small- to medium-sized cells with scant cytoplasm and hyperchromatic nuclei (Fig. 6.32b). Similar to pulmonary small cell NEC, nuclear molding, crushing, and necrosis are prominent; frequent mitoses are present. Large cell NEC shows cells with abundant cytoplasm, and vesicular nuclei with coarse chromatin and prominent nucleoli, arranged in nests and trabeculae. Frequent mitoses and comedo necrosis are identified. Both small cell and large cell NEC show positivity for at least one neuroendocrine marker, i.e. chromogranin, synaptophysin (Fig. 6.32c), CD56. Cytokeratin shows a characteristic paranuclear dot-like staining pattern. TTF-1 is frequently positive in small cell NEC, and should not be mistaken as evidence of pulmonary origin. Well-differentiated (carcinoid) and moderately differentiated (atypical carci-

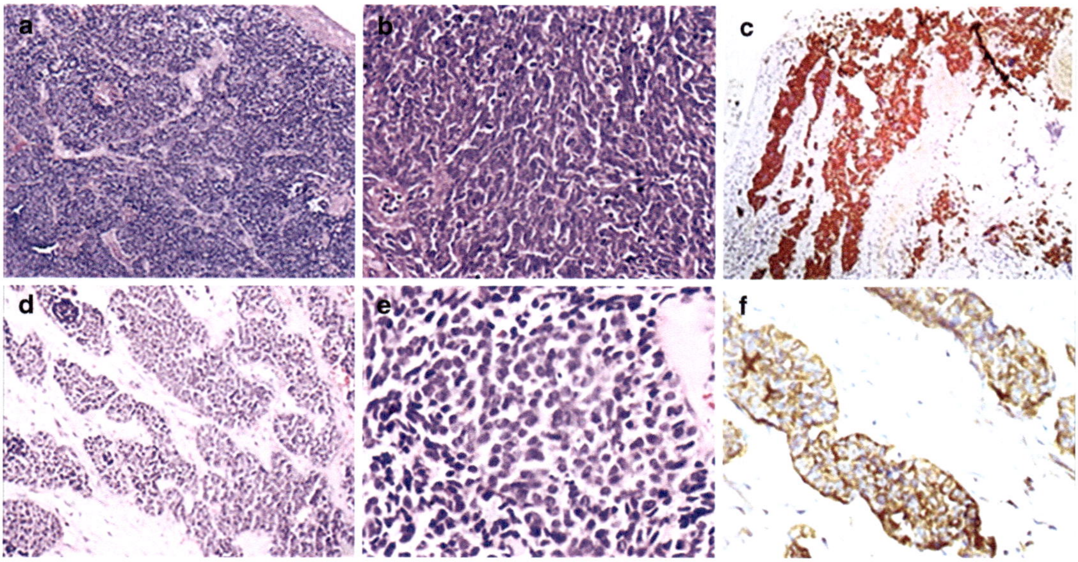

Fig. 6.32 Small cell neuroendocrine carcinoma showing lobular architecture (**a**), sheets of cells with scant cytoplasm, stippled chromatin, and nuclear molding (**b**) that are positive for synaptophysin (**c**); sinonasal undifferentiated carcinoma with nests and trabecular arrangement (**d**) of monomorphic malignant cells with brisk mitoses (**e**) and cytokeratin positivity (**f**)

noid) NEC are extremely rare in the sinonasal tract. Pituitary adenoma, ectopic or extending from the sella, should be excluded prior to making this diagnosis [100].

6.5.2.6 Sinonasal Undifferentiated Carcinoma (SNUC)

SNUC is a high-grade undifferentiated epithelial malignancy lacking specific differentiation, i.e. without glandular or squamous features by histological or immunohistochemical examination. It is a highly aggressive carcinoma with uncertain histogenesis and morphological overlap with other malignant tumours (Table 6.9). It is postulated that the cell of origin of this neoplasm may be related to both the Schneiderian membrane and olfactory epithelium. SNUC is now considered a diagnosis of exclusion and has become less common with the description of specific genetically defined tumour entities, such as SMARCB1-deficient carcinoma, SMARCA4-deficient carcinoma, and NUT carcinoma.

SNUC is composed of atypical, overtly malignant cells lacking squamous or glandular differentiation, which are arranged in sheets, lobules, or trabeculae (Fig. 6.32d). Cells have scant to moderate amount of cytoplasm, ill-defined cytoplasmic borders, large round vesicular to hyperchromatic nuclei, prominent nucleoli, and brisk mitotic activity (Fig. 6.32e). However, they are relatively isomorphic appearing. There usually is abundant necrosis and apoptosis. Surface dysplasia is not present. Tumour cells are immunoreactive with pan-cytokeratin (Fig. 6.32f), CK7, CK19, and epithelial membrane antigen, while CK5/6 and CK14 are negative. Focal positivity with neuroendocrine markers and p63 may be present. However, p40, a more specific marker of squamous differentiation is negative or maybe seen in occasional cells only. Neuroendocrine markers like chromogranin and synaptophysin may show focal positivity. Tumour cells are negative for NUT, INI1 expression is retained, and p16 may be positive, regardless of HPV status. A subset of SNUCs have recently been found to show mutation in *IDH1 and 2* genes, which can be identified by IDH immunohistochemistry and sequencing [101].

Table 6.9 Differential diagnosis of undifferentiated tumours of the sinonasal tract

Neoplasm	Morphological features	Immunohistochemistry
Non-keratinising SCC	Basaloid cells with nuclear pleomorphism; focal keratinisation, intercellular bridges	PanCK +; p63/ p40 +; INI1 retained
Basaloid SCC	Basaloid cells with peripheral palisading	PanCK +; p63/ p40 +; INI1 retained
Olfactory neuroblastoma	Lobular or diffuse architecture, fibrillary background, ganglionic differentiation	NSE, CG, synaptophysin, calretinin +; S100 + in sustentacular cells; PanCK may be positive, EMA negative
NUT carcinoma	Primitive basaloid cells Abrupt keratinisation +/–	PanCK, p63, p40 +; NUT1 +; INI1 retained
SMARCB1-deficient sinonasal carcinoma	Variable admixture of basaloid, plasmacytoid, rhabdoid cells; no true keratinisation; relatively uniform nuclei	PanCK +; p63, p40, CD34, neuroendocrine markers +/–; INI1 loss
Small cell neuroendocrine carcinoma	High N:C ratio with nuclear molding; abundant mitoses, necrosis, apoptosis	Neuroendocrine markers +; PanCK dot-like +; INI1 retained
Large cell neuroendocrine carcinoma	Organoid nesting pattern, trabeculae; large cells, coarse salt-and-pepper chromatin, prominent nucleoli +/–	Neuroendocrine markers +; PanCK dot-like +; INI1 retained
HPV-related multiphenotypic sinonasal carcinoma	Biphasic: Basal & ductal cells; cribriform architecture frequent; surface dysplasia present	S100, p40, p63 + in basal cells; CK7, CD117 + in ductal cells; p16, HR HPV ISH +; INI1 retained
Adenoid cystic carcinoma, grade III	Basaloid cells in solid sheets; focal cribriform pattern; small cells with angulated nuclei; surface dysplasia absent	CD117, p40, MYB +
Sinonasal undifferentiated carcinoma	Large round nuclei of uniform size; mitoses, apoptosis ++	p63, p40, NE markers focal +/–; PanCK +; INI1 retained
Ewing sarcoma	Small to medium cells with scant vacuolated cytoplasm, fine chromatin; necrosis	CD99, FLI1, NKX2.2 +; PanCK negative
Adamantinoma-like Ewing sarcoma	Basaloid cells with peripheral palisading; basement membrane-like material seen	PanCK, p40, CD99, FLI1, NKX2.2 +; INI1 retained
Rhabdomyosarcoma	Primitive round to spindle cells; rhabdomyoblasts; multinucleated cells	Myogenin, desmin, MyoD1 +
Lymphoma (Extranodal NK/T cell lymphoma, nasal type)	Dispersed cells; angiocentricity, angiodestruction; abundant necrosis	Leukocyte common antigen, lineage-specific markers (CD3, CD56) +; EBV EBER +
Mucosal melanoma	Pleomorphic, with epithelioid, plasmacytoid, and spindled cells; peritheliomatous pattern; melanin may be present	S100,SOX10,HMB-45,Melan-A+;PanCK-

6.5.3 Sinonasal Papillomas

Sinonasal papillomas are benign epithelial neoplasms arising from sinonasal mucosa. They are also known as Schneiderian papillomas, as they originate from the Schneiderian epithelium lining the nasal cavity. While they are benign tumours, they may be locally destructive, may recur, and on occasion may even undergo malignant transformation. Sinonasal papillomas are of three types viz. inverted (Fig. 6.33a–c), exophytic, and oncocytic, whose features are summarised in Table 6.10.

Malignant transformation of sinonasal papillomas follows a papilloma–dysplasia–carcinoma sequence. Dysplasia may be keratinising or non-keratinising, with the latter being more subtle and difficult to identify. Histological features indicative of malignant transformation in a papilloma include the presence of extensive exophytic pap-

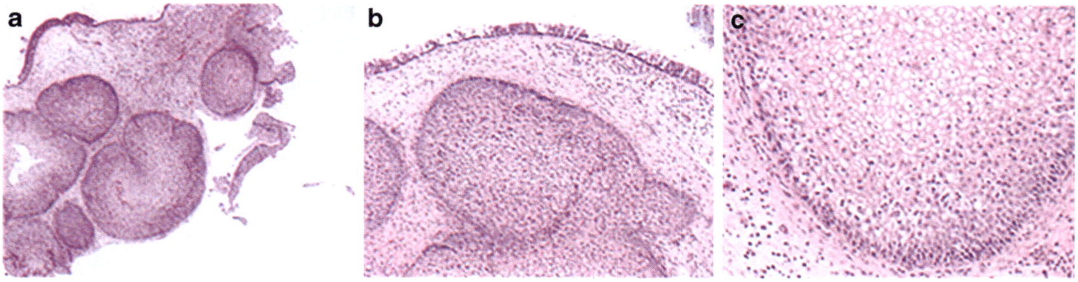

Fig. 6.33 Sinonasal inverted papilloma with endophytic submucosal proliferation of rounded nests (**a**) of immature squamous cells lacking atypia (**b**); transmigrating neutrophils are prominent (**c**)

Table 6.10 Salient features of different types of sinonasal papillomas

Inverted type	Exophytic type	Oncocytic type
Most common type	Rare	Least common
Lateral nasal wall, paranasal sinuses	Nasal septum	Lateral nasal wall, paranasal sinuses
Endophytic growth pattern	Exophytic polypoid growth	Exophytic and/or endophytic growth
Nests, ribbon-like growth pattern; edematous stroma	Papillary structures with delicate fibrovascular cores	Nested and papillary architecture
Multilayered non-keratinising immature squamous cells, with variable respiratory epithelial cells and mucocytes; transmigrating neutrophils are prominent	Multilayered squamous or respiratory epithelial cells, with mucocytes; rare transmigrating neutrophils; koilocytic change may be seen	Multilayered cuboidal to columnar epithelial cells with abundant eosinophilic cytoplasm; intraepithelial mucous cysts, neutrophilic microabscesses
Mutually exclusive *EGFR* mutations and low-risk HPV association	Association with low-risk HPV types 6 and 11	KRAS mutations
Low to intermediate risk of malignant transformation	Very low risk of malignant transformation	Low to intermediate risk of malignant transformation

illomatous growth in an inverted papilloma, decreased transmigrating neutrophils, atypical mitoses, necrosis, bone invasion, increased Ki-67 expression, and p53 expression in >25% of tumour cells [92, 94].

6.5.4 Mesenchymal Neoplasms

Biphenotypic sinonasal sarcoma is a recently described entity. It is a low-grade malignancy with a distinctive genetic signature and propensity for local recurrence but not metastasis, which is exclusive to the sinonasal region. It is characterised by t(2;4) resulting in fusion of the *PAX3* gene with *MAML3*, *NCOA1/2*, *FOXO1*, or *WWTR1* genes. These tumours are seen most commonly in females in the fourth to sixth decades of life. They are histologically characterised by infiltrating monomorphic spindle-shaped cells arranged in fascicles, herringbone, and storiform pattern in a collagenous background. At places, tumour cells may show evidence of Schwannian or rhabdomyoblastic differentiation. Entrapped epithelial invaginations with or without squamous metaplasia is a typical feature of this tumour. Tumour cells have minimal nuclear pleomorphism; mitoses are infrequent. These tumours display dual neural and myogenic differentiation histologically and immunohistochemically, hence the nomenclature "biphenotypic." Differential diagnosis of biphenotypic sinonasal sarcoma includes all spindle cell tumours that may occur in this region, as shown in Table 6.11 [102–104].

6.5.4.1 Rhabdomyosarcoma (RMS)

Rhabdomyosarcoma is a malignant soft tissue tumour with skeletal muscle differentiation.

Table 6.11 Differential diagnosis of common spindle cell neoplasms of the sinonasal tract

Tumour	Histopathological features	IHC	Genetics
Biphenotypic sinonasal sarcoma	Spindle cells in short fascicles Elongated nuclei Epithelial invaginations Staghorn vasculature	S100, SMA, muscle-specific actin, calponin, desmin/myogenin (patchy), PAX3, β-catenin (focal)	*PAX3* rearrangements
Glomangiopericytoma	Plump oval/spindle cells in short fascicles, syncytium Round to oval nuclei Staghorn vasculature Perivascular hyalinisation	β-Catenin, SMA, cyclinD1	*CTNNB1* mutations
Solitary fibrous tumour	Bland spindle cells in patternless pattern Alternating hypo- and hypercellular areas Ropey collagen Malignant: Increased cellularity, atypia, mitoses	STAT6, CD34, bcl2, CD99	*NAB2-STAT6* fusion
Monophasic synovial sarcoma	Plump oval to spindle cells in fascicular/herringbone pattern, scant cytoplasm; branching vasculature	CD99, bcl2, TLE1, cytokeratins, EMA	*SSX-SS18* fusion
Malignant peripheral nerve sheath tumour	Spindle cells with tapered nuclei, myxoid background Nuclear atypia, necrosis, mitoses	SOX10, S100 (focal), H3K27me3 loss	Neurofibromatosis type 1
Spindle cell rhabdomyosarcoma	Herringbone, fascicular architecture Greater atypia, mitoses	Desmin (more diffuse than BSNS), myoD1; PAX3 negative	*MYOD1* mutations
Leiomyosarcoma	Spindled cells in long fascicles Bright eosinophilic cytoplasm Cigar-shaped nuclei	SMA, SMMHC, desmin, caldesmon	
Fibromatosis	Spindled cells in broad fascicles Collagenised/myxoid matrix Infiltrating margins	Nuclear β-catenin	*CTNNB1* mutation
Fibrosarcoma	Cellular spindle cell tumour in fascicular/ herringbone pattern	Vimentin	
Inflammatory myofibroblastic tumour	Spindle cells admixed with inflammatory cells	ALK1, SMA	*ALK* translocations
Schwannoma	Cellular Antoni A and hypocellular Antoni B areas Benign spindle cells with fibrillary cytoplasm Wavy, buckled nuclei Verocay bodies Cystic, hemorrhagic areas	S100, SOX10, GFAP, NSE	
Meningioma	Whorled architecture, cells in syncytium, intranuclear inclusions, calcification	EMA, vimentin, progesterone receptor	
Phosphaturic mesenchymal tumour	Stellate to spindled cells with vesicular nuclei; smudgy matrix; grungy calcification; staghorn vessels; osteoclastic giant cells	Vimentin, FGF-23, somatostatin receptors (SSTR)	*FGFR1* gene fusions

RMS is the most common sinonasal sarcoma in children and young adults. There are three histological subtypes of RMS, viz. embryonal, alveolar, and spindle cell/sclerosing RMS.

Embryonal RMS is seen in young patients, i.e. the first decade of life. It is composed of small round, polygonal and spindle cells with scant cytoplasm and hyperchromatic nuclei in a myxoid to collagenous stroma. There is variable evidence of rhabdomyoblastic differentiation in the form of cells with bright pink cytoplasm and eccentric nuclei. Strap cells and, rarely, cytoplasmic cross-striations may also be seen. The botryoid variant of embryonal RMS presents as a polypoidal mass with linear condensation of tumour cells beneath the surface epithelium, forming a hypercellular "cambium" layer. Embryonal RMS shows diffuse strong desmin positivity and variable reactivity with myogenin and myoD1. *FGFR4/RAS/AKT* pathway mutations have been identified in embryonal RMS.

Alveolar RMS is seen in adolescents and young adults. It displays small to medium round blue cells arranged in an alveolar pattern with intervening fibrovascular septa. Multinucleated tumour cells are frequent, and are a clue to the diagnosis; rhabdomyoblasts may also be seen. The solid variant of alveolar RMS does not show the alveolar pattern with fibrovascular septa but has sheet-like growth of tumour cells. Alveolar RMS are diffusely positive for myogenin and stain positively at least focally with desmin. Alveolar RMS harbour *PAX3FOX01* (in 70–90% of cases) or *PAX7-FOX01* (in 10% of cases) gene fusions. These are of prognostic significance, with the former having worse outcomes than the latter. Fusion-negative alveolar RMS have a prognosis similar to embryonal RMS.

Spindle cell/sclerosing RMS are the rarest RMS subtypes and occur at all ages. In adults, they frequently occur at head and neck locations. They are comprised of intersecting fascicles of spindle-shaped cells with eosinophilic cytoplasm. Those with prominent stromal hyalinisation and nested or cord-like arrangement of tumour cells are designated as sclerosing RMS. Desmin and myogenin show variable staining but myoD1 is strongly positive in this RMS subtype. *MYOD1* mutations are seen in spindle cell/sclerosing RMS.

All RMS may aberrantly express CK, EMA, synaptophysin, chromogranin, INSM1, and CD99; hence, immunohistochemistry should be interpreted with caution [105].

6.5.4.2 Schwannoma

Schwannomas are benign nerve sheath tumours that originate from Schwann cells. They are unencapsulated tumours, with cellular Antoni A and hypocellular Antoni B areas. Antoni A areas are composed of elongated spindled cells with wavy, buckled nuclei having tapered ends. Nuclear palisading and Verocay bodies are present. Antoni B areas consist of a hypocellular, myxoid stroma with reticular appearance and infiltration by inflammatory cells, particularly by histiocytes. Perivascular hyalinisation and degenerative changes such as haemorrhage, cystic areas, and nuclear atypia are commonly seen. Schwannomas show diffuse strong S100 positivity.

6.5.4.3 Nasopharyngeal Angiofibroma

These are benign, locally aggressive fibrovascular neoplasms seen almost exclusively in adolescent males. They arise from a nidus in the posterolateral wall of the nasal cavity. The growth of these tumours is believed to be testosterone hormone-dependent. They are characterised by submucosal haphazard proliferation of thin- and thick-walled blood vessels which are surrounded by spindled to stellate shaped fibroblasts in a collagenous stroma (Fig 6.34a, b). There is minimal nuclear atypia, and mitoses are rare. Necrosis may be seen

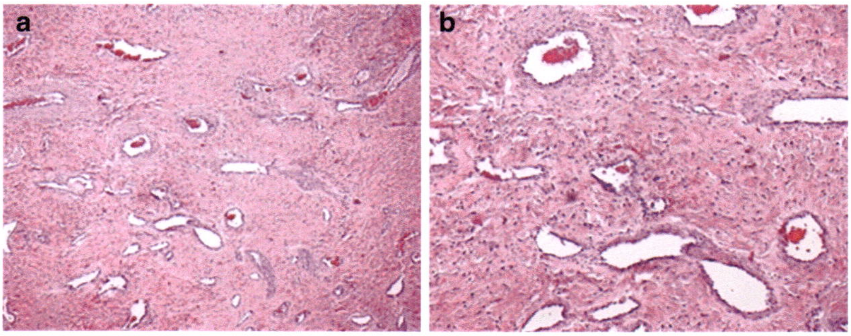

Fig. 6.34 Nasopharyngeal angiofibroma showing a spindle cell tumour with many blood vessels (**a**) from which the spindle cells emanate (**b**)

following embolisation, accompanied by intravascular foreign material. On immunohistochemistry, the tumour cells are immunopositive for androgen receptor and beta-catenin. The display genetic alterations are including loss of the Y chromosome and mutations in exon 3 of the *CTNNB1* (beta-catenin) gene in the majority of cases. Patients with familial adenomatous polyposis having a germline *APC* gene mutation are more likely to develop angiofibromas [106].

6.5.5 Other Malignant Neoplasms

6.5.5.1 Olfactory Neuroblastoma

Olfactory neuroblastoma, previously also known as esthesioneuroblastoma, originates from the specialised sensory olfactory neuroepithelium present near the cribriform plate of ethmoid. On histology, ONB shows a wide morphological spectrum, based on the grade of the tumour. Hyams grade is the most accepted grading system. Low-grade tumours (grade 1 and 2) consist of monomorphic small round blue cells with stippled/"salt and pepper" chromatin arranged in lobules separated by fibrovascular septae that are richly vascularised [62]. A variable amount of neurofibrillary matrix is interspersed between the tumour cells. Sustentacular cells are present at the periphery of the lobules. High-grade tumours show tumour cells arranged in sheets. Atypia and mitoses are increased, and necrosis may be present. Rosettes may be seen in ONB: Homer Wright pseudorosettes are identified in Hyams grades 1 and 2, and Flexner–Wintersteiner true rosettes in Hyams grades 3 and 4. Calcification may be present. ONBs stain positively with synaptophysin, chromogranin, INSM1, and neuron-specific enolase. Calretinin positivity has also been documented and may be helpful in diagnosis. While cytokeratin may be positive focally, EMA is usually negative. p63 and p40 are also usually negative. S100 stains the sustentacular cells. Dense core neurosecretory granules are present on ultrastructural examination of the tumour cells [107, 108].

6.5.5.2 Sinonasal Teratocarcinosarcoma

Sinonasal teratocarcinosarcoma (SNTCS) is an extremely uncommon malignant neoplasm with aggressive behaviour. It is characterised by the presence of a combination of ectodermal, mesenchymal, and neuroectodermal components in varying proportion. The ectodermal component consists of squamous or glandular epithelium; "fetal"-appearing squamous epithelium with clear polygonal cells is typical of SNTCS. The mesenchymal component consists of malignant spindle cells; differentiation along various lineages can be seen, including osteoid, cartilage, smooth muscle, and skeletal muscle differentiation. The neuroectodermal component consists of small round blue cells resembling ONB. The divergent differentiation seen in SNTCS is attributed to its origin from a multipotential adult somatic stem cell. The presence of individual components in small biopsies frequently leads to misdiagnosis and delay in management, which further worsens the outcome of this highly malignant tumour [109].

6.5.5.3 Extranodal NK/T Cell Lymphoma, Nasal Type

Extranodal NK/T cell lymphoma, nasal type (ENKTL) is the most frequently encountered lymphoma in the sinonasal tract. It has a strong association with Epstein–Barr virus (EBV). Biopsies show diffuse infiltrates of abnormal lymphoid cells of variable size with irregular, folded nuclei. Angiocentricity, angioinvasion, angiodestruction, and necrosis are prominent and serve as clues to the diagnosis when present. Variable cellularity, presence of necrosis, and admixed inflammatory cells can cause overlap with inflammatory processes, and obscure the diagnosis. The most common immunophenotype of the tumour cells is positivity for cytoplasmic CD3, CD56, CD57, TIA-1, perforin, and granzyme B. EBV detection by in situ hybridisation for EBV-encoded RNA (EBER) can be used for confirmation [107].

6.5.6 Fibroosseous Lesions

6.5.6.1 Ossifying Fibroma

Ossifying fibromas are benign fibroosseous lesions of the jaw and craniofacial bones. They are classified into three specific variants viz. Cemento-ossifying fibroma, Juvenile trabecular ossifying fibroma (JTOF), and Juvenile psammomatoid ossifying fibroma (JPOF).

Cemento-ossifying fibromas (COFs) are tumours of odontogenic origin, which occur in the third and fourth decades of life, with a female preponderance. The mandible is more frequently involved than the maxilla. Microscopically, COF demonstrates a variably cellular, fibroblastic proliferation in a fibrotic stroma, accompanied by deposition of mainly woven and scant lamellar bone, osteoid and cementum-like material arranged in irregular islands, trabeculae, and spheroids. The fibroblastic cells are bland, stellate to spindle-shaped, with normo- to hyperchromatic nuclei that lack atypia and mitoses. The bone shows osteoblastic rimming. Osteoclastic giant cells and secondary cyst formation are rare. COFs are associated with mutations in *CDC73* (*HRPT2*) gene. Multiple lesions occur in patients with hyperparathyroidism-jaw tumour syndrome attributed to this mutation. *GNAS* mutations, characteristic of fibrous dysplasia, are absent.

Juvenile trabecular ossifying fibroma (JTOF) occurs in the first and second decades of life with equal sex distribution and involves the maxilla more frequently than the mandible. JTOF is composed of a hypercellular stellate to spindle cell proliferation with minimal atypia and occasional mitoses. Stroma shows sparse collagen. Elongated curved and branched trabecular deposits of osteoid which mineralise at the centre and lack osteoblastic rimming are present. These may ossify and form lamellar bone. Clusters of osteoclastic giant cells may be seen and secondary cyst formation is not uncommon and can aid in distinction from COF.

Juvenile psammomatoid ossifying fibroma (JPOF) occurs over a wide age range with mean age in second to fourth decades of life and equal sex distribution. The paranasal sinuses and periorbital bones, i.e. ethmoid and frontal bones are more frequently affected than the gnathic bones. JPOFs consist of compact stellate to spindle-shaped cells with scant stroma, accompanied by numerous rounded, bluish deposits of woven bone known as psammomatoid bodies or ossicles, as they resemble psammoma bodies. Similar to JTOF, osteoblastic rimming is absent. Larger bone deposits may fuse to form irregular angulated trabeculae. Cystic degeneration and secondary cyst formation may be seen [110].

6.5.6.2 Fibrous Dysplasia

Fibrous dysplasia (FD) is a benign condition in which normal bone is replaced by disorganised immature bone and fibrous tissue. Clinical types include monostotic FD, polyostotic FD, and McCune–Albright syndrome characterised by polyostotic fibrous dysplasia, café-au-lait spots, and multiple endocrinopathies. The maxilla is involved more frequently than the mandible. FD is slightly more common in females and occurs in young adults. Histologically, FD shows replacement of the medullary cavity of normal bone by a cellular fibroblastic stroma containing narrow curvilinear (C shaped) and irregularly shaped (Chinese letter pattern) trabeculae of woven bone that lack osteoblastic rimming. FD is characterised by activating missense mutations in the *GNAS* gene, which is seen in all three forms [111].

6.5.7 Nasal Polyps

6.5.7.1 Inflammatory Nasal Polyp

These are polypoid Inflammatory swellings of the sinonasal mucosa with multifactorial aetiology. They are lined by respiratory mucosa on three sides, which may undergo squamous metaplasia. The basement membrane of the epithelium is thickened and hyalinised. The underlying lamina propria is expanded, edematous, and contains seromucous glands. Fibroblasts and small blood vessels may be seen in the stroma. A mixed chronic inflammatory cell infiltrate is usually present. Secondary changes may be identified, including ulceration, formation of granulation tissue, fibrosis, infarction, nuclear atypia in stromal fibroblasts, cartilaginous or osseous metaplasia, and mucous gland hyperplasia.

6.5.7.2 Antrochoanal Polyp

AC polyp is a distinct clinical type of inflammatory polyp arising from the maxillary sinus and extending into the nasal cavity through the maxillary ostium. It is histologically similar to inflammatory polyps, but seromucous glands are diminished or absent, and they lack eosinophils. Atypical stromal cells are more frequent, as is infarction, accompanied by neovascularisation.

6.5.7.3 Allergic Nasal Polyp

These are an inflammatory response of sinonasal mucosa to inhaled fungal allergens, mediated by eosinophils. They present as polypoid mucosal fragments with inflammation. Abundant separately lying mucinous material containing degranulated eosinophils and Charcot Leyden crystals, i.e. allergic mucin is found, which may contain fungal hyphae that are difficult to identify. Fungal elements are not seen within tissue fragments or blood vessels, unlike in invasive fungal sinusitis. Histochemical stains like PAS-D and Gomori methenamine silver may be used to highlight the fungal hyphae. It is not required to identify fungal elements to give the diagnosis.

References

1. Barnes L, Eveson JW, Reichart P, Sidransky D, eds. Pathology and Genetics of Head and Neck tumors.
2. Wood JW, Casiano RR. Inverted papillomas and benign nonneoplastic lesions of the nasal cavity. Am J Rhinol Allergy. 2012 Mar-Apr;26(2):157–63.
3. Sham CL, Lee DL, van Hasselt CA, et al. A case-control study of the risk factors associated with sinonasal inverted papilloma. Am J Rhinol Allergy. 2010;24:e37–40.
4. Dietmer T, Wiener C. Is there an occupational etiology of inverted papilloma of the nose and sinuses. Acta Otolaryngol (Stockh). 1996;116:762–5.
5. Kashima HK, Kessis T, Hruban RH, Wu TC, Zinreich SJ, Shah KV. Human papillomavirus in sinonasal papillomas and squamous cell carcinoma. Laryngoscope. 1992;102:973–6.
6. Ringert N. Pathology of malignant tumors arising in the nasal and paranasal cavities and maxilla. Acta Otolaryngol (Stockh). 1938;27(suppl):31–42.
7. McLachlin CM, Kandel RA, Colgan TJ, Swanson DB, Witterick IJ, Ngan BY. Prevalence of human papillomavirus in sinonasal papillomas: a study using polymerase chain reaction and in situ hybridization. Mod Pathol. 1992;5:406–9.
8. McKay SP, Grégoire L, Lonardo F, Reidy P, Mathog RH, Lancaster WD. Human papillomavirus (HPV) transcripts in malignant inverted papilloma are from integrated HPV DNA. Laryngoscope. 2005;115:1428–31.
9. Cheung FM, Lau TW, Cheung LK, Li AS, Chow SK, Lo AW. Schneiderian papillomas and carcinomas: a retrospective study with special reference to p53 and p16 tumor suppressor gene expression and association with HPV. Ear Nose Throat J. 2010;89:E5–E12.
10. Kraft M, Simmen D, Casas R, Pfaltz M. Significance of human papillomavirus in sinonasal papillomas. J Laryngol Otol. 2001;115:709–14.
11. Jenko K, Kocjan B, Zidar N. In inverted papillomas HPV more likely represents incidental colonization than an etiological factor. Virchows Arch. 2011;459:529–38.
12. Krause JH. Development of a staging system for inverted papilloma. Laryngoscope. 2000;110:965–8.
13. Ojiri H, Ujita M, Tada S, et al. Potentially distinctive features of sinonasal inverted papilloma on MR imaging. AJR Am J Roentgenol. 2000;175(2):465–8.
14. Lawson W, Patel ZM. The evolution of management for inverted papilloma: an analysis of 200 cases. Otolaryngol Head Neck Surg. 2009;140:330–5.
15. Lee TJ, Huang SF, Huang CC. Tailored endoscopic surgery for the treatment of sinonasal inverted papilloma. Head Neck. 2004;26:145–53.
16. Sham CL, Woo JK, van Hasselt CA, et al. Treatment results of sinonasal inverted papilloma: an 18-year study. Am J Rhinol Allergy. 2009;23:203–11.
17. Mendenhall WM, Hinerman RW, Malyapa RS. Inverted papilloma of the nasal cavity and paranasal sinuses. Am J Clin Oncol. 2007;30:560–3.
18. Eller R, Sillers M. Common fibro-osseous lesions of the paranasal sinuses. Otolaryngol Clin N Am. 2006;39:585–600.
19. Fu YS, Perzin KH. Non-epithelial tumors of the nasal cavity, paranasal sinuses, and nasopharynx. A clinicopathologic study. Cancer. 1974;33:1289–305.
20. Alexander AA, Patel AA, Odland R. Paranasal sinus osteomas and Gardner's syndrome. Ann Otol Rhinol Laryngol. 2007;116:658–62.
21. Speight PM, Carlos R. Maxillofacial fibro-osseous lesions. Curr Diagn Pathol. 2006;12:1–10.
22. Eversole R, Su L, Elmofty S. Benign fibro-ossous lesions of the craniofacial complex a review. Head Neck Pathol. 2008;2:177–202.
23. Waldron CA. Fibroosseous lesions of the jaws. J Oral Maxillofac Surg. 1993;51:828–35.
24. Kransdorf MJ, Moser RP Jr, Gilkey FW. Fibrous dysplasia. Radiographics. 1990;10:519–37.
25. Stompro BE, Wolf P, Haghihi P. Fibrous dysplasia of bone. Am Fam Phys. 1989;39:179–84.

26. Moore AT, Buncic JR, Munro IR. Fibrous dysplasia of the orbit in childhood. Clinical features and management. Ophthalmology. 1985;92:12–20.
27. Angelopoulos AP. Pyogenic granuloma of the oral cavity: statistical analysis of its clinical features. J Oral Surg. 1971;29:840–7.
28. Cawson RA, Binnie WH, Speight PM, Barrett AW, Wright JM. Lucas pathology of tumors of oral tissues. 5th ed. Missouri: Mosby; 1998. p. 252–4.
29. Zarrinneshan A, Zapanta P, Wall S. Nasal pyogenic granuloma. Otolaryngol Head Neck Surg. 2007;136:130–1.
30. Patil K, Mahima VG, Lahari K. Extragingival pyogenic granuloma. Indian J Dent Res. 2006;17:199–202.
31. Marx RE, Stern D. Oral and maxillofacial pathology: a rationale for diagnosis and treatment. Chicago: Quintessence Publishing Co; 2003. p. 21–3.
32. Herrington H, Adil E, Moritz E, et al. Update on current evaluation and management of pediatric nasal dermoid. Laryngoscope. 2016;126(9):2151–60. https://doi.org/10.1002/lary.25860.
33. Szymańska A, Szymański M, Czekajska-Chehab E, Szczerbo-Trojanowska M. Two types of lateral extension in juvenile nasopharyngeal angiofibroma: diagnostic and therapeutic management. Eur Arch Otorhinolaryngol. 2015;272(1):159–66. https://doi.org/10.1007/s00405-014-2965-y.
34. Gołąbek W, Szymańska A, Szymański M, Czekajska-Chehab E, Jargiełło T. Juvenile nasopharyngeal angiofibroma with intracranial extension–diagnosis and treatment. Otolaryngol Pol. 2019;74(2):1–7. https://doi.org/10.5604/01.3001.0013.5275.
35. Nicolai P, Schreiber A, Villaret AB. Juvenile Angiofibroma: evolution of management. Int J Pediatr. 2012;412545:11. https://doi.org/10.1155/2012/412545.
36. Schick B, Kahle G. Radiological findings in angiofibroma. Acta Radiol. 2000;41(6):585–93.
37. Szymańska A, Szymański M, Czekajska-Chehab E, Szczerbo-Trojanowska M. Invasive growth patterns of juvenile nasopharyngeal angiofibroma: radiological imaging and clinical implications. Acta Radiol. 2014;55(6):725–31. https://doi.org/10.1177/0284185113506189.
38. Lloyd G, Howard D, Lund VJ, Savy L. Imaging for juvenile angiofibroma. J Laryngol Otol. 2000;114(9):727–30.
39. Thakar A, Sakthivel P, Prashanth A, Bhalla AS, Sharma SC, Kumar R. Comparison of 68Ga-PSMA PET/CT and contrast-enhanced MRI on residual disease assessment of juvenile nasal Angiofibroma. Clin Nucl Med. 2020 Feb 11; https://doi.org/10.1097/RLU.0000000000002951.
40. Overdevest JB, Amans MR, Zaki P, Pletcher SD, El-Sayed IH. Patterns of vascularization and surgical morbidity in juvenile nasopharyngeal angiofibroma: a case series, systematic review, and meta-analysis. Head Neck. 2018;40(2):428–43. https://doi.org/10.1002/hed.24987.
41. Snyderman CH, Pant H, Carrau RL, Gardner P. A new endoscopic staging system for angiofibromas. Archives of Otolaryngology—Head and Neck Surgery. 2010;136(6):588–94.
42. Schuon R, Brieger J, Heinrich UR, Roth Y, Szyfter W, Mann WJ. Immunohistochemical analysis of growth mechanisms in juvenile nasopharyngeal angiofibroma. Eur Arch Otorhinolaryngol. 2007;264(4):389–94.
43. Thompson LDR, Fanburg-Smith JC. Update on select benign Mesenchymal and Meningothelial Sinonasal tract lesions. Head Neck Pathol. 2016;10(1):95–108. https://doi.org/10.1007/s12105-016-0697-6.
44. Boghani Z, Husain Q, Kanumuri VV, et al. Juvenile nasopharyngeal angiofibroma: a systematic review and comparison of endoscopic, endoscopic-assisted, and open resection in 1047 cases. Laryngoscope. 2013;123(4):859–69. https://doi.org/10.1002/lary.23843.
45. Nicolai P, Villaret AB, Farina D, et al. Endoscopic surgery for juvenile angiofibroma: a critical review of indications after 46 cases. American Journal of Rhinology and Allergy. 2010;24(2):e67–72.
46. Gates GA, Rice DH, Koopmann CF Jr, Schuller DE. Flutamide-induced regression of angiofibroma. Laryngoscope. 1992 Jun;102(6):641–4.
47. Thakar A, Gupta G, Bhalla AS, Jain V, Sharma SC, Sharma R, Bahadur S, Deka RC. Adjuvant therapy with flutamide for presurgical volume reduction in juvenile nasopharyngeal angiofibroma. Head Neck. 2011 Dec;33(12):1747–53.
48. Mallick S, Benson R, Bhasker S, Mohanti BK. Conformal radiotherapy for locally advanced juvenile nasopharyngeal angio-fibroma. J Cancer Res Ther. 2015;11(1):73–7. https://doi.org/10.4103/0973-1482.150349.
49. Mallick S, Benson R, Bhasker S, Mohanti BK. Long-term treatment outcomes of juvenile nasopharyngeal angiofibroma treated with radiotherapy. Acta Otorhinolaryngol Ital. 2015;35(2):75.
50. Goldenberg D, Golz A, Fradis M, et al. Malignant tumors of the nose and paranasal sinuses: az retrospective review of 291 cases. Ear Nose Throat J. 2001;80:272–7.
51. Shah UK, Hybels RL, Dugan J. Endoscopic management of low-grade papillary adenocarcinoma of the ethmoid sinus: case report and review of the literature. Am J Otolaryngol. 1999;20:190–4.
52. Suárez C, Ferlito A, Lund VJ, et al. Management of the orbit in malignant sinonasal tumors. Head Neck. 2008;30(2):242–50. https://doi.org/10.1002/hed.20736.
53. Lyon BM, Donald PJ. Radical surgery for nasal cavity and paranasal sinuses. Otolaryngologic Clincs of North America. 1991;24:1499–521.
54. Madani G, Beale TJ, Lund VJ. Imaging of sinonasal tumors. Semin Ultrasound CT MR. 2009;30(1):25–38. https://doi.org/10.1053/j.sult.2008.10.013.

55. Kraus D, Sternman BM, Levine HL, et al. Factors inuencing survival in ethmoid sinus cancer. Arch Otolaryngol Head Neck Surg. 1992;118:367–72.
56. Lloyd G, Lund VJ, Howard D, Savy L. Optimum imaging for sinonasal malignancy. J Laryngol Otol. 2000;114(7):557–62. https://doi.org/10.1258/0022215001906174.
57. Bishop JA. Recently described neoplasms of the sinonasal tract. Semin Diagn Pathol. 2016;33(2):62–70. https://doi.org/10.1053/j.semdp.2015.12.001.
58. Andreasen S, Kiss K, Mikkelsen LH, et al. An update on head and neck cancer: new entities and their histopathology, molecular background, treatment, and outcome. APMIS. 2019;127(5):240–64. https://doi.org/10.1111/apm.12901.
59. Lydiatt WM, Patel SG, O'Sullivan B. Head and neck cancers- major changes in the American joint committee on cancer eighth edition cancer staging manual. CA Cancer J Clin. 2017;67:122–7.
60. Morita A, Ebersold MJ, Olsen KD, et al. Esthesioneuroblastoma: prognosis and management. Neurosurgery. 1993;32:706–15.
61. Dulguerov P, calcaterra T. Esthesioneuroblastoma: the UCLA experience 1970-1990. Laryngoscope. 1992;102:843–9.
62. Hyam VJ, Batsakis JG. Michaels. Tumour of the upper respiratory tract and ear. Washington DC: air force institute of. Pathology. 1988:240–8.
63. Sarradin V, Siegfried A, Uro-Coste E, Delord JP. WHO classification of head and neck tumours 2017: Main novelties and update of diagnostic methods. Bull Cancer. 2018;105(6):596–2.
64. Jemal A, Bray F, Center MM, et al. Global cancer statistics. CA Cancer J Clin. 2011;61:69–90.
65. Huang TR, Zhang SW, Chen WQ, et al. Trends in nasopharyngeal carcinoma mortality in China, 1973–2005. Asian Pac J Cancer Prev. 2012;13:2495–2.
66. Yu MC, Yuan JM. Epidemiology of nasopharyngeal carcinoma. Semin Cancer Biol. 2002;12:421–9.
67. Henle G, Henle W. Epstein-Barr virus–specific IgA serum antibodies as an outstanding feature of nasopharyngeal carcinoma. Int J Cancer. 1976;17(1):1–7.
68. Miller WE, Earp HS, Raab-Traub N. The Epstein-Barr virus latent membrane protein 1 induces expression of the epidermal growth factor receptor. J Virol. 1995;69:4390–8.
69. Paine E, Scheinman RI, Baldwin AS Jr, et al. Expression of LMP1 in epithelial cells leads to the activation of a select subset of NF-kappa B/Rel family proteins. J Virol. 1995;69:4572–6.
70. Simons MJ, Wee GB, Chan SH, et al. Probable identification of an HLA second-locus antigen associated with a high risk of nasopharyngeal carcinoma. Lancet. 1975;1:142–3.
71. Ung A, Chen CJ, Levine PH, et al. Familial and sporadic cases of nasopharyngeal carcinoma in Taiwan. Anticancer Res. 1999;19:661–5.
72. Hildesheim A, Dosemeci M, Chan CC, et al. Occupational exposure to wood, formaldehyde, and solvents and risk of nasopharyngeal carcinoma. Cancer Epidemiol Biomark Prev. 2001;10:1145–3.
73. Peng JC, Sheen TS, Hsu MM. Nasopharyngeal carcinoma with dermatomyositis: analysis of 12 cases. Arch Otolaryngol Head Neck Surg. 1995;121(11):1298–1.
74. Chang MC, Chen JH, Liang JA, et al. Accuracy of whole-body FDG-PET and FDG-PET/CT in M staging of nasopharyngeal carcinoma: a systematic review and meta-analysis. Eur J Radiol. 2013;82:366–3.
75. Simo R, Robinson M, Lei M, Sibtain A, Hickey S. Nasopharyngeal carcinoma: United Kingdom National Multidisciplinary Guidelines. J Laryngol Otol. 2016;130:97–3.
76. Al-Sarraf M, LeBlanc M, Giri PG, et al. Chemoradiotherapy versus radiotherapy in patients with advanced nasopharyngeal cancer: phase III randomized intergroup study 0099. J Clin Oncol. 1998;16(4):1310–7.
77. Version 3.2019, 06/09/19 © National Comprehensive Cancer Network, Inc. 2019.
78. Peng H, Tang LL, Liu X, Chen L, Li WF, Mao YP. Anti-epidermal growth factor receptor therapy concurrently with induction chemotherapy in locoregionally advanced nasopharyngeal carcinoma. Cancer Sci. 2018;109:1609–6.
79. Tsang RK, To VS, Ho AC, Ho WK, Chan JY, Wei WI. Early results of robotic assisted nasopharyngectomy for recurrent nasopharyngeal carcinoma. Head Neck. 2015;37(6):788–3.
80. Castelnuovo P, Nicolai P, Turri-Zanoni M, Battaglia P, Bolzoni Villaret A, Gallo S, Bignami M. Dallan endoscopic endonasal nasopharyngectomy in selected cancers. Otolaryngol Head Neck Surg. 2013;149(3):424–30.
81. Ho AS, Kaplan MJ, Fee WE, et al. Targeted endoscopic salvage nasopharyngectomy for recurrent nasopharyngeal carcinoma. Int Forum Allergy Rhinol. 2012;2(2):166–3.
82. Wei W, Lam K, Ho C, et al. Efficacy of radical neck dissection for the control of cervical metastasis after radiotherapy for nasopharyngeal carcinoma. Am J Surg. 1990;160(4):439–2.
83. Yan H, Mo Z, Xiang Z, Rong D, Zhang Y, Chen G, et al. CT-guided ^{125}I brachytherapy for locally recurrent nasopharyngeal carcinoma. J Cancer. 2017;8(11):2104–3.
84. Jain A, Chia WK, Toh HC. Immunotherapy for nasopharyngeal cancer-a review. Chin Clin Oncol. 2016;5(2):22.
85. Stoker SD, Indrasari SR, Herdini C, Hariwiyanto B, Karakullukcu B, Dhamiyati W, Widayati K, Romdhoni AC, Fles R, Haryana SM, Wildeman MA, Tan IB. Photodynamic therapy as salvage therapy for patients with nasopharyngeal carcinoma experiencing local failures following definitive radiotherapy. Photodiagn Photodyn Ther. 2015;12(3):519–5.
86. Lee AWM, Ng WT, Chan LK, et al. The strength/weakness of the AJCC/UICC staging system

(7th edition) for nasopharyngeal cancer and suggestions for future improvement. Oral Oncol. 2012;48(10):1007–3.
87. Liu TR, Yang AK, Guo X, et al. Adenoid cystic carcinoma of the nasopharynx: 27-year experience. Laryngoscope. 2008;118:1981–8.
88. Wang X, Yan H, Luo Y, Fan T. Low-grade nasopharyngeal papillary adenocarcinoma: a case report and review of the literature. Onco Targets Ther. 2016;9:2955–9.
89. Zhang WL, Ma S, Havrilla L, Cai L, Yu CQ, Shen S. Primary thyroid-like low-grade nasopharyngeal papillary adenocarcinoma: a case report and literature review. Medicine. 2017;96:47.
90. Crapanzano JP, Ali SZ, Ginsberg MS, Zakowski MF. Chordoma: a cytologic study with histologic and radiologic correlation. Cancer. 2001;93(1):40.
91. Fernandez-Miranda JC, Gardner PA, Snyderman CH, Devaney KO, Mendenhall WM, Suárez C, Rinaldo A, Ferlito A. Clival chordomas: a pathological, surgical, and radiotherapeutic review. Head Neck. 2014;36(6):892–6.
92. Tumors of the nasal cavity, paranasal sinuses and skull base. In: El-Naggar AK, JKC C, Grandis JR, Takata T, Slootweg PJ, editors. WHO classification of head and neck tumors. IARC: Lyon; 2017. p. 11–61.
93. Nasal cavity and paranasal sinuses. In: LDR T, Wenig BM, Muller S, Nelson B, editors. Diagnostic pathology: head and neck. Philadelphia: Elsevier; 2016. p. 2–189.
94. Weindorf SC, Brown NA, McHugh JB, Udager AM. Sinonasal Papillomas and carcinomas: a contemporary update with review of an emerging molecular classification. Arch Pathol Lab Med. 2019;143:1304–16.
95. Kakkar A, Antony VM, Pramanik R, Sakthivel P, Singh CA, Jain D. SMARCB1 (INI1)- deficient sinonasal carcinoma: a series of 13 cases with assessment of histological patterns. Hum Pathol. 2018;83:59–67.
96. Agaimy A, Hartmann A, Antonescu CR, Chiosea SI, El-Mofty SK, Geddert H, et al. SMARCB1 (INI-1)-deficient Sinonasal carcinoma: a series of 39 cases expanding the morphologic and Clinicopathologic Spectrum of a recently described entity. Am J Surg Pathol. 2017;41:458–71.
97. Kakkar A, Antony VM, Irugu DVK, Adhikari N, Jain D. NUT midline carcinoma: a series of five cases, including one with unusual clinical course. Head Neck Pathol. 2018;12:230–6.
98. Bishop JA, Westra WH. NUT midline carcinomas of the sinonasal tract. Am J Surg Pathol. 2012;36:1216–21.
99. Rampinelli V, Ferrari M, Nicolai P. Intestinal-type adenocarcinoma of the sinonasal tract: an update. Curr Opin Otolaryngol Head Neck Surg. 2018;26:115–21.
100. Leivo I. Sinonasal adenocarcinoma: update on classification, Immunophenotype and molecular features. Head Neck Pathol. 2016;10:68–74.
101. Montone KT. The differential diagnosis of Sinonasal/ nasopharyngeal neuroendocrine/ Neuroectodermally derived tumors. Arch Pathol Lab Med. 2015;139:1498–507.
102. Agaimy A, Franchi A, Lund VJ, Skálová A, Bishop JA, Triantafyllou A, Andreasen S, Gnepp DR, Hellquist H, Thompson LDR, Rinaldo A, Ferlito A. Sinonasal undifferentiated carcinoma (SNUC): from an entity to morphologic pattern and Back again-a historical perspective. Adv Anat Pathol. 2019 Dec 24; https://doi.org/10.1097/PAP.0000000000000258.
103. Kakkar A, Rajeshwari M, Sakthivel P, Sharma MC, Sharma SC. Biphenotypic sinonasal sarcoma: a series of six cases with evaluation of role of β-catenin immunohistochemistry in differential diagnosis. Ann Diagn Pathol. 2018;33:6–10.
104. Gross J, Fritchie K. Soft tissue special issue: Biphenotypic Sinonasal sarcoma: a review with emphasis on differential diagnosis. Head Neck Pathol. 2020 Jan 16; https://doi.org/10.1007/s12105-019-01092-4.
105. Kane SV, Kakkar A, Oza N, Sridhar E, Pai PS. Phosphaturic mesenchymal tumor of the nasal cavity and paranasal sinuses: a clinical curiosity presenting a diagnostic challenge. Auris Nasus Larynx. 2018;45:377–83.
106. Kohashi K, Kinoshita I, Oda Y. Soft tissue special issue: skeletal muscle tumors: a Clinicopathological review. Head Neck Pathol. 2020 Jan 16; https://doi.org/10.1007/s12105-019-01113-2.
107. Purgina B, Lai CK. Distinctive head and neck bone and soft tissue neoplasms. Surg Pathol Clin. 2017;10:223–79.
108. Rooper LM, Bishop JA. Sinonasal small round blue cell tumors: an Immunohistochemical approach. Surg Pathol Clin. 2017;10:103–23.
109. Agaimy A. Poorly differentiated sinonasal tract malignancies: a review focusing on recently described entities. Cesk Patol. 2016;52:146–53.
110. Sable M, Kakkar A, Garg K, Suri V. Sinonasal Teratocarcinosarcoma: an underdiagnosed entity posing diagnostic challenges. Turk Neurosurg. 2017;27:468–71.
111. Hameed M, Horvai AE, Jordan RCK. Soft tissue special issue: gnathic fibro-osseous lesions and osteosarcoma. Head Neck Pathol. 2020 Jan 16; https://doi.org/10.1007/s12105-019-01094-2.

Extended Procedures 7

Pankuri Mittal, Hitesh Verma, Amit Kesari, R. S. Virk, Kshitiz Charya, Smriti Panda, Alok Thakar, Rajesh Kumar Meena, Ramesh S. Doddamani, Manish Gupta, Rohit Verma, Vikas Gupta, Ganakalyan Behera, Amit Shanker, Namrita Mahmi, M. Ravi Sankar, and Arulalan Mathialagan

Contents

P. Mittal · H. Verma (✉) · S. Panda · A. Thakar
N. Mahmi
Department of ENT, AIIMS, New Delhi, India
e-mail: drhitesh10@gmail.com

A. Kesari · M. R. Sankar · A. Mathialagan
Neurootology, SGPGIMS, Lucknow, UP, India

R. S. Virk
ENT, PGIMER, Chandigarh, India

K. Charya
Indus Hospital, Mohali, Punjab, India

R. K. Meena · R. S. Doddamani
Neurosurgery, AIIMS, New Delhi, India

M. Gupta
ENT, MMIMSR, MMU, Ambala, Haryana, India

R. Verma
ENT, DMC, Ludhiana, Punjab, India

V. Gupta · G. Behera
ENT, AIIMS, Bhopal, MP, India

A. Shanker
ENT, Brighton and Sussex University Hospital NHS, Brighton, UK

H. Verma, A. Thakar (eds.), *Essentials of Rhinology*, https://doi.org/10.1007/978-981-33-6284-0_7

Good radiology, better-quality visualization, advances in technology and in-depth anatomical knowledge allows removal of central skull base lesion by transnasal route. CECT and MRI scan in all planes at 1 mm interval is required to map the extent of the lesion. The diagnostic cerebral angiography (DSA) is indicated in selected cases, to obtain information regarding vascularity of the lesion and possible involvement of surrounding major neurovascular bundle. Extended endoscopic approaches are divided into median and paramedian type. Median approaches are for midline lesions. It is further divided on the basis of site of involvement such as frontal sinus, cribriform plate, planum sphenoidalis, etc. Paramedian approaches are for lateral lesions. It is further divided into anterior, middle and posterior approaches. Intraorbiral and transorbital comes under the anterior subtype. Cavernous sinus, petrous apex and infratemporal area lesions are managed by the middle approach. Condylar, hypoglossal canal and jugular fossa lesions are delt by posterior approach. Pituitary gland lies behind and above the sphenoid sinus. Number of hormones are secreted by the pituitary gland. Pituitary adenomas are dealt by both medical and surgical ways. These adenomas are the most common lesions managed by extended endoscopic approaches. Tumours involving the skin, extending beyond the mid-pupillary line, tumour infiltration into the orbital tissue and palatal bone erosion are the indications for open approaches. Open extra-cranial approaches are further subdivided into soft tissue and bony approaches. Moure's Lateral Rhinotomy Incision and Weber–Ferguson incisions are the most commonly used soft tissue approaches. Transcranial approaches to the anterior skull base are divided into anterior and anterolateral approaches depending upon the tumour extensions. The lacrimal system is for sucking the tears. The obstruction of nasolacrimal duct requires the creation of new communication between the sac and nasal cavity. Dacryocystorhinostomy is of two types: endoscopic and external. The endoscopic method provides almost equal results with an open approach. The endoscopic approach is devoid of complications of external approach such as lacrimal pump mechanism violation and external scar. The proper surgical technique and regular follow-up reduces the risk of restenosis. Choanal atresia is the stenosis/atresia of the posterior choana. It can present in isolation or as a part of the syndrome. It can be bony, membranous or mixed types. Endoscopic direct visualization is the gold standard way to confirm the diagnosis. Transnasal and transpalatal are the most accepted approaches.

CSF rhinorrhea is developed by the abnormal communication of the nasal cavity with the cranial cavity. The aetiology is broadly classified into traumatic and non-traumatic types. The numbers of haematological and biochemical parameters are mentioned for confirmation of the presence of CSF fluid within the nasal cavity but β-2-transferrin is the most specific for CSF. HRCT temporal bone with MR cisternography is the most accepted radiological investigation combination to localize the site of leak. Traumatic ones are mainly managed by a conservative approach but non-traumatic ones require surgical repair. Optic nerve comes in a lateral relationship with the posterior ethmoid and sphenoid sinus. Direct and indirect injuries are the types of optic nerve injury. No management option is available for direct injury. The indirect optic neuropathy is managed by both medical and surgical way. The extended surgical approaches create a large surgical cavity and iatrogenic communication of the nasal cavity with the cranial cavity. The flaps are used to separate these cavities and to improve the outcome of repairs.

7.1 Part A: Extended Endoscopic Approach

Extended endoscopic endonasal approaches (EEAs) have come up as a good substitute to traditional open approaches. Advance technology allows superior visualization and better control of instruments with precision in disease clearance. The extent of EEAs is from cribriform plate to clivus and C2 vertebrae. The major drawback of open approaches is the manipulation of the cerebrum, blood vessels and cranial nerves. The other disadvantages of traditional approaches are

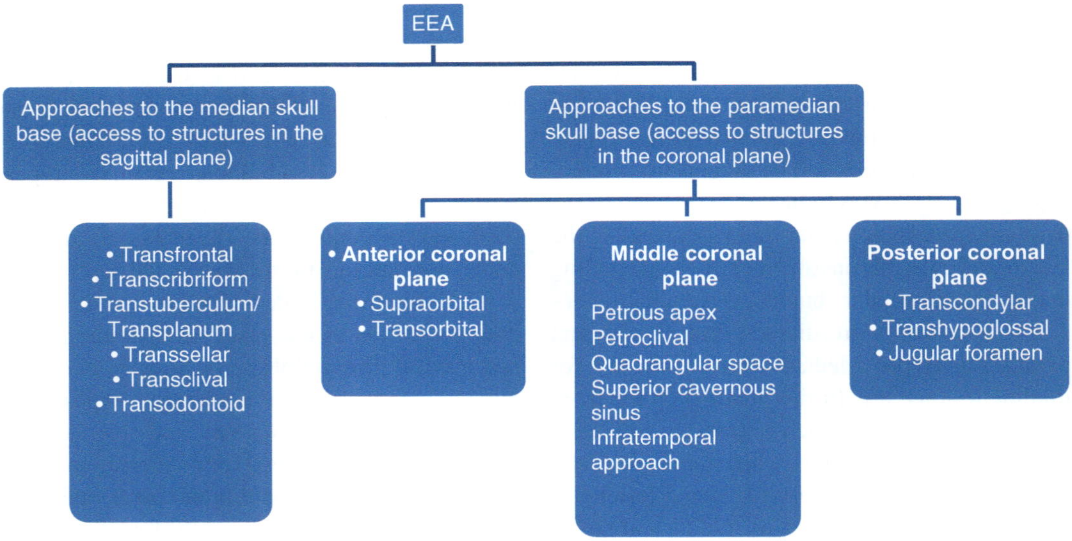

Fig. 7.1 Extended endoscopic approaches

large incision size, prolonged exposure time, bleeding, frontal lobe symptoms, prolonged hospitalization and medical care, etc. The rate of complications is drastically reduced by endoscopic approaches. In the last two decades, more and more centres have moved towards endoscopic approaches to the skull base and intracranial lesion because of the improvement in knowledge in endoscopic anatomy, hi-tech endoscopic equipment, micro-instruments, refining the expertise of the surgeon and EEAs have a lack of disadvantages of open approaches. Sphenoid sinus is the entry route for the majority of skull base lesions. Internal carotid artery, cavernous sinus, optic nerve and maxillary division of trigeminal nerve are the close-by vital structures, so good preoperative radiological assessment and selection of correct instruments with copious saline irrigation to prevent thermal trauma is the key for surgical success in EEAs. The complexity of lesion is the deciding factor for two-hands or four-hands technique.

EEA can be classified into approaches to median skull base and paramedian skull base, according to the orientation of the surgical field (target area) under two main categories and are further defined based on the anatomy of the corridor and target areas and their relationship with critical structures (Fig. 7.1) [1, 2]. The choice of approach is based on the extent of the lesion and in a number of situations; a combination of close-by approaches is required.

1. **Access to the median skull base (sagittal plane): anterior to posterior direction**

   (A) **Transfrontal Approach** (Fig. 7.2)

   The indications are chronic refractory frontal sinusitis not responding to other management, fibro-osseous lesions of frontal sinus, posterior table CSF rhinorrhoea, recurrent mucoceles, and other lesions of frontal sinus like dermoid. The surgery starts with complete exposure of bilateral frontal recesses. Superior septal window is created anterior to anterior attachment of middle turbinate and anterior to cribriform plate area to visulaized both frontal sinuses. The final step is the removal of the interfrontal sinus septum to create one large frontal sinus. It provides wide access to remove the disease and to deal with posterior table.

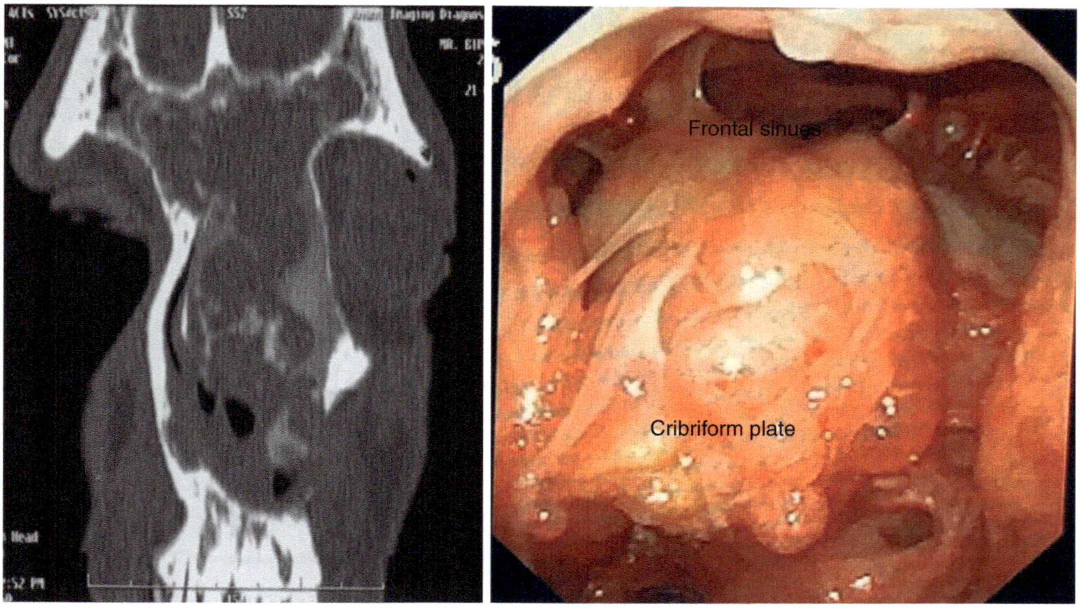

Fig. 7.2 CT scan of nose & PNS revealing heterogenous mass filling fronal sinuses, nasal cavity with surrounding osteogenesis. Right figure is showing healed postoperative cavity after transfrontal approach

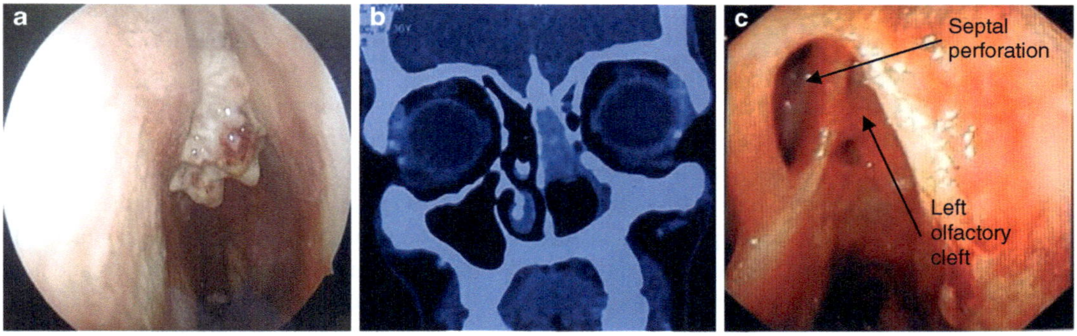

Fig. 7.3 Recurrent adenocarcinoma of left olfactory cleft. (**a**) endoscopic photo, (**b**) contrast-enhancing mass in the left nasal cavity and olfactory cleft, (**c**) healed postoperative cavity

(B) **Transcribriform Approach** [3]

Indications

It is indicated for tumours involving the central part of the frontal lobe and the olfactory bulb region (e.g. olfactory groove meningioma, esthesioneuroblastoma, adenocarcinoma) (Fig. 7.3).

Steps

(i) Debulking of intranasal mass may required to expose the cribriform plate region.

(ii) Complete anterior and posterior ethmoidectomy with wide sphenoidotomy and middle turbinate removal for exposure of the entire skull base is done to define the posterior limit of the lesion. Anterior and posterior ethmoid arteries are cauterized to de-vascularize the lesion. In selected cases, preservation of olfaction is possible on the other side.

(iii) An endoscopic modified Lothrop procedure (Draf III) is performed to label the anterior limit.

(iv) Bone lateral to tumour is drilled out and removed from frontal

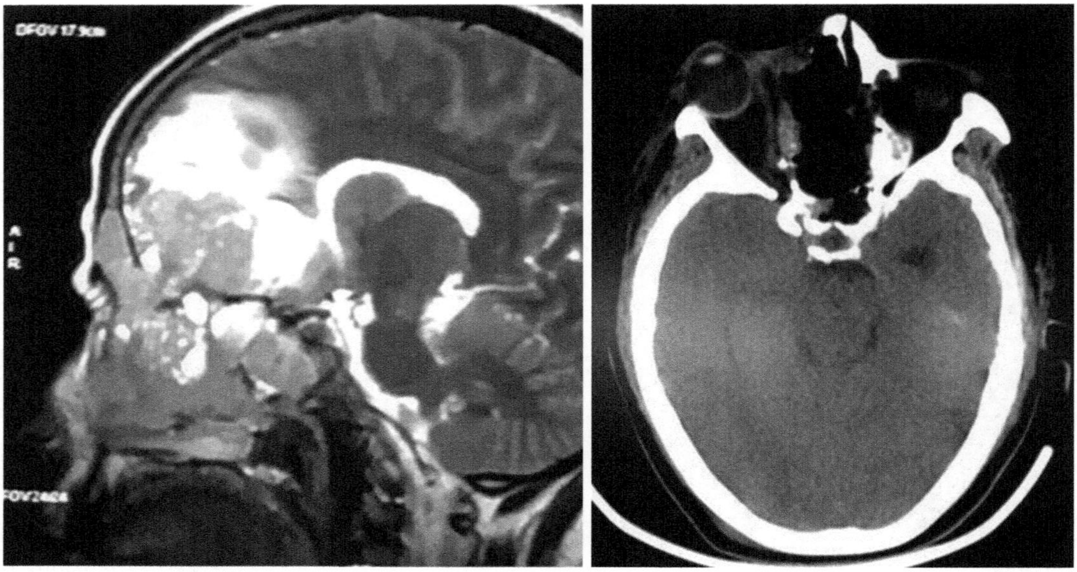

Fig. 7.4 Esthesioneuroblastoma. (**a**) sagittal MRI T2 images (Kadish stage 3 lesion), (**b**) surgical cavity (NCCT head) after combined transcribriform and transplanar approach

sinus posterior wall to planum sphenoidalis. Lateral limit of drill is orbital medial wall.

(v) Nasal septum is removed with 1 cm healthy margin from tumour to sphenoid sinus posteriorly and cribriform plate superiorly.

(vi) Dura mater is cauterized peri-tumourally with preservation of deep cortical vessels. Crista galli, olfactory nerve fibres, and falx are separated from tumour by inferior displacement.

(vii) The final defect is from the median orbital margin on both sides and from the posterior table of the frontal sinus till planum sphenoidalis in anteroposterior direction.

(viii) Closure of defect in layers with vascularized flap.

(C) **Transplanar Approach**

The limit of the corridor is from fovea ethmoidalis over posterior ethmoid and cribriform plate anteriorly. The posterior limit is the sella and the lateral limit is the optic nerve. It can combine with anterior or posterior extended approaches for surgical exposure (Fig. 7.4). Suprasellar lesions are managed by this approach by cauterization of superior inter-cavernous sinus.

(D) **Trans-sphenoidal Approaches**

The sphenoid sinus is the entry point for a number of trans-sphenoid approaches. Sphenoid bone is located in the centre of the cranial base in intimate contact with many important arterial, venous and neural structures. The pneumatization of the sphenoid bone creates a natural corridor. The next step is the identification of sphenoid ostium. The nasal septum is separated from the sphenoid rostrum. The anterior wall of the sphenoidal sinus is enlarged circumferentially and sphenoidal septae is drilled. The posterior and lateral walls of the sphenoidal sinus should be visible laterally; the sellar floor inferiorly, the sphenoethmoid planum above (Fig. 7.5) [4–6].

(i) **Trans-sellar Approach**

Indications

It allows access to pathologies of the pituitary gland such as pituitary adenomas, Rathke's cleft cysts, etc.

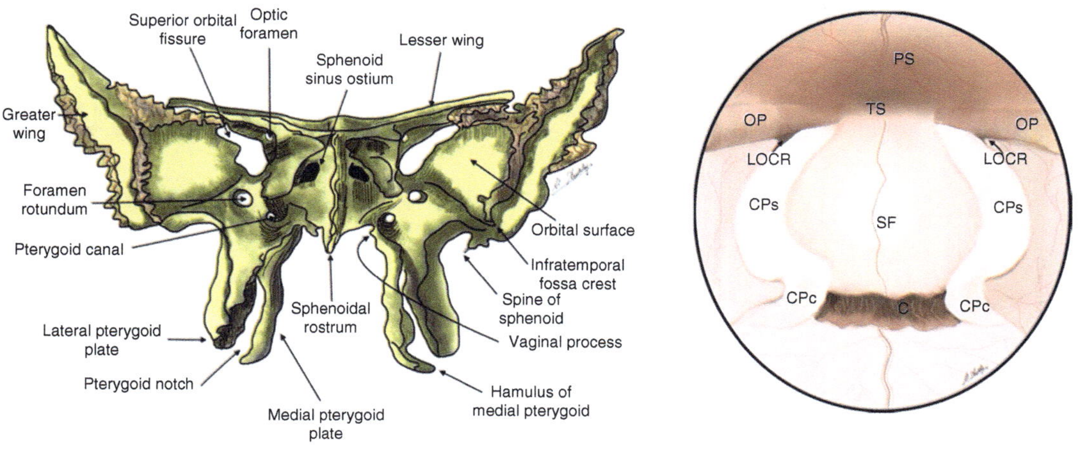

Fig. 7.5 The natural anatomy of sphenoid bone and endoscopic view of sphenoid sinus after wide sphenoidotomy and removal of posterior septum (Courtesy for line diagram—Dr. Arulalan Mathialagan- Senior Resident SGPGI, Lucknow)

It provides access to the medial cavernous sinus for pituitary adenomas that extend laterally behind the cavernous ICA. The first step is the completion of the trans-sphenoidal approach. Bone removal over the sellar face extends laterally beyond the medial aspect of the cavernous sinuses (CS) and superiorly and inferiorly to expose both the intercavernous sinuses. Further extended approaches require the creation of a wider surgical corridor to expose and work in the different areas around the sella (Fig. 7.6).

(ii) **Trans-tuberculum/Transplanum Approach**

Indications

The indications are extracellular pituitary adenomas with suprasellar extension, meningiomas and select craniopharyngiomas. The access is obtained through a more anterior trajectory compared with the one used to reach the sellar region. This route requires a wider opening of the anterior wall of the sphenoidal sinus, which is obtained by removing the superior (supreme) turbinates and the posterior ethmoid air cells. Above the sellar floor, the angle formed by the convergence of the sphenoid planum with the sellar floor is recognizable; from the intracranial view, this corresponds to the tuberculum sellae. As one moves the endoscope in an anterior direction, the sphenoid planum is visible. The opening of the planum starts with the removal of the tuberculum sellae, extended bilaterally in the direction of the optico-carotid recesses. The lateral extension of the opening is limited by the protuberances of the optic nerves (Fig. 7.6).

(iii) **Trans-clival Approach**

The surgical corridor is extending from dorsal sellae to the foreman magnum. It provides a head-on view to the brainstem and vertebrobasilar vascular network. It can further be divided into superior, middle and inferior approaches by location of dural opening of abducent and glossopharyngeal nerve. The internal carotid artery is the lateral limit for middle and inferior approaches. Vidian artery, intraoperative navigation system with carotid doppler helps in identification of carotid artery [6]. The limit of bone removal

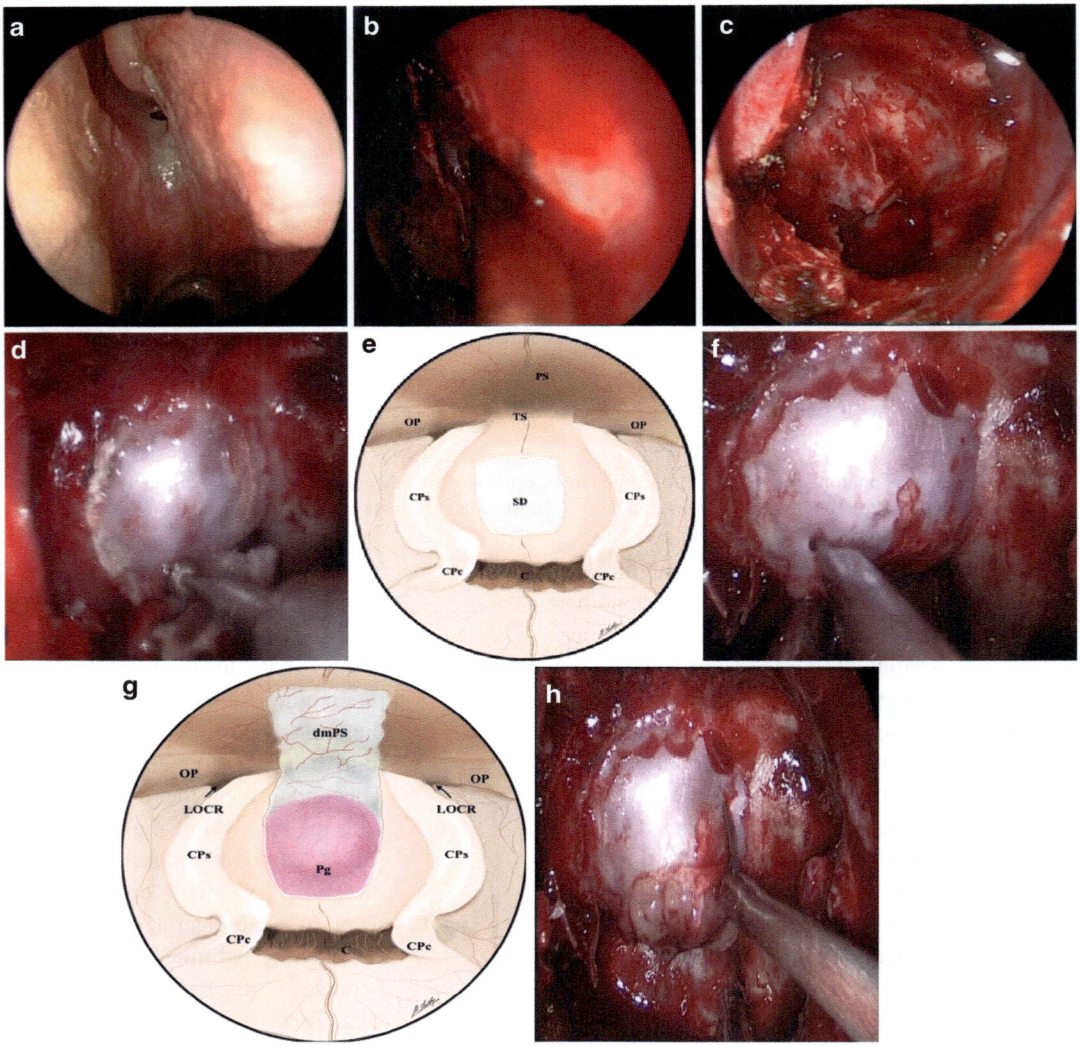

Fig. 7.6 Extended endoscopic trans-seller approach (courtesy—Dr. Ramesh Doddamani, Associate Professor, AIIMS, New Delhi). (**a**) Endoscopic view of right sphenoid ostium, (**b**) separation of posterior septum from rostrum of sphenoid sinus, (**c**) wide sphenoidotomy, (**d**) drilling of intersphenoid septum with bone over sella, (**e**) line diagram of figure **d**, (**f**) entry into sella turcica and flap creation, (**g**) line diagram of figure **f**, (**h**) adenomatous tissue is visible through entry site

can be tailored. Abducent nerve is at risk while working in the region of paraclival carotid [7].

(iv) **Transodontoid Approach**

The indications are decompression of the brainstem in rheumatoid arthritis and disintegration of the upper cervical spine. The limit of the surgical corridor is anterior limit of the foramen magnum to the body of C2 cervical vertebrae. Access is achieved by removal of nasal septum till floor of nasal cavity. Nasopharyngeal mucosa with underlying muscles is removed from one side eustachian tube opening to the other side [8]. C1 vertebral ring is removed after elevation of fascia and clival bone drilling.

2. **Access to Paramedian Corridor (Coronal Plane)**
The most critical and defining structure is ICA in this plane. The paramedian skull base may be divided into anterior (corresponding to the orbit and anterior cranial cavity), middle (corresponding to the middle cranial, pterygopalatine and infratemporal fossae) and posterior (includes the craniovertebral junction lateral to the occipital condyles and the jugular foramen) segments.
(A) **Anterior Coronal Plane**
It is further divided into the supraorbital and transorbital approaches [9–11]. Supraorbital approach provides access to anterior cranium lesion extending laterally over orbit. Transorbital is designed to reach both extraconal and intraconal lesions. The indications for the extraconal approach are the sinonasal lesions that displace, erode or invade the medial wall of the orbit and for orbital/optic nerve decompression in Graves' disease or trauma. The intraconal approach is indicated to address intraorbital benign space-occupying lesions, such as schwannomas, haemangiomas and meningiomas. The steps include complete ethmoidectomy and exposure of lamina papyracea in full extend. The next step is the removal of lamina. For supraorbital lesions, periorbita is lifted off from the cranium base with cauterization of ethmoid vessels. Binostril approach can be performed by superior septectomy. For intraconal compartment access, periorbita is incised to expose the medial and inferior rectus muscles. The gap between these two muscles represents the window for intraconal access (Fig. 7.7). As ophthalmic arteries and the optic nerves cannot be mobilized, they constitute the lateral limits of the approach.
(B) **Middle Coronal Plane**
It is further divided into five different zones, according to their relationship with specific segments of the ICA. Zone 1 is the boundary to approach the lesions found medial to petrous apex, zone 2 is corridor for infrapterous access, zone 3 is passage for suprapetrous access, zone 4 is for lateral cavernous sinus access and zone 5 is for middle fossa and infratemporal fossa. Except for zone 1, all zones start with a transpterygoid approach using the maxillary sinus as the working corridor [12–15]. These approaches provide access to skull base lesions posterior to the maxillary sinus (e.g. middle cranial, pterygopalatine and infratemporal fossae, lateral sphenoid recess, petrous apex, cavernous sinus). Common pathologies include schwannomas, juvenile nasopharyngeal angiofibromas, sinonasal malignancy and meningoencephaloceles.
(i) **Transpterygoid Approach**
The pterygopalatine fossa (PPF) is bound by the pterygoid process posteriorly, the palatine bone anteromedially and the maxilla anterolaterally. The ITF is an anatomic space located under the floor of the middle cranial fossa and posterior to the maxilla. It communicates medially with the pterygopalatine fossa through the pterygomaxillary fissure, anteriorly ITF is continuous with the inferior

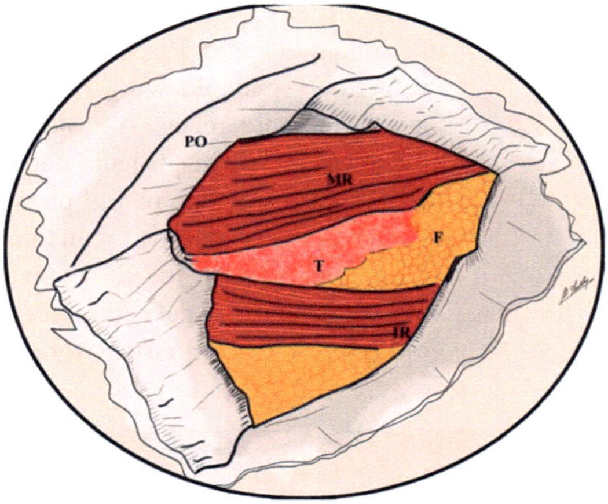

Fig. 7.7 Right transorbital intraconal approach. (Courtesy Dr. M. Arulalan, Senior Resident, Neuro-Otology, Department of Neurosurgery, SGPGIMS, Lucknow)

orbital fissure. Pneumatization of the sphenoid sinus extending into the greater sphenoid wing bears a lateral sphenoid recess (i.e. pterygoid recess), which projects under the middle fossa. The paired pterygoid processes comprise medial and lateral plates, fused at their anterior cephalic aspect, the pterygoid base. Three important foramina located from superolateral to infero-medial: foramen rotundum, vidian canal and palatovaginal canal.

The surgery begins with uncinectomy, anterior ethmoidectomy and wide middle meatus antrostomy (Fig. 7.8). The sphenopalatine and posterior nasal arteries are then identified at the sphenopalatine

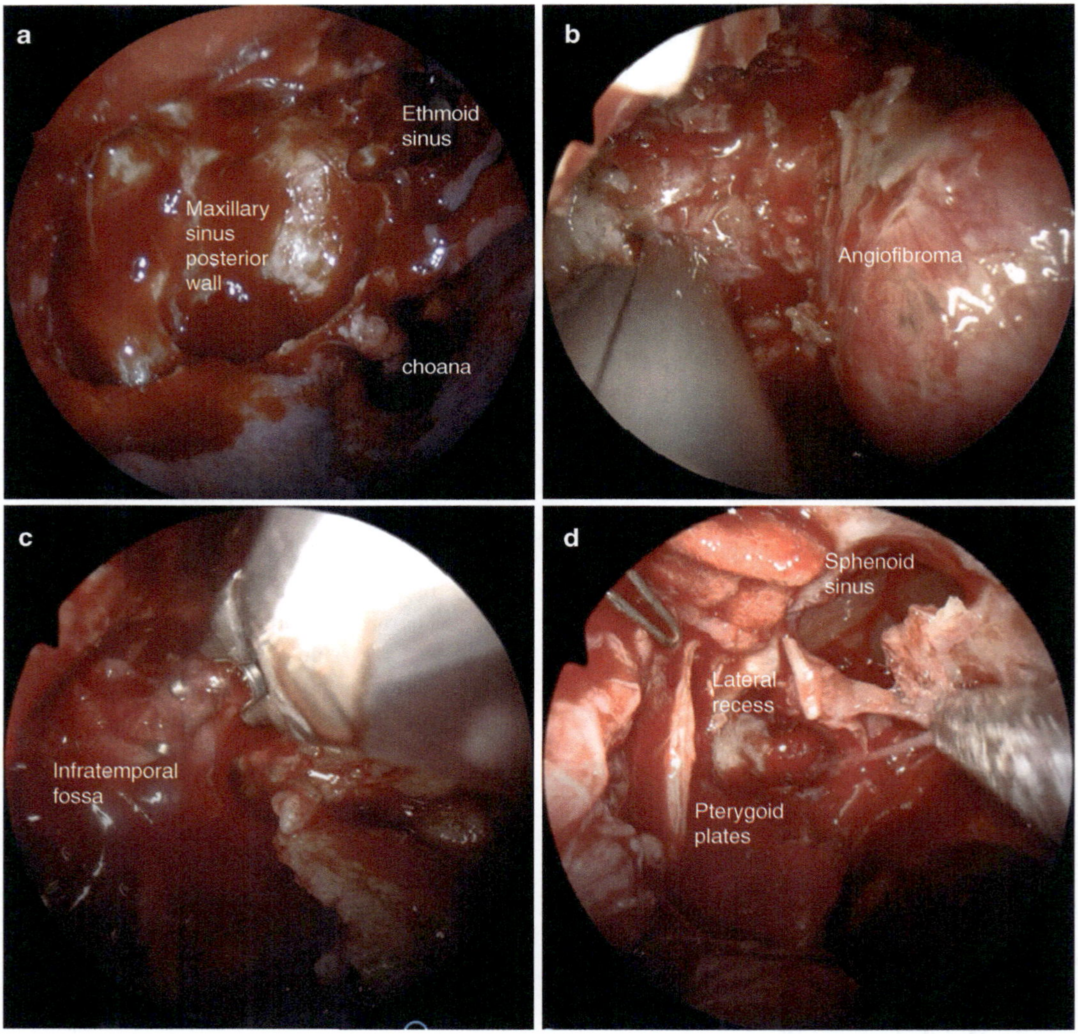

Fig. 7.8 Right middle coronal plane. (**a**) Complete exposure of posterior and part of the lateral wall of right maxillary sinus, (**b**) complete removal of posterior wall, (**c**) ligation of terminal branches of maxillary artery, (**d**) complete removal of pterygopalatine fossa content and displacement of tissue laterally after ligation of vessels, (**e**) line diagram is showing surgical field after removal of posterior maxillary sinus wall (Courtesy Dr. M. Arulalan, Senior Resident, Neurootology, Department of Neurosurgery, SGPGIMS, Lucknow)

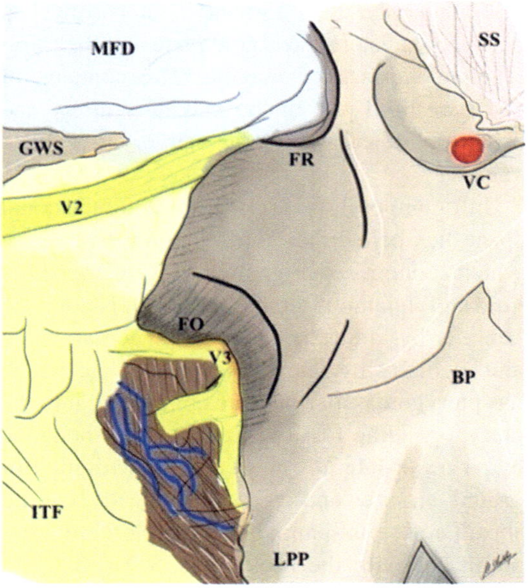

Fig. 7.8 (continued)

foreman. The posterior wall of the antrum is removed, revealing the contents of the PPF covered with periosteum. The sphenopalatine and posterior nasal arteries can be divided and mobilized laterally which exposes the vidian canal. The location of the vidian canal is usually at the insertion of the medial pterygoid plate on the pterygoid process of the sphenoid bone. The vidian nerve and artery inside the canal can be coagulated and divided, allowing for the subsequent lateralization of the contents of the pterygopalatine fossa and identification of the pterygoid base as well as the foramen rotundum. The base of the pterygoid plate is drilled, and the lateral sphenoid recess is opened. The infratemporal approach is discussed in the next section. The objective behind reconstruction is to restore the natural isolation of the intracranial structures from the sinonasal cavity, avoiding a CSF leak and secondary complications, such as infection or meningitis. A vascularized reconstruction (e.g. nasoseptal flap) is favoured. The reconstruction options are mentioned in the last section.

(ii) **Trans-cavernous Approach** [13]
It allows access lateral to cavernous carotid. Pituitary macroadenomas extending posterior to cavernous carotid is the only indication for the trans-cavernous approach. It allows lateral displacement of the carotid artery.

(iii) **Petrous Apex Approach** [10, 12]
Petrous apex lesions extending towards the sphenoid sinus can be accessed by this approach. Extended sphenoidotomy and drilling of bone over the petrous apex allows access.

(iv) **Suprapetrous Approach**
It starts with complete exposure of the course of internal carotid artery. Lesion extending into trigeminal nerve and Meckel's cave are managed by suprapetrous approach.

Infra-petrous, trans-condylar and parapharyngeal are the posterior coronal approaches. The surgical exposure in posterior coronal approaches is improved by Denker's approach, septal window and by wide maxillectomy. Zone 5 is discussed in the next section.

7.1.1 Contraindications of EEAs

Contraindications to an endoscopic approach to the skull base include tumour extending lateral to the midline of orbital roof, or lateral to optic nerve, cases where an oncological resection mandates a total maxillectomy, orbital exenteration or resection of facial skin, and most importantly lack of progressive experience in surgical team [16].

7.1.2 Limits of EEAs

Certain limitations to EEAs are significant posterior fossa extension with the tumour located behind the ICA, institutional limitations (lack of transnasal Doppler, stereotactic neuronavigation, specialized endo-bipolars and extraocular EMG monitoring) and tumours that circumferentially encase the carotid, so the endoscopic endonasal approach cannot achieve a gross total resection [16, 17].

7.2 Part B: Anatomy and Surgical Approaches to Pterygopalatine Fossa, Pterygomaxillary Fissure and Infratemporal Fossa

The pterygopalatine fossa (PPF), pterygomaxillary fissure (PMF) and infratemporal fossa (ITF) are continuous compartments that lie lateral to the sphenopalatine foramen with a greater wing of sphenoid forming their roof. Pterygomaxillary fissure (PMF) is a communication between the pterygopalatine fossa medially (which in turn communicate with the nasal cavity via the sphenopalatine foramen) and infratemporal fossa (ITF) laterally. It is formed by a narrow gap between the lateral pterygoid plate and the infratemporal surface of maxilla. The contents of PMF are third part of the maxillary artery and posterior superior alveolar nerve, artery and veins.

Infratemporal fossa is a three-dimensional space lies below the middle cranial fossa base which comprises of greater wing of the sphenoid and squamous temporal bone. It is bounded laterally by ramus of mandible, zygomatic arch and medially by lateral pterygoid plate which has pterygomaxillary fissure connecting it to the pterygopalatine fossa. Anteriorly, it is bounded by posterior-lateral wall of maxilla with inferior orbital fissure and posteriorly with carotid sheath and styloid apparatus. Inferiorly, it communicates with the neck (Figs. 7.9 and 7.10). Infratemporal fossa contents lie in three planes from superficial-to-deep in the axial plane. The first layer immediately posterior to periosteum of posterior wall of maxillary sinus consists of branches of maxillary artery. Second layer formed by various branches and anastomosis of V2 and V3 and third layer is consist of muscles of ITF. This surgical anatomy is important while dealing with the pathology of PPF and ITF (Fig. 7.11) [18–21].

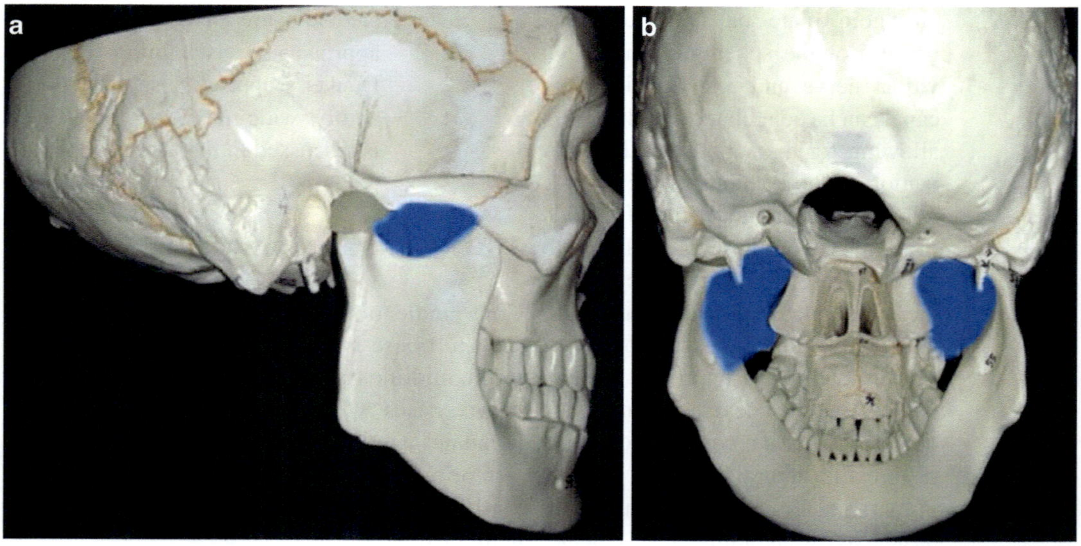

Fig. 7.9 Infratemporal fossa—bony outlines. (**a**) Lateral view and (**b**) posterior view

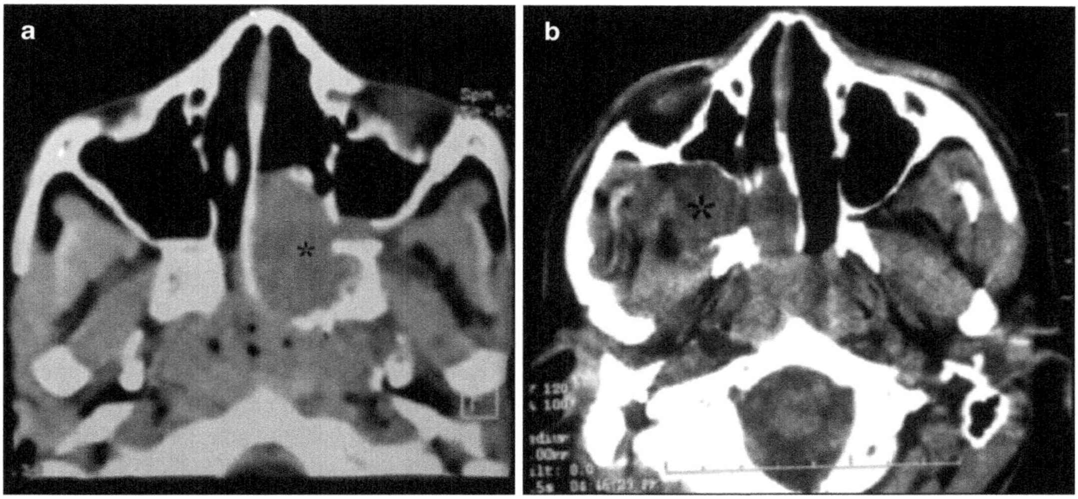

Fig. 7.10 Computed tomography Axial sections (**a**) showing tumour (asterisk) involving sphenopalatine foramen and pterygomaxillary fissure and (**b**) involving infratemporal fossa

The surgical approach to PPF and ITF can be either an endoscopic approach or an open approach. The endoscopic approach is mainly the anterior approach to ITF and suited for SPF, PPF and medial ITF which can combined with endoscopic Denker's approach or anterior maxillotomy for lateral ITF pathology. Open approaches can be either anterolateral like maxillary swing and midfacial degloving or lateral like Fisch's ITF approach C and infratemporal fossa approach D (preauricular transzygomatic approach).

7.2.1 Surgical Approach to PPF and ITF

Surgery of PPF and ITF can be done by either an endoscopic approach or by an open approach. The endoscopic approach is mainly an anterior approach to ITF and suited for SPF, PPF and Medial ITF which if combined with endoscopic Denker's approach or maxillotomy can be used for lateral ITF pathology. Open approaches can be either anterolateral like maxillary swing and midfacial degloving or lateral like Fisch's ITF approach C and D. Surgical approach to PPF and ITF are decided mainly by the type of lesion, its extension and experience of the surgical team.

1. **Endoscopic Approach to SPA, PPF and ITF**
   It is indicated for sphenopalatine artery ligation, maxillary artery ligation, vidian neurectomy, juvenile nasopharyngeal angiofibroma (Fisch Stage I, II and III JNA). Schwannomas of PPF and ITF are commonly arising from the maxillary nerve and mandibular nerve, paranasal sinus tumours (non-squamous) with extension into the SPA, PPF or ITF. Temporal lobe meningo-encephalocele is extending into the infratemporal fossa. Lesions of the middle cranial skull base, which are lying (intradural/extradural) lateral to cavernous sinus.
   Contraindications of Endoscopic Approach: Tumours are extending to the masseteric space and gingivobuccal sulcus. Large juvenile nasopharyngeal angiofibroma is receiving significant feeders from the internal carotid artery and other tumours encasing ICA. Tumours extending to the cavernous sinus, in around optic nerve and orbital apex, middle fossa and para-sellar extension are the relative contraindications.

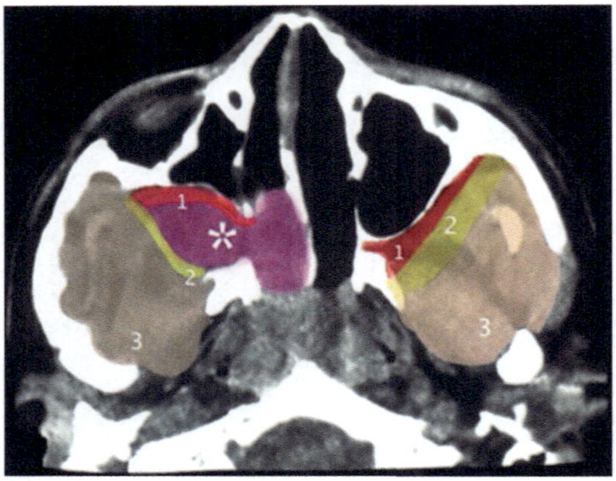

Fig. 7.11 Contents of infratemporal fossa in three planes. (1) Vascular layer (with branches of internal maxillary artery), (2) neural layer (with branches of maxillary and mandibular nerves) and (3) muscular layer. Right side (asterisk) is the tumour arising from the sphenopalatine foramen involving the nasopharynx and entering infratemporal fossa causing splaying of the vascular and neural layers

Surgical Steps (Fig. 7.12):

Endoscopic large meatal antrostomy is the first step of the endoscopic approach as this exposes the posterior-medial wall of the maxillary sinus, which lies anterior to SPF, PPF and ITF. Wider access can be gained by a medial maxillectomy. Removal of the lower part of middle turbinate creates more space for instrumentation. This is followed by an anterior and posterior ethmoidectomy. Pathologies in the SPA, PPF and medial ITF can be accessed after removal of posterior wall of maxilla with a Kerrison's rongeurs or drill starting from the anterior lip of SPA taking care to prevent injury to the periosteum of posterior wall of maxillary sinus, as maxillary artery and its branches lie directly posterior to it. The sphenopalatine artery can be identified just posterior to cristae on the posterior part of medial wall of maxilla and maxillary artery

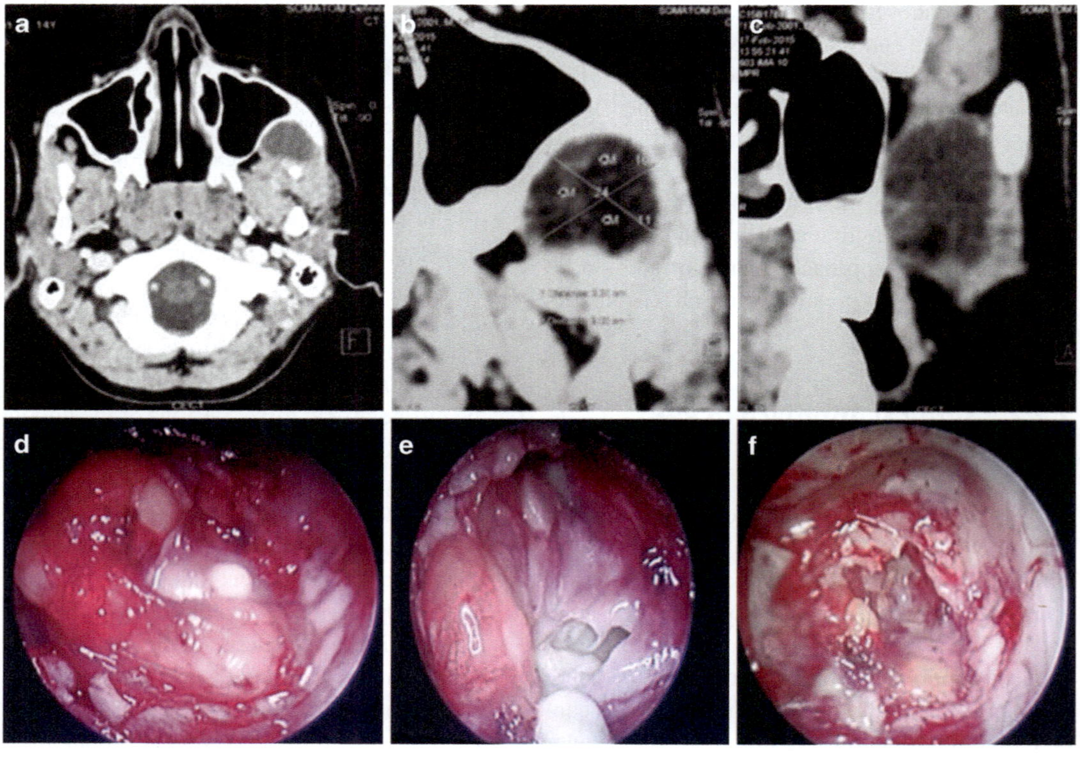

Fig. 7.12 Endoscopic excision of the infratemporal fossa tumour. (**a**) Axial CT showing hypodense lesion in left ITF, (**b**) zoomed image, (**c**) coronal section for the same lesion, (**d**) endoscopic exposure after removal of posterior wall of maxillary sinus, (**e**) tumour dissection from surrounding tissue, (**f**) postoperative cavity

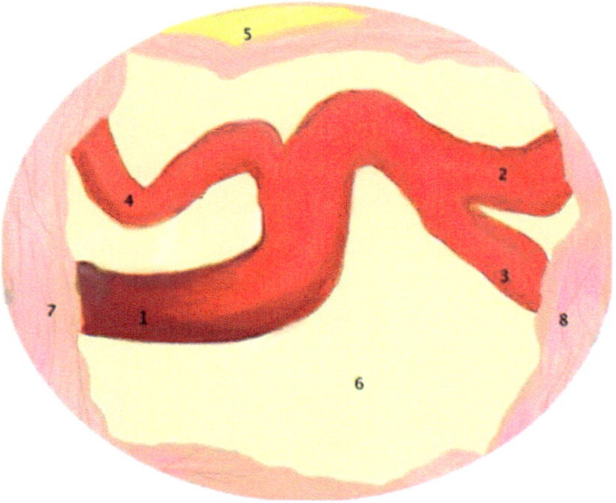

Fig. 7.13 Endoscopic view of right internal maxillary artery in the infratemporal fossa. (1) Internal maxillary artery, (2) sphenopalatine artery, (3) descending palatine artery, (4) infraorbital artery, (5) infraorbital nerve, (6) infratemporal fossa fat, (7) lateral wall of the maxillary sinus, (8) medial wall of the maxillary sinus

and its branches by careful dissection of periosteum of posterior wall of maxilla to expose contents of PPF, PMF and ITF (Fig. 7.13).

The maxillary artery dissection and the control is important as it is the major vascular supply to the tumours arising or located in this area. Preoperative embolization can reduce the vascularity in vascular tumours like JNA and hemangiopericytoma.

Lateral exposure of ITF by endoscope is limited by Piriform aperture, which can be removed by modified Denker's approach or by wide anterior wall maxillotomy to gain access to the lateral compartment of ITF. Single surgeon endoscopic approach can be converted into a two surgeon 4 handed technique after making a septal window anytime during surgery for better visualization, dexterity, dissection, for controlling the vessels and for tumour removal. For pathology located in the middle fossa and surrounding skull base, a greater wing of sphenoid and pterygoids can be drilled to access the middle fossa above, the petrous carotid from cavernous sinus to lateral part of temporal bone after either displacing the maxillary artery and its branches downward and clipping it [14, 15].

Complications

Bleeding can occur intraoperatively due to injury to the maxillary artery or its branches and rarely from feeders of ICA. Injury to the nasolacrimal duct is evident after surgery with complaints of epiphora. Injury to V2, sphenopalatine ganglia can lead to dry eye and numbness of the face. Orbital injury can occur during dissection of tumours, dissection around orbital fissure and optic nerve can lead to visual deterioration, if the optic nerve is injured and extraocular muscle injury can lead to diplopia. CSF leak can occur from the middle cranial fossa after tumour removal and repair of encephaloceles. Intracranial bleeding can also occur during tumour removal from the intradural compartment. Complications can happen due to removal of normal structures like piriform aperture leading to numbness of the vestibular area, nasal obstruction from crusting in nasal cavity and septal perforation. Postoperative epistaxis can occur leading to blood loss or aspirations [19, 22]. So, each and every step of the procedure has to be meticulously performed and the possible complication has to be anticipated and avoided.

2. **Open Approach to PPF and ITF**

Indications

It is indicated for the tumours of ITF with extensions to masticator space, buccinators space and Zygomatic space. Malignant lesions of the maxillary sinus with ITF involvement are managed by open anterior approach. It is also advised for gross extension of lesion to middle cranial fossa through foramen rotundum or ovale. Parotid gland, mandible and zygomatic bone can be involved by lateral extension of ITF lesions. Inferior extension of ITF lesions into parapharyngeal space is also managed by an open approach. Jugular foramen lesion with ITF extension is also handled by open approaches [23, 24]. Approaches for malignant lesions of the nose and PNS are mentioned in Part D (Sect. 7.4).

Contraindications

There is no absolute contraindication to the open approach to ITF as this approach can be extended or combined with other open or endoscopic approaches for tumour removal. Being a lateral vector, this approach is not suited for lesion crossing midline to other sides like contralateral sphenoid sinus and nasopharynx. Extensive malignant tumour like squamous cell carcinoma and tumour having extensive involvement of ICA or vertebral artery are deemed inoperable.

Surgical Steps

Open approaches to PPF and ITF are many. Most commonly performed open approaches are transmaxillary like midface degloving and maxillary swing approach which works in an anterior vector (Fig. 7.14), while commonly performed lateral approaches are preauricular transzygomatic (Fig. 7.15) approach for ITF lesions and a preauricular fronto-temporal orbitozygomatic for ITF lesions having major intracranial extension.

For a preauricular transzygomatic approach, a curvilinear incision is made in the preauricular region staying above the lower attachment of tragus coursing superiorly and then anteriorly in the frontal scalp to end superior to the supraorbital notch near the midline. Scalp incision is elevated by giving incision in the superficial layer of deep temporal fascia to prevent injury to the frontal branch of facial nerve. Temporal muscle is incised to gain exposure of zygomatic arch and lateral orbital rim in

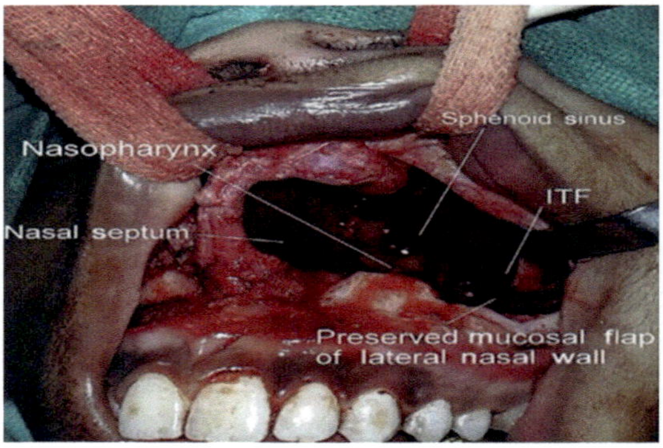

Fig. 7.14 Midfacial degloving for left ITF lesion

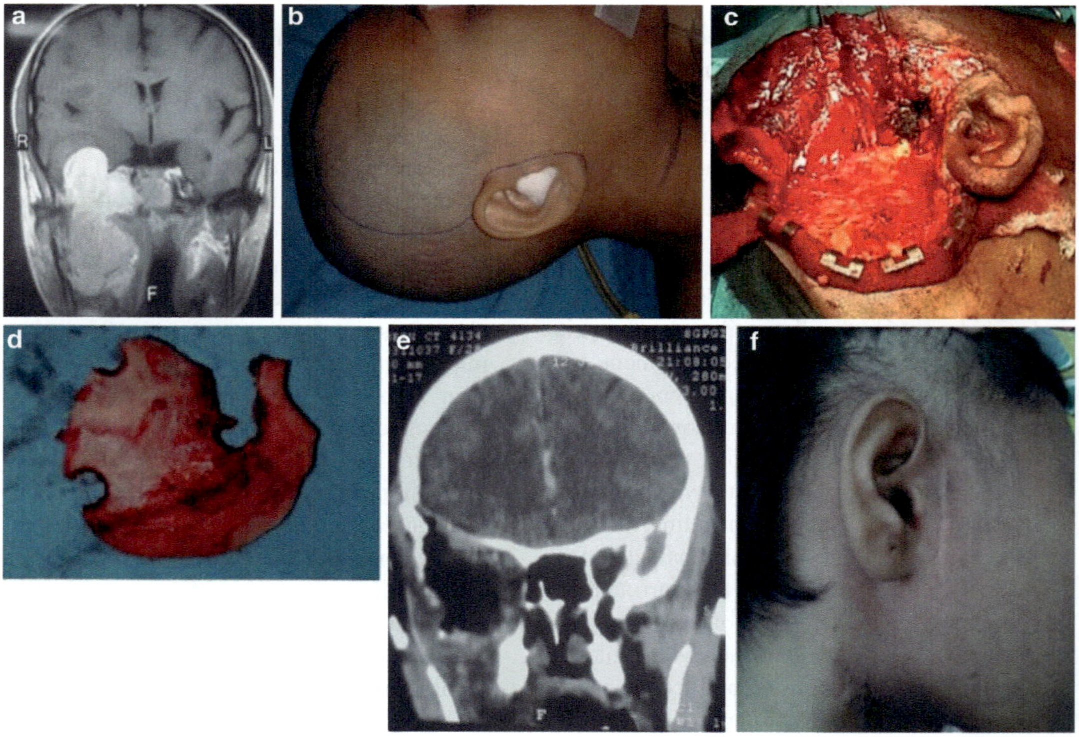

Fig. 7.15 Preauricular transzygomatic approach. (**a**) MRI is showing dumbbell tumour with ITF involvement of right side, (**b**) preauricular incision is marked with temporal extension, (**c**) flaps elevated, (**d**) temporal craniotomy bone, (**e**) postoperative CT scan and (**f**) healed wound

selected cases where zygomatic arch needs removed and in more advanced case orbitozygomatic osteotomy is required. Combining this with pterional craniotomy, middle cranial fossa can be approached. The middle fossa skull base is drilled to expose the V2, V3 and Middle meningeal artery which can be mobilized or sacrificed combining ITF and middle fossa. This approach can provide access for tumour removal medially from sphenoid sinus to cavernous sinus, superiorly from middle cranial fossa, laterally up to skin mandible and parotids, inferiorly till parapharyngeal space and lower neck if skin incision is extended below. Control of great vessels in the neck can be taken for lesions involving the petrous ICA.

Complications

Mandibular nerve needs to be sacrificed sometimes leading to hypoesthesia. Temporomandibular joint dysfunction can occur due to drilling, leading to varying degrees of trismus. Injury to ICA can occur if vertical petrous carotid is involved by lesion, as this approach does not give access to gain control over it. Injury to facial nerve and branches can lead to facial nerve palsy [25].

Conclusion

PPF and ITF have a complex anatomy and contain many neurovascular structures and a clear understating of this anatomy is important for surgery in this area. Medial and medium-size lesions are better suited by endoscopic approach while laterally based extensive tumours are better suited by open approach. Both approaches can be combined in selected cases for complete resection of lesions (Fig. 7.16).

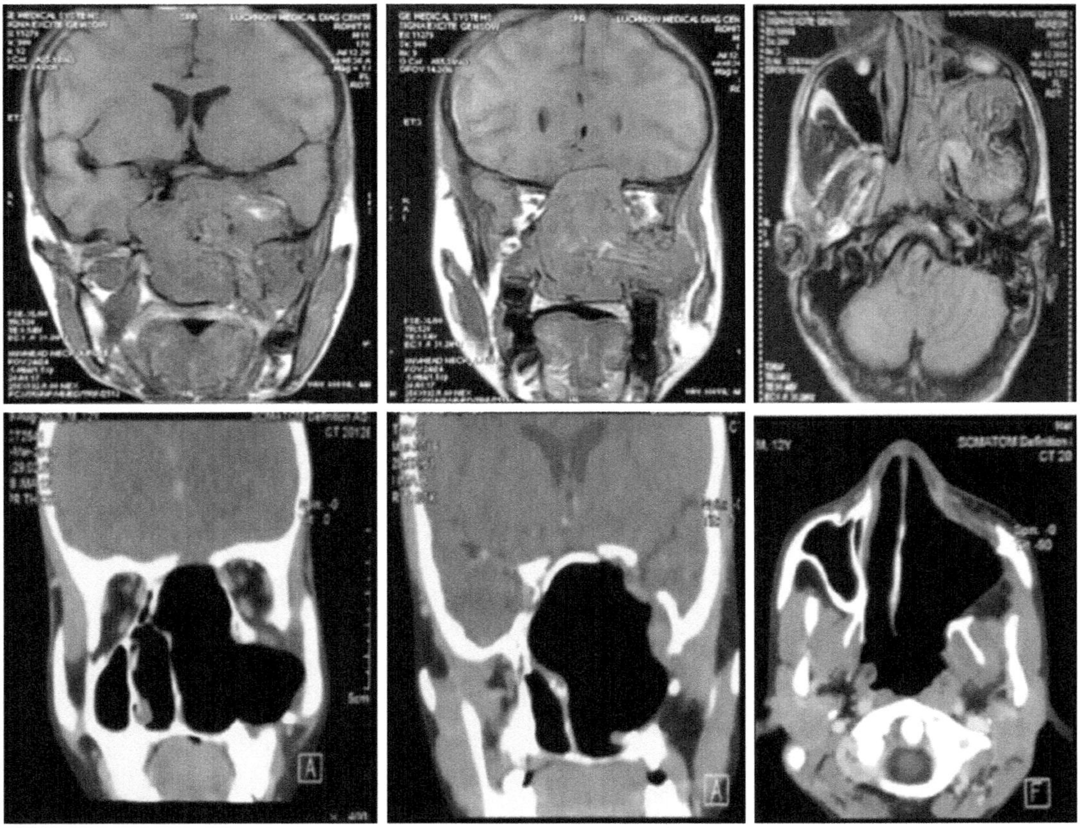

Fig. 7.16 Endoscopic and midfacial degloving approach is used to excise the lesion (pre- and postoperative radiology)

7.3 Part C: Pituitary Tumours and Surgical Management

Pituitary adenoma is the most common tumour of the sellar region (90–95%). The adenomas constitute 10–15% of all intracranial tumours [26]. The preoperative assessment, indication of surgery, selection of approach and postoperative care are jointly done by neurosurgeon, otolaryngologist, neuro-radiologist, endocrinologist and neuro-anaesthetist for a better patient outcome [27]. The presenting symptoms are based on the type of adenoma. Except prolactinoma, surgery remains the treatment of choice. The endoscopic transnasal trans-sphenoidal approach is the gold standard due to the panoramic view, preservation of normal function and reduced hospital stay. The use of newer technologies like plasma ablation provides a relatively bloodless field. An expertise in endoscopic techniques and the ability to use angled endoscopes is required. Detailed anatomical knowledge is the prerequisite as the margin of error is very less. During postoperative monitoring in ICU, one should look out for diabetes insipidus, CSF leak, meningitis and visual disturbance among other complications.

The endoscopic endonasal approach is the standard surgical approach for pituitary tumours; hence, it will be discussed in detail in this chapter. Transcranial approaches are mentioned in Part E (Sect. 7.5).

7.3.1 Anatomy

The pituitary gland is projected from inferior part of the hypothalamus and it maintains the functional connections via the infundibulum (pituitary stalk). The gland has an anterior lobe called adenohypophysis derived from the ectoderm of Rathke's pouch and a posterior lobe called neurohypophysis derived from neuroectoderm prosencephalon. The intermediate lobe is rudimentary in humans and degenerates after birth. The gland resides in the sella turcica and is covered by diaphragmatic sella (dural fold). Laterally it is bound by cavernous sinus and its contents (ICA, CN III, IV, V1,V2 VI) and anterior and inferiorly by the sphenoid sinus (Fig. 7.17).

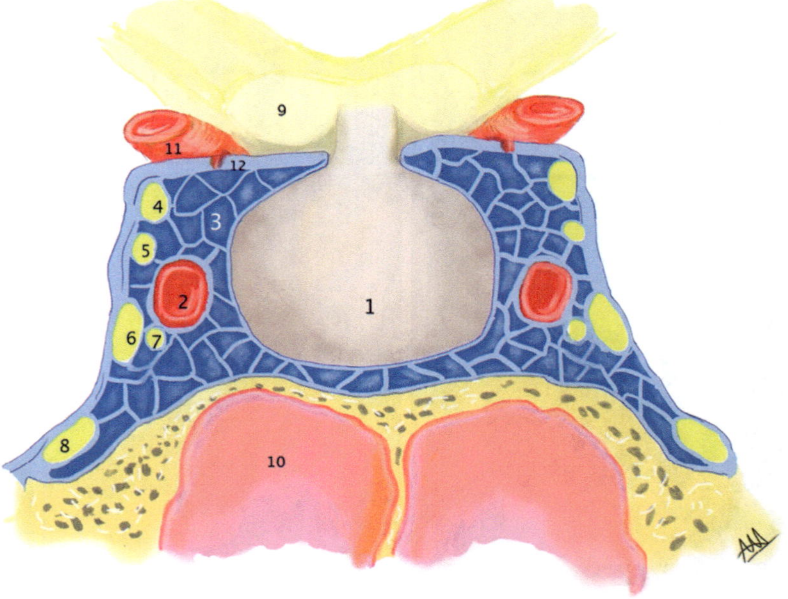

Fig. 7.17 Anatomical location and relations of pituitary gland (1) pituitary gland, (2) ICA (cavernous part), (3) cavernous sinus, (4) oculomotor nerve (III), (5) trochlear nerve (IV), (6) ophthalmic nerve (V_1), (7) abducent nerve (VI), (8) maxillary nerve (V_2), (9) optic chiasm, (10) sphenoid sinus, (11) ICA (clinoidal part), (12) posterior communicating artery

7.3.2 Physiology

Anterior pituitary secrets the hormones under the influence of the hypothalamus. The main hormones are growth hormone (GH), adrenocorticotrophic hormone (ACTH), thyroid-stimulating hormone (TSH), prolactin (PRL), gonadotropins (Luteinising hormone, LH and Follicular-stimulating hormone, FSH). Posterior pituitary secrets oxytocin and vasopressin (Figs. 7.18 and 7.19).

The list of pituitary tumours is long and differential diagnosis of sellar lesions is listed in Table 7.1.

(A) **Pituitary Adenoma**

It is the most common type of pituitary lesion. The classification of adenoma is based on the size of the tumour and immunohistochemical expression (Table 7.2) [28]. The incidence of incidentalomas is 10% [29, 30].

1. **Non-functional Pituitary Adenoma**

   No hormone is secreted and symptoms are usually due to pressure effects. The common clinical features include headache, visual disturbance, features of hypopituitarism and hydrocephalus. Indication of surgery in these patients is to relieve and to prevent the mass effect of the tumour and pituitary apoplexy [31]. As far as treatment is concerned, surgery remains the mainstay with radiotherapy in recurrent and invasive cases.

2. **Functional Pituitary Adenoma**

   The types of pituitary function adenoma are based on the hormone secreted by adenoma.

   (i) **Prolactinoma**

   This is the most common type (40%) of functional adenoma [28] with clinical features depending upon the gender. Females present as secondary oligomenorrhoea and/or galactorrhoea whereas males present with galactorrhoea, impotence, headache and visual disturbance. This tumour is unique because the medical treatment is the mainstay in more than 90% of the patients and includes dopamine agonists like bromocriptine and cabergoline. Surgical management, although rarely required, has specific indications like failure of medical treatment, patient preference, pituitary apoplexy, CSF leak during medical therapy [32] and pregnancy-related issues [33].

   (ii) **Acromegaly**

   These are the growth hormone-secreting tumours and about 10% of these tumours occur before adulthood and lead to gigantism. Clinical features include enlarged nose, chin, hands and feet and endocrine abnormalities include increased GH, insulin-like growth factor (IGF I) levels in serum. The morbidity and mortality in this subset of tumours is related to cardiovascular complications. As far as the treatment is concerned, surgery remains

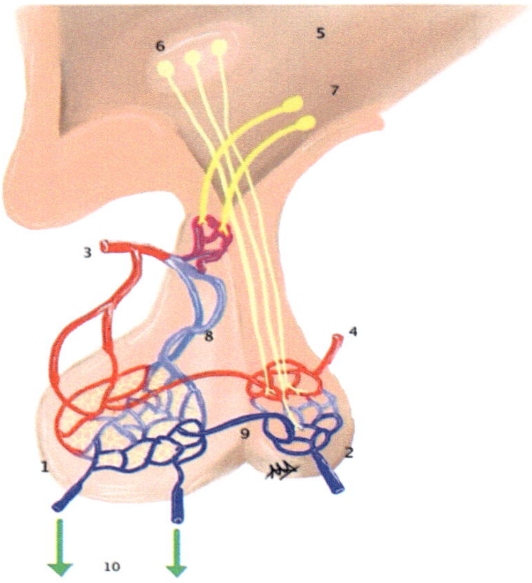

Fig. 7.18 Blood supply—Hypothalamic—Pituitary axis (1) anterior pituitary, (2) posterior pituitary, (3) superior hypophyseal artery, (4) inferior hypophyseal artery, (5) third ventricle, (6) neuroendocrine nuclei, (7) hypothalamus, (8) long portal vessels, (9) short portal vessels and (10) hormone release

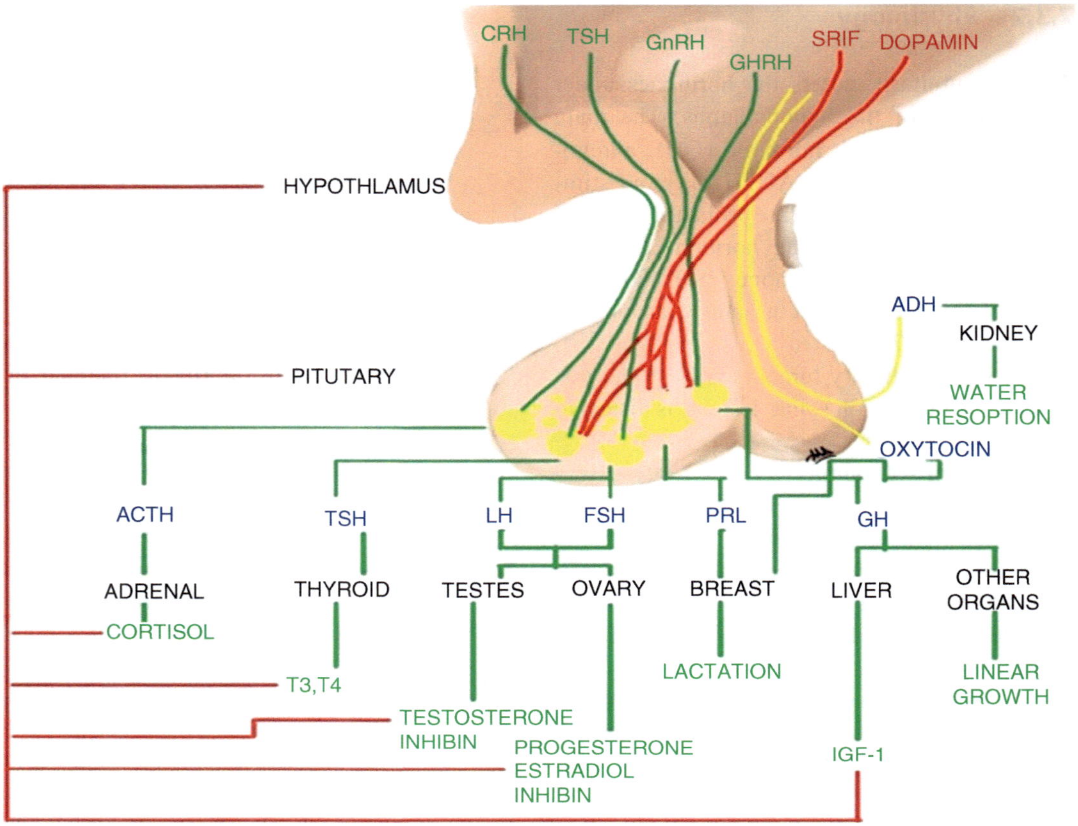

Fig. 7.19 Hypothalamic pituitary axis—regulation of hormone secretion

Table 7.1 Differential diagnosis of sellar lesions

Tumours	Pituitary adenoma Craniopharyngioma Meningioma Glioma Chordoma Lymphoma Metastasis
Cyst	Rathke's cyst Dermoid cyst
Inflammatory conditions	Bacterial Abscess Tuberculosis Sarcoidosis Langerhans cell histiocytosis Hypophysitis
Others	Pituitary apoplexy Hypothalamus hamartoma ICA aneurysms

Table 7.2 Classification of pituitary adenoma

Based on size	Based on character
Microadenoma (<1 cm) • Enclosed • Invasive	Non-functional Clinically no function (hypopituitarism due to pressure)
Macroadenoma (>1 cm) • Enclosed • Invasive • Expanding	Functional • Prolactinoma (Prolactin) • Acromegaly (GH) • Cushing disease (ACTH) • Gonadotropin-producing adenoma (LH, FSH) • Thyrotropin-producing adenoma (TSH) • Mixed (GH with PRL)
Mesoadenoma (1 cm)	

the mainstay with medical management aiming at correcting the hormonal abnormalities. The medical agents include somatostatin analogue, dopamine agonist and GH receptor antagonist. Radiotherapy is reserved for invasive and recurrent cases [34].

(iii) **Cushing Disease**
These tumours are usually ACTH-secreting microadenoma and have pronounced clinical features usually secondary to endocrine disturbances. These include truncal obesity, hypertension, hirsutism, glycosuria, osteoporosis and psychosis. Surgery remains the mainstay of treatment with medical therapy aiming to correct the endocrine imbalances. In rare cases, radiotherapy and bilateral adrenalectomy have also been used [35].

(iv) **Gonadotropin-Secreting Adenoma**
These are LH- and FSH-secreting tumours and their symptoms are usually due to mass effects; hence, surgery is the main choice of treatment.

(v) **Thyrotropin-Secreting Tumours**
These tumours secrete TSH and patients usually present with central hyperthyroidism features (palpitation, tremors, neck swelling, weight loss, sweating, etc.). Treatment is medical with somatostatin analogue if compressive effects are not prominent; otherwise, surgical removal of the tumour along with medical therapy must be taken into consideration.

(B) **Pituitary Apoplexy**
It is the sudden pituitary haemorrhage or haemorrhage in adenomas and usually presents with dramatic clinical features like sudden visual loss, headache and vomiting. Treatment is surgical removal of the tumour with evacuation of haematoma in order to relieve the pressure.

Preoperative Work-Up
Apart from relevant history, e.g. nasal surgery and co-morbid conditions, one should look for features of various endocrine conditions like Cushing, acromegaly, hyperthyroidism and hypopituitarism. Special examination includes ophthalmological work-up (visual acuity, visual field and proptosis evaluation), neurologic examination (e.g. cranial III, IV, V and VI), endocrine assessment (hormonal assessment and electrolyte evaluation), nasal endoscopic examination—to look for abnormal anatomy and adequacy for nasal septal flap. Imaging studies include delayed post-contrast MRI, which is the modality of choice. MRI helps in determining the extent of tumour, cavernous sinus involvement, ICA involvement (signal void in T2 MRI), identification of normal pituitary gland (neurohypophysis shows increased signal intensity in T1 non-contrast) and optic chiasm. CT paranasal sinus must also be done as it helps in surgical planning, anatomical study (sinuses, skull base, optic nerve, Onodi cell) and also helps in differential diagnosis (calcification in craniopharyngioma).

Aims and Principles of Pituitary Surgery
They include elimination of mass effect, restoration of pituitary function, prevention of recurrence, complete histopathological diagnosis, and if possible, normalization of hormonal production.

Operative Procedure

(i) **Anaesthesia**
General anaesthesia with orotracheal intubation is standard. The anaesthetist is requested for hypotensive anaesthesia (Mean Arterial Pressure between 60 and 80 mmHg, Heart rate less than 70) in order to get a clean surgical field and minimize the blood loss.

The patient is placed in a supine position with 30° head up (reverse Trendelenburg position) and ceftriaxone 2 g I.V. or clindamycin 600 mg IV/vancomycin 1 g iv in cases of beta-lactam allergy, is injected before starting the surgery.

(ii) **Instruments and Equipment**

A three-chip or preferably HD camera with a large LED monitor of 20 inches or larger (easier on the eyes) is required for visualizing the structures clearly. A complete Functional Endoscopic Sinus Surgery set with various sized straight and angled up-cut and down-cut rongeurs along with high-speed drill is essential. Among the optional instruments are microdebrider, plasma ablation and doppler for identification of para-sellar carotid artery. Neuro-navigation, if available, is recommended in cases of extensive tumour with distorted anatomy or revision surgery to identify the landmarks.

(iii) **Surgical Approaches**

The surgical approaches can be either transseptal, trans-ethmoidal or transnasal [36–38]. Endoscopic transnasal trans-sphenoidal approach is usually considered the standard approach for pituitary surgery because of the following advantages: good panoramic view, preservation of normal function, reduced hospital stays and improved patient outcome. The surgery can be divided into the following steps:

- **Position:** The surgery is started with the proper positioning of the patient. We use a reverse Trendelenburg position.
- **Nasal phase:** Nasal cavity is decongested with commercially available sponges or by cotton pledgets soaked in 1:10,000 Adrenaline. The surgical corridor used is the space between the middle turbinate and nasal septum. Inferior turbinate is out fractured to create space (not always needed), the Middle turbinate is lateralized and the superior turbinate is identified and gently lateralized to reveal the natural sphenoid ostia. Many times the sphenoid ostia is oedematous and not clearly visible, decongestion usually will expose it. If a Hadad flap is planned, then it has to be harvested before the septectomy is done.
- **Septal phase**: Using the plasma ablation, the mucosa around the ostia and the nasal septum is ablated away and steps are repeated on the opposite side. Septectomy is performed and the sphenoidal phase of surgery is started.
- **Sphenoidal phase:** Sphenoid ostias are widened on both sides using a rongeur and the keel of sphenoid drilled away using a high-speed cutting burr. Any bleeding from the bone is taken care of with a diamond burr (Figs. 7.20 and 7.21). With the sphenoid sinus wide open, the mucosa from the sinus is elevated and removed completely. After this, the intersinus septum is drilled away or cut with a through-cut. The bone over the sella is drilled using a diamond burr; if the bone is thick, a cutting burr is used. The thin bone is then taken away with a rongeur and the dura is exposed.
- **Sellar phase:** Using the coagulation mode of the plasma ablator, the dura

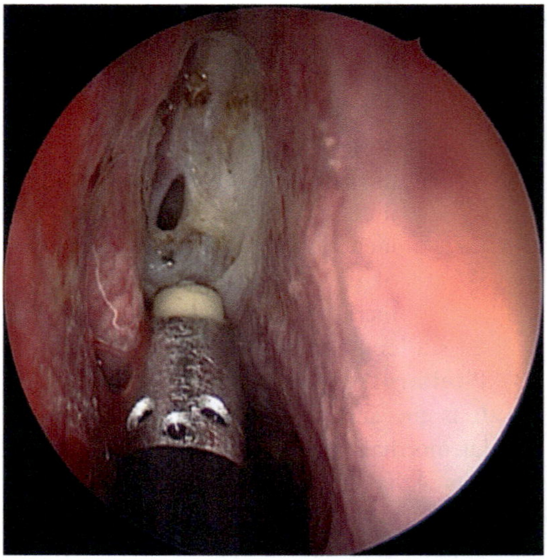

Fig. 7.20 Sphenoid ostia identified and area being plasma ablated

is coagulated and at this point, it becomes a four-hand technique with the neurosurgeon joining the surgery.

- **Neurosurgical removal of tumour:** An incision is made over the dura and using saline, hydro-dissection is done. If the tumour is soft and suckable, a major part of it just bulges out with hydro-dissection. Biopsy is taken and using curettes and suction, the neurosurgeon clears the tumour. Suprasellar and lateral extensions require angled endoscopes (30° or 45°). After ensuring complete tumour removal and examination of the sella, the defect is repaired.
- **Reconstruction of the defect:** The fat is wrapped in oxidized cellulose polymer. We have found that this makes it easier to manipulate the fat. A fascia lata graft is used by overlay, underlay or interlay fashion and fibrin glue is applied over it. A small piece of gel foam is then applied over the glue. No nasal packs are used. Readers can access the author's surgical video via the following link: https://youtu.be/L-YEssDFGGQ

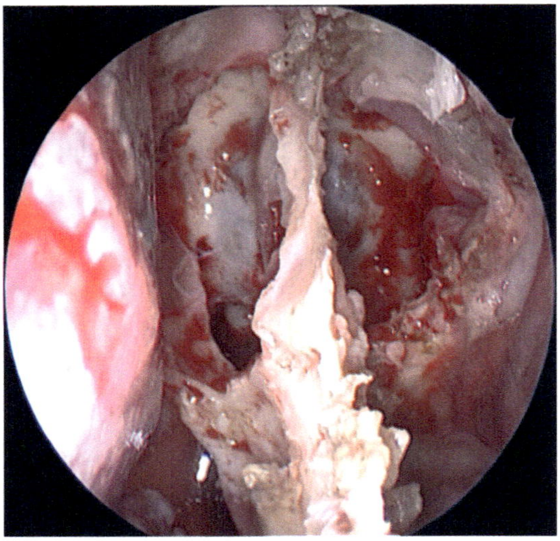

Fig. 7.21 Owls eye appearance, the ostia have been widened and septectomy done

7.3.3 Postoperative Care

The choice of antibiotics and analgesics is depending upon the institution's preference. The patient should spend his first 24–48 h in an ICU with physicians experienced in monitoring important signs like CSF leak, visual disturbance, nasal bleed, etc. The ICU team should be able to manage possible conditions like diabetes insipidus and meningitis. Routine advise includes bed rest, head-end elevation and stool softener along with copious saline drops to prevent crusting. The patient should be advised strict follow-up to prevent crusting.

7.3.4 Pearls of Pituitary Surgery

Superior turbinate, superior margin of choana are key landmarks for sphenoidal ostium identification. Adequate removal of the anterior wall of sphenoid is essential for good visualization of sella. Recognition of medial and lateral optico-carotid recesses are important. The need for vascularized nasoseptal flap is to be considered prior to sphenoidotomy. The drilling of tuberculum and planum is considered in suprasellar extension. The delineation of carotid in cavernous sinus extension is important and attention to superior and inferior inter-cavernous sinus is important.

7.4 Part D: Open Techniques for Nose and Paranasal Sinuses

The surgical approaches for the nose and paranasal sinuses range from endoscopic to conventional open techniques. The contemporary indications for endoscopic approaches to the paranasal sinuses and skull base have been expanded making conventional open techniques less frequent [39]. Absolute indications necessitating either a transfacial or a transpalatal incision include skin and subcutaneous tissue invasion, extensive involvement of the orbital fat, extraocular muscles and eyelid skin and palatal involvement. Traditionally, intracranial extension, cavernous sinus involvement [40] and extension beyond the mid-pupillary line were considered to preclude endoscopic approaches. With advancements in neuro-navigation and endoscopic surgical armamentarium, properly selected cases with the above-mentioned disease extension can be dealt without resorting to conventional open approaches. Open approaches in this chapter have been classified into bone and soft tissue approaches. Soft tissue approaches and incisions like the Moure's incision with lateral rhinotomy also serve as a precursor for bony approaches like the medial maxillectomy. Bony approaches can further be classified into midline, paramedian and lateral approaches based on the trajectory to the skull base. Strictly midline approaches include transpalatal, lateral rhinotomy, medial maxillectomy and Le Fort's Osteotomy approach. Paramedian approaches additionally target the infratemporal fossa with the maxillary swing being the best example. Lateral approach to the paranasal sinus and the skull base as in the case of a preauricular subtemporal approach provides excellent visualization of the lateral part of the infratemporal fossa, para-sellar, cavernous sinus and lesions located lateral to the cavernous internal carotid artery. Craniofacial resection pertains to a combination of transfacial or transpalatal approach to the paranasal sinus and a bicoronal incision with frontal craniotomy for the intracranial component. Choosing the best approach requires detailed preoperative radiological assessment and an understanding of tumour biology.

7.4.1 Indications for Open Approaches

These vary for inflammatory disease and for neoplastic disease. For inflammatory disease, mere drainage of sinus contents and partial removal of polypoid mucosa is appropriate and the contraindications to endoscopic approaches are few. Frontal sinus disease extending beyond the mid-pupillary line can however be a relative contraindication as it can be inaccessible even with the modified Lothrop technique. The prime focus of this chapter is on neoplastic disease (benign or malignant), the indications for open approaches may be listed as the following:

- Lesion extending beyond mid-pupillary line
- Skin involvement
- Extensive involvement of orbital fat, extraocular muscles and skin of the eyelid
- Involvement of the bone of the hard palate or paranasal sinuses
- Significant intracranial extension

7.4.2 Relative Contraindications for Surgical Resection of Nose/Paranasal Sinus Tumours

Surgical resection with open technique with or without endoscopic guidance can be attempted but resection may not offer oncological clearance of the disease [41]:

- Orbital apex involvement
- Infratemporal fossa involvement
- Erosion of pterygoid plates
- Cavernous sinus involvement
- Intradural/brain parenchymal involvement
- Involvement of nasopharynx and sphenoid sinus
- Cranial nerve involvement other than I, II and infraorbital nerve
- Encasement of internal carotid artery

Tumour extension to the above-mentioned sites are technically resectable. Resection can be attempted in case of benign tumours like nasopharyngeal angiofibroma and inverted papilloma, and similarly, low-grade sinonasal malignancies like olfactory neuroblastoma (Hyams grade 1 and 2), epithelial–myoepithelial carcinoma, biphenotypic sinonasal sarcoma and adenoid cystic carcinoma [42]. It is to be noted that although adenoid cystic carcinoma is a high-grade malignancy, it has a protracted course with disease recurrence and metastasis occurring after as long as 10 years, justifying the radical resection. Moreover, many of these tumours are relatively non-responsive to radiation or chemotherapy. Therefore, radical surgical excision followed by adjuvant therapy offers the best chance of cure [43, 44].

7.4.3 Preoperative Work-Up

Before embarking on the surgical aspects of treating sinonasal tumours, detailed preoperative evaluation is of paramount importance. This broadly includes radiologically mapping the tumour followed by biopsy from representative areas and screening for distant metastasis in case of malignant tumours:

- **Contrast-enhanced computed tomography (CECT)** should preferably be high-resolution 1 mm cuts in the axial, coronal and sagittal planes. This provides information with regard to bony involvement, intraorbital extension, skull base erosion, major vessel encasement.
- **MRI** provides information complimentary to that of CECT with better soft tissue delineation. Hyperintense signal in any of the paranasal sinuses on T2 will differentiate accumulated secretions from tumour. Invasion of periorbita can be identified on T1-weighted contrast sequences. Fat suppression allows one to establish orbital fat involvement. This facilitates preoperative decision-making with regard to management of the orbit. Perineural invasion can be inferred from a widened or destroyed of neural foramina on a CT scan. This can be confirmed on fat-suppressed contrast-enhanced T1-weighted sequences as enhancement along the course of the nerve or atrophy of the muscles seen as hyperintensity on T2-weighted sequences. MRI provides detailed information with regard to the extent of intracranial invasion. Extensive intraparenchymal invasion with surrounding oedema usually precludes curative-intent treatment.
- Histopathological information is obtained by means of an endoscopic biopsy. Radiology should precede biopsy as this helps to undertake a directed biopsy, and also the tissue oedema consequent to a biopsy may lead to overestimation of tumour extent if radiology is undertaken after. Open biopsy or sublabial biopsy should be avoided as this may lead to tumour seeding in the biopsy tract.
- Preoperative digital subtraction angiography with or without embolization can be considered for vascular lesions (angiofibroma, hemangiopericytoma and vasoformative tumours). This is also indicated in cases where radiology shows encasement, narrowing or irregularity of the internal carotid artery. Information gathered from DSA and cerebral cross-circulation will guide the management of carotid artery involvement.

7.4.4 Classification of Approaches to Nose and PNS

1. Soft Tissue Approaches (**Surgical Incisions Pertaining to the Nose and PNS**) (Fig. 7.22)
    - Moure's Lateral Rhinotomy Incision
    - Modified Moure's incision.
    - Weber–Ferguson incision.
    - Modified Weber–Ferguson incision.
    - Lynch–Howarth extension to Moure's incision.
    - Weber–Ferguson with subcilliary Dieffenbach Extension.
    - Midfacial degloving.
    - *Classical Moure's and Weber–Ferguson incisions provide excellent exposure but a facial scar. Modifications were introduced to incorporate the concept of nasal and facial aesthetic subunits.
    - *Lip-split in a Weber–Ferguson incision can be avoided in case of small tumours of the lateral wall of the nasal cavity.
2. Bony Approaches:
    - Maxillary swing
    - Le Fort I osteotomy
    - Transpalatal Approach
    - Denker's Approach
    - Facial Translocation

7.4.5 Soft Tissue Approaches

1. Moure's Lateral Rhinotomy incision is useful for **e**xcision of tumours located in the nasal cavity, maxillary sinus, ethmoid sinus

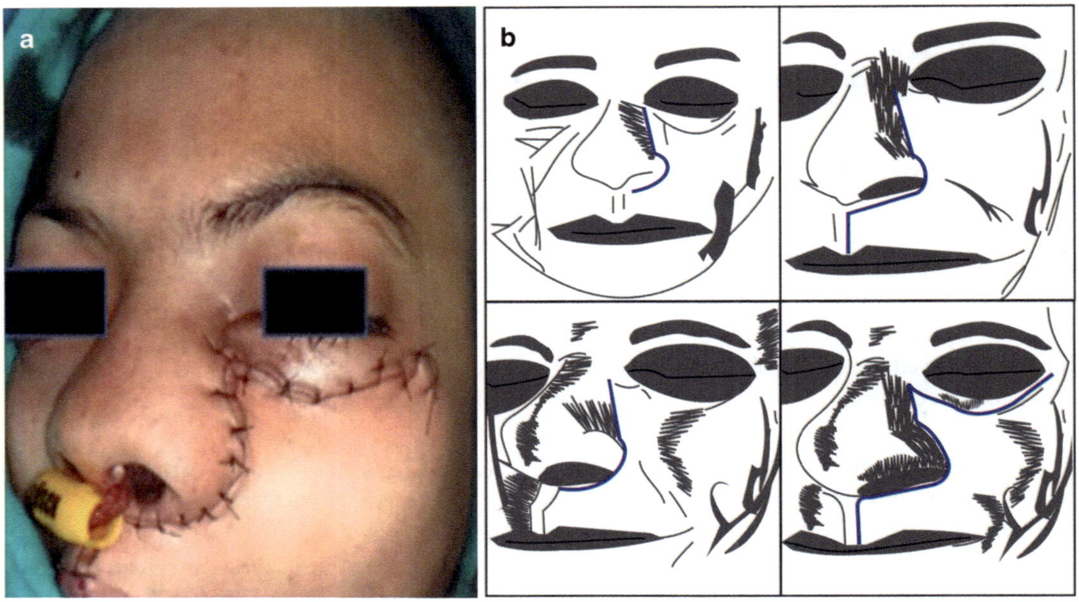

Fig. 7.22 Surgical incisions pertaining to the nose and PNS. (**a**) Weber–Ferguson–Longmire incision, (**b**) lateral rhinotomy, lateral rhinotomy with lip splitting incision, modified lateral rhinotomy, Weber–Ferguson–Longmire with subcilliary Dieffenbach Extension (Courtesy—Dr. Harsha Yadav, JR, ENT, AIIMS, New Delhi, India)

and orbit. Lynch–Howarth extension is helpful to access the frontal sinus. Weber–Ferguson with or without lip-split provides access to the lateral extension of the tumour to the pterygopalatine fossa or the infratemporal fossa. Soft tissue approaches can be part of more extensive procedures like medial maxillectomy, orbital exenteration and craniofacial resection

Limitations

The lateral rhinotomy approach is best suited for midline tumours with minimal paramedian extension. Therefore, exposure to the contralateral side or infratemporal fossa extension form an important limitation of this approach.

Technique

After making the incision, the flap is elevated in a subperiosteal plane. Close to the orbit, the flap is elevated superficial to the orbicularis oculi muscle. This is done to prevent ectropion. Lateral limit of dissection for Moure's Lateral Rhinotomy approach is the infraorbital foramen and the nerve. Modifications can be made to this step to include skin or subcutaneous tissue if involved by the disease process. Entry into the nasal cavity is facilitated by the use of a Kerrison rongeur to remove the bone at the naso maxillary suture line. Soft tissue connecting the nasal mucosa to the vestibule can be divided at the pyriform aperture to complete exposure.

Complications:

- Bleeding and haematoma can occur from the external carotid system, mainly the internal maxillary artery. This complication can be minimized by either preoperative embolization or by identifying and ligating the internal maxillary artery preemptively.
- Suture line dehiscence can occur especially if acute angulations are created while designing the incision. One should always place incisions on a bony framework especially near the medial canthus.

2. **Midfacial Degloving** (Figs. 7.14 and 7.23)
   This approach provides excellent exposure without the need for a facial incision. With regard to the indications, it serves as an alternative to the lateral rhinotomy. Additionally, tumours crossing the midline can also be approached. This technique can only be extended to lesions situated inferior to the infra-

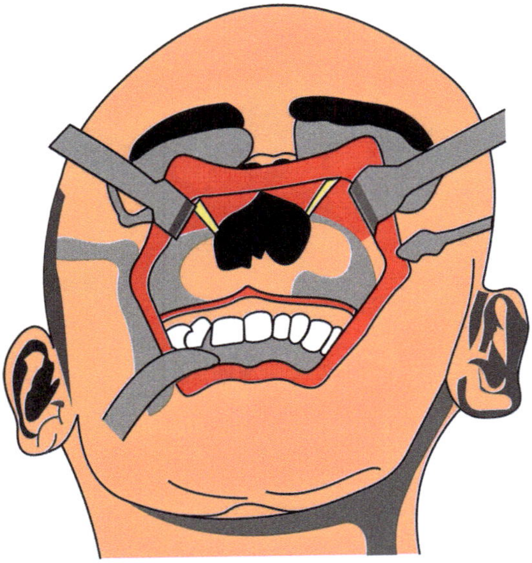

Fig. 7.23 Midfacial degloving (Courtesy—Dr. Harsha Yadav (JR (ENT), AIIMS, New Delhi)

orbital foramen. Moreover, skin and orbital invasion are not suitable for this technique.

Technique

Midfacial degloving entails elevation of the midface in a subperiosteal plane. To accomplish this, a sublabial incision is made from one maxillary tuberosity to the other. To elevate the cartilaginous external nasal framework off the pyriform aperture, a complete transfixion incision and an intercartilaginous incision is made. Once the vestibule is freed from the pyriform aperture, the flap elevation is completed till the infraorbital foramen.

Complications

A complication unique to this approach is vestibular stenosis.

7.4.6 Bony Approaches

1. **Maxillary Swing** (Fig. 7.24, Fig. 6.16 (Chap. 6))
Displacing the maxilla anteriorly as an osteoplastic flap with the overlying skin and soft tissue based on the greater palatine artery exposes the skull base posterior to the posterior wall of the maxilla.

Indications

Tumour extending to the following anatomical sites can be accessed using maxillary swing:

- Nasopharynx
- Infratemporal fossa
- Sphenoid sinus
- Pterygoid plates
- Cavernous sinus, clivus and foramen magnum

Limitations

This approach is ideally suited for midline and paramedian lesions. Therefore, one should not consider maxillary swing in case of tumour extension posterior to the carotid artery or extension to the contralateral skull base.

Technique

The soft tissue approach can either be a Weber–Ferguson or a midfacial degloving. One should be careful in not elevating beyond what is required to place the osteotomies to prevent devascularization of the osteoplastic flap. Preplating is performed at the following sites of osteotomy:

- Frontal process of maxilla extending from the pyriform aperture to the inferior orbital fissure
- Zygomatic process of the maxilla to the inferior orbital fissure

Palatal incision is the modified Owen's incision placed close to the alveolar process. Mucoperiosteal flap is elevated based on the contralateral greater palatine artery. Midline osteotomy is performed over the hard palate. The last osteotomy is placed between the maxillary tuberosity and the attachment of the pterygoid plates using a curved osteotome. After completion of the osteotomies, the entire maxilla with the overlying skin and soft tissue can be swung laterally exposing the pterygomaxillary fissure and the infratemporal fossa.

Complications

- Palatal fistula: This complication can be minimized by avoiding the superimposition of the mucosal and the hard palatal incision. One way to go about this is the modified Owen's incision and placement of a palatal prosthesis to keep the muco-

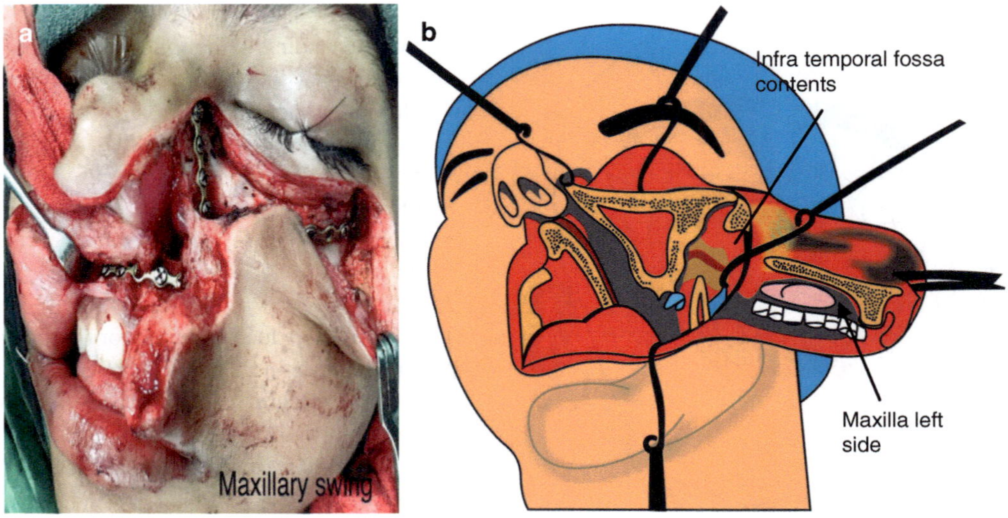

Fig. 7.24 Left maxillary swing. (**a**) Miniplates are fixed at the site of osteotomies (Courtesy—Dr. Kuldeep Thakur, MCh student (Head and Neck cancer), AIIMS, New Delhi, India), (**b**) Maxilla swung on left side which allows exposure of infratemporal fossa contents (Courtesy—Dr. Harsha Yadav (JR (ENT), AIIMS, New Delhi)

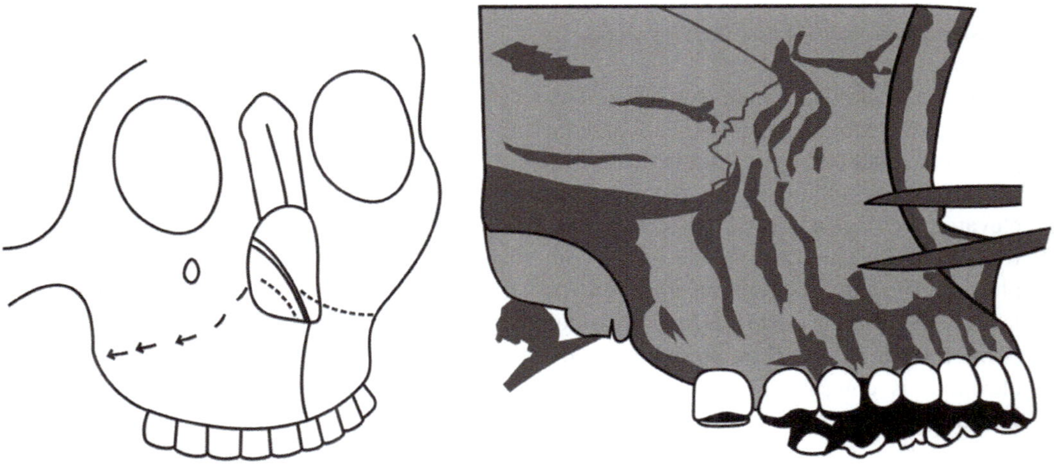

Fig. 7.25 Le Fort I Osteotomy (Courtesy—Dr. Harsha Yadav (JR (ENT), AIIMS, New Delhi)

periosteal flap in close proximity to the bone.
- Dental malocclusion: Preplating prior to osteotomy helps in maintaining postoperative occlusion.

2. **Le Fort I Osteotomy** (Fig. 7.25)
Following a sublabial incision, a transverse facial osteotomy is created along the lines of Le Fort I fracture displacing the palate inferiorly.
Indications
This is a strictly midline approach for selected cases of nasopharyngeal angiofibroma, clival chordoma and nasopharyngeal carcinoma. If combined with medial maxillectomy, it can provide some paramedian extension also.

Limitations
Exposure anterior to the pituitary and posterior to the carotid artery is not possible with this approach.
Complication
The risk of devascularization of the alveolar ridge leading to palatal necrosis is a potential complication.

3. **Transpalatal Approach**
This is another midline approach with the following variants:
   - **Palatal Retraction**—Retracting the soft palate anteriorly provides exposure for adenoidectomy, biopsy and excision of small tumours from the nasopharynx.
   - **Palatal Split**—Vertical division of the soft palate allows exposure from the lower third of clivus to C2. Can be used for basilar artery aneurysm.
   - **Palatal Drop**—Owen's inverted U incision is placed on the palate about 1 cm medial to the alveolar ridge, separating the hard and soft palate for choanal atresia and angiofibroma.
   - **Sardana's Approach**—S-shaped incision with three segments, a peroral palatal drop approach (Owen's incision), an ipsilateral sublabial incision and a connecting U-shaped incision curving behind the maxillary tuberosity and connecting the previous two incisions. Especially indicated for tumours extending from the nasopharynx to the infratemporal fossa via the pterygomaxillary fissure.

Limitation
The transpalatal approach and its modification allow excision of midline tumours from the nasopharynx to C2. Exposure anterior to choana and sphenoid sinus, lateral to Eustachian tube and posterior to foramen magnum and brainstem are not accessible.
Complication
Palatal fistula is a potential complication.

4. **Denker's Approach**
Trans-naso-maxillary approach—Involves a large Caldwell–Luc antrostomy through sublabial route followed by removal of lateral nasal wall and frontal process of maxilla. Essentially a medial maxillectomy is undertaken via the sublabial route.

5. **Preauricular Subtemporal Approach** ((Fig. 6.17, Chap. 6), Figs. 7.13 and 7.26)
Unlike maxillary swing which provides a direct anterior approach to the infratemporal fossa, preauricular subtemporal offers a lateral approach to the same. It is indicated in case of tumour involvement lateral and posterior to cavernous part of ICA. One can approach the entire skull base from the nasopharynx to the petrous apex and clivus with minimal brain retraction.

6. **Facial Translocation Approach**
This approach is based on the concept of "Modular-Disassembly" of facial subunits by Janecka et al. [45]. This means that the face is divided into subunits each with its own neurovascular supply. It is divided into:
(a) Limited facial translocation
(b) Standard facial translocation
(c) Extended facial translocation
An example of standard facial translocation is provided here. To approach the nasopharynx as well as infratemporal fossa and middle cranial fossa, the entire maxilla, lateral orbital wall and zygoma can be swung laterally as one single unit.

7. **Maxillectomy**
Maxillectomy can be classified as either total if all six walls are removed or partial if it involves preservation of any of the six walls. Examples of partial maxillectomy include: medial maxillectomy, subtotal maxillectomy (preserving orbital floor) and palate preserving maxillectomy. Sometimes orbital exenteration is performed along with total maxillectomy. In this case, the appropriate term would be a radical maxillectomy.
(a) Total maxillectomy (Fig. 7.27)
Indicated in malignancy arising from the maxillary sinus, invasive fungal disease causing destruction of the maxillary sinus. The soft tissue approach preceding a maxillectomy can either be a Weber–Ferguson incision or a sublabial incision. It involves excision of the maxillary sinus, one half of the hard palate, floor of

the orbit, palatine bone, lateral wall of nose and the inferior turbinate. The following osteotomies are performed to mobilize the maxilla:

(i) Superomedially—Nasal process of maxilla.
(ii) Superolaterally—Between maxilla and zygomatic arch.
(iii) Inferiorly—Between lateral incisor and canine till midline of palate.

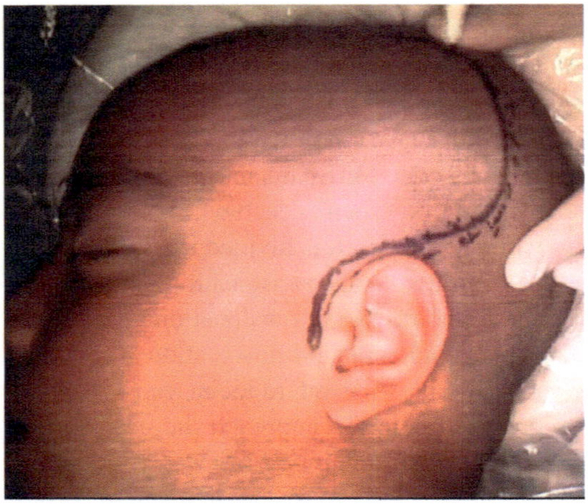

Fig. 7.26 Left side marked Preauricular Subtemporal Approach

(iv) Inferolaterally—The maxilla is separated from the pterygoid plates.
   - May be accompanied by ethmoidectomy or sphenoidotomy

(b) Partial Maxillectomy: Medial maxillectomy: with or without ethmoidectomy. Involves resection of medial wall of maxillary sinus from the floor of orbit to floor of nasal cavity. The most common nasal pathology where this is indicated is inverted papilloma.
Osteotomies:
   (i) Supromedially—From pyriform aperture towards inferior orbital fissure, inferiorly and parallel to fronto-ethmoidal suture line
   (ii) Laterally—Vertically along anterior wall of maxilla towards inferior orbital fissure along floor of orbit
   (iii) Inferiorly—Above the alveolar arch
   (iv) Infero-medially—Parallel to floor of nasal cavity floor inferior to inferior turbinate

8. **Craniofacial Resection** (Fig. 7.28)
Involves resection of intracranial as well as extra-cranial parts of a sinonasal tumour extending to the anterior skull base. Paranasal sinuses are approached either by a lateral rhi-

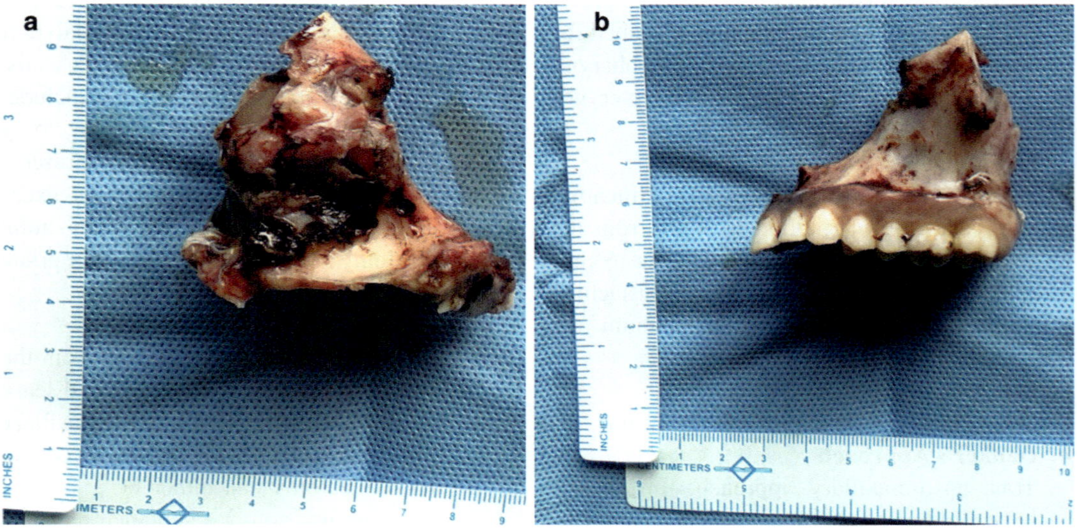

Fig. 7.27 Maxillectomy specimen. Cuts are made the same as maxillary swing but anterior soft tissue flap is separated from underlying bone as showed in Fig. 6.16 of Chap. 6.

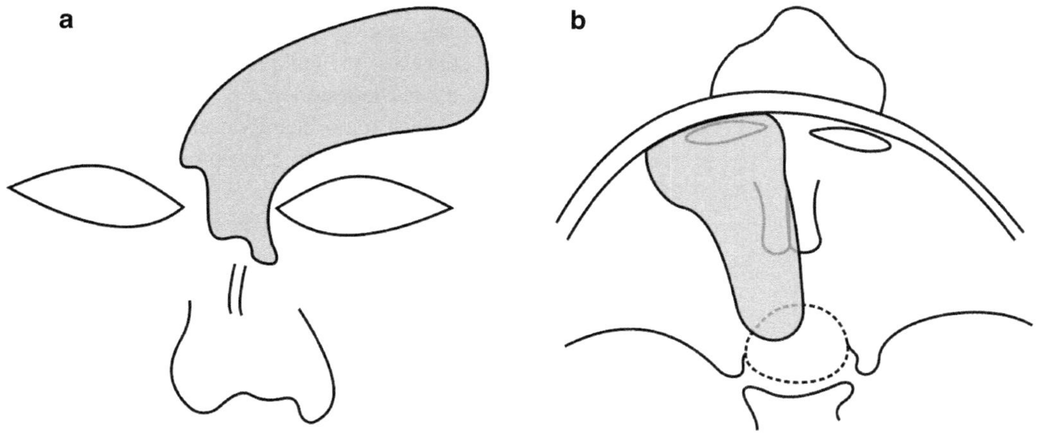

Fig. 7.28 Craniofacial resection

notomy or a midfacial degloving. Tumour may also be approached by a nasal endoscopic approach. For the purpose of anterior skull base exposure, a bifrontal craniotomy is performed using a bicoronal incision. Cheesman and Reddy [46] have classified craniofacial resection into three types:

- Type I: It is an extended medial maxillectomy with limited resection of the anterior part of the skull base without resorting to a craniotomy.
- Type II: Here the intracranial component is approached through a window craniotomy.
- Type III: This is the traditional craniofacial resection where bicoronal incision is made followed by bifrontal craniotomy.

9. **Transbasal Approach**
   The difficulties and potential complications related to a craniofacial resection are mitigated to a certain extent by the transbasal approach. The soft tissue approach can be either a bicoronal incision or a brow incision or a spectacle incision. Instead of performing a bifrontal craniotomy, the frontonasal unit is elevated as a free bone flap. The advantages in doing so are limited brain retraction while approaching lesions, extending posteriorly towards the clivus. If approached through traditional craniofacial resection, the resulting brain retraction produces significant perioperative morbidity.

7.5 Part E: Open Anterior Skull Base Approaches: Indications and Complications

The anterior cranial base has an endocranial surface, which faces the brain, and an exocranial surface, which faces the nasal cavity and sinuses, orbits, pharynx, infratemporal and pterygopalatine fossae, and the parapharyngeal and infrapetrosal spaces. Canals, foramina and fissures through which numerous neural and vascular structures passes connect both the surfaces. On the endocranial side, the border between the anterior and middle cranial bases is the sphenoid ridge joined medially by the chiasmatic sulcus. On the exocranium side, the anterior and middle cranial bases are divided at the level of a transverse line extending through the pterygomaxillary fissures and the pterygopalatine fossae at the upper level and the posterior edge of the alveolar process of the maxilla at a lower level. Medially, this corresponds to the anterior part of the attachment of the vomer to the sphenoid bone.

The pathological conditions affecting the anterior cranial base are highly heterogeneous groups. They can be classified according to the site of tumour origin as described below:

1. **Basal neurovascular structures and meninges**
    - Meningiomas: Olfactory groove, Planum Sphenoidale, Tuberculum sella
    - Schwannomas
    - Pituitary adenoma
    - Craniopharyngiomas
    - Paraganglioma
    - Hemangiopericytoma
2. **Cranial base**
    - Chordoma
    - Chondrosarcoma
    - Osteosarcoma
    - Plasmacytoma
    - Metastasis
3. **Subcranial with upward extension**
    - Sinonasal carcinomas
    - Olfactory neuroblastoma
    - Juvenile angiofibroma
    - Nasopharyngeal carcinoma
    - Adenoid cystic carcinoma
    - Primary sarcomas

Anosmia, frontal lobe dysfunction, increased intracranial pressure, nasal obstruction, CSF rhinorrhoea, epistaxis, visual changes and endocrine dysfunction are the list of symptoms with intracranial connection of mass lesion of the nose and paranasal sinuses.

7.5.1 Diagnostic Work-Up

The clinical examination is focused on complete evaluation with special attention to the head and neck region. Supplemental information regarding the extent of the tumour can be obtained by ophthalmoscopy, indirect laryngoscopy or flexible fibreoptic nasopharyngoscopy. The imaging battery includes contrast-enhancing computerized tomography (CECT) scan, magnetic resonance imaging (MRI) with contrast scan. The diagnostic cerebral angiography (DSA) is indicated in selected cases to obtain information regarding vascularity of the lesion and possible involvement of surrounding major neurovascular bundle. Elective preoperative angiographic embolization is advised in highly vascular cases to reduce intraoperative blood loss. Quantitative assessment of visual acuity and visual field charting is required to document the preoperative status of vision. Endocrine work-up is for tumours extending to the sellar/suprasellar region. The approaches for anterior skull base are tabulated in Fig. 7.29 [47, 48].

Transcranial approaches indicated for lesions restricted to the intracranial compartment. They are divided into anterior and anterolateral approaches depending upon the tumour extensions [49–51]:

1. **Anterior:**
    - Bifrontal craniotomy
    - Unifrontal craniotomy
    - Transbasal craniotomy

    Anterior craniotomy approaches are indicated for midline lesions like meningiomas of olfactory groove, planum sphenoidale, tuberculum sella, esthesioneuroblastomas without lateral extensions. Large midline lesions are approached using bifrontal craniotomy whereas small lesions can be approached using either unifrontal/bifrontal craniotomy. The incision is bicoronal or unilateral frontal curvilinear incision. Following the incision, a bifrontal (large lesions) or unifrontal (small lesions) craniotomy is performed. Dura is opened based on superior sagittal sinus (SSS) and the sinus ligated and cut. Sinus ligation is done in large lesions involving the cribriform plate. Smaller lesions may not require sinus ligation (Fig. 7.30).
2. **Anterolateral**—Five types of anterolateral approaches are described:
    (a) Fronto-orbital
    (b) Fronto-temporal craniotomy
    (c) Pterional craniotomy (Frontosphenotemporal)

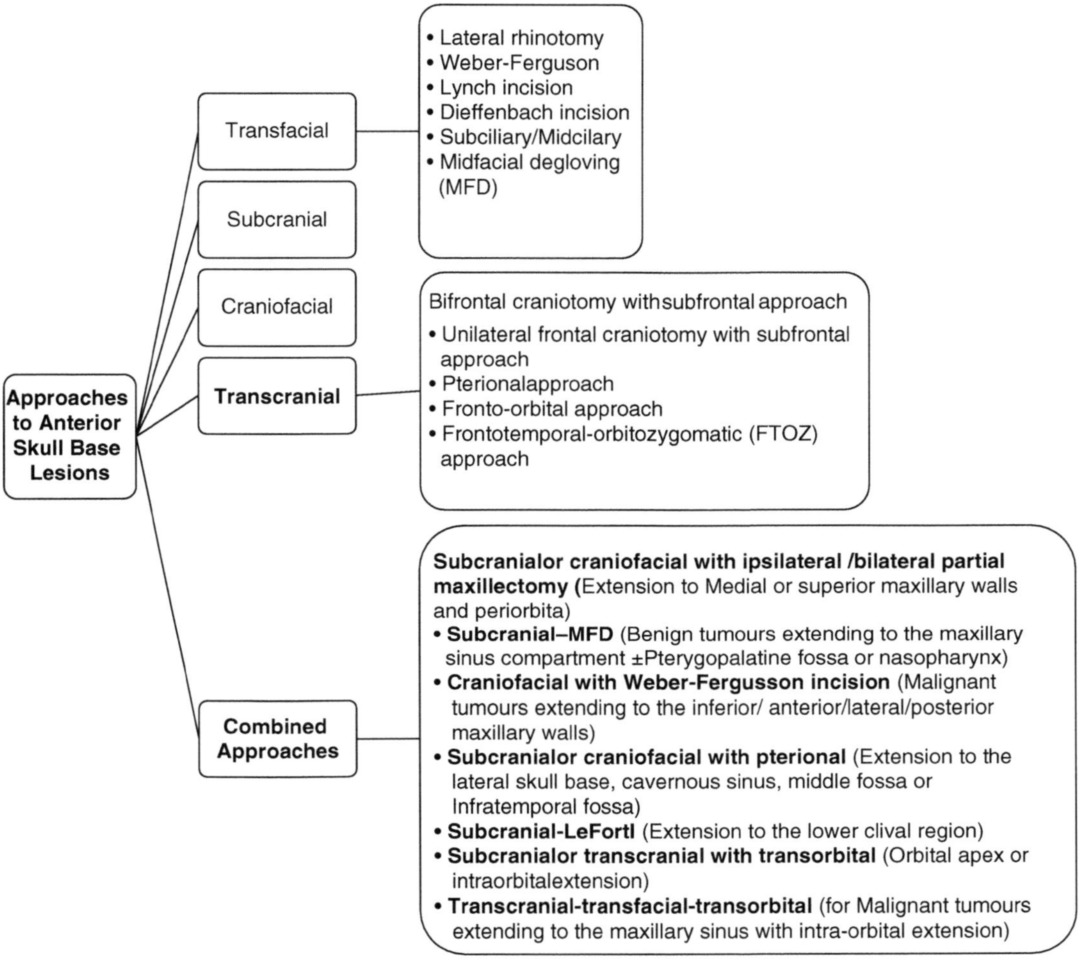

Fig. 7.29 Approaches to anterior skull base

(d) Fronto-temporo-orbito-zygomatic (FTOZ): An extension of pterional craniotomy
(e) Supraorbital keyhole craniotomy

Fronto-orbital is useful for lesions with orbital extensions. Fronto-temporal craniotomy is used for lesions with lateral and middle cranial fossa extensions. Pterional craniotomy is the workhorse of neurosurgery as most of the lesions can be approached with this craniotomy.

It is for midline lesions of anterior as well as middle fossa lesions like meningiomas, sellar/suprasellar and para-sellar lesions. FTOZ is an extension of the pterional craniotomy with additional removal of orbit and zygomatic bones (Fig. 7.31). FTOZ is useful for lesions involving cavernous sinus and suprasellar lesions reaching up to the third ventricle.

Supraorbital keyhole is the mini frontolateral craniotomy (Fig. 7.32). It starts with an eyebrow incision and it is cosmetically acceptable, includes frontal-orbital and part of the zygomatic process. The indications are anterior skull base lesions, sellar suprasellar lesions and aneurysms of anterior circulation.

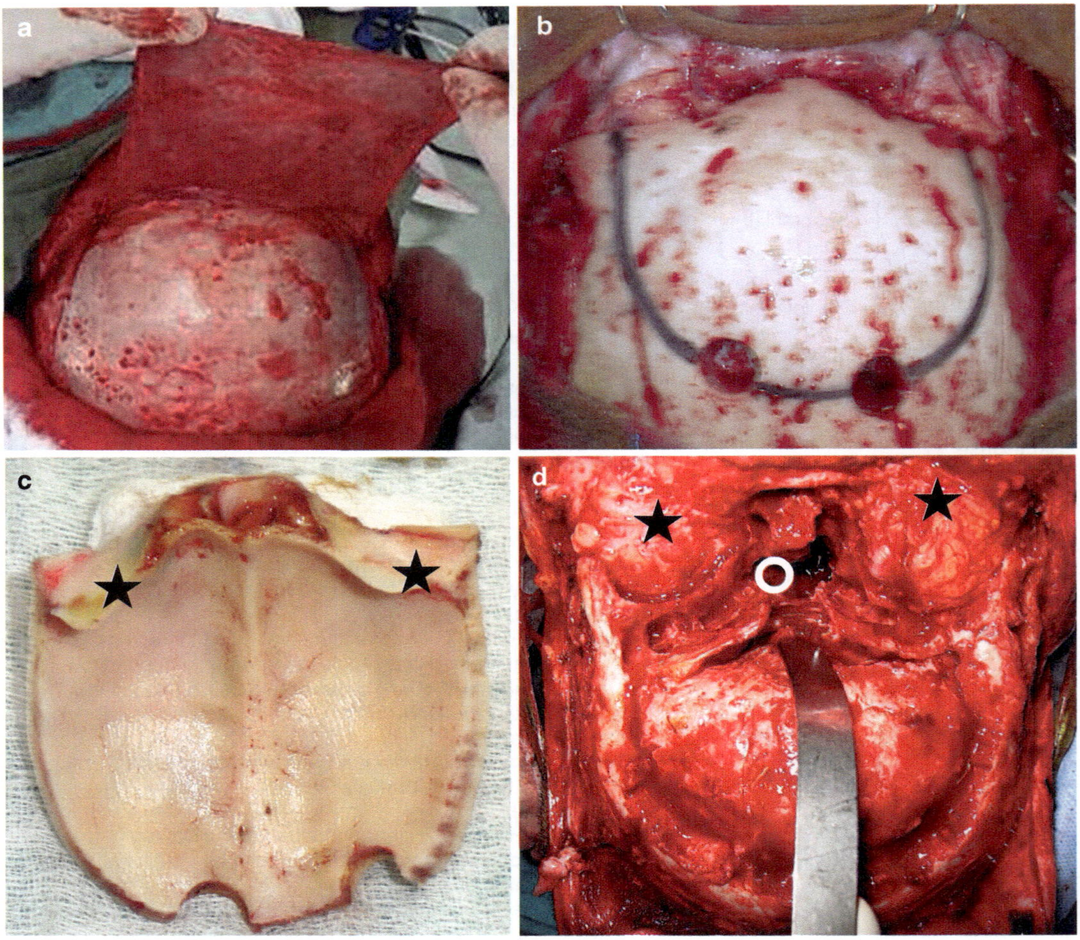

Fig. 7.30 Stepwise demonstration of transbasal approach: (**a**) Bicoronal skin incision and elevation of subgaleal flap separately for skull base carpeting later, (**b**) Burr holes on either side of SSS, (**c**) Single-piece craniotomy with intact bilateral superior orbital walls and nasion, (**d**) Exposed bifrontal dura, spatula in midline over SSS, bilateral orbit (Star), bilateral frontal sinus and ethmoids (Donut) along with nasion

It is contraindicated in well-pneumatized frontal sinus and lesions involving cribriform plate (relative contraindication).

7.5.2 The Subcranial Approach

It is a single-stage procedure used for tumours involving the anterior skull base [52, 53]. It involves coronal incision and osteotomy of the naso-fronto-orbital bone segment. It allows access to the intra- and extra-cranial compartments of the anterior skull base. The advantages are direct exposure of the anterior skull base from anterior to posterior, allows simultaneous intradural and extradural tumour removal from anterior to posterior, does not require facial incisions and minimal frontal lobe manipulation. The disadvantage of this approach is osteonecrosis, especially following radiotherapy (RT).

7.5.3 Reconstruction

The aim is to create watertight dural closure and secure barrier between the nasal cavity and the

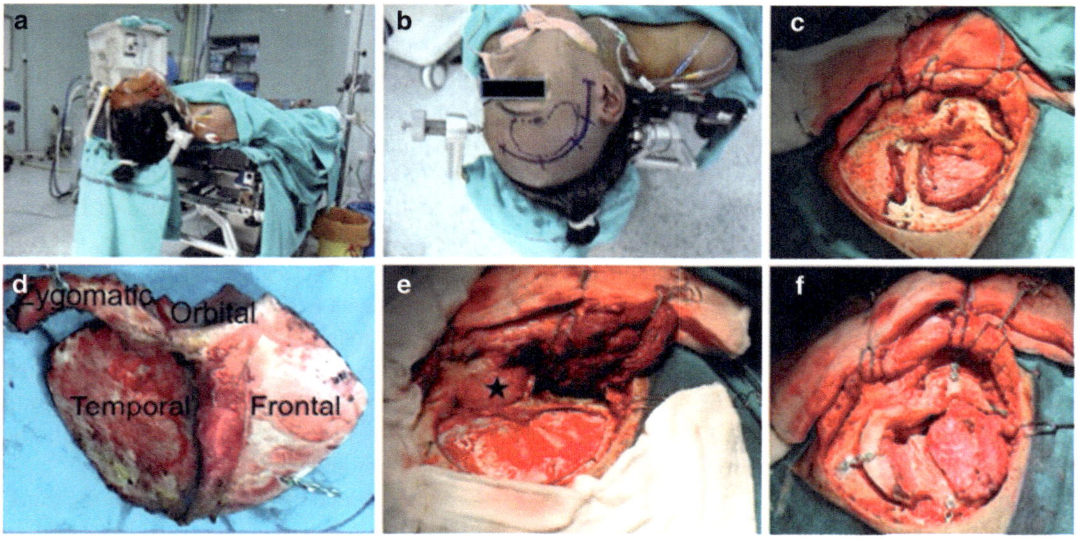

Fig. 7.31 Stepwise demonstration of FTOZ craniotomy. (**a**) Positioning with malar eminence as the highest point, (**b**) Curvilinear hairline incision, (**c**) Fronto-temporo zygomatic bony exposure with cuff of muscle left attached along the superior temporal line, (**d**) Single-piece craniotomy with the temporalis muscle cuff, (**e**) Exposed orbit (Star) and the fronto-temporal dura, (**f**) Bone fixed with miniplates and screws

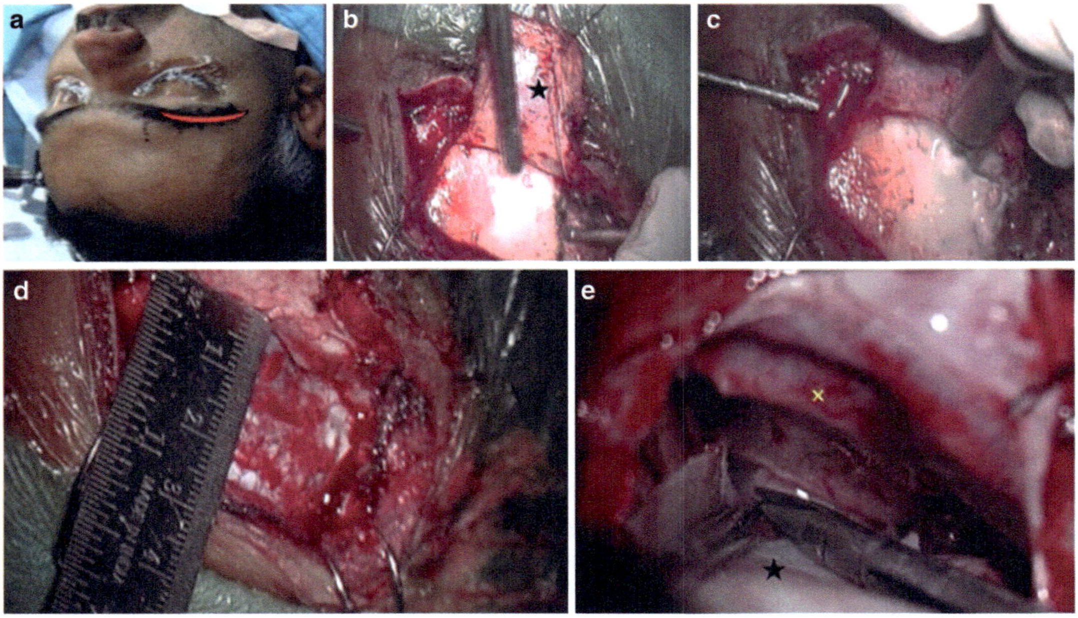

Fig. 7.32 (**a**) Eyebrow incision shown as red, (**b**) elevation of periosteal flap (star) separately, suction pointing on the supraorbital frontal bone, (**c**) fashioning the craniotomy (2.5 × 2.5 cms) using the footplate drill, (**d**) exposed dura, (**E**) after dural opening using suction and scissors and suction as dynamic retractors resting on the basifrontal lobe covered with cotton (star) and basal dura of anterior cranial base (yellow asterisk)

cranial cavity. It can be done by curetting of mucosa of frontal, ethmoidal and sphenoidal sinus and packed with fat. The dura defects should be closed primarily with sutures or with a fascial graft. Basal repair performed by placing a pedicled galea aponeurotica-pericranial-frontalis muscle flap based on the supraorbital–supratrochlear vessels along the anterior cranial fossa base (Fig. 7.28a). Further posterior reinforcement of fascia lata graft with temporalis muscle rotation is required to obliterate the dead space. Bony segments secured in their respective anatomical positions using sutures or miniplates + autologous temporal or frontal bone to reinforce the skull base bony reconstruction. Additionally, musculocutaneous and free flaps based on the pectoralis major and trapezius as well as free omental flaps for basal repair.

7.5.4 Complications

Transcranial surgery has a long list of complications such as cerebral edema, frontal lobe signs (mainly due to retraction)—deficits of speech, memory, cognitive and intellectual function, seizures, CSF leak, subdural or extradural haematoma, pneumocephalus, CNS Infections like meningitis and brain abscess, vascular complications like carotid, anterior/middle cerebral artery injuries, hormonal dysfunction and cranial nerve deficits [54].

7.6 Part F: Lacrimal Sac Anatomy and DCR

The lacrimal gland has a tubule-acinar structure and secretes serous tears in superior fornix. The secretomotor fibres are from the VII nerve through the pterygopalatine ganglion. The lacrimal system starts from the lacrimal puncta and consists of vertical and horizontal canaliculi (upper and lower), a common canaliculus, lacrimal sac and nasolacrimal duct. Lacrimal sac is 12–15 mm long, situated in lacrimal fossa formed by frontal process of maxilla and lacrimal bone, anterior to posterior. The superior border of the lacrimal sac is above the middle turbinate's anterior attachment and is lateral to the agger nasi cells. The anterior attachment of the uncinate process is regarded as the posterior limit of bone removal. The lacrimal sac and nasolacrimal duct slopes down backward and inward. Chronic dacryocystitis is more common in females than males because of the narrow nasolacrimal duct in women. On blinking the orbicularis muscle alternate contraction and relaxation creates negative pressure in the lacrimal sac; this tear pump helps in sucking tears into the sac. Capillary action carries most of the tears (70%) into the lower punctum and canaliculus, while the rest is carried through the upper punctum and canaliculus.

As demonstrated on Scintillography, the transfer of fluid from the canaliculi to the sac is an active process, while the flow of tears into the nasolacrimal duct is the passive process.

7.6.1 Pathology—Dacryocystitis

The most common cause is blockage of the nasolacrimal duct, leading to inflammation of the sac. It occurs due to:

- Structural limitation—congenital incomplete canalization (Hasner's valve), narrow osseous nasolacrimal duct, grossly deviated nasal septum, inferior turbinate hypertrophy, polyp or tumour.
- Infection from surrounding structures—nasal infection, ethmoidal inflammation, conjunctival infection, long-standing nasal packs.
- General infection—Influenza, chickenpox.

7.6.2 Preoperative Tests/ Investigations

1. ROPLAS—"Regurgitation on pressure over the lacrimal sac" area—the positive test indicates the blockage of the nasolacrimal duct (Fig. 7.33).
2. Jones dye test—Fluorescein dye is instilled in the eye. The presence of dye in the nasal cavity in 5 minutes is considered as normal

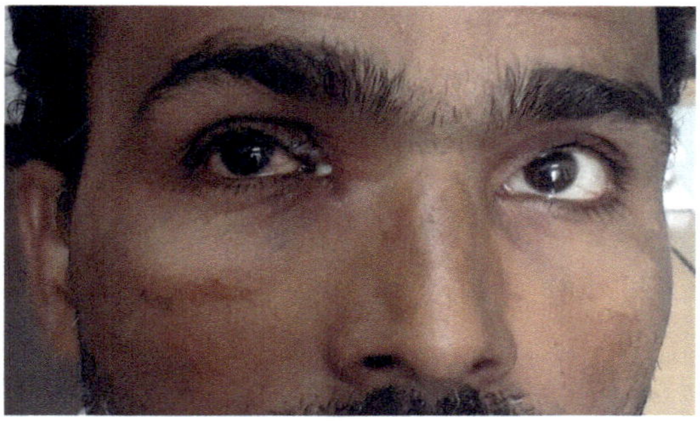

Fig. 7.33 Positive ROPLAS test on right side

functioining lacrimal pump system in the nasal cavity is considered as normal functioning lacrimal pump system [55].

(a) Positive primary Jones test—no obstruction.
(b) If dye is not detected in the nose, syringing is done and then fluorescein detected, is labelled positive secondary Jones test, which signifies functional obstruction in the nasolacrimal duct.
(c) If no fluorescein is detected in the nose even after syringing, it is labelled negative secondary Jones test, which signifies stenosis of puncta or canalicular system.

3. Probing—4% lignocaine drops are instilled in the eye. The punctum is dilated with Nettleship's punctual dilator and Bowman's probe. Soft block indicates a canalicular or common canalicular block whereas hard stop indicates that the probe is in the lacrimal sac and is touching the bone.
4. Syringing—the punctum is cannulated with a soft cannula and saline is injected. No regurgitation is considered as normal functioning drainage system. Canalicular block is considered when the fluid is regurgitated from the same punctum. Regurgitation through the opposite punctum is either due to common canalicular blockage or NLD blockage. In NLD blockage fluid is mixed with mucoid or purulent secretion. In common canalicular blockage, fluid is clear.
5. Radiology—T2-weighted images of MRI is helpful in detecting obstruction site exactly within nasolacrimal duct and thus planning for correct endoscopic procedure [56]. The sensitivity of CT and MRI can be improved by injection of contrast (Dacrocystrography). In dacroscintigraphy, technetium 99 is placed on the ocular surface. The canaliculi and sac are visible within 10–15 s. The dye appears in the nasal cavity after 10–30 min intervals. Dacroscintigraphy is not useful because of poor resolution and poor anatomical detailing.

The indications for dacryocystorhinostomy (DCR) is obstruction of the nasolacrimal duct not responding to conservative treatment (like hot compresses, massage, probing and intubation) in children [57], dacryocystitis with NLD obstruction, mucocele with NLD obstruction, congenital fistula and posttraumatic NLD obstruction with epiphora. DCR can be done by endoscopic or open approach. ENT surgeons are more familiar with endoscopic DCR. The advantages of Endoscopic DCR are scarless surgery, preservation of orbicularis oculi pump mechanism. It also allows simultaneous correction of intranasal pathology and results of endoscopic DCR are comparable with external DCR [58]. The prerequisite for success endo DCR is correct identification of lacrimal sac and prevention of restenosis. Pre-existing anatomical variations such as concha bullosa, septal deviation, agger nasi cells and lateralization of uncinate process can increase the risk of failure as they require more excision of mucosa for exposure. Bony window can be mal-positioned or incomplete due to anatomical variations [59].

7.6.2.1 Surgical Technique for Endoscopic DCR

The key landmark is the ridge formed by the frontal process of maxilla at the anterior attachment of the middle turbinate, anterior to uncinate process, on the lateral nasal wall [60]. The sac is located at and anterior to the axilla of middle turbinate or maxillary line in around 95% of cases (Fig. 7.34).

The flap elevation is started with two separate incisions 8 mm above and below the axilla of middle turbinate or it can be started with a vertical curved anterior incision given 1 to 1.5 cm to the base of uncinate process vertically down till the anterior end of the middle turbinate than two horizontal incision (Fig. 7.35).

The overlying mucosa is separated using a blunt dissector and this strip of mucosa is removed using a pair of through-cut forceps. The Kerrison's bone punch is hooked against the posterior part of the anterior lacrimal crest (Fig. 7.36) and bone removed working from posterior thin bone to anterior thick bone. A wide bony window is made of the size of approximately 12–15 mm (Fig. 7.36). Bone can also be removed by drilling, chisel and hammer or laser. The use of powered instruments has not shown an added advantage on surgical success with cold instruments [61, 62]. Periosteum and sac wall incised vertically using sickle knife or 12 number blade, pus drained, suction cleaning done (Fig. 7.36). The whole of the medial wall of the sac can be removed or anterior-based flap can be created to minimize mucosal trauma. Nasal mucosal flap can be joined with posterior wall of

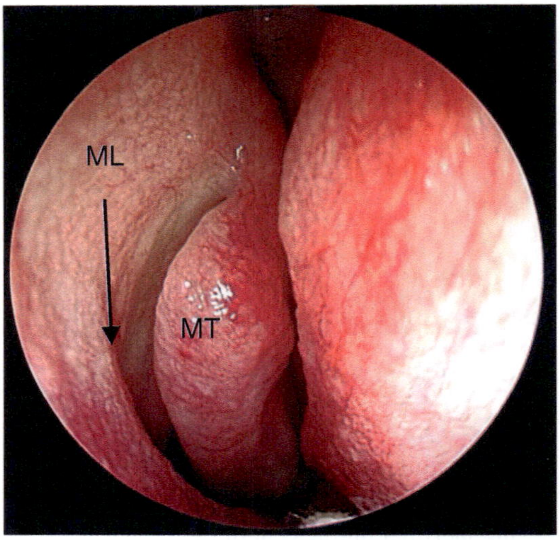

Fig. 7.34 Relationship of sac with maxillary line (ML) and anterior end of the middle turbinate (MT) (Courtesy—Dr. Hitesh Verma, Associate Professor, AIIMS, New Delhi, India)

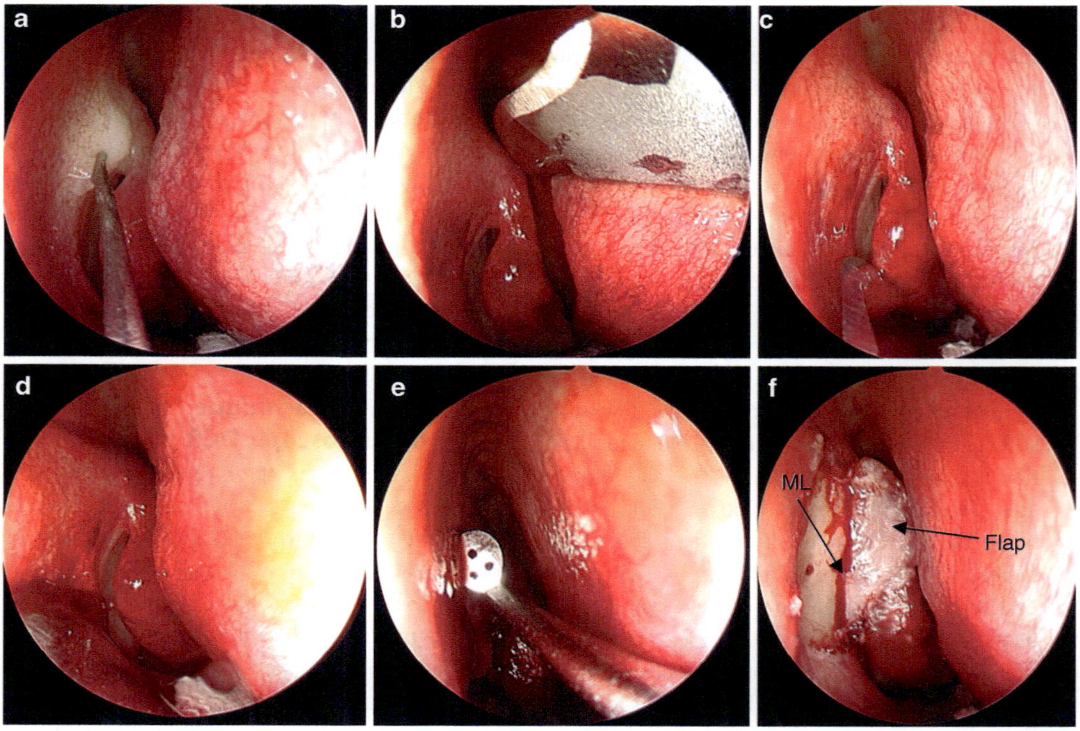

Fig. 7.35 The surgical steps of flap elevation. (**a**) local infiltration, (**b**) site of upper incision, (**c**) site of lower incision, (**d**) two horizontal incision lines, (**e**) joining of horizontal incision, (**f**) posterior-based flap. Maxillary line (ML) (Courtesy—Dr. Hitesh Verma, Associate Professor, AIIMS, New Delhi, India)

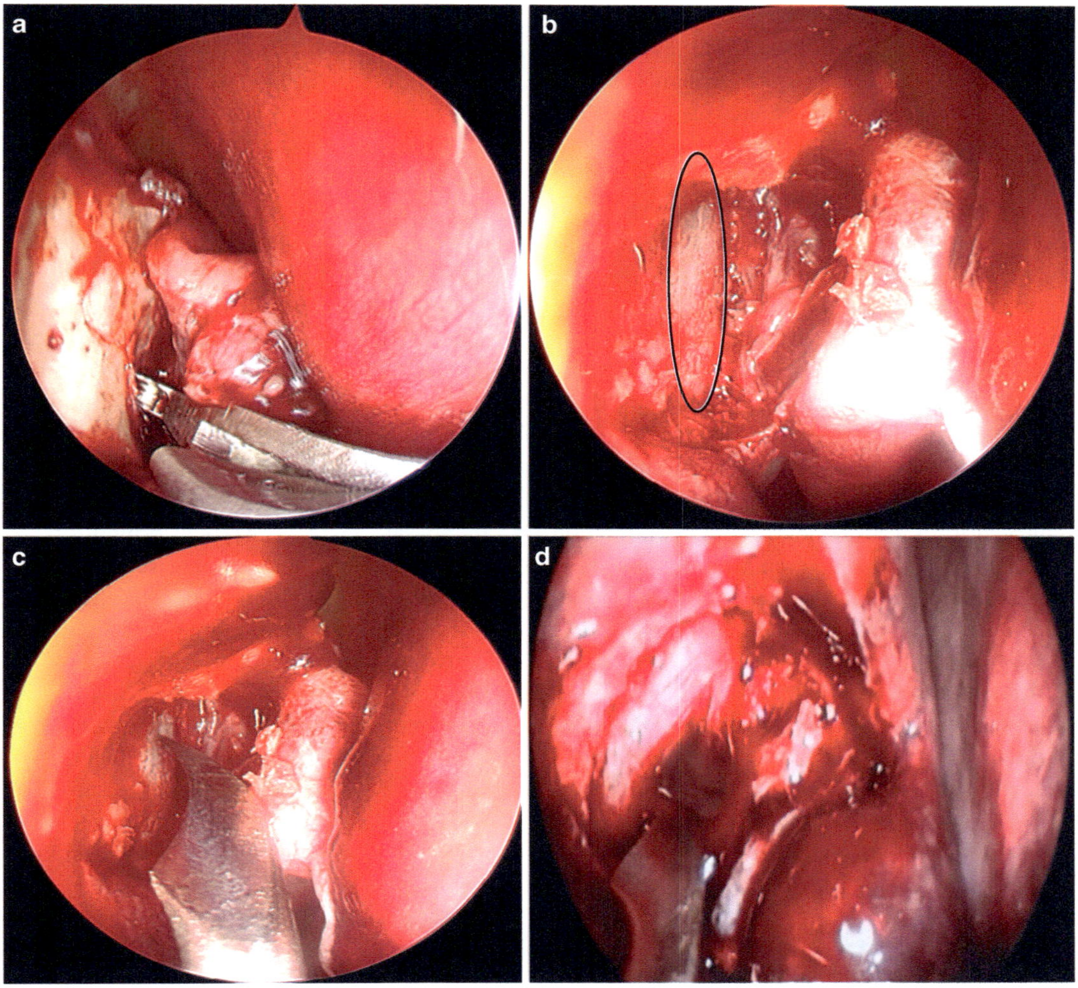

Fig. 7.36 (**a**) Kerrison's punch is engaged for bone removal, (**b**) lacrimal sac exposure, (**c**) sharp instrument is projected over lacrimal sac, (**d**) straw colour fluid coming out after puncturing of sac (Courtesy—Dr. Hitesh Verma, Associate Professor, AIIMS, New Delhi, India)

sac window and anterior-based sac flap can be joined with nasal mucosa to reduce the chances of granulation formation, scarring and risk of restenosis. Nasal mucosal flap can be double posterior based or bipedicled to cover a major area of exposed bone to reduce granulation formation [63, 64]. Tissue glue can be applied at mucosal junction to prevent retraction and separation of approximated flaps.

Grommet, t sheet, hydrogel, otogenic T tube, proline and silicone tube are the materials mentioned in literature for stenting. Silicone tube is used by most of the surgeon. Silicon tube stenting in selected cases [65], covering of exposed bone with nasal or lacrimal sac mucosal [66] application of Mitomycin C [67] are the techniques to prevent restenosis. Silicon tube with metal probes at both ends is placed through upper and lower punctum and pulled out of the sac into the nose and knot tied to secure it. The tube is removed after 6 weeks by cutting the loop at the medial canthus. Stenting is indicated when the surgeon is suspecting poor outcomes of surgery like excessive mucosal trauma, significant flap damage, poor anatomy of the sac, revision cases, etc. [68] The meta-analysis showed that silicone stenting is not affecting the surgical success and postoperative complications rate [69].

Points to Remember Poor localization of sac, incomplete osteotomy, inadequate opening on medial wall of sac, significant iatrogenic mucosal injury and circumferential cicatrization are the most common causes of failure [70]. The surgical success can be improved by proper tissue handling, good flaps approximation with good cavity care (Fig. 7.37).

Follow-Up Any nasal pack placed should be removed after 24–48 h. Medical management is indicated for a week. Look for any regurgitation from punctum, crusting, granulations, stenosis at rhinostomy site or displacement of tube at weekly intervals for a month.

Surgical Technique of External DCR

A curvilinear skin incision is made at the level of the medial canthus. Orbicularis oculi muscle is separated and the anterior lacrimal crest is identified. Periosteum is cut and lacrimal sac is lifted from lacrimal fossa. Bony window is created with burr or chisel hammer and widened with Kerrison punch. The punctum is cannulated and the sac is tented medially. Sharp scissors are used to create openings and flaps in the medial sac wall and nasal mucosa. Corresponding cut ends of sac wall and mucosa sutured together to create a new pathway for drainage and wound closed in layers. The advantages are direct visualization, the creation of an adequate bony window and suturing of mucosa. The disadvantages are scar and disruption of the pump mechanism.

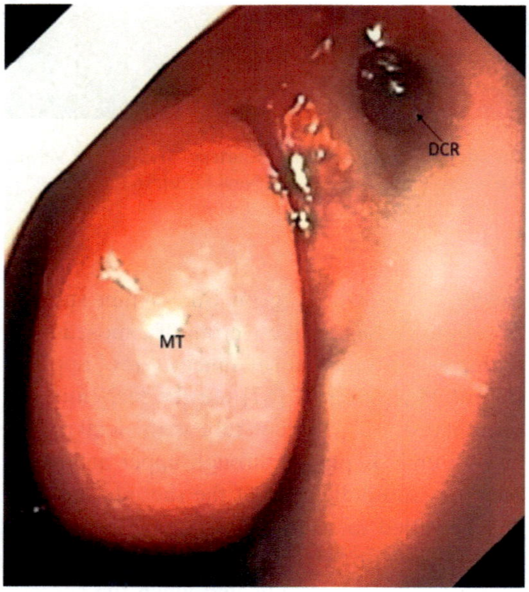

Fig. 7.37 Wide-open nasolacrimal sac (courtesy—Dr. Karan Agarwal, skull base fellow, AIIMS, New Delhi, India)

Recent Development

- Intranasal laser Dacryocystorhinostomy—KTP-YAG laser helps in precise coagulation and vaporization of soft tissue, and thus blood loss and scarring are minimal.
- Transcanalicular laser-assisted Dacryocystorhinostomy—The passing of a laser probe through the upper punctum and canaliculi down the nasolacrimal duct and firing the laser to open up the sac wall. Methylcellulose viscous is used along to dilate the sac and lubricate the passage of laser fibre. The advantages are fast technique, laser passed towards the nose, so no risk of injury to the eye. The disadvantages are that the membrane formation may occur due to charring and cause blockage, sump syndrome may not be addressed, there is a risk of canalicular injury and success rate is low due to small-sized window placed at a higher level [71].
- Balloon Dacryoplasty—It is indicated in children with failed probing or silicone intubation. In this, the nasolacrimal duct is dilated in its distal portion using a balloon catheter inserted through the upper punctum. The balloon is inflated by injecting water and is retained for one and a half minutes. After deflation, it is withdrawn and again inflated for half a minute at the junction of the lacrimal sac and nasolacrimal duct.
- Ultrasonic endoscopic dacryocystorhinostomy is a new emerging technique. It utilizes specific ultrasonic vibrations with irrigation to

emulsify and cut bone tissue with precision and is less damaging to the surrounding soft tissue [72].
- Microcanalicular endoscopes allow high-resolution dacryoendoscopy, giving a direct, clear view of luminal obstruction, better understanding and decision-making for probing or DCR. But, due to the small diametre of dacryoendoscope, image quality is limited [73].

Limitations of EndoDCR

In patients with epiphora due to lacrimal system dysfunction above the sac, like canalicular stenosis, Dacryocystorhinostomy is not useful. These patients need Conjunctivodacryocystorhinostomy with insertion of Lester Jones glass bypass tube [74]. Elderly patients and patients with proximal obstruction of lacrimal system have a poor prognosis with endoscopic DCR [75].

7.7 Part G: Sinus Mucocele

Mucoceles are epithelial lined, mucus containing sacs filling any of the paranasal sinuses [76]. They are caused by obstruction of the sinus ostium or obstruction of a mucous secreting gland in the lining of the sinus. In paranasal sinuses, they most commonly involve frontal and ethmoid sinuses. They result from obstruction to the drainage pathway of the sinus. The common presenting symptoms are nasal obstruction, swelling, visual abnormalities, headache and neurological effects. Significant morbidity is usually secondary to ophthalmological or neurological involvement. Computed tomography is the radiological investigation of choice. It shows expansile, homogenous mass, with remodelling of the bony walls of the involved paranasal sinus. On magnetic resonance scan, mucocele is iso-/hypointense on T1 and hyperintense on T2-weighted images. Surgical exploration is the standard treatment with the endoscopic approach being preferred nowadays.

7.7.1 Aetiology

Almost one-third of the cases do not have any predisposing factor. In others, the cause of obstruction may be inflammation, polyps, trauma, surgery or mass lesion [77]. Cystic degeneration of glandular tissue has been postulated to account for mucocele, but a classical double wall is invariably not found in these lesions [78]. Various bone-resorbing factors like PGE2, leukotrienes, IL-1, TNFa have been found in mucoceles [79, 80]. So, it can be assumed that in mucocele, obstruction is followed by some other event to initiate the production of these bones resorbing cytokines resulting in bony expansion. The extended endoscopic procedures and obliteration of sinuses have more chances of mucocele formation [81].

7.7.2 Pathology

Histopathologically, mucoceles have pseudostratified ciliated columnar epithelium. Chronic cases may show squamous metaplasia. Additional findings may include cholesterol granuloma, haemorrhage, fibrosis and granulation tissue.

7.7.3 Clinical Features

Mucoceles are most common in the third or fourth decade of life with a slight male predilection. Fronto-ethmoidal region is involved in almost 90% of cases followed by ethmoids, sphenoid and maxillary sinus. Symptoms vary depending on the location of the mucocele and may be classified as rhinological, neurologic or most frequently ophthalmologic. Fronto-ethmoidal mucoceles present with proptosis, hypophthalmos, diplopia and periorbital swelling. Sphenoid mucocele may present with occipitoparietal headache, visual disturbance, diplopia, ptosis. 3, 4, 6 cranial nerves may be involved. Pituitary may be involved rarely. Nasal endoscopic examination may reveal a mass in the nasal cavity or a bulge in the region of the sinus drainage area.

7.7.4 Imaging

Computed tomography (CT) is the most relevant radiological investigation. It provides basic anatomical detail of the mucocele, its relation with the surrounding structures and helps in surgical planning. CT shows an expansile, homogenous mass with remodelling of the surrounding bone (Figs. 7.38 and 7.39). The appearance of mucocele on magnetic resonance imaging (MRI) depends on the contents. In general, mucoceles are hypo/iso-intense on T1W1 and hyperintense on T2W2 (Fig. 7.40). MRI is superior to CT for the evaluation of intracranial and orbital extension [82].

Benign and malignant neoplasms of sinonasal origin, fungal sinusitis, odontogenic cyst (maxilla) and cholesterol granuloma are the differentials for mucocele.

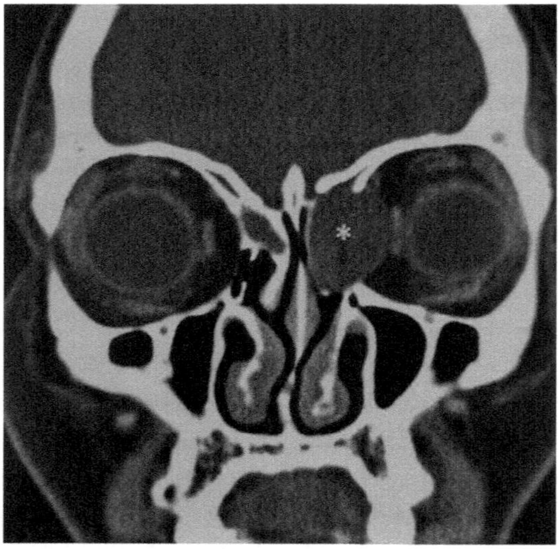

Fig. 7.38 Coronal CT scan showing mucocele left fronto-ethmoid region with erosion of lamina papyracea

7.7.5 Treatment

Early surgical intervention is the treatment of choice. An endonasal endoscopic approach is almost always feasible and involves wide marsupialization (Figs. 7.41, 7.42, and 7.43). This has the advantage of no scar, no interference with periorbital structures and excellent visualization. It also provides better restoration of normal sinus function. Virtually all ethmoidal, sphenoidal, frontal and maxillary mucoceles can be managed endoscopically [83–88]. However, the bone remodelling after endoscopic surgery may take a long time to recover. So, it is essential to counsel the patient that cosmetic results may not be achieved immediately.

External approaches may include a Lynch–Howarth, Caldwell–Luc or osteoplastic flap approach. These may be relevant in cases with a history of previous surgery with significant scarring or in presence of significant pathology in the frontal region [89]. Both external and endonasal approaches may be combined when endonasal approach is not possible.

7.7.6 Results

The overall recurrence rates are reported to be less than 10%. Periodic nasal endoscopy in the office is recommended to assess the patency of ostium. Visual outcomes are usually good after early surgical intervention (Fig. 7.44).

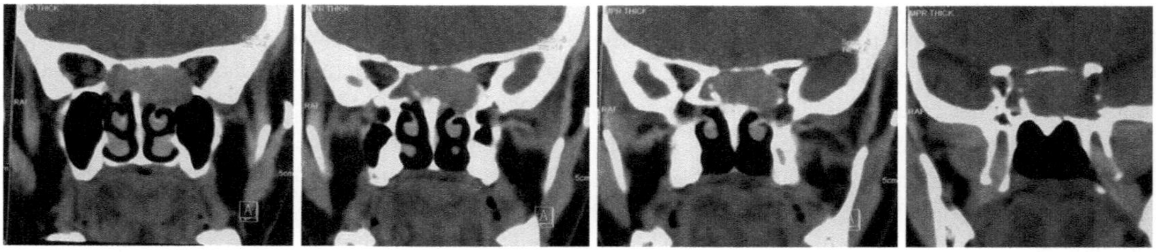

Fig. 7.39 Coronal CT scan showing mucocele involving posterior ethmoid and sphenoid sinus with erosion of sphenoid walls

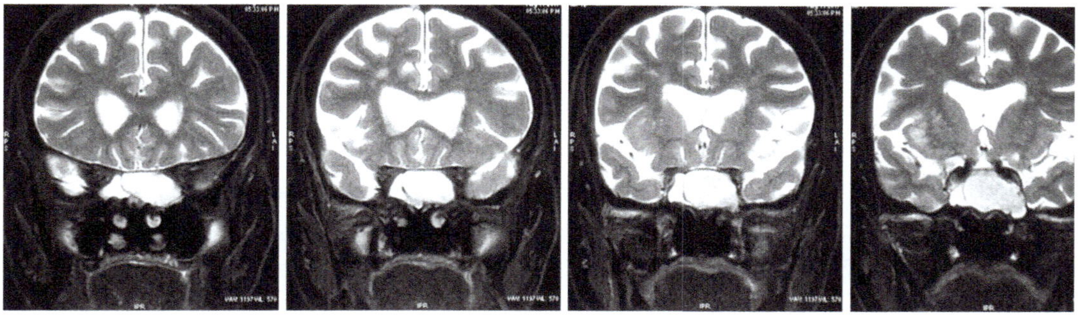

Fig. 7.40 T2 MRI demonstrating hyperintense signal in sphenoid sinus consistent with mucocele

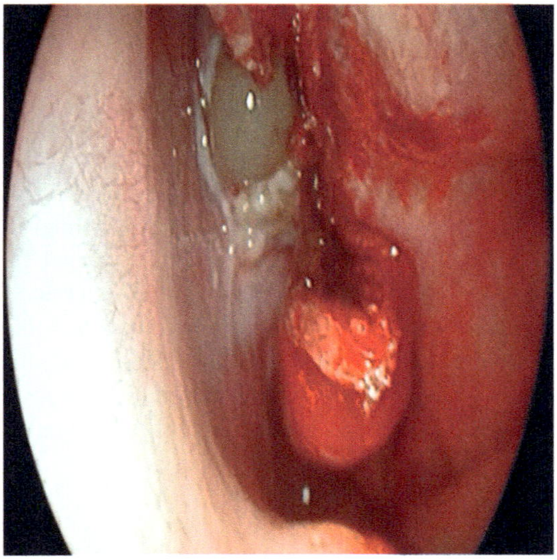

Fig. 7.41 Endoscopic view of sphenoid mucocele after sphenoidotomy showing mucoid contents

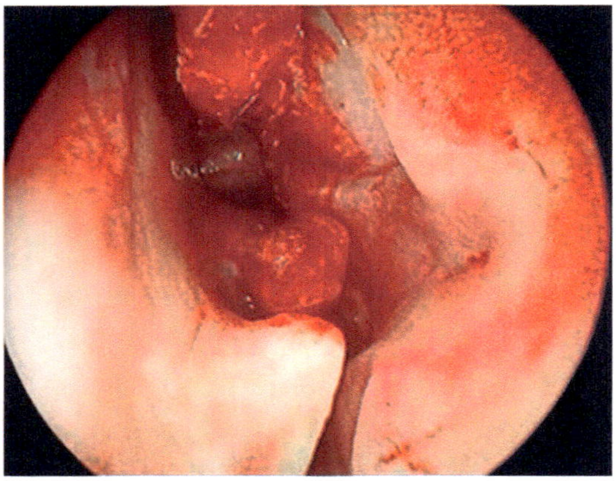

Fig. 7.42 Endoscopic view after evacuation of sphenoid and wide sphenoidotomy

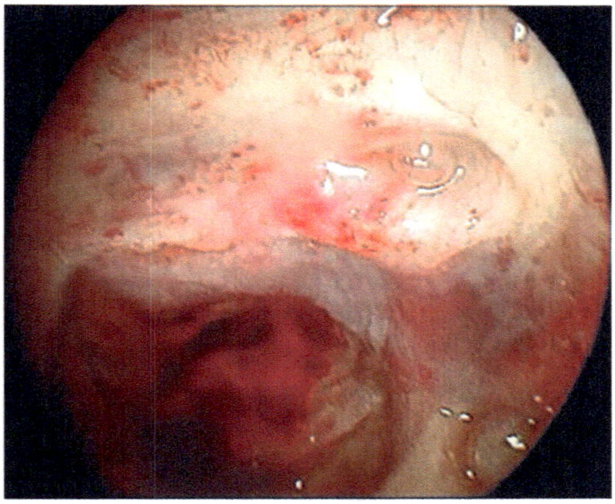

Fig. 7.43 View of sphenoid sinus showing expansion of its walls and erosion of skull base

7.7.7 Complications

Haemorrhage, cerebrospinal fluid rhinorrhea and injury to the orbit can occur at surgical exploration. These complications have become uncommon with the advent of endoscopic techniques.

7.8 Part H: Choanal Atresia and Management

Nasal choana are the paired opening in the posterior part of the nasal cavity which communicate anterior nasal cavity with the nasopharynx. Each choana is bounded superiorly by the inferior surface of the sphenoid body, inferiorly by the horizontal portion of the palatine bone, laterally by medial pterygoid lamina and medially by vomer.

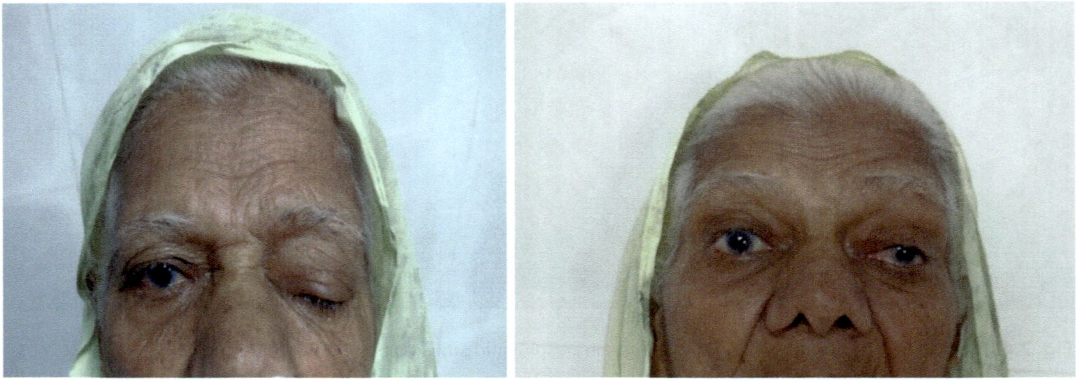

Fig. 7.44 Patient with left sphenoid mucocele exhibiting proptosis and ptosis (preoperative image). Ocular symptoms in the immediate postoperative period

The absence of a normal opening is called atresia. Choanal atresia was first described by Roederer in 1755. Choanal opening(s) may be occluded by soft tissue (membranous), bone or both. Recent data based on CT shows mixed bony and membranous atresia to be the most common (70%) and pure bony to be forming the almost 30% percentage of atresia. Pure membranous atresia is rarest in radiology [90]. The incidence of choanal atresia is 1:5000 to 1:8000 live births [91, 92]. It is more commonly encountered in females (2:1). Choanal atresia may be unilateral or bilateral; unilateral presentation being more common than bilateral (65–70%). In unilateral cases, right choana involvement is more common than left. The closure part of the nasal cavity is roomy. Choanal atresia is not interfering with the development of the face. Three-fourth cases of bilateral atresia are associated with other congenital anomalies like CHARGE syndrome, Crouzon's syndrome, Treacher Collins syndrome, Polydactyly, craniosynostosis, cleft lip/palate and nasal/palatal deformities.

7.8.1 Aetiology

Various theories are proposed for the origin of choanal atresia. Some of the popular ones are the persistence of the buccopharyngeal membrane, persistence of the nasobuccal membrane of Hochstetter, medial outgrowth of vertical and horizontal processes of the palatine bone, incomplete resorption of the nasopharyngeal mesoderm. The most popular theory is the local misdirection of neural crest cell migration. The reason behind it, Treacher Collins syndrome which is caused by abnormal neural crest migration has a high rate of choanal atresia. Certain external factors like Retinoic acid deficiency [93] and the use of antithyroid drugs (methimazole, carbimazole, propylthiouracil) during pregnancy are linked to choanal atresia [94].

7.8.2 Patho-physiology

Neonates are obligate nose breathers as the larynx is placed at a higher level which descends at 4–6 weeks of life and mouth breathing is established. In bilateral choanal atresia, neonate experiences episodes of asphyxia and severe distress with or without cyanosis in quiet respiration when the mouth is closed, especially during sleep or feeding. Cyanosis is relieved by crying or gasping when the child opens the mouth widely, releasing air obstruction.

7.8.3 Clinical Presentation

Clinical presentation in choanal atresia cases depends on the laterality, character and severity of atresia. Bilateral choanal atresia is a life-threatening condition. It may cause acute respiratory distress and cyanosis in a newborn. Distress and cyanosis are relieved with crying and there happens return of cyanosis with rest (paradoxical cyanosis). Difficulty in feeding is obvious in these newborns. Unilateral choanal atresia presents later in life. Presenting complaints in unilateral cases are unilateral chronic nasal discharge with nasal obstruction and the child shows thick nasal discharge on examination. A child with unilateral choanal atresia presents rarely with respiratory distress.

Differential diagnosis includes pyriform aperture stenosis, nasolacrimal duct cyst (dacryocystocele), turbinate hypertrophy, septal dislocation and deviation, antrochoanal polyp, nasal neoplasm, meningocele, encephalocele.

7.8.4 Diagnosis and Evaluation

1. *Clinical Tests/Examination*—A confirmatory diagnosis of choanal atresia is made only by transnasal endoscopic examination of the posterior choana. Endoscopic examination with 2.7 mm rigid or flexible nasal endoscope after nasal decongestion and mucous suctioning allows direct visualization of choanal atresia (Fig. 7.45). Decreased fogging on placing a metallic tongue depressor just below the nostril may be used as the initial bedside test. No sound of breathing when the bell of the stethoscope over nostril raised the possibility of atresia. A more frequently used screening test is an attempt to pass an infant feeding tube or suction catheter (6–8 F) through the nostril into the child's oral cavity. Failure to pass the catheter into the oral cavity calls for transnasal endoscopic examination. Cotton wisp test and methylene blue dye test are the two other infrequently used screening tests.

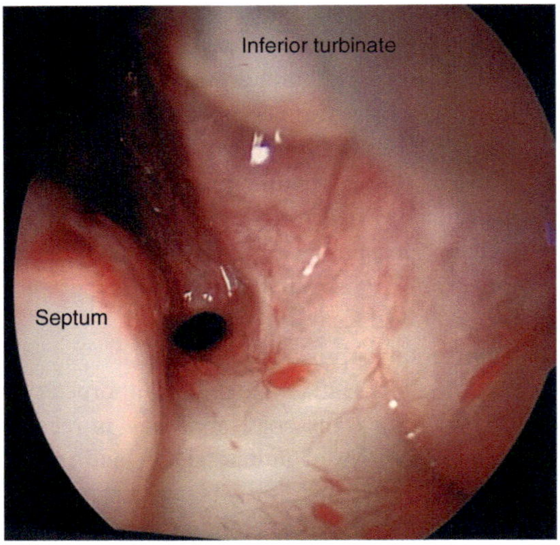

Fig. 7.45 Left partial choanal atresia with roomy nasal cavity (Courtesy—Dr. Hitesh Verma, Associate Professor, AIIMS, New Delhi, India)

Radiological Tests—Computed Tomography (non-contrast) is the radiological investigation of choice. One-mm thick coronal and axial cuts of nose and paranasal sinuses in both bony and soft tissue windows are requested (Fig. 7.46). The indications of CT scan are to characterize the type of atresia (bony/membranous/mixed), delineate thickness of atresia, estimate mean choanal air space and to differentiate from other causes of nasal obstruction.

7.8.5 Treatment

The treatment of choice is surgery. The timing or urgency of surgery depends upon laterality. In cases of bilateral choanal atresia, an immediate preliminary airway management is warranted followed by elective surgery. In unilateral atresia

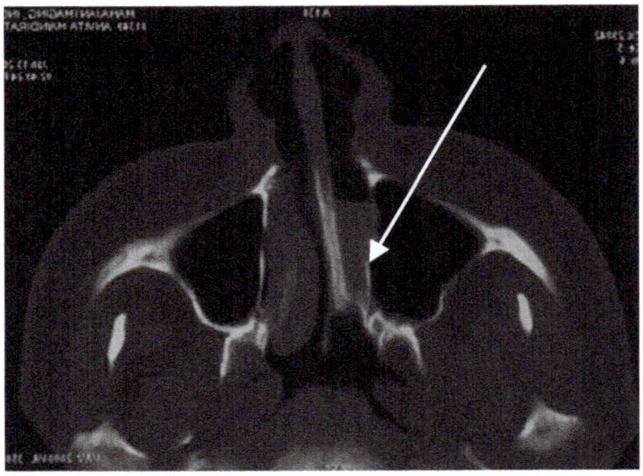

Fig. 7.46 Axial CT scan, unilateral left mixed choanal atresia

cases, definitive surgery can be postponed to later school-going age group.

7.8.6 Preliminary Airway Management

Bilateral choanal atresia is an emergency requiring immediate airway intervention. Inserting an oral airway is the best initial airway management in such cases. *McGovern nipple* is also a viable option. It is an intraoral nipple with a large opening made by cutting its end off and is secured in the mouth with ties around the infant's head. If, in spite of this, the patient fails to maintain an adequate airway, endotracheal intubation is the other alternative. If the patient is having associated comorbidities such as cardiopulmonary instability and multilevel airway obstruction tracheostomy may be needed [95].

7.8.7 Definitive Surgical Management

Over the years, various surgical procedures have been proposed. An ideal surgical procedure should maintain the patency of choana; it should not interfere with normal craniofacial development with minimal invasiveness and less risk of recurrences.

7.8.7.1 Surgical Approaches

1. Transnasal Endoscopic Approach
   It is the most preferred surgical approach because of better surgical outcomes and fewer complication rates [96]. This approach was first demonstrated by Stankiewicz and later modified by other authors [97, 98]. This surgery is completed in the following steps:
   (a) Adequate nasal decongestion.
   (b) Rigid nasal endoscope (2.7 mm) is introduced for visualization of atretic plate.
   (c) A laterally based mucosal flap is raised to expose the bony part.
   (d) The best point of entry into nasopharynx is at the thinnest part of the atretic plate, found usually at the junction between the hard palate and vomer which is at the most infero-medial point of the atretic plate. It is the safest site to enter into the nasopharynx.
   (e) Starting from this most infero-medial portion of the atretic plate, bone is removed sequentially, superiorly and laterally. Powered instruments are used for the bone removal (microdebrider or diamond drill). Spacious single neo-choana with removal of all intervening tissue and covering of bony defect with mucosal flap is the key to success (Fig. 7.47).

   The primary success rate is between 67 and 88% (Mean = 85.3%) [99, 100]. Frequent postoperative use of nasal saline irrigation and periodic endoscopic surveillance or second-look procedure is required. If the nasal passage is too narrow to pass both endoscope and drill, a 120° endoscope from nasopharyngeal side may be used for visualization (Retropalatal approach). The rest of the procedure is performed transnasally.
2. Transpalatal Approach
   This approach was first described by Owens. Greater palatine vessels-based, U-shaped mucosal flap is elevated posteriorly beyond the hard and soft palate junction. The palatine bones posterior to the greater palatine foramina, the atresia plates, the posterior vomer and the medial pterygoid plates are carefully drilled using a diamond burr [95]. It carries the risk of significant complications including palatal flap breakdown and fistula formation, palatal muscle dysfunction, velopharyngeal insufficiency and effect on maxillary growth causing crossbite and high palatal arch deformity. The transpalatal approach is not preferred nowadays.
3. Transseptal Approach
   Described by Hall et al. and Osquthorpe et al. in 1982, the transseptal approach is recommended in case of unilateral CA and in age >8 years [101]. It permits better correction of any deviations of the septum, resection of the posterior part of the vomer and preservation of mucosal flaps for coverage of the bleeding area.

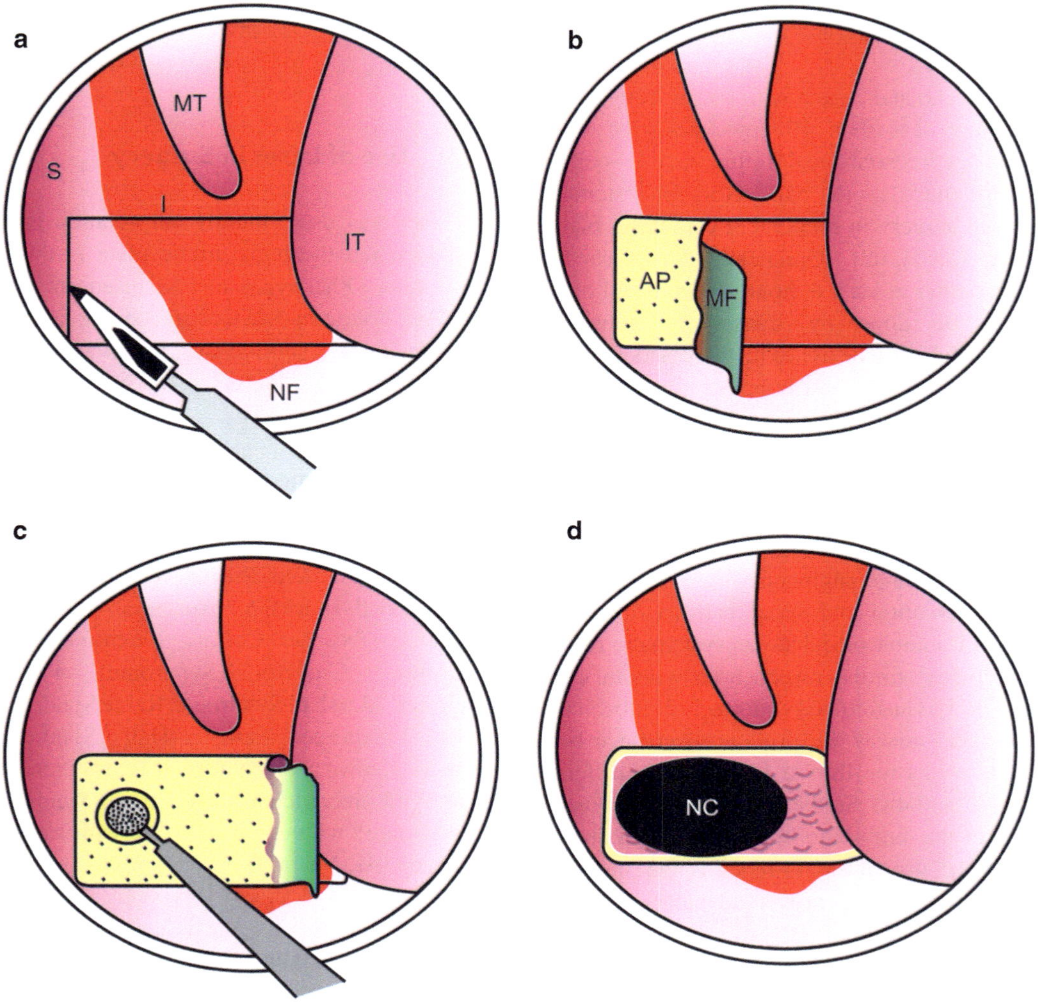

Fig. 7.47 Transnasal endoscopic approach for choanal atresia repair, from left nostril. Similar for the right side also *S* septum, *I* incision line, *IT* inferior turbinate, *MT* middle turbinate, *NF* nasal floor, *AP* atretic plate, *MF* mucosal flap, *NC* neo choana

4. Trans-antral Approach
   The trans-antral approach is only of historical interest. By providing adequate exposure to the surgical field, this approach permits an adequate and prompt control of any bleeding with a lesser risk of damaging the sphenopalatine arteries, veins and nerves. But this approach can significantly increase the risk of deformities of growing structures such as the maxilla and upper teeth.
   Sublabial-transseptal approach is also described. Transnasal, transpalatal and transseptal approaches are mostly used but the Cochrane review has not shown advantage of one surgical approach over other [102].

7.8.8 Prevention of Restenosis After Surgery

Bilateral choanal atresia with purely bony atretic plate, age less than 10 days, nasopharyngeal reflux, gastroesophageal reflux and associated malformations are the risk factors for restenosis. Delayed surgery in bilateral atresia has a higher failure rate [103]. Unilateral atresia can be delayed after at least 6 months of age and repair should be done by transnasal endoscopic approach [104]. The use of microbebrider, micro-drills reduces the surrounding trauma which reduces the risk of scarring. After a successful repair, a close and long follow-up at 2, 4 and 8 weeks with endoscope-assisted cleaning of the nasal cavity and surgical site should help in reducing restenosis. Use of Mitomycin C (inhibits fibroblasts and angiogenesis), stents, mucosal flap preservation and serial balloon dilatations are still a matter of debate as systematic review has depicted similar results even without using them [105]. Customized endotracheal tube, nasopharyngeal airway and Teflon sheet have been used as stents for 48 h to 12 months in different series (Fig. 7.48). Studies favour either no use of stents or use limited to bilateral choanal atresia. Today, the use of stents remains the surgeon's choice in absence of proven advantage. Stenting is less likely required for older patients. Surgery with navigation is preferred in syndromic association.

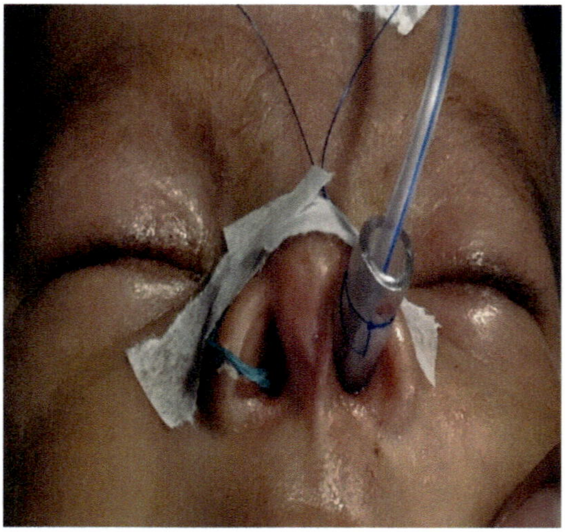

Fig. 7.48 Postoperative stenting (Courtesy—Dr. Hitesh Verma, Associate Professor, AIIMS, New Delhi, India)

7.8.9 Use of Laser in Surgery

CO_2 laser was used initially but ablation is not possible when the bony atretic plate is thicker than 1 mm. Other types of laser used are KTP, Nd-YAG, holmium-YAG, contact diode laser but they lack a significant advantage over microdebrider.

7.8.10 Syndromes Associated with Choanal Atresia

CHARGE, Axenfeld–Rieger Syndrome—Type 1, Diamond–Blackfan Anaemia, DiGeorge Syndrome, Treacher Collins Syndrome, Apert Syndrome, Crouzon Syndrome, Pfeiffer Syndrome, Marshall Syndrome, Raine Syndrome, Fraser Syndrome, Pallister–Hall Syndrome, Burn–McKeown Syndrome, Cat Eye Syndrome, Fryns Syndrome, McKusick–Kaufman Syndrome are associated with choanal atresia with variable frequency [91, 106].

7.9 Part I: Cerebrospinal Fluid Rhinorrhea

Cerebrospinal fluid (CSF) leak occurs as a result of an abnormal communication between the subarachnoid space and a pneumatized area in the skull base that includes the sinonasal tract. This communication or fistula must involve a breach of the arachnoid and dura matter, the bone of skull base and the underlying mucosa. Spinal fluid leak from the intracranial space to the nasal respiratory tract is potentially very serious because of the risk of an ascending infection which could produce fulminant meningitis. CSF rhinorrhea commonly occurs following head trauma (fronto-basal skull fractures), as a result of surgery, or destruction of lesions. In cases where a confirmatory test is needed, the beta-2 transferrin assay is the test of choice because of its high sensitivity and specificity. Various combinations of planar tomography and CT, contrast-enhanced CT cisternography, and radionuclide cisternography, and, more recently, MR cisternography have been used in the diagnosis of CSF leak. MRI with NCCT is a very useful and specific diagnostic and localizing technique.

Traumatic CSF rhinorrhea is managed by conservative measures in 70–80% of cases. In cases of iatrogenic and spontaneous leaks, it is less likely to heal with conservative measures. It is currently accepted that endoscopic intranasal management of CSF rhinorrhea is the preferred method of surgical repair, with higher success rates and less morbidity than intracranial surgical repair. Uncomplicated CSF fistula, located at the posterior wall of frontal sinuses can be repaired extradurally with osteoplastic frontal sinusotomy. Intracranial approaches should be reserved for more complicated CSF rhinorrhea. The timing for surgery and CSF drainage procedures must be decided with great care and with a clear strategy. This chapter reviewed the applied anatomy and physiology, causes, diagnosis and treatment of CSF leakage.

7.9.1 Applied Physiology

The total volume of CSF in adults is 90–150 ml. CSF is produced in the choroid plexus and ependyma at a rate of 0.35 ml/min (500 ml/d). It is absorbed in arachnoid villi, total volume turned over 3–5 times per day. CSF circulates from the lateral ventricle to the third ventricle via the aqueduct of Sylvius. From the third ventricle, the fluid circulates into the fourth ventricle and out into the subarachnoid space via the foramina of Magendie and Luschka. After circulating through the subarachnoid space, CSF is reabsorbed via arachnoid villi.

CSF consists of a mixture of water, electrolytes (Na^+, K^+, Mg^{2+}, Ca^{2+}, Cl^-, and HCO_3^-), glucose (60–80% of blood glucose), amino acids and various proteins (22–38 mg/dL). CSF is colourless, clear and typically devoid of cells such as polymorphonuclear cells and mononuclear cells (<5/μL). CSF represents the end product of the ultrafiltration of plasma across epithelial cells in the choroid plexus lining the ventricles of the brain. Circulation of CSF is maintained by the hydrostatic differences between its rate of production and its rate of absorption. Normal CSF pressure is approximately 10–15 mmHg, and elevated pressure constitutes an intracranial pressure (ICP) greater than 20 mmHg.

7.9.2 Applied Anatomy

The most common anatomic sites of spontaneous cerebrospinal fluid (CSF) leaks are the areas of congenital weakness of the anterior cranial fossa and areas related to the type of surgery performed. The lateral lamella of the cribriform plate appears to be involved in approximately 40% of the cases, the frontal sinus in 15% whereas sella turcica and sphenoid sinus are involved in 15%. Common sites of injury secondary to endoscopic sinus surgery include the lateral lamella of the cribriform plate and the posterior ethmoid roof near the anterior and medial sphenoid wall. Rarely, the leak can originate in the middle or posterior cranial fossa and can reach the nasal cavity by way of the middle ear and eustachian tube. These patients typically present with aural fullness due to a serous middle ear effusion.

7.9.3 Classification

It is classified by Ommaya et al. (1960) [107]. It is grossly divided into traumatic, non-traumatic and congenital types. Both entities can be further classified:

(A) Traumatic
  (i) Non-surgical
  (ii) Surgical
(B) Non-traumatic
  (i) Normal pressure
  (ii) High pressure
(C) Congenital

Traumatic CSF leak can be divided on the basis of aetiology:

(A) Trauma—it is the most common type and anterior cranial fossa is the most common site (cribriform and roof of ethmoid). It is further classified into non-surgical and surgical. Non-surgical (accidental) accounts for ~80% of all CSF leaks result of blunt or penetrating head trauma. 2–3% of major head trauma results in CSF leaks. CSF leak occurs in 15–30% of cases of skull base fracture. Leak may be either immediate (within 48 h) or delayed and in ~95% of cases of delayed leaks occur within 3 months. Surgical (Iatrogenic) CSF leak accounts for 16% of CSF leaks. Endoscopic sinus surgery is the most common cause (0.5% of ESS cases). The most common site of injury is the lateral lamella of the cribriform plate.

(B) Non-traumatic—it is 4% of cases of CSF rhinorrhea. It can be further classified into high, normal pressure leaks. High-pressure leak is 45% of non-traumatic cases. The pathophysiology is persistent high intracranial pressure (ICP), that leads to remodelling and thinning of the skull base and creates communication (theorized to be due to ischemia from compression of vessels). The causes of high ICP are intracranial tumour growth (typically pituitary tumours) and hydrocephalus secondary to obstruction of the normal pathway of CSF fluid drainage. Normal pressure leaks are 55% of non-traumatic cases. The causes are true spontaneous leaks (usually seen in adults). Tumours and other osteolytic lesions of skull base erodes the boundary of the nasal and cranial cavity (nasopharyngeal carcinoma, inverted papilloma, etc.)

(C) Congenital—It may be either increased ICP or normal ICP. The reason for congenital CSF leak is the failure of closure of the normal linings which separates the cranial and nasal cavity. It typically involves the foramen cecum and fonticulus frontalis. The persistent cricopharyngeal canal creates a vertical midline defect connecting the middle cranial fossa to the sphenoid. Primary empty sella syndrome is developed by congenital widening of the diaphragma sella.

7.9.4 Patient Evaluation

Presenting symptoms are clear, watery discharge from the nose (more on bending forward). The fluid is non-sticky and has a salty taste in the mouth. Patients are not able to sniff back the fluid. The other presentation is the history of recurrent meningitis. The history should be focused on duration, onset, associated symptoms. History should also include the severity, laterality and quantity of rhinorrhea. The important questions are history of trauma, symptoms of meningitis, recent sinus surgery or neurosurgery. The physical examination includes complete ENT examination, weight and BMI, site of leak by banding forwards.

7.9.5 Differential Diagnosis

Autonomic dysfunction, allergic rhinitis, CSF oto-rhinorrhoea are the differentials for CSF rhinorrhoea.

7.9.6 Investigations

(A) **Bed Side Test**

1. Halo or Ring Sign—blood will separate out from CSF when nasal discharge is placed on a filter paper (central blood with clear ring). The ring sign is not specific to bloody CSF. Blood mixed with water, saline, and other mucus will also form a ring sign.
2. Reservoir sign—Morning rise showed gush of CSF leak. It is because of fluid collection in paranasal sinuses.
3. A handkerchief is not stiff when soaked with CSF fluid.

(B) **Laboratory Tests**

1. **Glucose testing**—It is a rapid but highly unreliable test. CSF glucose level is two-third of blood glucose level. Glucose oxidase paper colour is changed with glucose concentrations of 5+ mg/dL. In recent trauma, the presence of blood gives false-positive results. Recent men-

ingitis or other intracranial infections cause a lower concentration of glucose in CSF (false-negative). False-positive results with lacrimal secretions or nasal mucus. Negative glucose virtually eliminates a diagnosis of CSF fluid.

2. **Beta-trace protein**—It is also known as prostaglandin D synthase. It is synthesized primarily in arachnoid cells, oligodendrocytes and choroids plexus (CNS). It is also found in human testis, heart and serum. It is not routinely ordered as it may be altered in many cases like renal insufficiency, multiple sclerosis, cerebral infarctions and some CNS tumours. Fluid with a concentration >2.0 mg/L is usually positive for CSF. Concentration <1.5 mg/L is not likely to contain CSF. Sensitivity and specificity are not high as beta-2-transferrin.
3. **Beta-2-transferrin—**It is currently the single best test for identifying the presence of CSF [108]. It is a protein produced by neuraminidase in CNS located only within the CSF, perilymph and aqueous humour. The assay has a high sensitivity (94–100%) and specificity (98–100%). It is rapid and is a non-invasive test and it requires only 0.5 cc of fluid. It is stable at room temperature for approximately 4 h, so immediate refrigeration following collection is recommended. Specimen should not be frozen. If assay facility is available, one can get results within 3 h. Sensitivity is about 100% with specificity of 95%.

(C) **Imaging Studies**

1. **High-Resolution CT Scans** [109]—It is the imaging modality of choice for identifying a skull base defect associated with a CSF leak (Fig. 7.49). It may demonstrate skull base defects resulting from accidental or iatrogenic trauma, and underlying anatomic or developmental abnormality, or an erosive lesion such as neoplasm. It should have 1 mm cuts with axial, sagittal and coronal views. Pneumocephalus on a CT scan may indicate a dural tear. A deviated crista galli is a radiological sign supporting primary CSF rhinorrhea. However, it may reveal defects in the skull base that do not leak or are not sites of active leaking, making the diagnosis more difficult.

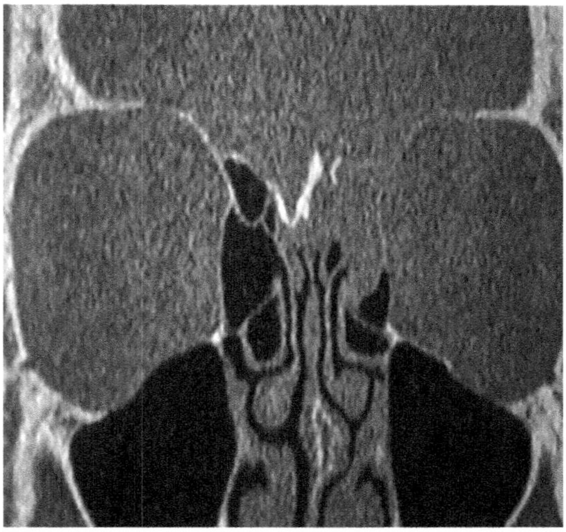

Fig. 7.49 CT PNS showing left roof of ethmoid bony defect post-trauma

2. **CT Cisternography**—It is more invasive, not very frequently used. Intrathecal contrast dye is injected and a CT scan is obtained. It is more accurate especially those with active leaks (Fig. 7.50). Sensitivity for detecting leaks drops from nearly 100% with active leaks to 60% with intermittent leaks. It may miss cribriform or ethmoid sinus defects. It can be associated with nausea, headaches and acute organic psychosyndromes.
3. **Magnetic resonance imaging (MRI)**—It is not recommended as a first-line imaging modality unless an encephalocele is suspected. It demonstrates soft tissue abnormalities and pooling of CSF (high signal intensity on T2). It is not good at defining bony defects, unlike a CT scan. Contrast helps in the differentiation of sinus inflammation from CSF fluid. It is more expensive and time-consuming.
4. **MR Cisternography**—Avoidance of intrathecal injection of contrast is the key

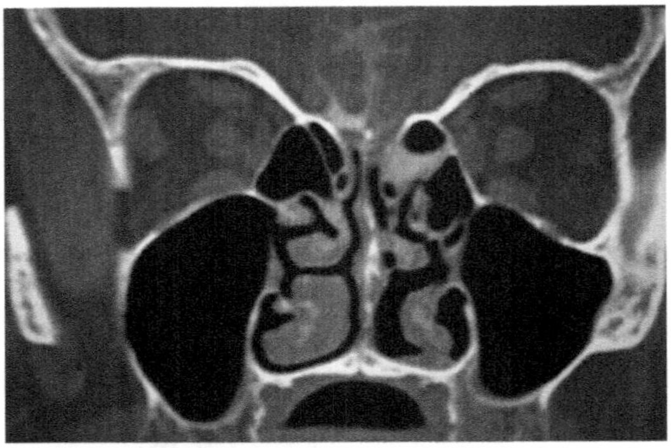

Fig. 7.50 CT cisternography showing left lateral lamella of cribriform plate defect

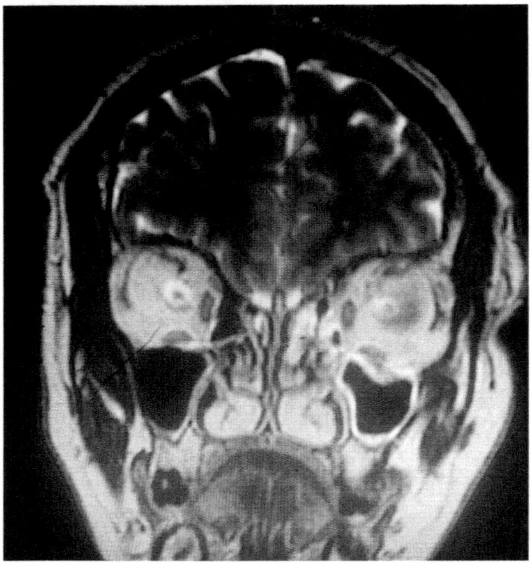

Fig. 7.51 MRI cisternography (T2 with Cg) in spontaneous CSF rhinorrhea, defect in left cribriform plate

benefit of it. T2-weighted imaging can be used to detect CSF in the sinonasal cavity (Fig. 7.51). Pulse sequence can be designed to enhance the detection probability. As with CT cisternography, false-negative studies may result in intermittent leaks. MR cisternography and HRCT of nose PNS is the most accepted modality to diagnose the site of leak.

5. **Nuclear medicine tests (radionuclide cisternography)**—Intrathecal injection of radioactive tracers (technetium-99, I-131, Indium 111) is done and pledgets placed at areas suspected of leak and scintigrams of the skull are obtained. Pledgets are then removed and measured for radioactive tracer. The test is positive only with active leak (70% detection when active, 30–40% in inactive) and it has poor localization. Radioactive isotope is absorbed into the circulatory system and deposited into normal tissues.

(D) **Diagnostic Procedures**

Intrathecal injection of Fluorescein dye: It is good at locating active CSF leaks. After lumbar puncture or drain placement, 10 ml of CSF is withdrawn and about 0.1 ml of 10% fluorescein solution is mixed with withdrawn CSF. The mixture is then re-injected into the subarachnoid space over 10 min period. In most cases, dye can be seen without filters. Smaller defects may require filters or black light (yellow filter on endoscope, blue on light source). It is important to keep a low concentration of fluorescein; high doses can lead to severe side effects (500 + mg) like seizure, pulmonary edema, coma and death.

7.9.7 Treatment

(A) **Medical Therapy**

1. **Conservative management:** It has been advocated in immediate-onset CSF rhinorrhea following accidental trauma. It consists of a 7–10 day trial of bed rest with the head end elevation by 15–30 degrees. The patient should avoid coughing, sneezing, nose-blowing and heavy weight lifting. Stool softeners should be used to decrease the strain associated with bowel movements. 75–80% of traumatic CSF leaks will spontaneously resolve with this management.
2. **Lumbar drain** [110]**:** Lumber drain can be considered if CSF leak does not resolve after 5–7 days of conservative management, mainly in large skull defects or iat-

rogenic CSF leaks. Continuous drainage is recommended over intermittent drainage (prevents spikes in CSF pressure). The usual rate of drain is 10–15 cc/h. Risks involve headaches, nausea and emesis, pneumocephalus, infection, coma.

3. **Antibiotics:** Role is controversial. The reason for use is to prevent intracranial infections. Brodie et al. concluded that there is no significant difference in the incidence of meningitis with prophylactic antibiotic therapy [111]. It can be used in iatrogenic CSF leak following skull base injuries during FESS.
4. **Diuretic:** It is utilized in the presence of a CSF leak with increased ICP [112]. Acetazolamide inhibits the conversion of water and CO_2 to bicarbonate and H+. Loss of H+ slows the action of the Na+/K+ ATPase enzymes that are responsible for the production of CSF results in decreased ICP.

(B) **Surgical Therapy**

1. **Intracranial Approach:** (mostly done via frontal craniotomy, rarely middle or posterior fossa)
   The indications include comminuted skull fractures with displaced fragments requiring reduction, extensive skull base fractures associated with intracranial haemorrhages or contusions that require craniotomy for treatment [113]. It is also indicated when co-existing surgically amenable mass lesion is laying inside the cranium, more than 3 cm cranial defect, multiple defects, multiple failed endoscopic repairs and when site of leak is not visible by all investigations. Dural defects may be closed primarily with or without the use of grafts which could be free or pedicled periosteal or dural flaps (Fig. 7.27a), muscle plugs, mobilized portions of the falx cerebri, fascia grafts or many commercial grafts. It should be reinforced with fibrin glue. Advantages include direct visualization of defect, inspection of adjacent cerebral cortex with a better chance of patching a defect in the face of increased ICP. Disadvantages comprise increased morbidity, increased hospital time, injury to the brain from retraction (haematoma, seizures, cognitive dysfunction and risk of permanent anosmia). It is not good for visualization of the sphenoid sinus. Failure rates for this approach are 40% for the first attempt and 10% overall.
2. **Extracranial Approach: It can be further divided into external and endoscopic types.**
   (a) **External approach:** These procedures are infrequently chosen in current practice, given the high success rates and low morbidity associated with the endoscopic approach. However, they should be part of every skull base surgeon's armamentarium.
   - **External ethmoidectomy**—Begins with the tarsorrhaphy on the ipsilateral eye. Incision is made halfway between the medial canthus and the midline of the nose down to the bone. Lateral elevation of the periosteum exposes the anterior lacrimal ridge and the lacrimal fossa. The lacrimal sac is elevated and retracted out of the fossa. The anterior ethmoidal artery which will be encountered 2–2.5 cm posterior to the lacrimal crest should be ligated. The fronto-ethmoid suture line marks the level of fovea ethmoidalis (dissection should never be superior to this line). The posterior ethmoidal artery is found approximately 1.2 cm posterior to the anterior ethmoidal artery in the fronto-ethmoid suture line and the optic nerve lies 5–6 mm posterior to the posterior ethmoidal artery. A complete dissection of

the ethmoid labyrinth should be done and the skull base defect is then identified.

- **Trans-ethmoidal sphenoidotomy**—First an external ethmoidectomy is carried out as above, the sphenoid sinus opening is then identified and enlarged; the anterior wall of the sinus is removed to reach the sella region.
- **Sublabial-transseptal sphenoidotomy**—Can be carried out using sublabial or transnasal incision with exposure of pyriform aperture and nasal spine is made free. Left or right septal mucoperichondrial flap is elevated laterally and inferiorly along the nasal floor in the subperiosteal plane. The cartilaginous septum is dislocated from the maxillary crest and the contralateral nasal floor mucoperiosteal flap is elevated. The contralateral nasal septum is not elevated off the cartilage. The bony–cartilaginous junction is disarticulated and the opposite posterior flap is elevated. The bony septum is removed to expose the sphenoid rostrum, which is widely removed via osteotomies or a drill to expose the entire sinus.
- **Trans-antral approach**—It offers wide access to the anterior sphenoid, ethmoids, pterygopalatine fossa and maxilla. A gingivobuccal sulcus incision is made to expose the anterior wall of the maxilla. The periosteum is elevated superiorly as far as the infraorbital nerve and canine fossa osteotomy performed to enter into the maxillary sinus. The ethmoidal bone can then be approached medially and superiorly through the maxilloethmoidal angle. When needed, the pterygopalatine fossa can be accessed via the posterior wall of the maxillary sinus.
- **Osteoplastic flap**—Indicated for the defect in the posterior table of the frontal sinus especially if more than 2 cm and above the floor and lateral to the lamina papyracea and is approached via coronal incision or eyebrow incision (Fig. 7.52).

(b) **Endoscopic Approach:** It is the most common and successful approach (90–95% success rate) [114]. The advantages are better magnified visualization, angled visualization, no external incisions and minimized intranasal mucosal injuries. It is of many types:

- **Transfrontal approach** (Lothrop or Draf III procedure)—It allows access to the floor and posterior wall of the frontal sinus. The main advantage is it avoids obliteration of the frontal sinus with the osteoplastic flap. The frontal sinus outflow tract must be preserved to avoid mucocele. It is not effective for the defects in the most lateral or superior aspects of the sinus. It begins by performing a complete ethmoidectomy followed by identification and dissection of frontal recess with removal of superior septum and interfrontal septum.
- **Transcribriform approach**—Exposes the medial anterior cranial fossa from the medial aspect of the middle turbinate to the olfactory groove (Fig. 7.53). Posteriorly, it extends to the anterior aspect of the planum sphenoidale. Crita galli is exposed by removal of the perpedicular plate of ethmoid bone. Care should be

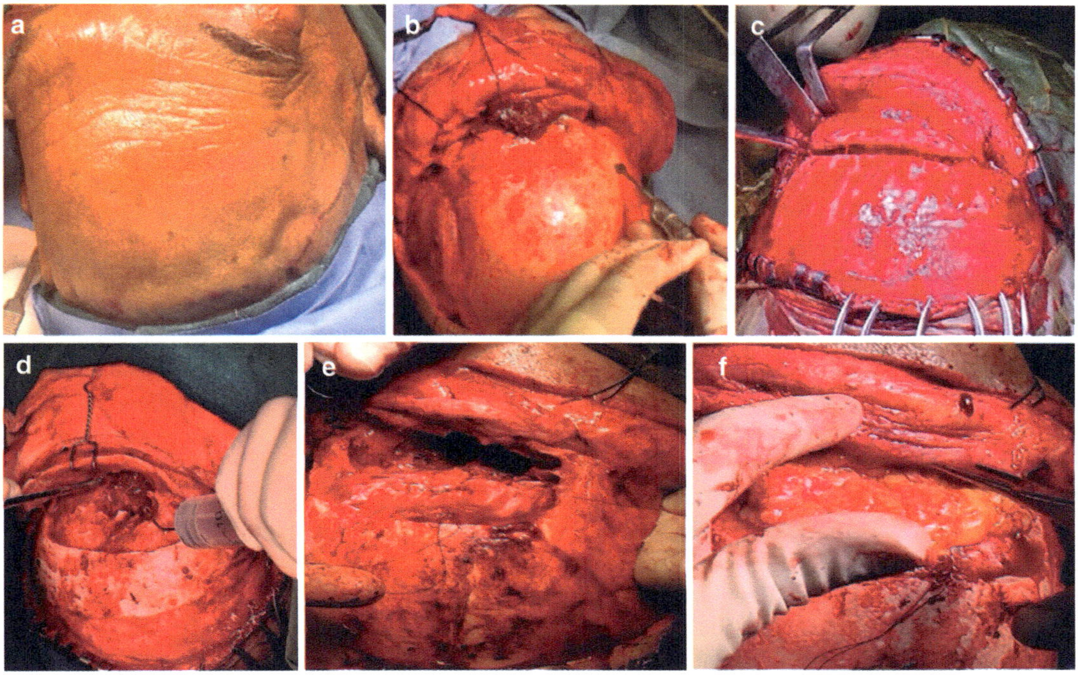

Fig. 7.52 (**a**) Incision marking, (**b**) drilling the outline of frontal sinus after marking with X-ray templet, (**c**) anterior frontal sinus wall is elevated, (**d**) view of frontal sinus, (**e**) repair of dural defect with fascia lata and secured with suturing, (**f**) obliteration of frontal sinuses (Courtesy—Dr. Hitesh Verma, Associate Professor, AIIMS, New Delhi, India)

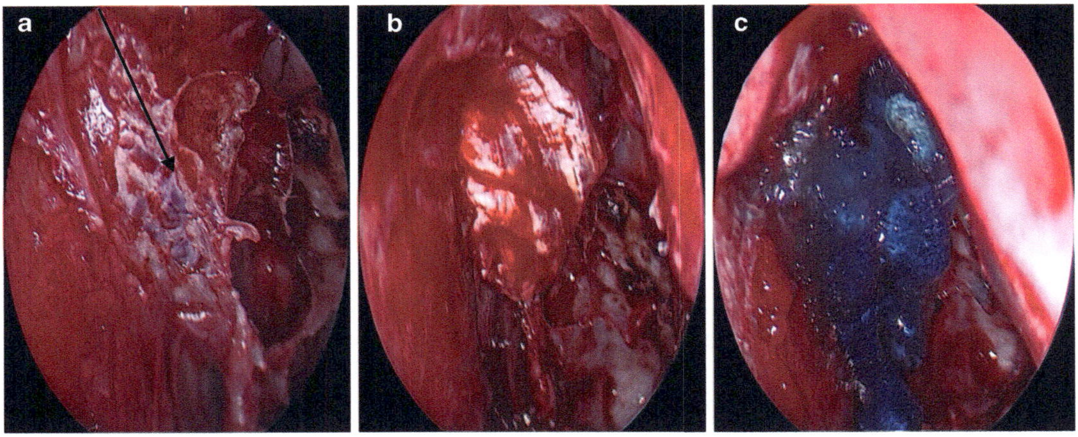

Fig. 7.53 (**a**) Showing bony defect of left cribriform plate with dura exposed in spontaneous leak (black arrow), (**b**) facia lata composite grafting, (**c**) showing fibrin glue/dura seal in situ

taken while doing dissection near the olfactory groove.

- **Transfovea approach**—For getting access to the lateral aspect of the anterior cranial fossa. The dissection extends from the middle turbinate to the lamina papyracea. The frontal sinus marks the anterior limit and the sphenoid marks the posterior limit. In some

cases, the middle turbinate is removed and the transfovea and transcribriform approaches are combined.
- **Transplanum approach**—Allows exposure of skull base defects along the planum sphenoidale and those with significant involvement of the suprasellar region. Anterior and posterior ethmoidectomy is performed first, which provides access to the most anterior aspect of the planum. The anterior seller wall is taken down to provide posterior exposure.
- **Trans-sellar approach**—The route of choice can be medial or lateral to middle turbinate for defects on the sella turcica. It is part of extended endoscopic procedure for pituitary lesion excision. Complete ethmoidectomy is followed by the opening of sphenoid sinus ostia. If bilateral access is needed, the posterior bony septum and the intersinus septum can be removed.
- **Transpterygoid approach**—First an endoscopic modified medial maxillectomy is performed. The infraorbital nerve is then identified and its trajectory followed. A complete sphenoethmoidectomy is then performed. The crista ethmoidalis is isolated and the main branch of the sphenopalatine artery (SPA) is identified. The pterygopalatine ganglion which lies posterior to the SPA should be preserved. The fat in the pterygopalatine fossa may be dissected or cauterized until the pterygoid bones are identified. Anterior wall of the lateral recess of the sphenoid sinus, pterygoid base is drilled. It is good to access any defect in the middle fossa floor that occurs in this vicinity lateral to the Sternberg canal and the foramen rotundum.

The key to endoscopic repair of a CSF leak is good visualization and exposure of the defect. If an encephalocele is present, it should be cauterized at its stalk with bipolar cautery prior to reduction into the anterior cranial fossa to prevent intracranial haemorrhage. For good exposure, the surgeon should elevate the surrounding mucosa to provide 2–5 mm of bone exposure around the defect. Any mucosa remaining in the defect should be removed prior to repair to avoid poor adhesion of graft with bed and to prevent future mucocele formation.

There are many types of grafts utilized, but it should be noted that the graft should be roughly 30% larger than the defect to account for postoperative shrinkage. Types of grafting material utilized are cartilage, bone (septum, mastoid tip, middle turbinate), mucoperichondrium, septal mucosa, turbinate mucosa and/or bone, fascia (temporalis, fascia lata), abdominal fat, and pedicled septal or turbinate flaps. It should be noted that pedicled flaps tend to tint, fold and contract when utilized.

7.9.8 Grafting Techniques

1. Overlay technique—a graft is placed directly over the defect.
2. Underlay technique—the graft is placed between the dura and bony defect.
3. The combined technique utilizes both underlay and overlay grafts.
4. Bathplug technique, where a fat plug with a specifically secured vicryl suture into the intradural space [115].

In addition to these techniques, we may reinforce the repair with fibrin glue to provide an improved seal. The placement of absorbable (gel foam) and/or non-absorbable packing can further improve the seal. Non-absorbable pack removal may lead to the displacement of the graft when removed. In the face of increased ICP, it is recommended that a multilayered graft be utilized.

The size of the defect also plays a role in the grafting technique utilized. If the defect is <2 mm, the type of grafting technique utilized typically does not make much difference as most techniques will be successful in repairing the CSF leak. If the defect is 2–5 mm, one must note whether comminuted bone segments or significant dural injury is present. If they are not present, the use of an overlay grafting technique is sufficient. However, if either is present, one should utilize a composite graft or a separately harvested bone plus mucosa grafting technique where the bone is placed in an underlay fashion while the mucosa is placed in an overlay fashion. If the defect is >5 mm, the repair should be performed with a composite graft or separate bone plus mucosa grafting technique as described above. Meningitis (0.3%), brain abscess (0.9%), subdural haematoma (0.3%), smell disorders (0.6%), headache (0.3%) are the complications of endoscopic technique (much lesser than craniotomy) [116].

Postoperative care includes bed rest with the head of the bed set at 15–30 degrees for 3–5 days. The blood pressure should be maintained at a normal level. Stool softeners and cough suppressants to prevent straining, coughing. The patients should be advised to avoid blowing the nose and any heavy lifting. If a lumbar drain is utilized postoperatively, it should be left 3–5 days with a maximum drainage of 10–15 cc/h. If non-absorbable packing is utilized, antibiotics should be given.

7.10 Part J: Optic Nerve Anatomy and Management

Orbit is pyramidal in shape with apex posteriorly and base directed anteriorly. The optic canal rests in the sphenoid bone and lies at the apex of the orbit. Optic nerve injury is classically divided into direct and indirect types. Direct optic nerve injury is caused by penetrating injuries to the optic nerve whereas indirect optic nerve injury occurs due to blunt impact to head or face which further sets a shearing force damaging the optic nerve or its blood supply. Direct and indirect injuries both cause mechanical and ischemic damage to the optic nerve. CT scanning helps in delineating fractures of bones and is critical for surgical planning. MRI is superior in delineating soft tissue involvement. Both corticosteroids and surgical decompression alone or in combination helps in improving visual prognosis.

Orbital and Optic Nerve Anatomy [117]

Optic nerve is 3–4 mm in diametre, 35–50 mm in length from retina to optic chiasma. It is basically divided into four segments. The first segment named as intraocular segment is around 1 mm in length. The second segment is intraorbital with 20–30 mm length, third and fourth segments are intracanalicular (5–11 mm) and intracranial (3–16 mm), respectively, as depicted in Fig. 7.54. The optic canal is approximately 6.5 mm in diametre and 8–10 mm in length. Figure 7.55 depicts relations of intracanalicular part of the optic nerve. Relations of intraorbital part of optic nerve are shown in Fig. 7.56. Optic canal contains optic nerve axons, their supportive glia, the ophthalmic artery and branches of the carotid sympathetic plexus of the autonomic nervous system. Axons of the optic nerve arise from the ganglion cell layer of the retina and extend beyond chiasma and optic tracts just before synapsing in the lateral geniculate body.

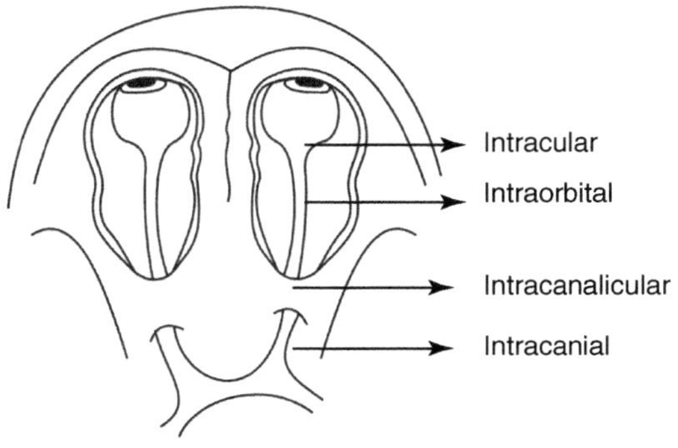

Fig. 7.54 Parts of optic nerve

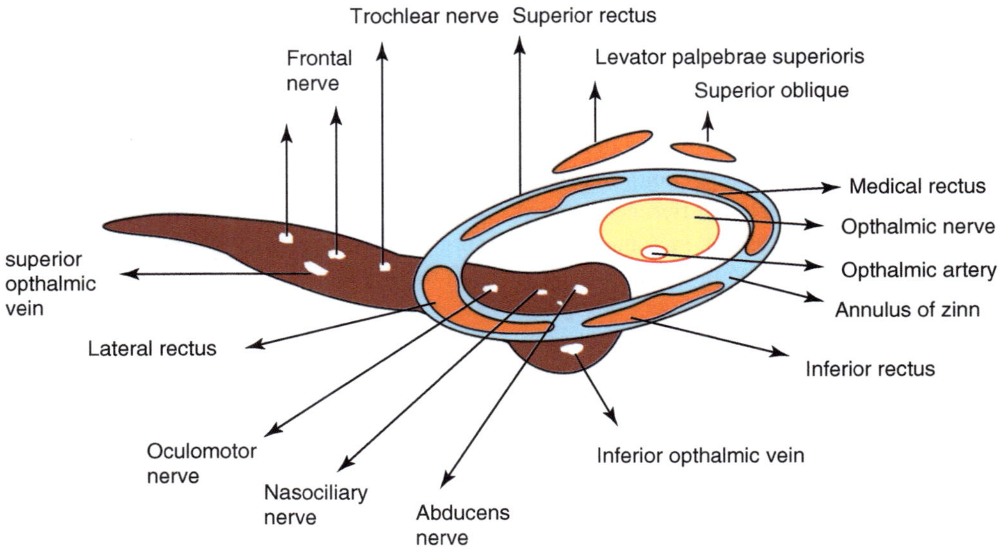

Fig. 7.55 Relationship of intracanalicular segment of optic nerve

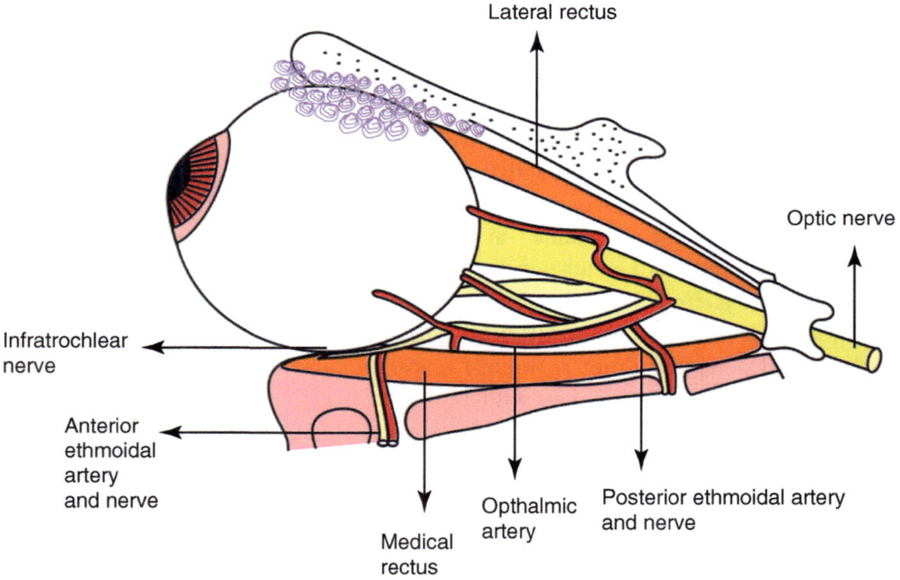

Fig. 7.56 Relationship of intraorbital part of optic nerve

The optic nerve is surrounded by pia, arachnoid and dura mater in its intraorbital and intracanalicular part which forms the optic sheath. In the intracanalicular part, the dura is fused to sphenoid periosteum and at the posterior end of the optic canal, the optic nerve sheath is fused to dura lining calvaria. Thus, intracranial part lies in subarachnoid space. Intraocular optic nerve is supplied by arterial circle of Zinn–Haller with contributions from posterior ciliary arteries, the pial arterial network and the peripapillary choroidal vasculature. Perforating branches derived from the ophthalmic artery supplies intraorbital part of the optic nerve and intracanalicular part is supplied by small pial branches from ophthalmic artery. On the other hand, intracranial part is supplied by pial branches of the internal carotid, anterior cerebral and anterior communicating arteries.

Traumatic optic nerve injury is basically of two types: direct and indirect optic nerve injury. Direct Optic Nerve injury is caused by penetrating objects impinging directly on the optic nerve. Direct optic nerve injuries have a worst prognosis than indirect optic nerve injuries. Indirect optic nerve injuries are further divided based on anatomical site into anterior and posterior. Anterior indirect optic nerve injuries are the injuries anterior to where the central retinal artery enters the optic nerve 8–12 mm posterior to insertion of nerve into globe whereas posterior indirect optic nerve injuries are posterior to this site.

Initial ocular examination should be done including visual acuity using Snellen's chart, colour vision and visual field charting [118]. Swinging Flashlight test should be used to elicit Relative Afferent Pupillary Defect (RAPD) which is positive in traumatic optic neuropathy but may be absent in bilateral cases. Ophthalmoscopic examination will help to evaluate the retinal and choroidal circulation, optic nerve head morphology and to rule out any intraocular foreign body. Visual evoked potentials (VEP) are usually not required to establish the diagnosis but may be used in questionable cases. Flash VEP amplitude ratio greater than 0.5 appears predictive of a favourable, long-term visual outcome in unilateral traumatic optic neuropathy. It has diagnostic value in patients having suspicion of bilateral optic neuropathy where RAPD may not be evident. Thin Section CT Scanning is the main modality to see fractures of the optic canal and to plan for any surgical intervention. MR imaging is useful in chiasmal trauma and should be done after the metallic orbital foreign body is being ruled out.

Diagnosis of Indirect over Direct TON [119] is made on the following findings:

1. Variable visual loss ranging from normal to no light perception in indirect TON; direct TON causes immediate and severe visual loss.
2. Relative afferent pupillary defect is present except in cases of symmetric B/L TON.
3. Impairment of colour vision.
4. Variable visual field defects.

Optic disc appearance in anterior indirect TON is associated with disc swelling and retinal haemorrhages whereas in posterior indirect TON fundus looks normal. In direct TON, there could be avulsed optic nerve head or optic disc swelling with haemorrhages. CT findings can be suggestive of direct TON and excluding indirect TON. Although both direct and indirect mechanisms can cause optic nerve damage, a clear distinction between the two is difficult.

Other causes of optic neuropathy include:

1. Dysthyroid optic neuropathy is a consequence of Graves orbitopathy that results in decreased visual acuity, RAPD, disturbed colour vision, optic disc abnormalities and visual field defects. Diagnosis and management requires a multidisciplinary approach. Mechanism of dysthyroid optic neuropathy appears to be caused by direct compression of the optic nerve due to enlarged extraocular muscles, stretching caused by proptosis and inflammation. Treatment options are high dose i.v steroids followed by orbital decompression. The accepted dose regimen of these patients is once per week dose of 500 mg i.v methylprednisolone for 6 weeks followed by 250 mg per week for another 6 weeks. Total cumulative dose should not be more than 6–8 g [120].
2. Fibrous dysplasia [121]—Clinical low vision with radiological proven optic nerve encasement and documented progression of vision deterioration are the indications of optic nerve decompression in fibrous dysplasia.
3. Benign intracranial hypertension—the role of optic nerve fenestration can prevent further visual loss in patients of BIH with rapidly progressing vision loss but the risk of meningitis is increased.

Treatment Options—There are two main modalities of treatment including medical therapy and surgical decompression used alone or in combination:

(A) Medical therapy—Corticosteroids were considered as neuroprotective due to their antioxidant properties and inhibition of free radical-induced lipid peroxidation. This hypothesis was reinforced following National Acute Spinal Cord Injury Study 2 [NASCIS II]; a multicentre clinical trial that evaluated patients with acute spinal cord injury concluded that the use of methylprednisolone (30 mg/kg loading dose, followed by 5.4 mg/kg/h for 24 h) started within 8 h of injury was associated with a significant improvement in both motor and sensory function compared to patients treated with a placebo [122, 123]. There is no convincing evidence that steroids provide any additional benefit over conservative management as there is high rate of spontaneous visual recovery in TON [123].

(B) Surgical decompression—Due to the lack of Randomized controlled trials, the timing and outcome of surgery is still controversial. In a recent meta-analysis, they divided patients into two groups based on the timing of surgery, in which 57% of patients in the early group (patients who had surgery in <3 days) had visual improvement and 51% in the late group (>7 days) also improved. So, it concludes that even in delayed cases, surgical intervention should be done [124, 125]. In patients with partial vision loss, surgical decompression was beneficial even when surgery was performed after 1 year of onset of visual loss [126]. The surgical decompression can be done by endoscopic or external approaches:

1. Endoscopic optic nerve decompression [127]—This technique is less invasive and provides good exposure to the optic canal and orbital apex. This procedure is done under general anaesthesia. Adequate nasal decongestion is achieved using epinephrine and using a 4 mm 0 degree rigid endoscope, standard spheno-ethmoidectomy is performed. Fracture of lamina papyracea approximately 1 cm anterior to the optic canal is done and then lamina papyracea is removed in a posterior direction to expose the annulus of Zinn. Thin lamina is then replaced with a thick bone of lesser wing of sphenoid near optic canal, which is then removed after adequate thinning like eggshell. Removal of bone for a distance of 1 cm posterior to the face of the sphenoid sinus is usually sufficient. In acute conditions, incision of the optic sheath is recommended in case of intra-sheath haematoma or significant papilledema. Optic sheath incision showed better results in delayed decompression. Optic sheath is then incised with sickle knife in the superomedial quadrant to minimize risk of injury to ophthalmic artery (Fig. 7.57).

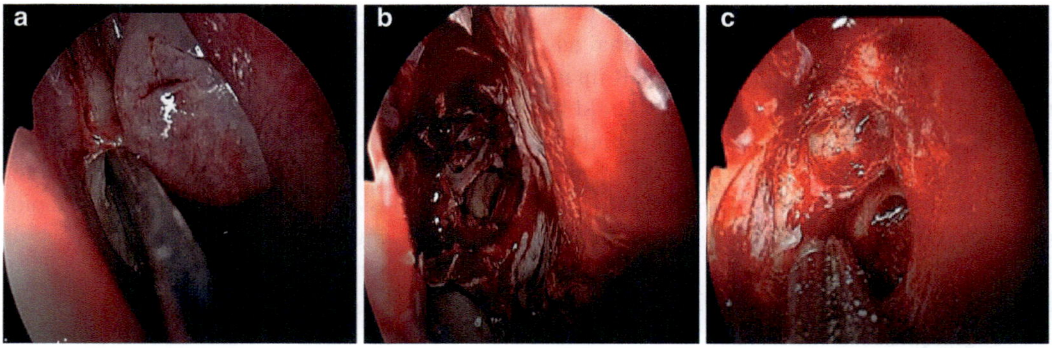

Fig. 7.57 Endoscopic optic nerve decompression. (**a**) Uncinectomy, (**b**) wide middle meatus antrostomy, ethmoidectomy and sphenoidotomy, (**c**) drilling of sphenoid bone, (**d**) exposure of optic nerve (ON), (**f**) incision on optic sheath

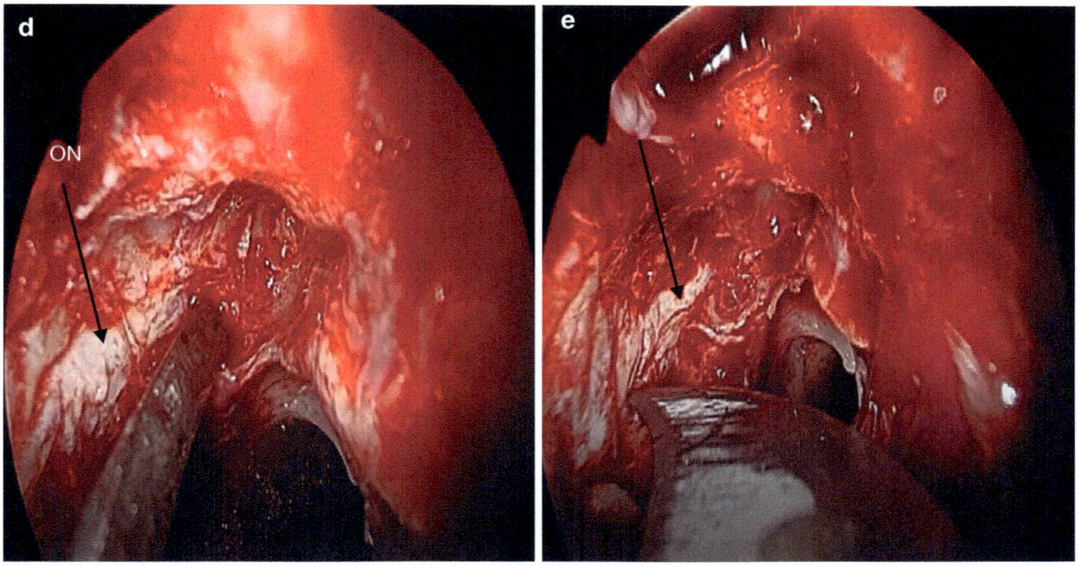

Fig. 7.57 (continued)

2. Extra-nasal Trans-ethmoidal Approach [124]—This technique provides access to the ethmoid sinus and medial wall of orbit. The incision is made along the medial canthus from the inferior margin of medial aspect of the eyebrow and then the periosteum is elevated followed by removal of lacrimal bone and lamina papyracea. Following which, the medial wall of the apex of orbit, optic canal and optic foramen is drilled using diamond burr. Then thinned-out OC ring is removed after tilting orbital contents to the lateral side (Fig. 7.58). Endoscopic-assisted medial transorbital approach is also used to overcome drawbacks of facial scar.
3. Transcranial approach [124]—This technique is more invasive than the endonasal approach as it requires brain retraction that can lead to serious complications. It can also alter cosmetic appearance as compared to the endonasal approach although it provides a familiar view to neurosurgeons and achieve wider decompression. Recently minimally invasive approaches like the supraorbital approach have been introduced but lack clinical data.

There are other agents who have experimental importance and little clinical evidence to support the effectiveness of these therapies [128]. These are:

1. Crystallins—these are the heat shock proteins which act as anti-inflammatory agents and are neuroprotective.
2. Erythropoietin—it increases retinal ganglion cell somata and survival of axon.
3. Glutamate inhibitors—it acts as an excitatory neurotransmitter in the eye.
4. Neurotropic factors—these factors help in the survival of existing neurons and growth and differentiation of newer ones. These include fibroblast growth factor-2 (FGF-2), brain-derived neurotrophic factor (BDNF) and ciliary neurotrophic factor (CNTF).
5. Tacrolimus—Protective role by inducing fibroblastic apoptosis and prevents loss of myelin.
6. Therapeutic hypothermia.
7. TNFα and NO synthase inhibitors—they enhance retinal ganglion cell survival.
8. Adipose tissue-derived stem cells are tried to repair ischemic optic neuropathy and optic nerve injury in rat models and showed success.

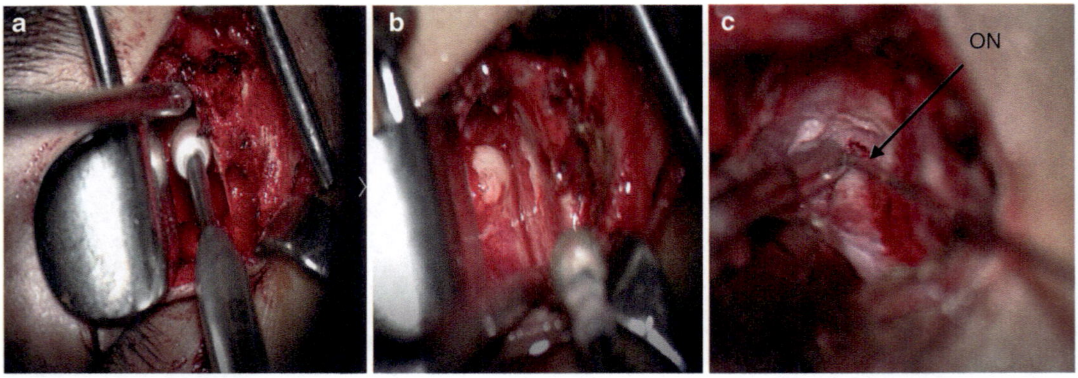

Fig. 7.58 External optic nerve decompression in fibrous dysplasia. (**a**) Drilling of medial orbital wall right side to gain posterior access. Self-retaining retractor is placed, (**b**) separation of orbital content from medial wall with wider posterior view, (**c**) optic nerve decompression in intracanalicular portion

7.11 Part K: Skull Base Reconstruction in Extended Endoscopic Approaches

With widespread application of extended endoscopic skull base procedures, the need for a robust reconstruction, preferably by the same approach and from the tissue in the vicinity, was the need of the hour. This necessity gave rise to the invention of the endonasal mucosal flaps. The endonasal flaps are designed based on the vascularity of the nasal mucosa. The nasal mucosa of both the septum as well as the lateral nasal wall is used along with its vascularity for the reconstruction of the defects. The choice of the endonasal mucosal flap is dictated by the site and size of the skull base defect. The Hadad–Bassagasteguy flap is the commonly used axial nasoseptal flap (NSF) based on the posterior septal branch of the Sphenopalatine artery. Flaps that can be harvested from the lateral nasal wall are the anteriorly based inferior turbinate endonasal flap which is a random Pattern flap based on the anterior ethmoidal artery. The posteriorly based Inferior turbinate endonasal flap which is an axial flap based on the inferior conchal artery. The middle turbinate flap which is again an axial flap based on the middle turbinate artery. Regional flaps can also be used for reconstruction like the temperoparietal facial flap, based on the anterior branch of the superficial temporal artery. The supraorbital and supratrochlear artery based Pericranial flap and the Palatal flap (Oliver flap) based on descending palatine artery can also be used based on the location and size of the defect.

7.11.1 Introduction

Recent advances in vascular reconstruction techniques in skull base procedures have led to extended endonasal endoscopic procedures as the gold standard for anterior skull base pathologies (Fig. 7.59). It reduces short- and long-term complications like CSF leak (reduced from 20–30% to <5%) [129–131], meningitis and postoperative mortality and morbidity [132, 133].

7.11.2 Principles of Skull Base Reconstruction

Preoperative anticipation of area and size of the defect, type of leak, type of reconstruction and type of tissue available for reconstruction, sound knowledge of nasal vascular anatomy and whether reconstruction is feasible as a part of the endoscopic procedure or not, is important. Attention to the flap harvesting, storage during tumour resection, positioning (Avoid kinking of

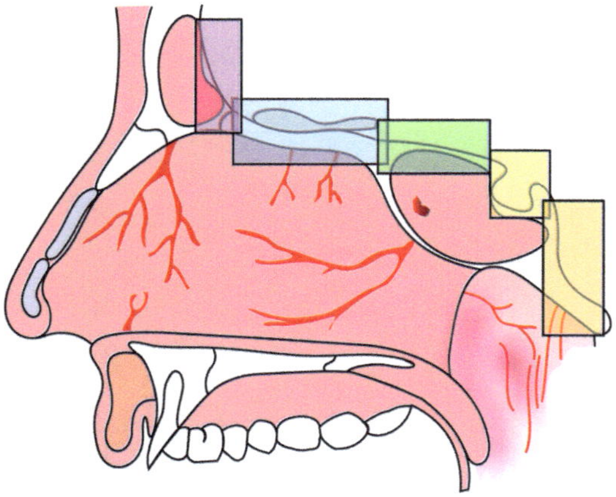

Fig. 7.59 Extended endonasal approach (1) transfrontal, (2) trans-cribriform, (3) transplanum, (4) trans-sellar, (5) trans-clival

the pedicle) and fixation over the defect is paramount for the best outcome. Flaps should be periodically removed from its stored position to reduce congestion. The flap should confound to the complex skull base defect by making the surrounding bone surface smooth and filling dead space with fat. Avoid burying of functional mucosa as this can lead to mucocele formation in the late postoperative period. Reconstruction should be robust and reliable enough to separate the nasal cavity from the cranial cavity. Small defects (CSF grades 0, 1, 2) are usually managed with non-vascularized graft [134]. Large defects (CSF grade 3, 4), defects with high central pressure, post-radiotherapy and those who need postoperative radiotherapy will need vascular reconstruction (Fig. 7.60 and Table 7.3). Restoration of normal nasal and cranial physiology as much as possible should always be attempted. Avoiding a tight nasal packing at the end of the procedure will help in retaining adequate vascularity to the harvested vascular flaps. CSF diversion can be considered in selected cases, like those where there is a direct communication of the defect with high-flow CSF pathways (communication with the third ventricle). In cases of lesion crossing lateral to pterygoid plan, contralateral falp is indicated. Covering of two contiguous areas of skull base defect is feasible with a single flap (NSF), when more than two contiguous areas involved plan more than one flap. A free mucosal graft can be used as a supplement for defect coverage along with vascularized flap. Postoperative adequate bed rest, bowel regime, head-end elevation, maintenance of airway pressure is important.

Nasal vascular anatomy (Fig. 7.61) About 40% have two branches of the posterior septal artery at sphenopalatine foramen and 70% have two branches of the posterior septal artery at the level of sphenoid ostium (Fig. 7.61c). Mean distance from sphenoid ostium is 9.3 mm (5–15 mm) [135, 136].

7.11.3 Endonasal Mucosal Flaps

1. **Nasoseptal flap (NSF)—(Hadad–Bassagasteguy flap)**—The NSF was designed by Gustavo Hadad and Luis Bassagasteguy from Argentina in 1996. It is an axial flap that is based on the posterior septal branch of the Sphenopalatine artery (Fig. 7.62b). The flap provides a large surface area and a wide arc of rotation which helps in covering defects from the frontal region till the lower Clivus (Fig. 7.62c). The side from which it should be harvested depends on anatomical variation (deviated nasal septum and turbinate anomalies), side and extent of tumour, visualization and space for instrumentation, surgeon preference, side and size of skull base defect. It is preferred to harvest the flap from the non-tumour side or from the side of the dural defect. In paediatric patients (till 14 years), due to the differential growth rate of facial skeleton with the cranium, the use of NSF is limited [131]. Contraindications for an NSF are if the tumour is involving the nasal septum or the sphenoidal rostrum and in patients in whom there is a history of previous septal surgery.

   Surgical Technique

   Adequate decongestion of the nasal mucosa as in any other endonasal surgery is essential before attempting any instrumentation and this is an essential initial step. Exposure of

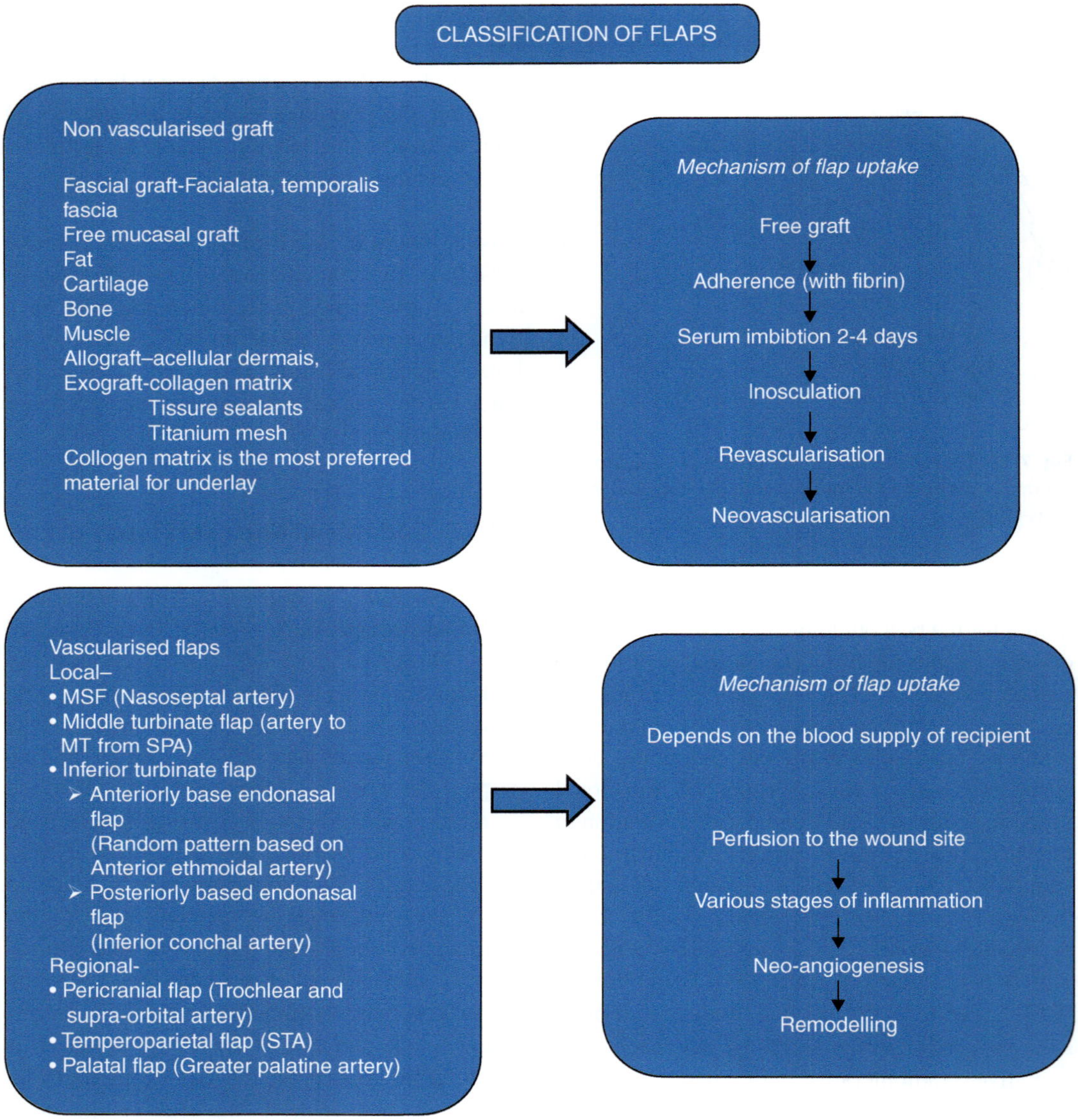

Fig. 7.60 Classification and mechanism of uptake of graft and flap

Table 7.3 Intraoperative CSF leak grading system

Grade of leak	Description
Grade 0	Absence of leak confirmed by Valsalva manoeuvre
Grade 1	Small "weeping" leak confirmed by Valsalva manoeuvre, without obvious or with only small diaphragmatic defect
Grade 2	Moderate CSF leak, with obvious diaphragmatic defect
Grade 3	Large CSF leak, resulting from dural defect that comprises the entire diaphragm or planum
Grade 4	Large CSF leak, resulting from a dural defect of: • Other single or multiple modules • Trans-sellar module and an adjacent module

Sphenoethmoidal recess is the next step, and this is done by lateralization of the middle turbinate (or partial resection) followed by resection of lower one-third of superior turbinate. This is followed by the exposure of mucosal bridge between sphenoidal ostium and upper choana. A fine tip mono-polar on 12–15 W setting is preferred for mucosal incision. The superior incision of the NSF starts just below the sphenoidal ostium and followed anteriorly 1 to 1.5 cm below the anterior skull base till the anterior end of the middle turbinate. Based on the need, it can be extended superiorly till the dorsum of the nose or anteriorly till the mucocutaneous junction. The inferior incision is made over the superior aspect of the posterior choana and extends towards the posterior part of septum and junction of septum and nasal floor, based on the need it can involve the nasal floor or the inferior turbinate (Fig 7.62a). The anterior incision is made to connect the superior and inferior incisions. The plane of dissection is in the sub-mucoperichondrial over the cartilaginous

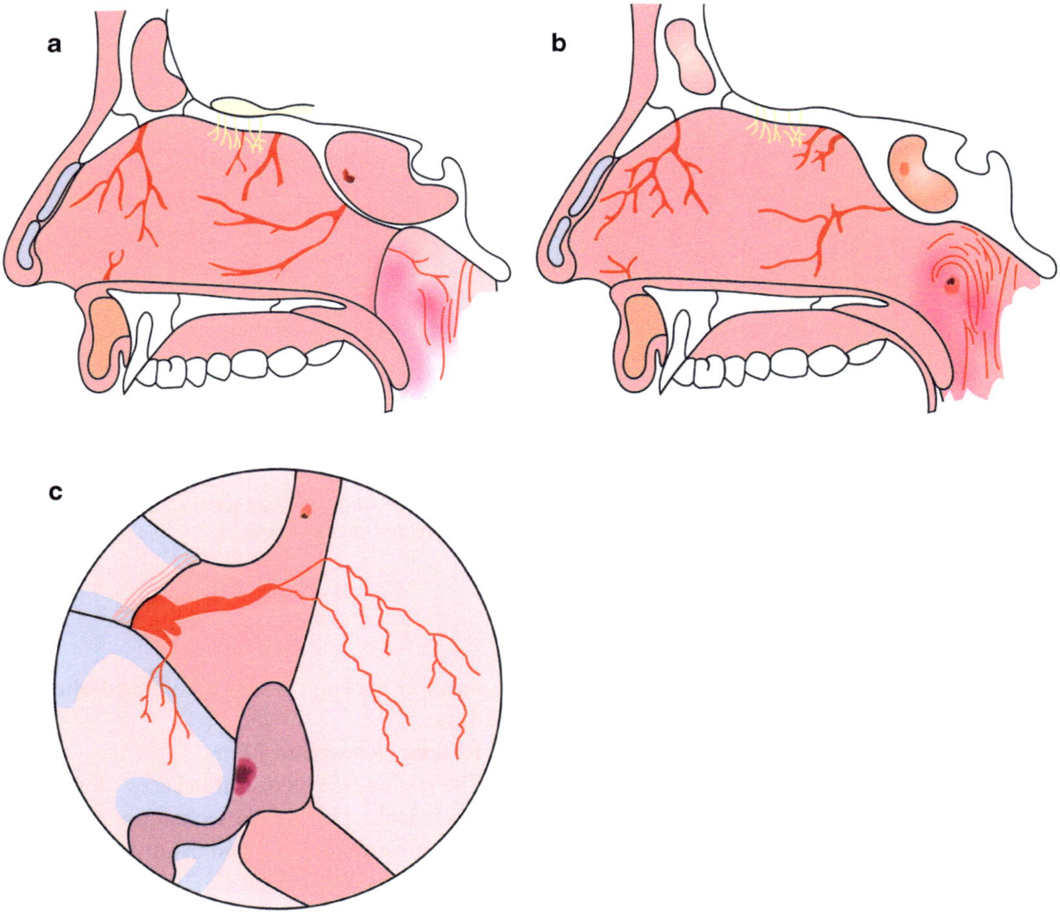

Fig. 7.61 Nasal vascular anatomy (**a**) Medial Nasal wall, (**b**) Lateral Nasal wall, (**c**) Endoscopic Posterior nasal cavity. (1) Anterior ethmoidal artery, (2) Posterior ethmoidal artery, (3) Nasoseptal branch of sphenopalatine artery (SPA), (4) Superior branch of posterior septal artery, (5) inferior branch of posterior septal artery, (6) Superior labial branch of facial artery, (7) SPA (main trunk), (8) Posterior lateral nasal artery, (9) Middle turbinate artery, (10) Inferior turbinate artery, (11) Superior turbinate, (12) Middle turbinate, (13) Inferior turbinate

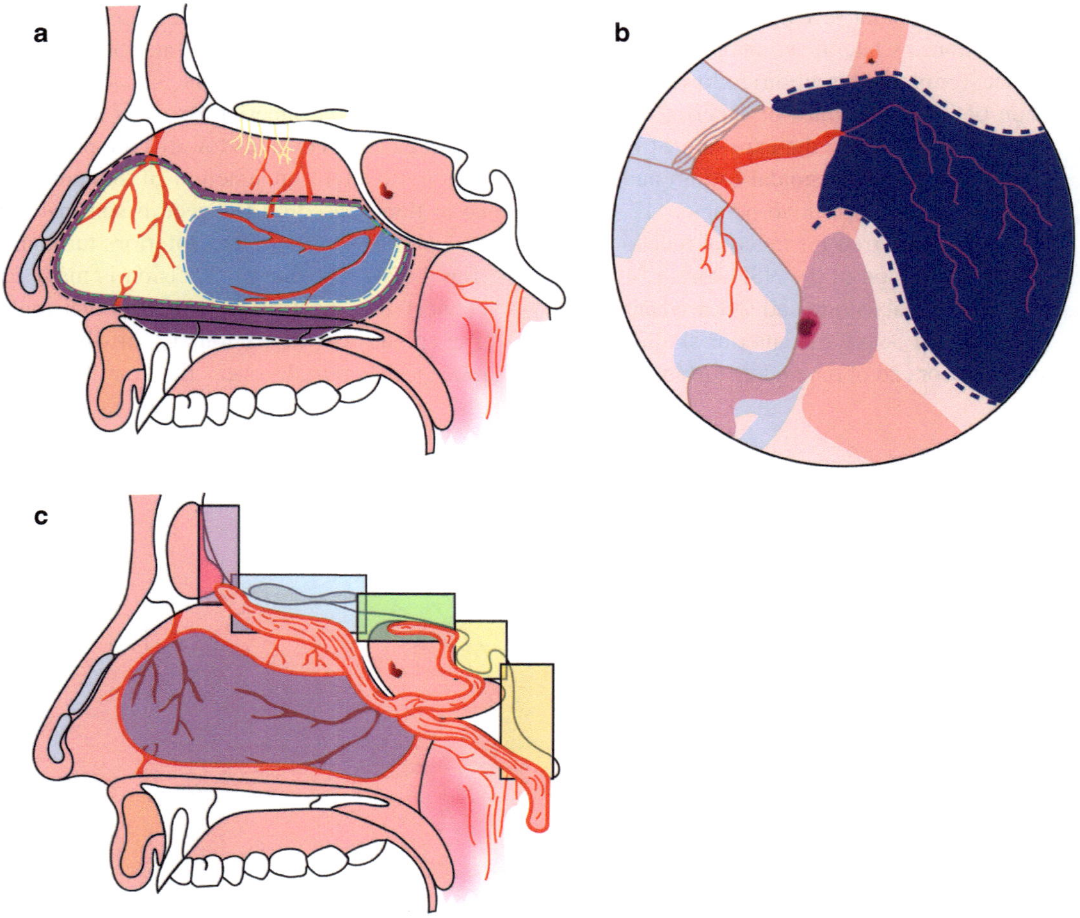

Fig. 7.62 Nasoseptal flap (NSF), (**a**) Types of NSF, (**b**) Incisions of NSF, (**c**) Uses of NSF. (1) Basic NSF, (2) anterior extension, (3) lateral extension (into floor with or without inferior turbinate mucosa), (4) superior incision, (5) inferior incision, (6) reconstruction of posterior table of the frontal sinus, (7) reconstruction of planum and sella, (8) reconstruction of clivus

nasal septum and sub-mucoperiosteal at its bony part.

After harvesting, the flap is stored in the nasopharynx or into the wide middle meatal antrostomy. Repair is preferably multilayered, inlay with collagen graft (preferred) or synthetic dural substitutes, autologous fascia, fat and onlay with vascularized flaps primarily covering the high-pressure areas and followed by layers of oxidized cellulose, tissue glue and gel foam. Final support for the reconstruction can be given using a Foley catheter or nasal packing, which is removed after 2–3 days.

2. **Rescue Nasoseptal Flap**

   The rescue NSF is useful in cases of unanticipated leaks [135]. The technique consists of identification of sphenoid ostium followed by short mucosal incision (1–2 cm) from ostium to superior septum, and this is followed by an inferior incision made over superior choana and vascular pedicle is dissected from anterior sphenoid space. Total mucosal flap elevation can be done at the end of the procedure if

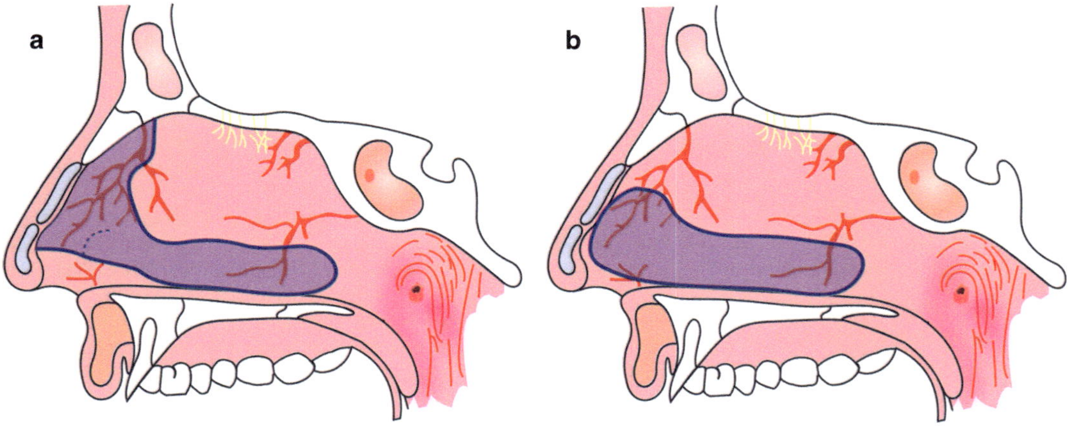

Fig. 7.63 Inferior turbinate nasal flap. (**a**) Anteriorly based flap, (**b**) posteriorly based flap

needed. The major concern about the rescue NSF is that the vascular pedicle is at risk throughout the procedure.

3. **Anteriorly Based Inferior turbinate endonasal flap** (Fig. 7.63a)
   The anteriorly based inferior turbinate endonasal flap is the random pattern flap based on anterior ethmoidal artery [137]. The Mucosa of the inferolateral nasal wall is used for the reconstruction. This flap is useful in reconstructing posterior frontal sinus defects.
4. **Posteriorly Based Inferior turbinate endonasal flap** (Fig. 7.63b)
   The posteriorly based inferior turbinate endonasal flap is an axial flap based on the inferior conchal artery. This artery enters 1–1.5 cm anterior to posterior end of inferior turbinate from the lateral side of the inferior turbinate [137]. This endonasal flap is useful in repairing small sellar and clival defects.
5. **Middle turbinate flap** (Fig. 7.64)
   The middle turbinate flap is an axial flap based on the middle turbinate artery [138]. This is useful in repairing cribriform area defects.
6. **Regional flaps**
   (a) **Temperoparietal facial flaps**
   The temperoparietal facial flap is based on the anterior branch of the superficial temporal artery. This regional flap is used for the reconstruction of defects from planum sphenoidale till the cranial–vertebral junction area. The only contraindication is any previous fronto-temporal procedures. Through a hemi-coronal incision, flap is raised between the subcutaneous tissue and superficial layer of the deep temporal facia and transported via the infratemporal fossa and the pterygopalatine fossa [139].
   (b) **Pericranial flap** (Fig. 7.30A)
   The Pericranial flap derives its vascular supply from the supraorbital and supratrochlear artery. It is used for the closure of defects from cribriform area, the sella

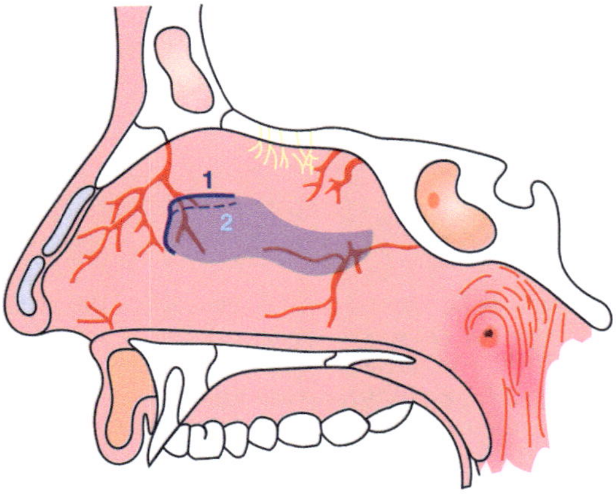

Fig. 7.64 Middle turbinate flap. (1) Anterior and medial incision, (2) lateral incision

and till the clivus. It cannot be harvested in patients who have undergone a previous fronto-temporal procedure. Through coronal incision or endoscope-assisted coronal incision pericranium flap is harvested [140].

(c) **Palatal flap (Oliver flap)**
The palatal flap or the Oliver flap is based on the descending palatine artery. It is useful for defect repair in planum, sella and clivus regions. In patients with previous palatal procedures, the flap cannot be used. The mucoperiosteal flap from the hard palate with preservation of one side greater palatine vessels is harvested transported into nasal cavity to reconstruct the skullbase defect [141].

(d) Other less commonly used flaps for skull base deconstruction are the occipital flap and the buccal flap [142].

References

1. De Lara D, Ditzel Filho LF, Prevedello DM, et al. Endonasal endoscopic approaches to the paramedian skull base. World Neurosurg. 2014;82(6 Suppl):S121–9. https://doi.org/10.1016/j.wneu.2014.07.036.
2. Kassam A, Snyderman CH, Mintz A, Gardner P, Carrau RL. Expanded endonasal approach: the rostrocaudal axis. Part I. Crista galli to the sella turcica. Neurosurg Focus. 2005;19(1):E3.
3. Cappabianca P, Cavallo LM, de Divitiis E. Endoscopic endonasal transsphenoidal surgery. Neurosurgery. 2004;55(4):933–41. https://doi.org/10.1227/01.neu.0000137330.02549.0d.
4. Goudakos JK, Markou KD, Georgalas C. Endoscopic versus microscopic trans-sphenoidal pituitary surgery: a systematic review and meta-analysis. Clin Otolaryngol. 2011;36(3):212–20. https://doi.org/10.1111/j.1749-4486.2011.02331.x.
5. Aydin S, Cavallo LM, Messina A, et al. The endoscopic endonasal trans-sphenoidal approach to the sellar and suprasellar area. Anatomic study. J Neurosurg Sci. 2007;51(3):129–38.
6. Vescan AD, Snyderman CH, Carrau RL, et al. Vidian canal: analysis and relationship to the internal carotid artery. Laryngoscope. 2007;117(8):1338–42. https://doi.org/10.1097/MLG.0b013e31806146cd.
7. Kassam A, Snyderman CH, Mintz A, Gardner P, Carrau RL. Expanded endonasal approach: the rostrocaudal axis. Part II. Posterior clinoids to the foramen magnum. Neurosurg Focus. 2005;19(1):E4.
8. Geltzeiler M, Turner M, Rimmer R, et al. Endoscopic nasopharyngectomy combined with a nerve-sparing transpterygoid approach. Laryngoscope. 2020;130:2343–8. https://doi.org/10.1002/lary.28479.
9. Locatelli D, Pozzi F, Turri-Zanoni M, et al. Transorbital endoscopic approaches to the skull base: current concepts and future perspectives. J Neurosurg Sci. 2016;60(4):514–25.
10. Kenyon B, Antisdel JL. Anatomic evaluation of endoscopic transnasal transorbital approach to the lateral orbital apex. Am J Rhinol Allergy. 2014;28(1):82–5. https://doi.org/10.2500/ajra.2014.28.4000.
11. Kong DS, Young SM, Hong CK, et al. Clinical and ophthalmological outcome of endoscopic transorbital surgery for cranioorbital tumors. J Neurosurg. 2018;131(3):667–75. https://doi.org/10.3171/2018.3.JNS173233.
12. Mehta GU, Raza SM. Endoscopic endonasal transpterygoid approach to petrous pathologies: technique, limitations and alternative approaches. J Neurosurg Sci. 2018;62(3):339–46. https://doi.org/10.23736/S0390-5616.18.04302-3.
13. Hardesty DA, Montaser AS, Carrau RL, Prevedello DM. Limits of endoscopic endonasal transpterygoid approach to cavernous sinus and Meckel's cave. J Neurosurg Sci. 2018;62(3):332–8. https://doi.org/10.23736/S0390-5616.18.04330-8.
14. Park HH, Hong SD, Kim YH, et al. Endoscopic transorbital and endonasal approach for trigeminal schwannomas: a retrospective multicenter analysis (KOSEN-005) [published online ahead of print, 2019 Jun 21]. J Neurosurg. 2019:1–10. https://doi.org/10.3171/2019.3.JNS19492.
15. Battaglia P, Turri-Zanoni M, Dallan I, et al. Endoscopic endonasal transpterygoid transmaxillary approach to the infratemporal and upper parapharyngeal tumors. Otolaryngol Head Neck Surg. 2014;150(4):696–702. https://doi.org/10.1177/0194599813520290.
16. Kasemsiri P, Carrau RL, Ditzel Filho LF, et al. Advantages and limitations of endoscopic endonasal approaches to the skull base. World Neurosurg. 2014;82(6 Suppl):S12–21. https://doi.org/10.1016/j.wneu.2014.07.022.
17. Watanabe K, Zomorodi AR, Labidi M, Satoh S, Froelich S, Fukushima T. Visualization of dark side of skull base with surgical navigation and endoscopic assistance: extended petrous rhomboid and rhomboid with maxillary nerve-mandibular nerve vidian corridor. World Neurosurg. 2019;129:e134–45. https://doi.org/10.1016/j.wneu.2019.05.062.
18. Joo W, Funaki T, Yoshioka F, Rhoton AL Jr. Microsurgical anatomy of the infratemporal fossa. Clin Anat. 2013;26(4):455–69. https://doi.org/10.1002/ca.22202.
19. Fortes FS, Sennes LU, Carrau RL, et al. Endoscopic anatomy of the pterygopalatine fossa and the transpterygoid approach: development of a surgical instruction model. Laryngoscope. 2008;118(1):44–9. https://doi.org/10.1097/MLG.0b013e318155a492.
20. Arya S, Rane P, D'Cruz A. Infratemporal Fossa, Masticator space and parapharyngeal space: Can the

radiologist and surgeon speak the same language? Otorhinolaryngol Clin. 2012;4(3):125–35.
21. Falcon RT, Rivera-Serrano CM, Miranda JF, et al. Endoscopic endonasal dissection of the infratemporal fossa: anatomic relationships and importance of eustachian tube in the endoscopic skull base surgery. Laryngoscope. 2011;121(1):31–41. https://doi.org/10.1002/lary.21341.
22. Hofstetter CP, Singh A, Anand VK, Kacker A, Schwartz TH. The endoscopic, endonasal, transmaxillary transpterygoid approach to the pterygopalatine fossa, infratemporal fossa, petrous apex, and the Meckel cave. J Neurosurg. 2010;113(5):967–74. https://doi.org/10.3171/2009.10.JNS09157.
23. Kim SM, Paek SH, Lee JH. Infratemporal fossa approach: the modified zygomatico-transmandibular approach. Maxillofac Plast Reconstr Surg. 2019;41(1):3. https://doi.org/10.1186/s40902-018-0185-x.
24. Sekhar LN, Schramm VL Jr, Jones NF. Subtemporal-preauricular infratemporal fossa approach to large lateral and posterior cranial base neoplasms. J Neurosurg. 1987;67(4):488–99. https://doi.org/10.3171/jns.1987.67.4.0488.
25. Jain R, Keshri A, Manogaran R, Kumar R, Keeranghat P. Preauricular transzygomatic approach for infratemporal fossa and surrounding skull base lesion: an institutional experience. Ann Otol Neurotol. 2018;01(02):094–9.
26. Parent AD, Brown B, Smith EE. Incidental pituitary adenomas: a retrospective study. Surgery. 1982;92(5):880–3.
27. Willemse RB, van Furth WR, Fokkens W, CG. Endoscopic approach to the sella. In: Georgalas C, Fokkens W, editors. Rhinology and skull base surgery from the lab to the operating room: an evidence-based approach. Thieme, New York. Stuttgart; 2013. p. 738–57.
28. Marcello D. Bronstein. Surgical indications for pituitarytumors. In: Stamm AIC, editor. Transnasal endoscopic skull base and brain surgery tips and pearls. New York: Thieme, Stuttgart; 2011. p. 224–7.
29. Teramoto A, Hirakawa K, Sanno N, Osamura Y. Incidental pituitary lesions in 1,000 unselected autopsy specimens. Radiology. 1994;193(1):161–4. https://doi.org/10.1148/radiology.193.1.8090885.
30. Hall WA, Luciano MG, Doppman JL, Patronas NJ, Oldfield EH. Pituitary magnetic resonance imaging in normal human volunteers: occult adenomas in the general population. Ann Intern Med. 1994;120(10):817–20. https://doi.org/10.7326/0003-4819-120-10-199405150-00001.
31. Dekkers OM, Pereira AM, Romijn JA. Treatment and follow-up of clinically nonfunctioning pituitary macroadenomas. J Clin Endocrinol Metab. 2008;93(10):3717–26. https://doi.org/10.1210/jc.2008-0643.
32. Bronstein MD, Musolino NR, Benabou S, Marino R Jr. Cerebrospinal fluid rhinorrhea occurring in long-term bromocriptine treatment for macroprolactinomas. Surg Neurol. 1989;32(5):346–9. https://doi.org/10.1016/0090-3019(89)90137-7.
33. Bronstein MD. Prolactinomas and pregnancy. Pituitary. 2005;8(1):31–8. https://doi.org/10.1007/s11102-005-5083-4.
34. Jallad RS, Musolino NR, Salgado LR, Bronstein MD. Treatment of acromegaly: is there still a place for radiotherapy? Pituitary. 2007;10(1):53–9. https://doi.org/10.1007/s11102-007-0002-5.
35. Pivonello R, De Martino MC, De Leo M, Lombardi G, Colao A. Cushing's Syndrome. Endocrinol Metab Clin N Am. 2008;37(1):135–149, ix. https://doi.org/10.1016/j.ecl.2007.10.010.
36. Sindwani R, Woodard TD, Recinos PF. Endoscopic cranial base and pituitary surgery. Otolaryngol Clin N Am. 2016;49(1):xix–xx. https://doi.org/10.1016/j.otc.2015.09.01.
37. Sethi DS, Leong JL. Endoscopic pituitary surgery. Otolaryngol Clin North Am. 2006;39(3):563. https://doi.org/10.1016/j.otc.2006.01.011.
38. Favier V, Boetto J, Cartier C, Segnarbieux F, Crampette L. Endoscopic transnasal transseptal pituitary surgery. Eur Ann Otorhinolaryngol Head Neck Dis. 2019;136(2):131–4. https://doi.org/10.1016/j.anorl.2018.10.005.
39. de Almeida JR, Zanation AM, Snyderman CH, et al. Defining the nasopalatine line: the limit for endonasal surgery of the spine. Laryngoscope. 2009;119(2):239–44. https://doi.org/10.1002/lary.20108.
40. Yasuda A, Campero A, Martins C, Rhoton AL Jr, de Oliveira E, Ribas GC. Microsurgical anatomy and approaches to the cavernous sinus. Neurosurgery. 2005;56(1 Suppl):4–27. https://doi.org/10.1227/01.neu.0000144208.42171.02.
41. Donald PJ. Skull base surgery for malignancy: when not to operate. Eur Arch Otorhinolaryngol. 2007;264(7):713–7. https://doi.org/10.1007/s00405-007-0268-2.
42. Svane-Knudsen V, Jørgensen KE, Hansen O, Lindgren A, Marker P. Cancer of the nasal cavity and paranasal sinuses: a series of 115 patients. Rhinology. 1998;36(1):12–4.
43. Loy AH, Reibel JF, Read PW, et al. Esthesioneuroblastoma: continued follow-up of a single institution's experience. Arch Otolaryngol Head Neck Surg. 2006;132(2):134–8. https://doi.org/10.1001/archotol.132.2.134.
44. Lin EM, Sparano A, Spalding A, et al. Sinonasal undifferentiated carcinoma: a 13-year experience at a single institution. Skull Base. 2010;20(2):61–7. https://doi.org/10.1055/s-0029-1236165.
45. Janecka IP, Sen CN, Sekhar LN, Arriaga M. Facial translocation: a new approach to the cranial base. Otolaryngol Head Neck Surg. 1990;103(3):413–9. https://doi.org/10.1177/019459989010300312.
46. Cheesman AD, Reddy K. Craniofacial resection: a 10 year experience. Proceedings of the 15th European Rhinologic Congress; 1995.
47. Abu-Ghanem S, Fliss DM. Surgical approaches to resection of anterior skull base and paranasal sinuses

tumors. Balkan Med J. 2013;30(2):136–41. https://doi.org/10.5152/balkanmedj.2013.9112.
48. Donald PJ. Frontobasal approach for trauma and tumor. Minim Invasive Neurosurg. 1994;37(2):37–41. https://doi.org/10.1055/s-2008-1053446.
49. Elbabaa SK, Al-Mefty O. Craniofacial approach for anterior skull-base lesions. Atlas Oral Maxillofac Surg Clin North Am. 2010;18(2):151–60. https://doi.org/10.1016/j.cxom.2010.08.007.
50. Hendryk S, Czecior E, Misiołek M, Namysłowski G, Mrówka R. Surgical strategies in the removal of malignant tumors and benign lesions of the anterior skull base. Neurosurg Rev. 2004;27(3):205–13. https://doi.org/10.1007/s10143-004-0323-z.
51. McCutcheon IE, Blacklock JB, Weber RS, et al. Anterior transcranial (craniofacial) resection of tumors of the paranasal sinuses: surgical technique and results. Neurosurgery. 1996;38(3):471–80. https://doi.org/10.1097/00006123-199603000-00009.
52. Raveh J, Laedrach K, Speiser M, et al. The subcranial approach for fronto-orbital and anteroposterior skull-base tumors. Arch Otolaryngol Head Neck Surg. 1993;119(4):385–93. https://doi.org/10.1001/archotol.1993.01880160029006.
53. Spektor S, Valarezo J, Fliss DM, et al. Olfactory groove meningiomas from neurosurgical and ear, nose, and throat perspectives: approaches, techniques, and outcomes. Neurosurgery. 2005;57(4 Suppl):268–80. https://doi.org/10.1227/01.neu.0000176409.70668.eb.
54. Abergel A, Fliss DM, Margalit N, Gil Z. A prospective evaluation of short-term health-related quality of life in patients undergoing anterior skull base surgery. Skull Base. 2010;20(1):27–33. https://doi.org/10.1055/s-0029-1242982.
55. Jones LT, Linn ML. The diagnosis of the causes of epiphora. Am J Ophthalmol. 1969;67:751–4.
56. Somma F, d'Agostino V, Tortora F, et al. Magnetic resonance imaging in the pre-operative evaluation of obstructive epiphora: true-FISP and VIBE vs gadolinium. Radiol Med. 2017;122(2):123–30. https://doi.org/10.1007/s11547-016-0696-4.
57. Savino G, Battendieri R, Traina S, et al. External vs. endonasal dacryocystorhinostomy: has the current view changed? Acta Otorhinolaryngol Ital. 2014;34(1):29–35.
58. Rudert H, Maune S, Mahnke CG. Komplikationen der endonasalen Chirurgie der Nasennebenhöhlen. Inzidenz und Strategien zu ihrer Vermeidung [Complications of endonasal surgery of the paranasal sinuses. Incidence and strategies for prevention]. Laryngorhinootologie. 1997;76(4):200–15. https://doi.org/10.1055/s-2007-997414.
59. Hashemi SM, Eshaghian A. Limited approach in endoscopic dacryocystorhinostomy of pediatrics. Adv Biomed Res. 2017;6:141. https://doi.org/10.4103/abr.abr_375_14.
60. Metson R. Endoscopic surgery for lacrimal obstruction. Otolaryngol Head Neck Surg. 1991;104(4):473–9. https://doi.org/10.1177/019459989110400408.
61. Herzallah I, Alzuraiqi B, Bawazeer N, et al. Endoscopic Dacryocystorhinostomy (DCR): a comparative study between powered and non-powered technique. J Otolaryngol Head Neck Surg. 2015;44:56. https://doi.org/10.1186/s40463-015-0109-z.
62. Khalifa MA, Ragab SM, Saafan ME, El-Guindy AS. Endoscopic dacryocystorhinostomy with double posteriorly based nasal and lacrimal flaps: a prospective randomized controlled trial. Otolaryngol Head Neck Surg. 2012;147(4):782–7. https://doi.org/10.1177/0194599812447759.
63. Mueller SK, Freitag SK, Lefebvre DR, Bleier BS. Endoscopic DCR using bipedicled interlacing mucosal flaps. Laryngoscope. 2018;128(4):794–7. https://doi.org/10.1002/lary.26730.
64. Tsirbas A, Wormald PJ. Endonasal dacryocystorhinostomy with mucosal flaps. Am J Ophthalmol. 2003;135(1):76–83. https://doi.org/10.1016/s0002-9394(02)01830-5.
65. Tabatabaie SZ, Heirati A, Rajabi MT, Kasaee A. Silicone intubation with intraoperative mitomycin C for nasolacrimal duct obstruction in adults: a prospective, randomized, double-masked study. Ophthalmic Plast Reconstr Surg. 2007;23(6):455–8. https://doi.org/10.1097/IOP.0b013e3181579795.
66. Tsirbas A, Davis G, Wormald PJ. Mechanical endonasal dacryocystorhinostomy versus external dacryocystorhinostomy. Ophthalmic Plast Reconstr Surg. 2004;20(1):50–6. https://doi.org/10.1097/01.IOP.0000103006.49679.23.
67. Selig YK, Biesman BS, Rebeiz EE. Topical application of mitomycin-C in endoscopic dacryocystorhinostomy. Am J Rhinol. 2000;14(3):205–7. https://doi.org/10.2500/105065800782102672.
68. Saeed BM. Endoscopic DCR without stents: clinical guidelines and procedure. Eur Arch Otorhinolaryngol. 2012;269(2):545–9. https://doi.org/10.1007/s00405-011-1727-3.
69. Kang MG, Shim WS, Shin DK, Kim JY, Lee JE, Jung HJ. A systematic review of benefit of silicone intubation in endoscopic dacryocystorhinostomy. Clin Exp Otorhinolaryngol. 2018;11(2):81–8. https://doi.org/10.21053/ceo.2018.00031.
70. Dave TV, Mohammed FA, Ali MJ, Naik MN. Etiologic analysis of 100 anatomically failed dacryocystorhinostomies. Clin Ophthalmol. 2016;10:1419–22. https://doi.org/10.2147/OPTH.S113733.
71. Joshi RS. Conventional dacryocystorhinostomy in a failed Trans-canalicular laser-assisted dacryocystorhinostomy. Indian J Ophthalmol. 2011;59(5):383–5. https://doi.org/10.4103/0301-4738.83617.
72. Sivak-Callcott JA, Linberg JV, Patel S. Ultrasonic bone removal with the Sonopet Omni: a new instrument for orbital and lacrimal surgery. Arch Ophthalmol. 2005;123(11):1595–7. https://doi.org/10.1001/archopht.123.11.1595.
73. Kato K, Matsunaga K, Takashima Y, Kondo M. Probing of congenital nasolacrimal duct obstruction with dacryoendoscope. Clin Ophthalmol. 2014;8:977–80. https://doi.org/10.2147/OPTH.S60377.

74. Lim C, Martin P, Benger R, Kourt G, Ghabrial R. Lacrimal canalicular bypass surgery with the Lester Jones tube. Am J Ophthalmol. 2004;137(1):101–8. https://doi.org/10.1016/j.ajo.2003.08.002.
75. Nomura K, Arakawa K, Sugawara M, Hidaka H, Suzuki J, Katori Y. Factors influencing endoscopic dacryocystorhinostomy outcome. Eur Arch Otorhinolaryngol. 2017;274(7):2773–7. https://doi.org/10.1007/s00405-017-4541-8.
76. Kuczkowski J, Narozny W, Stankiewicz C, et al. Sluzowiaki zatok przynosowych [Mucoceles of the paranasal sinuses]. Otolaryngol Pol. 2007;61(5):680–6. https://doi.org/10.1016/S0030-6657(07)70506-1.
77. Lund VJ. Anatomical considerations in the aetiology of fronto-ethmoidal mucoceles. Rhinology. 1987;25:83–8.
78. Benkhatar H, Khettab I, Sultanik P, Laccourreye O, Bonfils P. Mucocele development after endoscopic sinus surgery for nasal polyposis: a long-term analysis. Ear Nose Throat J. 2018;97(9):284–94. https://doi.org/10.1177/014556131809700918.
79. Lund VJ, Harvey W, Meghji S, Harris M. Prostaglandin synthesis in the pathogenesis of fronto-ethmoidal mucoceles. Acta Otolaryngologica. 1988;106:145–51.
80. Lund VJ, Henderson B, Song Y. Involvement of cytokines and vascular adhesion receptors in the pathology of fronto-ethmoidal mucoceles. Acta Otolaryngologica. 1993;113:540–6.
81. Hansen FS, van der Poel NA, Freling NJM, Fokkens WJ. Mucocele formation after frontal sinus obliteration. Rhinology. 2018;56(2):106–10. https://doi.org/10.4193/Rhin17.187.
82. Weissman JL, Tabor EK, Curtin HD. Magnetic resonance imaging of the paranasal sinuses. Top Magn Reson Imaging. 1990;2(4):27–38.
83. Kennedy DW, Josephson JS, Zinreich SJ, Mattox DE, Goldsmith MM. Endoscopic sinus surgery for mucoceles. Laryngoscope. 1989;99:885–95.
84. Facon F, Nicollas R, Paris J, Dessi P. La chirurgie des mucocèles sinusiennes: notre expérience à propos de 52 cas suivis à moyen terme [Surgery of mucocele of the paranasal sinuses: report of 52 cases with a middle term follow up]. Rev Laryngol Otol Rhinol (Bord). 2008;129(3):167–73.
85. Santos PLD, Chihara LL, Alcalde LFA, Masalskas BF, Sant'Ana E, Faria PEP. Outcomes in surgical treatment of mucocele in frontal sinus. J Craniofac Surg. 2017;28(7):1702–8. https://doi.org/10.1097/SCS.0000000000003224.
86. Venail F, Marlier F, Makeieff M, et al. Indications des voies combinées (endoscopique et externe) dans le traitement des mucocèles sinusiennes [Combined approach (endoscopic and external) for the treatment of sinusal mucoceles]. Rev Laryngol Otol Rhinol (Bord). 2003;124(3):165–70.
87. Khong JJ, Malhotra R, Selva D, Wormald PJ. Efficacy of endoscopic sinus surgery for paranasal sinus mucocele including modified endoscopic Lothrop procedure for frontal sinus mucocele. J Laryngol Otol. 2004;118(5):352–6. https://doi.org/10.1258/002221504323086534.
88. Courson AM, Stankiewicz JA, Lal D. Contemporary management of frontal sinus mucoceles: a meta-analysis. Laryngoscope. 2014;124(2):378–86. https://doi.org/10.1002/lary.24309.
89. Reale G, Ungari C, Riccardi E, et al. Fronto-ethmoidal osteoma. Open treatment. Ann Ital Chir. 2014;85(3):214–8.
90. Brown OE, Pownell P, Manning SC. Choanal atresia: a new anatomic classification and clinical management applications. Laryngoscope. 1996;106(1 Pt 1):97–101. https://doi.org/10.1097/00005537-199601000-00019.
91. Kurosaka H. Choanal atresia and stenosis: development and diseases of the nasal cavity. Wiley Interdiscip Rev Dev Biol. 2019;8(1):e336. https://doi.org/10.1002/wdev.336.
92. Ramsden JD, Campisi P, Forte V. Choanal atresia and choanal stenosis. Otolaryngol Clin North Am. 2009;42(2):339. https://doi.org/10.1016/j.otc.2009.01.001.
93. Dupé V, Matt N, Garnier JM, Chambon P, Mark M, Ghyselinck NB. A newborn lethal defect due to inactivation of retinaldehyde dehydrogenase type 3 is prevented by maternal retinoic acid treatment. Proc Natl Acad Sci U S A. 2003;100(24):14036–41. https://doi.org/10.1073/pnas.2336223100.
94. Barbero P, Valdez R, Rodríguez H, et al. Choanal atresia associated with maternal hyperthyroidism treated with methimazole: a case-control study. Am J Med Genet A. 2008;146A(18):2390–5. https://doi.org/10.1002/ajmg.a.32497.
95. Kwong KM. Current updates on choanal atresia. Front Pediatr. 2015;3:52. https://doi.org/10.3389/fped.2015.00052.
96. Holtmann L, Stähr K, Kirchner J, Lang S, Mattheis S. Die endonasale endoskopische Resektion von Choanalatresien – wie groß ist der Langzeiterfolg? [Endonasal endoscopic surgery of choanal atresia – long term results]. Laryngorhinootologie. 2018; https://doi.org/10.1055/s-0044-101464.
97. Saraniti C, Santangelo M, Salvago P. Surgical treatment of choanal atresia with transnasal endoscopic approach with stentless single side-hinged flap technique: 5 year retrospective analysis. Braz J Otorhinolaryngol. 2017;83(2):183–9. https://doi.org/10.1016/j.bjorl.2016.03.009.
98. Eladl HM, Khafagy YW. Endoscopic bilateral congenital choanal atresia repair of 112 cases, evolving concept and technical experience. Int J Pediatr Otorhinolaryngol. 2016;85:40–5. https://doi.org/10.1016/j.ijporl.2016.03.011.
99. De Freitas RP, Berkowitz RG. Bilateral choanal atresia repair in neonates--a single surgeon experience. Int J Pediatr Otorhinolaryngol. 2012;76(6):873–8. https://doi.org/10.1016/j.ijporl.2012.02.063.
100. Durmaz A, Tosun F, Yldrm N, Sahan M, Kvrakdal C, Gerek M. Transnasal endoscopic repair of choanal atresia: results of 13 cases and meta-analysis.

J Craniofac Surg. 2008;19(5):1270–4. https://doi.org/10.1097/SCS.0b013e3181843564.
101. Wormald PJ, Zhao YC, Valdes CJ, et al. The endoscopic transseptal approach for choanal atresia repair. Int Forum Allergy Rhinol. 2016;6(6):654–60. https://doi.org/10.1002/alr.21716.
102. Cedin AC, Atallah AN, Andriolo RB, Cruz OL, Pignatari SN. Surgery for congenital choanal atresia. Cochrane Database Syst Rev. 2012;2:CD008993. https://doi.org/10.1002/14651858.CD008993.pub2.
103. Murray S, Luo L, Quimby A, Barrowman N, Vaccani JP, Caulley L. Immediate versus delayed surgery in congenital choanal atresia: a systematic review. Int J Pediatr Otorhinolaryngol. 2019;119:47–53. https://doi.org/10.1016/j.ijporl.2019.01.001.
104. Moreddu E, Rizzi M, Adil E, et al. International Pediatric Otolaryngology Group (IPOG) consensus recommendations: diagnosis, pre-operative, operative and post-operative pediatric choanal atresia care. Int J Pediatr Otorhinolaryngol. 2019;123:151–5. https://doi.org/10.1016/j.ijporl.2019.05.010.
105. Bedwell JR, Choi SS. Are stents necessary after choanal atresia repair? Laryngoscope. 2012;122(11):2365–6. https://doi.org/10.1002/lary.23381.
106. Keller JL, Kacker A. Choanal atresia, CHARGE association, and congenital nasal stenosis. Otolaryngol Clin North Am. 2000;33(6):1343-viii. https://doi.org/10.1016/s0030-6665(05)70285-1.
107. Ommaya AK, Di Chiro G, Baldwin M, Pennybacker JB. Non-traumatic cerebrospinal fluid rhinorrhea. J Neurol Neu-rosurg Psychiatry. 1968;31:214–25.
108. Chan DT, Poon WS, IP CP, Chiu PW, goh KY. How useful is glucose detection in diagnosing cerebrospinal fluid leak? The rational use of CT and Beta-2 transferrin assay in detection of cerebrospinal fluid fistula. Asian J Surg. 2004;27(1):39–42. https://doi.org/10.1016/S1015-9584(09)60242-6.
109. Schuknecht B, Simmen D, Briner HR, Holzmann D. Nontraumatic skull base defects with spontaneous CSF rhinorrhea and arachnoid herniation: imaging findings and correlation with endoscopic sinus surgery in 27 patients. AJNR Am J Neuroradiol. 2008;29(3):542–9. https://doi.org/10.3174/ajnr.A0840.
110. Casiano RR, Jassir D. Endoscopic cerebrospinal fluid rhinorrhea repair: is a lumbar drain necessary? Otolaryngol Head Neck Surg. 1999;121(6):745–50. https://doi.org/10.1053/hn.1999.v121.a98754.
111. Brodie HA. Prophylactic antibiotics for post-traumatic cerebrospinal fluid fistulae. A meta-analysis. Arch Otolaryngol Head Neck Surg. 1997;123(7):749–52. https://doi.org/10.1001/archotol.1997.01900070093016.
112. Chaaban MR, Illing E, Riley KO, Woodworth BA. Acetazolamide for high intracranial pressure cerebrospinal fluid leaks. Int Forum Allergy Rhinol. 2013;3(9):718–21. https://doi.org/10.1002/alr.21188.
113. Scholsem M, Scholtes F, Collignon F, et al. Surgical management of anterior cranial base fractures with cerebrospinal fluid fistulae: a single-institution experience. Neurosurgery. 2008;62(2):463–71. https://doi.org/10.1227/01.neu.0000316014.97926.82.
114. Briggs RJ, Wormald PJ. Endoscopic transnasal intradural repair of anterior skull base cerebrospinal fluid fistulae. J Clin Neurosci. 2004;11(6):597–9. https://doi.org/10.1016/j.jocn.2003.09.011.
115. Wormald PJ, McDonogh M. 'Bath-plug' technique for the endoscopic management of cerebrospinal fluid leaks. J Laryngol Otol. 1997;111(11):1042–6. https://doi.org/10.1017/s0022215100139295.
116. Hegazy HM, Carrau RL, Snyderman CH, Kassam A, Zweig J. Transnasal endoscopic repair of cerebrospinal fluid rhinorrhea: a meta-analysis. Laryngoscope. 2000;110(7):1166–72. https://doi.org/10.1097/00005537-200007000-00019.
117. Steinsapir KD, Goldberg RA. Traumatic optic neuropathy. Surv Ophthalmol. 1994;38(6):487–518. https://doi.org/10.1016/0039-6257(94)90145-7.
118. Steinsapir KD, Goldberg RA. Traumatic optic neuropathy: a critical update. Compr Ophthalmol Updat. 2005;6(1):11–21.
119. Yu-Wai-Man P. Traumatic optic neuropathy-clinical features and management issues. Taiwan J Ophthalmol. 2015;5(1):3–8. https://doi.org/10.1016/j.tjo.2015.01.003.
120. Saeed P, Tavakoli Rad S, Bisschop PHLT. Dysthyroid optic neuropathy. Ophthalmic Plast Reconstr Surg. 2018;34(4S Suppl 1):S60–7. https://doi.org/10.1097/IOP.0000000000001146.
121. Abe T, Satoh K, Wada A. Optic nerve decompression for orbitofrontal fibrous dysplasia: recent development of surgical technique and equipment. Skull Base. 2006;16(3):145–55. https://doi.org/10.1055/s-2006-949517.
122. Levin LA, Beck RW, Joseph MP, Seiff S, Kraker R. The treatment of traumatic optic neuropathy: the International Optic Nerve Trauma Study. Ophthalmology. 1999;106(7):1268–77. https://doi.org/10.1016/s0161-6420(99)00707-1.
123. Yu-Wai-Man P, Griffiths PG. Steroids for traumatic optic neuropathy. Cochrane Database Syst Rev. 2013;6:CD006032. https://doi.org/10.1002/14651858.CD006032.pub4.
124. Oh HJ, Yeo DG, Hwang SC. Surgical treatment for traumatic optic neuropathy. Korean J Neurotrauma. 2018;14(2):55–60. https://doi.org/10.13004/kjnt.2018.14.2.55.
125. Dhaliwal SS, Sowerby LJ, Rotenberg BW. Timing of endoscopic surgical decompression in traumatic optic neuropathy: a systematic review of the literature. Int Forum Allergy Rhinol. 2016;6(6):661–7. https://doi.org/10.1002/alr.21706.
126. Thakar A, Mahapatra AK, Tandon DA. Delayed optic nerve decompression for indirect optic nerve injury. Laryngoscope. 2003;113(1):112–9. https://doi.org/10.1097/00005537-200301000-00021.

127. Metson R, Pletcher SD. Endoscopic orbital and optic nerve decompression. Otolaryngol Clin N Am. 2006;39(3):551–ix. https://doi.org/10.1016/j.otc.2006.01.004.
128. Kumaran AM, Sundar G, Chye LT. Traumatic optic neuropathy: a review. Craniomaxillofac Trauma Reconstr. 2015;8(1):31–41. https://doi.org/10.1055/s-0034-1393734.
129. Harvey RJ, Nogueira JF, Schlosser RJ, Patel SJ, Vellutini E, Stamm AC. Closure of large skull base defects after endoscopic transnasal craniotomy. J Neurosurg. 2009;111(2):371–9.
130. Kassam AB, Thomas A, Carrau RL, Snyderman CH, Vescan A, Prevedello D, et al. Endoscopic reconstruction of the cranial base using a pedicled nasoseptal flap. Neurosurgery. 2008;63(1 Suppl 1):ONS44–52; discussion ONS52–3
131. Shah RN, Surowitz JB, Patel MR, Huang BY, Snyderman CH, Carrau RL, et al. Endoscopic pedicled nasoseptal flap reconstruction for pediatric skull base defects. Laryngoscope. 2009;119(6):1067–75.
132. Harvey RJ, Smith JE, Wise SK, Patel SJ, Frankel BM, Schlosser RJ. Intracranial complications before and after endoscopic skull base reconstruction. Am J Rhinol. 2008;22(5):516–21.
133. Hadad G, Bassagasteguy L, Carrau RL, Mataza JC, Kassam A, Snyderman CH, et al. A novel reconstructive technique after endoscopic expanded endonasal approaches: vascular pedicle nasoseptal flap. Laryngoscope. 2006;116(10):1882–6.
134. Esposito F, Dusick JR, Fatemi N, Kelly DF. Graded repair of cranial base defects and cerebrospinal fluid leaks in transsphenoidal surgery. Oper Neurosurg. 2007;60(4 Suppl 2):295–304.
135. Pinheiro CD, Synderman CH. Nasoseptal flap. Adv Otorhinolaryngol. 2013;74:42–55.
136. Pinheiro-neto CD, Ramos HF, Peris-celda M, Fernandez-miranda JC, Gardner PA, Snyderman CH, et al. Study of the nasoseptal flap for endoscopic anterior cranial base reconstruction. Laryngoscope. 2011;121(12):2514–20.
137. Stamm AC, editor. 44 Management of skull base defects after extended endoscopic skull base surgery: from free grafts to vascularized flaps. In: Transnasal endoscopic skull base and brain surgery. Stuttgart: Georg Thieme Verlag; 2011.
138. Georgalas C, Fokkens W, editors. Reconstruction of the skull base and management of skull base surgery complications. In: Rhinology and skull base surgery. Stuttgart: Georg Thieme Verlag; 2013.
139. Fortes FSG, Carrau RL, Snyderman CH, Kassam A, Prevedello D, Vescan A, et al. Transpterygoid transposition of a temporoparietal fascia flap: a new method for skull base reconstruction after endoscopic expanded endonasal approaches. Laryngoscope. 2007;117(6):970–6.
140. Patel MR, Shah RN, Snyderman CH, Carrau RL, Germanwala AV, Kassam AB, et al. Pericranial flap for endoscopic anterior skull-base reconstruction. Neurosurgery. 2010;66(3):506–12.
141. Oliver CL, Hackman TG, Carrau RL, Snyderman CH, Kassam AB, Prevedello DM, et al. Palatal flap modifications allow pedicled reconstruction of the skull base. Laryngoscope. 2008;118(12):2102–6.
142. Patel MR, Taylor RJ, Hackman TG, Germanwala AV, Sasaki-Adams D, Ewend MG, et al. Beyond the nasoseptal flap: outcomes and pearls with secondary flaps in endoscopic endonasal skull base reconstruction. Laryngoscope. 2014;124(4):846–52.

Prevention and Management of Complications

8

Anupam Kanodia, Hitesh Verma, Avni Jain, Gopica Kalsotra, Sheetal Kumari, Sonu Kumari Agrawal, Hitender Gautam, Darwin Kaushal, Abhishek Gugliani, and Jaini Lodha

Contents

A. Kanodia · H. Verma (✉)
ENT, AIIMS, New Delhi, India
e-mail: drhitesh10@gmail.com

A. Jain
ENT, ESIC Medical College Faridabad, Faridabad, Haryana, India

G. Kalsotra · S. Kumari
ENT, GMC, Jammu, India

S. K. Agrawal · H. Gautam
Microbiology, AIIMS, New Delhi, India

D. Kaushal · A. Gugliani
ENT, AIIMS, Jodhpur, Rajasthan, India

J. Lodha
ENT, Seven Hills Hospital, Andheri East Mumbai, Maharashtra, India

H. Verma, A. Thakar (eds.), *Essentials of Rhinology*, https://doi.org/10.1007/978-981-33-6284-0_8

8.1 Part A: Cavity Management

Performance of FESS for a patient suffering from nasal polyposis or just chronic rhinosinusitis is only half the work done. Post-operative management of the patient is as important as the surgery itself. A good follow-up with endoscopic suction cleaning allows the cavity to heal with minimum scarring and adhesion formation. An ideal post-FESS nasal cavity is a cavity without scars or adhesions; with all the diseased sinuses adequately opened to allow medical therapy to penetrate them. A good cavity care decreases the chances of infection in the nasal cavity, prevents scar formation and hastens normal healing by enhancing mucosa to grow over the raw areas.

To achieve a healthy nasal cavity post-surgery, the patient should be religiously followed-up in the post-operative period (Fig. 8.1). The first follow-up in the post-operative period is pack removal. If absorbable nasal packing has been used, then the first follow-up can be after 3–7 days of surgery. However, if the conventional nasal pack has been placed, it should be removed with in 2–3 days, using liberal saline and glycerine irrigation. Following this, the patient needs to follow-up every week for at least 1 month, thereafter if the cavity has healed, he may be asked to follow-up every 3–6 months subsequently.

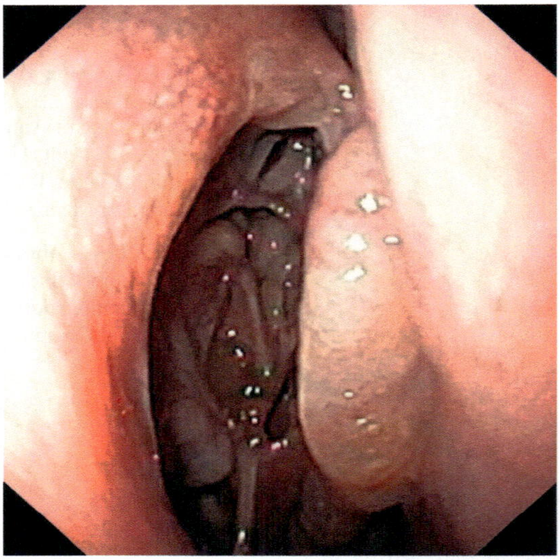

Fig. 8.1 Healed right nasal cavity with few adhesions

Saline irrigations are preferably continued lifelong [1, 2]. On follow-up visits, the patient undergoes nasal endoscopic evaluation of the cavity. Any blood clots, crusts or debris are cleaned. Any swelling around the nose or eyes needs to be examined, any deterioration in vision or double vision needs to be evaluated further.

The cavity care is similar for patients who undergo surgery for malignancy. However, during the follow-up visits, the operating surgeon needs to clean the cavity endoscopically, simultaneously looking for any evidence of recurrence of malignancy.

8.1.1 Nasal Packing Post-Surgery

Nasal tampons with smooth and fine pores have little tendency to adhere to tissues and hence cause decreased pain on removal. Cotton gauze strips cause the most discomfort, followed by the non-coated polyvinyl acetal packs, followed by the other types. Nasal packing should only be done when required and should be removed or replaced in 24–48 h depending on the extent of surgery.

Pack removal can be done in the sitting position, with the patient holding a bowl under his nose for holding the removed pack and to collect the discharge that occurs subsequently. Adequate lubrication of the pack needs to be done with normal saline, glycerine and lignocaine (2%). An analgesic can be administered 1 h prior to pack removal. Once the pack is adequately softened, it may be pulled out very slowly using the rotatory movement of the wrist and forearm. One pack should be removed at a time. After removal, topical nasal rinsing may be done using saline and glycerine. Xylometazoline may be added for better haemostasis. Posterior pharyngeal wall needs evaluation for any active bleeding.

Patient needs to be observed for 30–60 min after complete pack removal for any residual anterior or posterior bleeding. Thereafter patient can be discharged.

Post pack removal, nasal saline mist sprays should be used every 2–4 hours to prevent crust formation and clot deposition. Some bleeding might happen from the nasal cavity while doing nasal cavity irrigation with saline. However, it is rarely significant. It can be controlled by local pressure, dabbing the nose with a cloth or a tissue and breathing gently through the nose. Apart from saline irrigation, alkaline nasal douching needs to be done twice or thrice a day. It helps in removal of any debris and prevents crust formation. Steroids, when used topically and orally to block the pathway of inflammation, are beneficial in polyp disease, including AFRS, as they reduce the chances of recurrance [3].

Other important instructions are as follows:

(a) Avoid sneezing with mouth closed. Never suppress sneeze/cough.
(b) Do not blow your nose.
(c) Do not bend, lift or strain after surgery.
(d) Avoid aspirin and other NSAIDs for seven to ten days after surgery. If required, take paracetamol.
(e) If the patient is on blood thinners, like Clopidogrel and Aspirin, consult a physician for best time to restart the medications.

8.1.2 Post-Operative Assessment of Surgical Outcomes

Surgical outcomes can be measured subjectively and objectively. SNOT 22 score is widely used subjective scoring method for assesing CRS-related disease severity and quality of life [4]. SNOT-20 and SNOT-22 are validated Quality of Life (QoL) questionnaires, which are answered by the patient. They contain 20 and 22 subjective measures respectively based on which quality of life assessment can be done for sinonasal conditions. They can be used to gauge the subjective improvement following sinonasal surgeries [5].

Objectively endoscopic assessment needs to be done using Lund Kennedy scores. The LK Endoscopy Score consists of five parameters (polyposis, discharge, edema, scarring and crusting). Each parameter is given a score of 0, 1 or 2 based on its severity [6]. Table 8.1 demonstrates the LK scoring system.

Although Lund Kennedy is the commonly used scoring system, there is another scoring system—Philpott Javer Endoscopic System which is used to grade AFRS (Tables 8.2 and 8.3) [7].

Table 8.1 Lund Kennedy endoscopic grading

Characteristics	Score = 0	Score = 1	Score = 2
Polyposis	None	Confined to the middle meatus	Beyond middle meatus
Discharge	None	Clear and thin	Thick and mucopurulent
Crusting	Absent	Mild	Severe
Scarring	Absent	Mild	Severe
Edema	Absent	Mild	Severe

Table 8.2 Philpott Javer endoscopic staging system

Philpott Javer Endoscopic staging system for AFRS				
Frontal	0–9	1	0–9	1
Ethmoid	0–9	1	0–9	1
Maxillary	0–9	1	0–9	1
Sphenoid	0–9	1	0–9	1
Total	40		40	
Bilateral total	80			

Table 8.3 Philpott Javer endoscopic grading system

Grading	State of mucosa
0	No edema
1–3	Mucosal edema (mild/moderate/severe)
4–6	Polypoid edema (mild/moderate/severe)
7–9	Frank polyposis (mild/moderate/severe)

Table 8.4 Kupferberg staging system

Stage	Endoscopic findings
0 (A/B)	No mucosal edema
I (A/B)	Mucosal edema
II (A/B)	Polypoidal edema
III (A/B)	Sinus polyps

A without allergic mucin, *B* with allergic mucin

Another staging system that is used is Kupferberg staging system [7] (Table 8.4)

The most commonly used staging system remains Lund Kennedy staging system.

8.1.3 Nasal Douching

Traditionally, alkaline nasal douche has been prepared by taking a teaspoon of sodium bicarbonate, sodium diborate and sodium chloride (in a ratio of 1:1:2) and mixed in half a pint (280 ml) of lukewarm boiled water. The solution is stirred until all the salts have dissolved. Other agents are as follows:

- Hypertonic saline irrigation is also described.
- A recent randomized controlled trial favours the use of Ringer's lactate over hypertonic or isotonic saline [8].

However, to date the alkaline nasal douche remains the preferred douching solution. Home-made alkaline solutions are equally effective when compared to ready made dry preparations [9].

There are agents that can be used to prevent recurrent crusting, which are as follows:

- Twenty-five percent glucose in glycerine has been used locally for patients with atrophic rhinitis to inhibit the growth of proteolytic organisms. They can also be used by a person who is having recurrent crusting, after having done adequate nasal douching first.
- Manuka honey has been used in the same role as glucose-glycerine solution. Manuka honey is used as a topical antimicrobial agent in cases of chronic infections. In vitro studies show it is effective against biofilm-producing bacteria and fungi. There is still no firm level I evidence supporting the use of manuka honey, but the RCTs show marginal improvement in acute exacerbations of chronic rhinosinusitis [10]. There is however, no statistically significant improvement in SNOT 22 scores proven as yet. However, it may have a role in recalcitrant patients and needs further trials to prove its value.
- Steroid irrigations are the mainstay of topical treatment post endoscopic sinus surgery in eosinophilic chronic rhinosinusitis (eCRS). Eosinophilic CRS is defined histologically as the presence of 10 eosinophils per high power field. They are delivered in large volume posi-

tive pressure saline irrigations in a dilute form. They do not cause HPA axis suppression [11].

However, topical steroids have limited role in patients with AFRS.

The following steroidal preparations can be used for nasal irrigation for chronic rhinosinusitis and post-FESS cavity

- Fluticasone propionate
- Beclomethasone
- Budesonide (Pulmicort)

A comparative study by Neubauer et al. showed that Budesonide had greater improvements in SNOT-22 scores and Lund—Kennedy scores as compared to Fluticasone [12]. A clinical trial at Yale University is currently comparing the efficacy of Fluticasone and budesonide in controlling the symptoms of chronic rhinosinusitis. Nasal douching clears the mucus and crusts. It also curbs the urge to pick the nose or blow the crusts out. There is a lot of raw area after sinus surgery, which leads to the collection of debris, and the formation of crusting, which leads to increase in infection rate and synechiae formation. Nasal douching minimizes the collection of debris and mucus and accelerates the healing of the raw area.

Following methods can be employed for nasal douching:

- Pre-filled containers, neti pots or bulb syringes may be used for nasal douching. While breathing through the mouth, the solution is introduced in one nostril while tilting the head to the other side. This allows the solution to clear both the nasal cavities and post-nasal space while it flows out through the other nostril. The same procedure is to be repeated on the other nostril. Gentle blowing of the nose can be done after the procedure to remove any leftover soft crusts and debris. If it stings, one may reduce the amount of salt in the solution.
- 'Sniffing method': Taking the solution in a wide-mouthed mug, one can sniff the solution from one nostril while blocking the other nostril. The solution is then allowed to passively drain through the same nostril. Later the same process can be repeated with the other nostril. One must ensure not to sniff large quantities or to swallow the solution. The cupped hand can also be used in place of mug.
- Using a battery-powered pump or a medical squeeze bottle, which allows the solution to flow out from the other nostril, hence maximizing its effect [13].

Large volume low-pressure irrigations are the preferred method of douching when compared to sniffing method, like medical squeeze bottle, neti pots or bulb syringes [14]. There are various methods of delivery- sprays, rinses and respules. There is no level I evidence supporting the use of any of the three modalities. Please note, the positions for using nasal topical sprays, i.e. head back and head down positions are not described for douching.

8.1.4 Post-Operative Complications and Their Management

Recurrent crusting, occasional bleeding and synechiae formation are the most common post-operative problems faced by the patient and the operating surgeon. Crusting can be prevented by proper nasal douching and weekly cavity cleaning. Bleeding can be prevented by the proper technique of saline irrigations and nasal douching, also by not allowing the cavity to dry up. The forceful blowing of the nose should be avoided.

Synechiae formation can be prevented by minimizing the mucosal trauma intraoperatively and being regular and thorough with cavity cleaning on post-operative visits. It is best to avoid the formation of synechiae in the first place. However, once they form, they can be released using sharp instruments or cautery under local or general anaesthesia. The synechiae has a tendency to recur. To prevent their formation again, silastic sheet, X-ray plate or non adhesive nasal pack can be placed in the nasal cavity to prevent mucosal approximation.

8.1.5 Recent Advances

Following novel therapies have been introduced for improving SNOT 22 scores

(a) aPDT (Antimicrobial Photodynamic therapy)—Non-invasive non-antibiotic broad-spectrum antimicrobial treatment. It has been shown to be effective against biofilm-forming microorganisms [15]. This works on a simple principle, it introduces a non-toxic molecule that turns bactericidal on exposure to visible light, by forming free radicals.
(b) Steroid saline irrigations—Can be started immediately post-operatively for cavity cleaning purpose and to prevent recurrence of polyps. E.g., Budesonide preparation can be done as follows:
    2.5 mg/2 ml ampules are used; they are dissolved in 240 ml of water. Then nasal douching is done on either side thrice a day. It can be reduced to twice a day after the first week and once a day after the first month.
(c) Steroid stents—These stents are inserted in nasal cavities to keep the sinus openings patent. They gradually release a steroid that reduces local inflammation in post-operative period. However, their role in decreasing the symptoms and SNOT 22 scores in patients of CRS remains doubtful [16].
(d) Biologicals—omalizumab, dupilumab, mepolizumab. They are experimental expensive therapies. They have been successful in about 40% of recalcitrant cases.
(e) Personalized therapies using cytokines.
(f) Immunotherapy—Allergen immunotherapy has been shown to decrease post-operative exacerbations, decreases the need for revision surgery and lead to decreased dependence on steroids [17].

8.1.6 Other Therapies

The following therapies are described for AFRS patients that fail high concentration budesonide and budesonide irrigations. Tab Montelukast 10 mg OD—causes the significant improvement in some patients. It is symbiotic with budesonide irrigations. Betadine rinses, Itraconazole, aPDT are the other therapies. Short course of systemic steroids is good option for refractory cases. Biologicals and cytokine therapy are in experimental stage.

Oral itraconazole is proven to be beneficial in selected cases of AFRS. They are started at 200 mg BD and the responders are subsequently tapered to the lowest effective dose within 2 months. Non-responders are given a trial of 2 months after which the drug is stopped. Itraconazole therapy requires regular monitoring of liver function tests and cardiac function. The EPOS 2012 paper does not recommend routine use of systemic or topical antifungals like amphotericin B for routine management of AFRS, as there is insufficient evidence supporting its use [3].

8.2 Part B: Antifungal Therapy

8.2.1 Introduction

Surgical debridement is the preferred treatment modality for fungal sinusitis. Antifungals with surgical debridement are the treatment strategy for invasive fungal sinusitis. The incidence of invasive fungal infection increases because of widespread use of antibiotics, steroids and immunosuppressant drugs. With the advancement in knowledge and technology, the graph of organ transplantation and intervention is raised. Antifungals are used by some clinicians in extensive AFRS in pre-operative period or in follow-up period, when the surgeon is not sure for disease clearance or in patients with persistent symptoms after surgery, to reduce the recurrence rate. Fungal sinusitis occurs in different forms and due to various pathogens, each requiring a specific treatment regime aimed at the causative pathogen. Antifungal agents have varying toxicity and the benefit versus toxicity ratio needs to be weighed before starting treatment. The newer antifungal agents that are less toxic are very expensive. The management protocol for invasive fungal sinusitis is antifungal treatment and debridement of the involved part.

8.2.2 Classification of Antifungals [18]

1. Antibiotics:
   (a) Polyenes: Amphotericin B, Nystatin, Hamycin
   (b) Heterocyclic benzofuran: Griseofulvin
   (c) Echinocandins: Caspofungin, Micafungin, Anidulafungin
2. Antimetabolite: Flucytosine (5-FC)
3. Azoles:
   (a) Imidazoles:
      (i) Topical: Clotrimazole, Econazole, Miconazole, Oxiconazole
      (ii) Systemic: Ketoconazole
   (b) Triazoles (systemic): Fluconazole, Itraconazole, Voriconazole, Posaconazole
4. Allylamine: Terbinafine
5. Other topical agents: Tolnaftate, Undecylenic acid, Benzoic acid, Quiniodochlor, Ciclopirox olamine, Butenafine, Sodium thiosulfate

8.2.3 Antifungal Agents Used for Treatment of Fungal Sinusitis

1. Amphotericin B

   Amphotericin B, is most commonly used polyene antifungal agent and it remains the standard drug of choice for managing life-threatening systemic fungal infections [1]. It was isolated by Gold et al. in 1955 from *Streptomyces nodosus*. It is the standard drug for all types of invasive fungal infections, including invasive aspergillosis, zygomycosis and severe infections of blastomycosis, coccidioidomycosis, sporotrichosis and histoplasmosis. Amphotericin B is also proved to be effective in the treatment of candidemia and disseminated candidiasis. Local irrigation of amphotericin B is reported to be controversial treatment to control of invasive sino-orbital infections. Retrobulbar injection of amphotericin B is also used for the treatment of invasive sino-orbital Aspergillosis. Amphotericin B binds to sterols, more preferentially to ergosterol, which is a major component of the fungal cell membrane. This results in an increased permeability of the cell membrane, leading to leakage of intracellular components and eventually cell death [19, 20]. Owing to its lipophilic nature, amphotericin B also binds to cholesterol in the mammalian cell membrane, but to a lesser degree, which probably accounts for its toxicity. Also, its interaction with host cells can have a positive effect by activation of macrophages through an oxidation-dependent process.

   Amphotericin B is available in four formulations:

   (a) Amphotericin B Deoxycholate

   It is actually a colloidal suspension of amphotericin B, in which deoxycholate (bile salt) is used as solubilizing agent. This formulation has high toxicity. It has poor CNS penetration. The patient should be hydrated with 500–1000 mL of saline before starting the amphotericin infusion. This supplements the sodium required to maintain the intravascular volume and inhibits the tubuloglomerular feedback system, which reduces the risk of nephrotoxicity. Continuous administration versus 5 h administration of the drug is controversial therapy, continuous infusion have less toxicity profile whereas 5 h infusion have more fungicidal effect. The usual protocol is to administer test dose by diluting 10–15 mg of the drug in 50–100 mL of 5% dextrose, and given slowly intravenously over 20 minutes. If there is no reaction, then the complete dose can be administered. The standard dose ranges from 0.25 to 1 mg/kg/day given once daily, diluted in 5% dextrose, to be given slowly intravenously (over 2–6 h) [19, 21]. There are two ways to administer the drug. The first is to start with a low dose and titrate gradually till the maximum dose is achieved. This method is no longer recommended. The second method which is preferred is to start with a standard dose as per patients' body weight and maintain the same till total cumulative dose is achieved. The maximum daily dose in adults is 1.2 mg/kg, and in children is 1.5 mg/kg but more than 1 mg/kg body weight increases the chances of side effect drastically which in turn increases the treatment duration and hospital stay. The total cumulative dose ranges between 2 and 3 g given over 2–3 months. The renal function tests and serum electrolytes should be monitored twice weekly and complete haemogram once weekly. As amphotericin B is sensitive to light, the infusion bottle and tubing should be covered and protected from sunlight, to maintain drug effectiveness. The use of concomitant nephrotoxic drugs must be avoided.

Amphotericin B is highly toxic and has various side effects. The immediate side effects are infusion related and usually begin 1–1.5 h after starting the infusion. They are very common and occur in more than half of the patients. It is probably due to the release of cytokines (Interleukins and tumour necrosis factor α). The infusion-related side effects commonly include fever, chills, rigor, headache, nausea, vomiting. Acute anaphylaxis may rarely occur. These may be managed symptomatically by premedication with paracetamol, antihistamines and antiemetics. Hydrocortisone injection 0.6 mg/kg with the infusion may reduce the severity of the reaction. Thrombophlebitis is also commonly seen with amphotericin infusion. It can be reduced by slowing down the rate of infusion of amphotericin B, adding small amount of heparin to the infusion (1000 units/L), using a central line, or by diluting the concentration of the infused drug. Nephrotoxicity is another common side effect in patients receiving amphotericin B, occurring in up to 80% of patients. The contraindication of amphotericin is acute renal failure. Symptoms are a result of electrolyte wasting (potassium and magnesium) due to impaired urine concentrating ability [19, 21, 22]. It is also associated with renal tubular acidosis. Nephrotoxicity can be minimized by 500–1000 mL of normal saline infusion before and after amphotericin B infusion. If serum creatinine rises above 3 mg/dL, it should be temporarily discontinued or substituted with a lipid-based amphotericin formulation. Patients receiving a total dose greater than 4–5 g of amphotericin B deoxycholate may have permanent renal dysfunction. Amphotericin B has also been reported to directly suppress erythropoietin production leading to normochromic normocytic anaemia. Infrequently, neutropenia and thrombocytopenia may also be seen [19, 21].

(b) Lipid-Based Formulations of Amphotericin B

Recently, lipid-based formulations of amphotericin B have been made available, using various lipid carriers. These lipid-based formulations of the drug have fewer side effects as compared to amphotericin B deoxycholate. They are selectively delivered into the reticuloendothelial system, such as the liver and spleen, and to a lesser extent, the lungs. There are three lipid preparations: amphotericin B colloid dispersion (ABCD), amphotericin B lipid complex (ABLC) and liposomal amphotericin B (LAMB). Their standard doses are ABCD: 3–5 mg/kg, ABLC: 5 mg/kg and LAMB: 1–5 mg/kg. The standard cumulative dose is 5–7 g but it can exceed further which is depends on clinical condition and patient tolerance. The dose-related efficacy of lipid-based formulations is lower than conventional amphotericin B but, as higher doses can be used, it makes them more efficacious.

Lipid-based formulations of amphotericin B are particularly used for the treatment of invasive fungal infections in patients intolerant of or refractory to Amphotericin B deoxycholate. LAMB is used as empiric therapy for fungal infections in febrile neutropenic patients. It is also used in the treatment of patients with Aspergillus, Candida, Cryptococcus sp. infections refractory to or intolerant of Amphotericin B deoxycholate. It is the drug of choice for rhinocerebral mucormycosis, which requires administration of high dose of polyenes after debridement [23]. Liposomal Amphotericin B also has better CNS penetration than Amphotericin B deoxycholate or ABLC.

It has multiple advantages over amphotericin B deoxycholate and is well tolerated by the patient. It produces a milder reaction on infusion, causes minimal anaemia and nephrotoxicity. The only disadvantage of this drug is that it is expensive. Colloidal suspension creates more side effects than liposomal preparation by upregulation of the inflammatory gene.

2. Azoles

   Lately, azoles are gaining importance in the treatment of fungal rhinosinusitis as they are active against multiple fungal pathogens without the serious side effects of amphotericin B deoxycholate. They have also shown effectiveness in treatment of systemic mycoses. Azoles inhibit cytochrome P450 enzyme and thus impair ergosterol synthesis, which is an essential component of the fungal cell membrane [21, 24]. This leads to damage of cell membrane of fungus by increasing its permeability and causing cell death.

   These drugs include imidazoles (clotrimazole, miconazole, ketoconazole) and triazoles (itraconazole, fluconazole). Ketoconazole, given orally, has been used successfully for the treatment of invasive mycosis. However, its use has been mostly replaced by triazoles owing to their superior efficacy, pharmacokinetics and safety profile. Fluconazole is available in both oral and intravenous preparations. The daily dose varies between 200 and 800 mg, depending on the severity of infection. It is highly water soluble and its absorption is not affected by the presence of food or gastric pH[6]. It has excellent activity against most Candida species and is widely used for various fungal infections by *Candida albicans*. Fluconazole has better CNS penetration than itraconazole. Itraconazole is very effective against Aspergillus and black moulds, that typically cause fungal sinusitis. It is the drug of choice in these cases, unless there is extensive bone invasion where initial therapy is amphotericin B [23]. There have also been reports of the efficacy of itraconazole for the treatment of allergic fungal rhinosinusitis and fungal ball. Both oral and intravenous preparations are available. The daily dose is 100–400 mg/day depending on the indication. Its oral absorption and availability is highly variable and unpredictable. It is better absorbed when administered with food or acidic beverages. The side effects of azoles are gastritis, rash, headache, the elevation of liver enzymes, and aldosterone-like effects in high doses (itraconazole). Hepatotoxicity, peripheral neuropathy, pancreatitis and androgen related side effects (alopecia, gynecomastia, loss of libido, etc.) are side effect of long-term use [25].

3. Newer Drugs

   (a) Voriconazole: It is a synthetic derivative of fluconazole, a second-generation triazole. It is useful for the treatment of acute and chronic invasive aspergillosis. It is preferred over amphotericin B where the cause of fungal infection is not known. Both oral and intravenous preparations are available and it is good alternative to amphotericin B in invasive aspergillosis. It is given as loading dose of 6 mg/kg iv BD for 2 doses, followed by 3 mg/kg iv BD for 30 days. On signs of improvement, it can be changed to 200 mg BD orally to complete 24 weeks [26]. The side effects include mild elevation of liver enzymes and transient visual disturbances. The limiting factor is that the drug is expensive.

(b) Posaconazole: It is an azole, active against yeasts and moulds including zygomycetes, aspergillosis, candida and cryptococcal infection. It is used as salvage therapy in invasive fungal sinusitis after failure or intolerance to other antifungals [27]. It is available in oral preparations and the doses are 200 mg thrice daily as preventive management for invasive fungal infection. The therapeutic doses are 800 mg daily in divided doses for invasive fungal infection.

(c) Echinocandins: This class of antifungal agents acts by inhibiting 1, 3 β-glucan synthesis a critical component for maintenance of fungal cell wall integrity [21]. It is approved for treatment of invasive aspergillosis resistant to conventional antifungal and empirical management of neutropenic patients suspected of having fungal sinusitis. Drugs belonging to this class are caspofungin, micafungin, anidulafungin.

8.2.4 Antifungal Drug Resistance

Drug resistence is the major cause of treatment failure. This can occur in circumstances such as wrong diagnosis, multiple pathogens or immune reconstitution inflammatory syndrome, seen in patients receiving immune-modulating therapies, which may be confused with failure to control the fungal infection [27]. Also, in patients with severe immunosuppression, the antifungal cannot overcome the severe immunodeficiencies until the host immunity is improved. Recent studies have shown that early treatment of fungal infection with a lower burden of organisms reduces treatment failure [28, 29]. Some fungal strains possess more virulent characteristics than others and infection with such strains may have a poorer prognosis. Toxicity from polyenes (nephrotoxicity) and azoles (hepatitis) can be a cause of treatment failure [30, 31]. Drug-drug interaction, drug-target interaction, upregulation of drug transporters, biofilms and reduced cellular concentration can lead to morbidity and mortality by inducing drug resistance. Studies have shown that an increase in resistance to azole antifungal drugs may allow some cross-resistance to amphotericin B. The possible mechanism is azoles cause an alteration in ergosterol synthesis which consequently decreases the number of potential binding sites on the fungal cell membrane for amphotericin B or multiple drug resistance (MDR) pumps. In invasive mycoses, when the site of infection is necrotic with poor vascularity, debulking surgery is essential to overcome antifungal resistance and tissue samples should be evaluated for the sensitivity of drug against particular organism. A suboptimal length of treatment, prolong drug exposure, repeated and prophylactic treatment may also lead to drug resistance. Lastly, the underlying disease must be controlled or prevent fungal infections in high-risk patients. In vitro assessment of drug susceptibility, newer drugs are the alternatives in patients resistant to or not responding to conventional treatment. Failure to treatment is defined as no improvement or worsening of clinical or radiological features in 7–14 days after starting standard antifungal treatment.

8.2.5 Duration of Medical Therapy for Fungal Sinusitis

Treatment end point should be tailor made and multiple factors can be considered in each patient. Treatment should be continued till there is complete resolution of all symptoms of fungal sinusitis for at least 2 weeks, resolution of endoscopic findings, resolution of radiological findings, negative fungal culture and biopsy the suspected area. Serum biomarkers such as galactomannan, β-D-glycan and Aspergillus specific PCR can be considered as end point for treatment as they have high negative predication value. Sometime patient tolerance and co-morbidities are the major limiting factor for complete treatment [32].

8.2.5.1 Combination of Antifungal

Simultaneous administration of two or more antifungal drugs is a controversial topic in view of significant side effects, patient tolerance but it has shown advantages against certain organism and drug resistance. Flucytosine with amphotericin B combination demonstrated survival benefit in cases of *Cryptococcal meningitis*. Calcium—calcineurin signalling pathway plays a dominant role in immunity. Synergistic action of calcineurin inhibitors such as cyclosporine A, tacrolimus (FK 506) and pimecrolimus with azoles is helpful to kill resistant fungi. Glucocorticoid (dexamethasone, budesonide, hydrocortisone), antimetabolic agents (mycophenolic acid, mizoribine), the target of rapamycin and few traditional Chinese medications (tetrandrine, artemisinin, matrine) showed addictive effect with antifungal. These drugs are more studied with candida species. Hydrocortisone with amphotericin in human and rapamycin with azoles in rat showed some synergistic effectiveness against Aspergillus infection [33].

8.2.5.2 Recent Advances

Urea derivative of amphotericin B is showed more potent outcome with less adverse effects in the animal model. Isavuconazole is potent orally and intravenously available azole and it is approved by the US FDA for the invasive form of aspergillosis and mucor infections. Fungal sphingolipid, calcineurin, Hsp 90, etc. are the newer target sites for drugs. VT 1129, VT 1161 and VT 1598 are the newer tetrazoles and they claimed to be more specific for fungal cytochrome 51 and less for mammalian 450 cytochrome. Aminocandin (IP960 or HMR3270), CD 101, enfumafungin, etc. are the newer echinocandins against Aspergillus and candida species [34, 35].

8.3 Part C: Fess Complications

Functional Endoscopic sinus surgery is highly sophisticated type of surgery that aims at maintaining the physiological function and anatomical structure. Powered instrumentations and stereotactic image-guided surgery have improved efficacy and safety of this procedure and have revolutionized endoscopic sinus surgery and extended its applications. Because of the highly variable individual anatomy and the intimate relationship to the orbit, anterior cranial fossa and vascular structures, sinus surgery has many potential complications. Thorough knowledge of anatomy, detailed assessment of pre-operative imaging and advanced technology such as endoscopes, microdebrider and Image guidance with hypotensive anaesthesia can reduce the chance of complications drastically. Revision surgery, extensive nasal polyposis, dehiscence of sinuses lining wall, distorted anatomy are the common reason behind complications. Normal anatomical various such as hypoplastic or extensive pneumatized sinuses, long and high cribriform plate, asymmetrical low lying ethmoidal roof are the other factors. Dehiscent bony canal over optic nerve, internal carotid artery and anterior ethmoid artery can induce catastrophic complication.

Posterior choana, middle turbinate/ remnant of it, sphenoid sinus, skull base, septum and maxillary sinus roof are the stable intranasal landmarks to be considered especially in revision surgery. The factors with poorer outcomes include previous surgery, extensive disease, poor knowledge of anatomy and radiology. Outdated technology and the presence of risk factors such as smoking, asthma, aspirin sensitivity, allergies and in immune deficiency, etc. are the other factors for poor outcome. The list of complications is illustrated in Table 8.5. Nasal complications are the most common complications followed by orbital and intracranial complications.

8.3.1 Nasal Complications

8.3.1.1 Adhesion (Synechiae)

This is the most common complication of FESS and it is seen in 4–35% of cases [36]. Synechiae develop when two opposing raw mucosal surfaces remain in contact after the surgery. Gross septal deviation, revision surgery, and middle turbinate instability is the major causes of synechiae formation. The spacer should be placed under the vision to prevent instability of middle turbinate. Initially, micro fibrinous bands develop and forms a scar tissue. Synechiae at maxillary ostia and ethmoid cavity have worse effect as it affects

Table 8.5 Complications of Endoscopic Sinus Surgery

Nasal complications	Intracranial complications	Orbital complications
• Synechiae (adhesion) • Haemorrhage • Stenosis of ostium • Mucocele/Pyocele • Olfactory impairment • Injury to NLD	• CSF Rhinorrhea • Meningitis • Encephalocele	• Orbital subcutaneous emphysema • Fat prolapse • Extraocular muscle injury • Orbital hematoma • Optic nerve injury

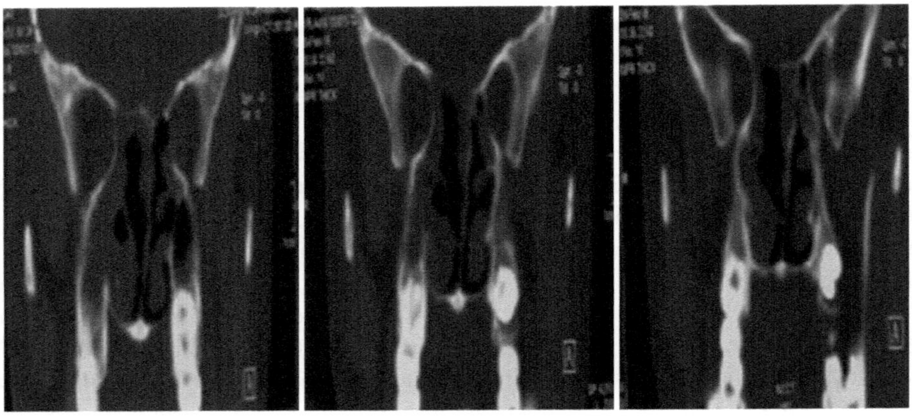

Fig. 8.2 NCCT PNS orbit is showing synechiae in between inferior turbinate and septum

the drainage of maxillary, ethmoid sinuses. It also interferes in post-operative cavity cleaning. To prevent this, surgery should be performed with care. Any kind of injury to healthy mucosa should be avoided. Loose hanging mucosa and bony chips should be removed during surgery and in post-operative care. Irrigation of the cavity is required to minimizing the effect of heat injury. Absorbable and non-absorbable spacer is placed in between two raw surfaces to prevent approximation and adhesion. Meta-analysis, review articles showed advantage of spacer placement against synechiae formation [37–39]. Bolgerization and suture medialization of middle turbinate are helpful in preventing synechiae formation when middle turbinate is destabilized (Fig. 8.2) [40]. Soft adhesion can be removed easily but hard adhesion requires sharp instruments to break it and raw surfaces are seperated by spacer placement. Regular follow-up with operative surgeon and proper cavity care can prevent synechiae formation.

8.3.1.2 Haemorrhage

Nasal bleeding can be divided into bothersome mucosal ooze, bleeding from a named vessel and life-threatening haemorrhage from maxillary and internal carotid artery. Surgeon's scale is proposed to qualify amount of blood in field [41]. The scale is ranged from 0 to 5 where score 2 means mild ooze and it requires minimal suctioning. In score 3, the field is improved with suctioning and in score 4, continue suctioning is required to see the surgical field. In score 5, the surgical field is not improved with continue suctioning.

1. *Mucosal Ooze*—It may limit the view of surgical field which leads to increase operative

time. It also increases the risk of complications and may lead to termination of procedure. Mucosal ooze can be reduced by avoidance of NSAIDS, platelet inhibitors. Pre-operative antibiotics and oral steroid reduces intraoperative bleeding by reducing edema, exudates and blood vessels trauma by reducing the load of inflammatory mediators [42]. Oral steroids also enhance the effect of vasoconstrictors by increasing the spasticity of smooth muscles. The doses were varied from 30–60 mg per day with 7 days duration with or without tapering [43]. Pre-operative steroid can generate serious side effects so it should be used cautiously [43, 44]. Pre-operative administration of tranexamic acid reduces periorbital edema and intraoperative bleeding [45, 46]. Hypotensive anaesthesia, reverse Trendelenburg position, intraoperative local infiltration in pterygopalatine fossa via greater palatine or sphenopalatine foramen and application of cotton pledgets with vasoconstrictor reduces mucosal ooze to some extent [47].

2. *Bleeding from Named Vessel*—Sphenopalatine artery is the major blood supply of the sinonasal region. Anterior ethmoidal artery is the branch of the ophthalmic artery. Anterior ethmoid artery can be injured while removal of antero-superior part of the anterior ethmoid cell. Low lying anterior ethmoid artery is found in cases with higher Keros, long cribriform plate, wide antero-posterior frontal recess and presence of supraorbital recess [48]. Abnormal course can be assessed by proper pre-operative radiology. Injury to the lateral part of the vessel can retract intra-orbitally and creates complications by rising intra-orbital pressure. Avoidance is the best way to prevent complications and if the dealing is required, it should be done in the middle part of intranasal course of anterior ethmoid artery so cauterization of injured vessel is possible. Once it retracts in orbit, external approach is required to control bleeding and the management of anterior ethmoid artery bleeding is mentioned in Chap. 9. The posterior branch of sphenopalatine artery is running just inferior to sphenoid ostium which can be injured by the inferior widening of ostium. Vessel injury can be avoided by separating the mucosa inferiorly before ostium widening. The management of sphenopalatine bleeding is mentioned in Chap. 9.
3. *Internal Carotid Injury*—Sellar type of pneumatization of the sphenoid sinus has thinnest bony wall over carotid or may even have dehiscent carotid. Sometimes accessory sphenoid septum is attached over the ICA bulge. Anomalies and aneurysms of the artery also predispose to the internal carotid artery injury. This can be avoided by pre-operative radiological assessment and without pulling or avulsion of septas in the sphenoid sinus. The management is mentioned in Chap. 9.

8.3.1.3 Sinus Ostium Stenosis

Sinus ostium stenosis is defined as loss of more than 50–60% of intraoperative size. Neo-osteogenesis at the ostium level can lead to stenosis (Fig. 8.3). Complex anatomy and narrow outflow tract of frontal sinus make it as most vulnerable sinus for recurrence of disease secondary

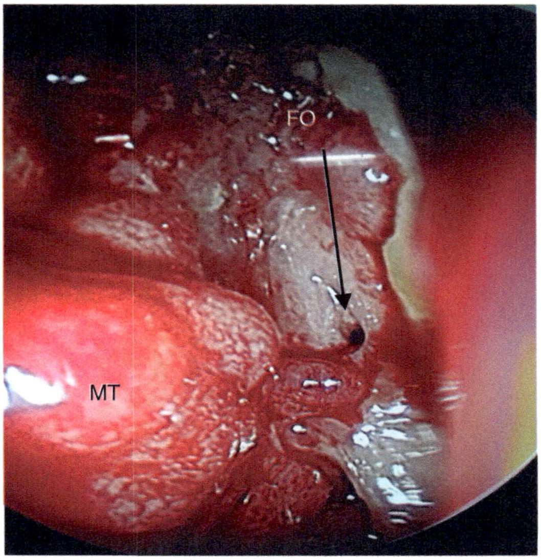

Fig. 8.3 Neo-osteogenesis with stenosis of left side frontal ostium (FO). *MT* middle turbinate)

to stenosis. It is found as high as 60% [49]. The final size of the frontal ostium is defined around 1 year of post-surgery period. The preservation of normal ostium wall at least at one side, carpeting of exposed bone by mucosal graft or flap, Mitomycin C application, steroid releasing sinus implants and proper cavity care can reduce the chances of stenosis [50–52].

8.3.1.4 Mucocele/Pyocele

It is a late complication of endoscopic surgery. Mucocele appears after years of surgery. The persistent mucosal inflammation and intraoperative trauma can lead to narrowing/obstruction of sinus cells outflow. The mucocele formation is ranged from 0 to 13% after endoscopic surgeries [53]. Frontal sinus is the most affected sinus because of its narrow drainage pathway. Ethmoid and sphenoid are the next common sinuses in sequence. With the expansion in the list of endoscopic procedures, the chances of mucocele formation are increasing (Fig. 8.4). Complete excision of mucosa is difficult in narrow and hidden part of sinuses. Mucoceles may be incidental finding or it may present with headache, orbital symptoms and facial disfiguring, etc. Extensive diseases have higher chances of mucocele formation because of significant damage to normal mucociliary function while disease clearing. The measurements mentioned in the mucosal ooze section and proper cavity care are also applicable to minimize the chances of mucocele formation. In extended endoscopic approaches, complete removal of mucosa under flap and the proper marking of mucosal surface of the flap is required for prevention of iatrogenic mucocele [54]. The regular follow-up and interval MRI helps in early diagnosis [55]. Majority are manageable by endoscopic approach. Complicated mucoceles require urgent intervention. The detailed management of mucoceles is mentioned in Chap. 7.

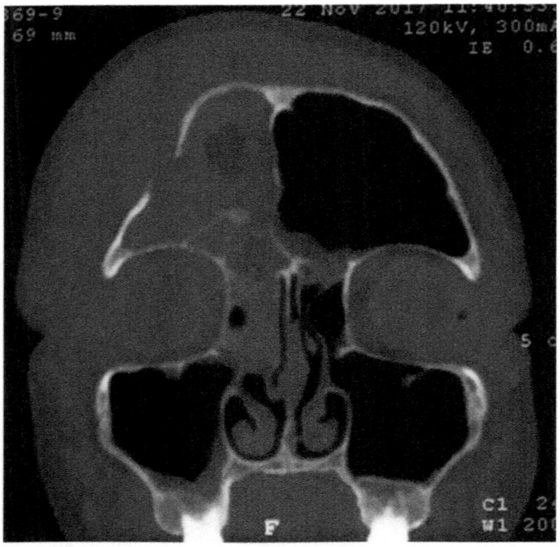

Fig. 8.4 Right iatrogenic frontoethmoidal mucocele. Hypodense area is the retained bone wax which is blocking the outflow tract of frontal sinus. Anterior wall of the frontal sinus is also breached which presented as fluctuation swelling on the frontal sinus (Pott's puffy tumour)

8.3.1.5 Nasolacrimal Duct Injury

Nasolacrimal duct is the continuation of nasolacrimal sac in the lateral nasal wall. The course is variable in the medial maxillary wall (Fig. 8.5). The distance between the duct and anterior maxillary sinus wall is found less than 7 mm in approximately 88% of cases [56] whereas in nasal endoscopic evaluation in cadavers, it runs at and anterior to the maxillary line in 95% of cases [57]. NLD can be injured while aggressive removal of uncinate bone, anterior enlargement of the maxillary ostium and in extended endoscopic approaches to pterygomaxillary fossa and infratemporal fossa. Not all NLD injuries are presented with tearing. Proper pre-operative knowledge of NLD course, anterior and posterior nasolacrimal duct approach can reduce the injury chances [58]. In extended endoscopic approaches, sharp cut to NLD or DCR is advised. Dacrocystostomy is the treatment option for symptomatic cases. The details of the procedure are mentioned in Chap. 8.

8.3.1.6 Empty Nose Syndrome

It is a late complication. It occurs after extensive and usually recurrent sinus surgeries with the removal of large areas of mucous membranes and resection of superior and middle turbinates. Patient will complain of paradox nasal obstruction in presence of objective wider nasal cavities

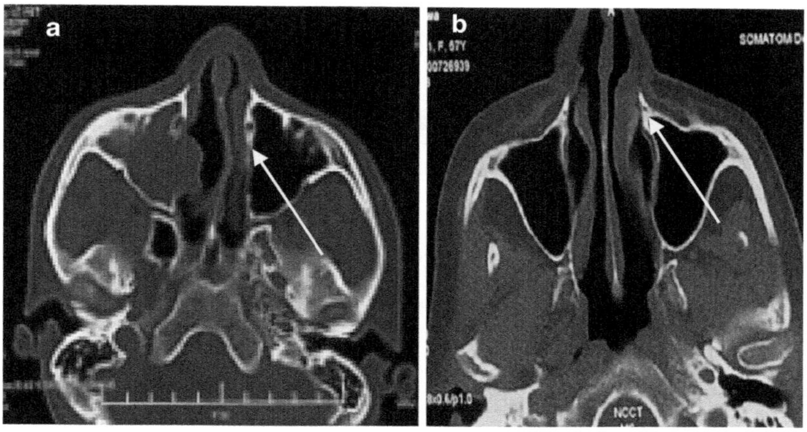

Fig. 8.5 Course of nasolacrimal duct canal. It is very much away from anterior maxillary sinus wall in (**a**) and in (**b**), no gap in between anterior maxillary wall and NLD canal

and irritating crust formation. The etiology and management of empty nose syndrome is mentioned in last section.

8.3.1.7 Olfactory Impairment

It may occur due to avulsion of olfactory neuroepithelium from olfactory cleft or over resection of superior turbinate. It can be prevented by avoiding unnecessary handling in the olfactory cleft region and if required, sharp cutting instruments should be used to prevent scarring.

8.3.2 Orbital Complications

The orbit comes in close relationship with all paranasal sinuses. Periorbita is the only soft tissue barrier in between orbit and paranasal sinuses. Pre-operative radiology is helpful in accessing bony anatomy, dehiscence's of periorbital wall, fat prolapsed, optic nerve course. The incidence of orbital complications is ranged from 0.5 to 5%. The list of orbital complications is mentioned in Table 8.5.

8.3.2.1 Subcutaneous Emphysema

It is characterized by the presence of air in orbital tissue. This occurs due to natural communications or by accidental or iatrogenic breach of partly wall. Orbital emphysema occurs due to forceful nose blowing, sneezing and mask ventilation. It is mostly seen in eyelids with the normal sclera and extraocular movement. Creaking and crepitating are the clinical findings on eyelids. It is generally self-limiting and reabsorbs in short period. Patient should be advised to avoid activities like nose blowing, etc. Progressive emphysema can create acute compartment syndrome. It is painful condition that can present with restriction of extraocular movement and impairment of vision. It requires urgent decompression of collected air to prevent permanent vision loss secondary to vascular compression and optic nerve stretching (Fig. 8.6) [59, 60].

8.3.2.2 Damage to Lamina Papyracea, Periorbita and Orbital Fat Prolapse

Median orbital wall is formed by frontal process of maxilla, lacrimal bone and lamina payracea from anterior to posterior direction. Lamina papyracea is the thinnest medial orbital bone and its thickness reduces with age advancement. Predisposing factors for fat prolapsed are dehiscent Lamina papyracea, revision surgery, extensive disease, distorted anatomy, excessive bleeding and hypoplastic Maxillary Sinus (Fig. 8.7). The preservation of median bony wall and periorbita in dehiscent bony wall is the key to prevent orbital complications. Fat is prolapsed when sickle knife inserted blindly while uncinectomy, dacrocystostomy and undue pulling of lateral attachment of middle turbinate. Periorbita touching is painful under local anaesthesia. Retrograde uncinectomy is the safer technique [58]. Powered instruments have damaging effect on orbital tissue than cold instruments by its

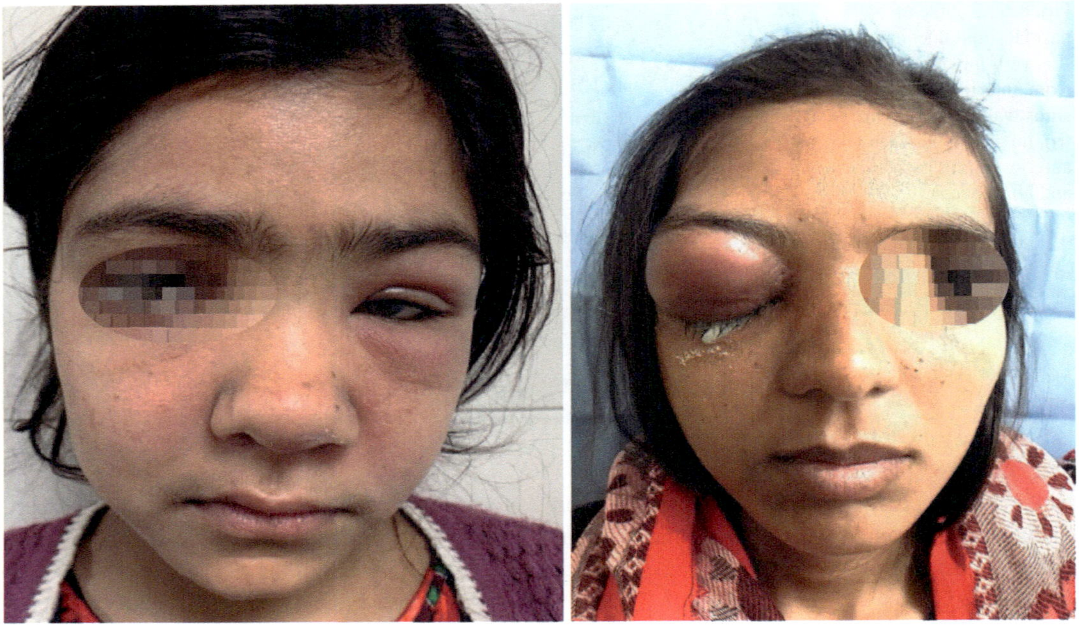

Fig. 8.6 Left side emphysema with normal-looking sclera. The right side picture is showing acute compartment syndrome

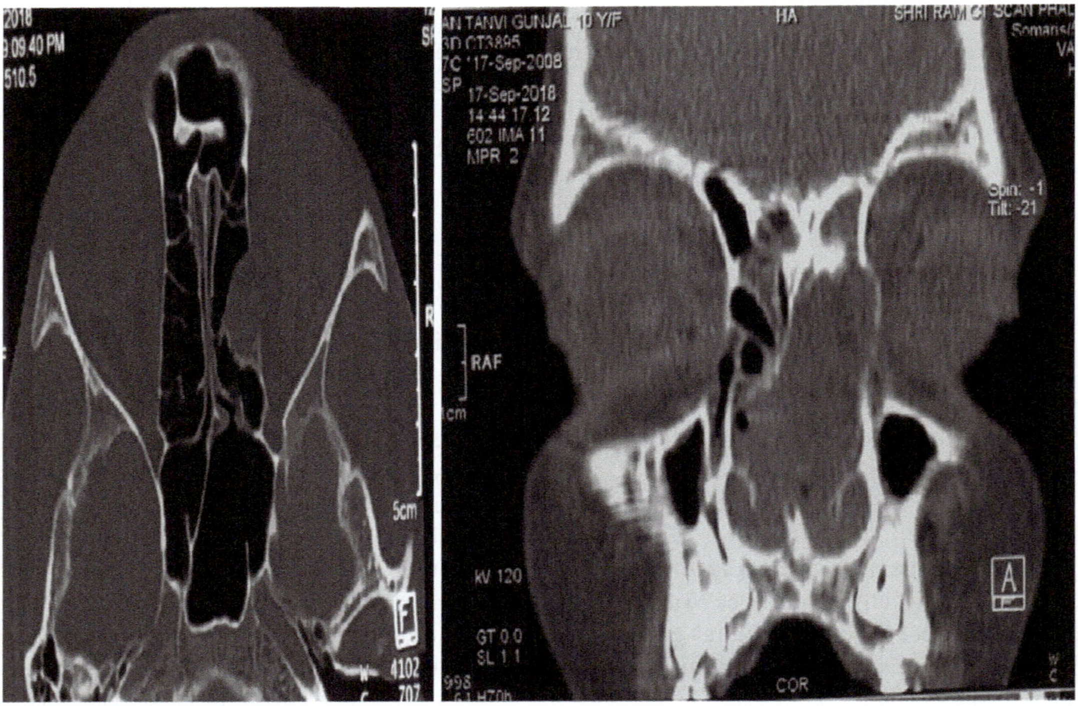

Fig. 8.7 NCCT PNS orbit (axial cut) is depicting the dehiscence of lamina with prolapsed orbital fat. The patient had history of trauma in childhood. Coronal cut is showing extensive S/T/D in the left side of nasal cavity and ethmoid sinus with pushed lamina papyracea

suctioning effect [61]. The Stankiewicz pressure test shows the movement of medial wall when injury occurs to lamina papyracea and periorbita [62]. In doubtful cases, fat float test can be done. Surgery can be completed by avoiding manipulation of prolapsed fat, gentle bipolar of fat obstructing the view and by avoid suctioning over it. Sinus ostium should be widened enough to prevent obstruction of the drainage pathway by prolapsed fat. Surgeon should avoid tight nasal packing. The patient should be advised not to blow nose post-operative.

8.3.2.3 Injury to Extraocular Muscles

The right eye injury is more common than the left eye probably due to right-handed surgeon's majority. The medial rectus is the most vulnerable extraocular muscle followed by inferior rectus and superior oblique. Strabismus and diplopia are the leading clinical features. For contusions, the treatment option is conservative treatment (observation, antibiotics and steroids). If the muscle is entrapped, the involved muscle should be released. Gross divergent squint and absent adduction are the sign of muscle transaction. ENT surgeon may seek the advice of ophthalmologist. The various management options include hang back suture (strabismus reduction), botulinum toxin in contra muscle, the recession of lateral rectus and transposition [63, 64].

8.3.2.4 Orbital Hematoma

The orbit is the close compartment. The Normal intraocular pressure (IOP) is 10–20 mmHg. Orbital hematoma is the post septal accumulation of blood. It accounts 0.05–0.5% of endoscopic surgery. The clinical features are progressive proptosis, severe retrobulbar pain and visual impairment. The signs are raised IOP and alter pupillary reflex. The intraoperative features are dilated fixed pupil and bradycardia. It is of two types, slow venous type and fast arterial type. In the slow venous type, intra-orbital veins are injured. Fast arterial type is mostly iatrogenic and ethmoidal arteries are injured. Increased tension in globe can cause irreversible visual impairment by inducing optic nerve stretching and vascular compression. It can lead to permanent blindness, if orbit is not decompressed within 100–120 min. The standard treatment policy for intraoperatively diagnosed orbital hematoma is urgent orbital and optic nerve decompression. When it is noticed in ward, the surgical decision on the basis of intraocular pressure (IOP) is controversial. The medical management includes eye massaging, i/v mannitol, i/v dexamethasone, and removal of nasal packing. If IOP is above 30–35 mmHg and in patients with IOP less than 20 with progressive proptosis, severe retro-orbital pain, RAPD, cherry red macula and no retinal artery pulsation, the management option is urgent canthotomy and or cantholysis in ward after local infiltration. Clamps are applied below and above lateral canthus for devascularization. Canthotomy is full thickness incision on lateral canthus towards the orbital rim. Cantholysis is the release of the lateral canthal ligament. Both procedures allow anterior prolapse of orbit and it can reduce pressure by 10–15 mmHg. In progressive cases, endoscopic or external orbital decompression with multiple parallel incisions on periorbita to suppress the effect of raised IOP [63, 64]. Some surgeons performed canthal procedures and orbital wall decompression in one go [65].

8.3.2.5 Injury to Optic Nerve

The optic nerve runs in the lateral relationship of the posterior ethmoid and sphenoid sinus. The various predisposing factors for direct optic nerve injury are the presence of Onodi cell, dehiscent optic nerve canal and attachment of accessory sphenoid septum with the optic canal [66]. Indirect damage can occur by compromising the blood supply of optic nerve [63, 64]. It is seen in orbital hematoma. Altered visual reflex is the sign of abnormality of function of optic nerve. Pre-operative radiological assessment of the course of optic nerve can minimize the chances of injury. Intraoperative diagnosed optic nerve injury should be managed by orbital and optic nerve decompression. Post-operatively diagnosed cases are managed by mega doses of i/v steroids (Methylprednisolone) and endoscopic optic nerve decompression. The prognosis is very poor even after all measures taken [67, 68].

8.3.3 Intracranial Complications

8.3.3.1 CSF Fistula

Extended endoscopic approaches increase the chances of CSF rhinorrhoea. Incidence varies from 0.2 to 16% in literature [69]. The patients with high BMI, revision surgery and history of radiotherapy are at more risk. It occurs due to damage to the skull base and dura. Lateral lamella of the cribriform plate, ethmoid roof are the most common site for CSF leak in FESS but in extended approaches, pituitary fossa is the most common site. Chances are increased by dehiscence in skull base by nasal pathology like polyposis, tumour, etc. Inadequate knowledge of radiology and undue manipulation of structures attached with skull base like middle turbinate, superior turbinate, etc. can lead to iatrogenic skull base damage. It is safe to identify skull base first by posterior to anterior approach especially in revision cases or in cases with distorted anatomy and if there is non-availability of navigation system. CSF rhinorrhoea is diagnosed by identifying the outflow of watery fluid from skull base. The preventive measures for failed dural repair in extended approaches is to avoid large surgical defect, achieve adequate haemostasis before the closure of defect with graft or flap, mucosa should be replaced back over multilayer repair where sinus obliteration is not planned, under vision nasal packing and smooth extubation. Intraoperatively diagnosed cases should be repaired in the same sitting by experienced surgeon. In post-operative diagnosed cases, conservative management includes i/v mannitol, stool softener, cough suppressants, head end elevation and restricted movement, etc. The use of lumber drain is based on the effect of conservative management and surgeon's choice [69]. The site of leak in persistent cases (1–2 weeks of conservative management) can diagnose by either single imaging or by combining of different modalities such as NCCT PNS orbit with MR cisternography and intra-thecal or topical application of fluorescein dye (Fig. 8.8) [70, 71]. Endoscopic multilayer closure of the defect is

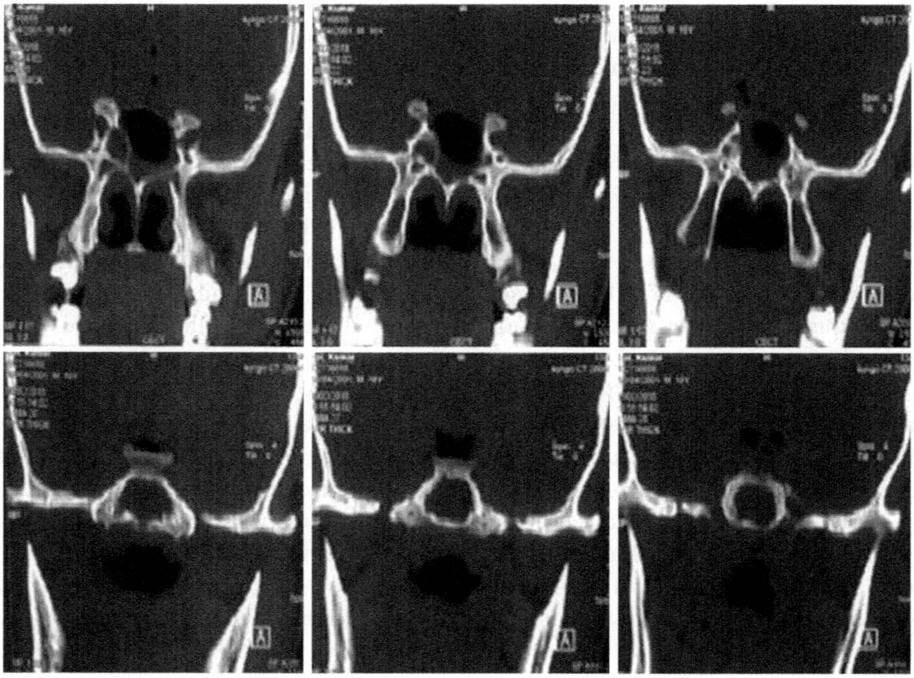

Fig. 8.8 NCCT coronal cut- skull base is damaged at sphenoid sinus superior wall with pneumocephalus

advised and naso-septal flap is most commonly used to repair skull base defect [72].

8.3.3.2 Meningitis

This is a relatively rare intracranial complication and incidence varies from less than 1 to 10%. Extended endoscopic approaches have relatively higher risk of meningitis. Intraoperative and post-operative CSF leak, perioperative lumber drain, prolong surgery, revision surgery in short span, missed prophylactic antibiotics are the common reason for meningitis in the post-operative period. Recent systemic review and meta-analysis are not supporting the utility of prophylactic lumber drain [73]. Sometimes, the infection may spread along perivascular and vascular or perineural spaces of the olfactory fibres. The meningitis trend is decreasing in the recent past because of improvement in endoscopic surgical expertise, advance instruments, better sealing materials and use of naso-septal flap [74, 75].

Patient presents with severe headache, high-grade fever, nuchal rigidity, vomiting, cranial nerve palsy, behavioural changes and seizures. Sometime dry cough, mild headache and raised TLC count is the only feature because of ongoing post-surgical medications. In such cases, CSF fluid analysis is helpful in creating the diagnosis. MR cisternography is good investigation in doubtful cases of CSF leak. Treatment includes targeted broad-spectrum antibiotics for 2 weeks and closure of the defect in persistent CSF rhinorrhoea patients.

8.3.3.3 Pneumocephalus

It occurs due to the presence of air in the cranial cavity due to communication between the extra-cranial and intracranial cavity. It is rare complication of sinus surgery. It is more common in patients with intraoperative and post-operative CSF leak. It is also common with extended endoscopic approaches for the removal of intradural lesions. Post-operative pneumocephalus is associated with greater risk of CSF leak and intracranial infection (Fig. 8.8). The mechanism is believed to be 'ball valve' mechanism or 'inverted bottle' mechanism. The patient can complain of dizziness, visual alterations, confusion, behavioural and personality change. NCCT head is good enough to pick air. Pneumocephalus requires no treatment in asymptomatic patients. Tension pneumocephalus requires prompt treatment, decompression of the aerocele followed by the closure of the defect [76, 77].

8.4 Part DA: Biofilms: Its Composition, Detection Methods and Role in Human Infections (Microbiologist Aspect)

Biofilms are defined as group of microbes in which cells adhere to each other or substratum irreversibly. Biofilms can be present everywhere in the environment. These biofilms have the potential to neutralize antibiotics and result in prolonged treatment. Due to its resistant properties to antimicrobials and infections associated with indwelling devices poses a problem for public health. Biofilms formation is a multi-step process in which adaptation occurs during a series of events under diverse nutritional and environmental conditions. Biofilms have been found to be involved in a wide variety of microbial infections in the body such as bacterial vaginosis, urinary tract infections, catheter infections, middle-ear infections, the formation of dental plaque, gingivitis, coating lenses and endocarditis, infection in cystic fibrosis, and infections of indwelling devices. The biofilms are significantly resistant to antibiotics and infection associated with them is difficult to eradicate. Microbiological diagnosis is important for the diagnosis of biofilms. The traditional methods like microscopy, culture techniques are not always suited for the understanding of biofilm science and are less sensitive for detection. Therefore, there is need of newer methods for the detection of biofilms. The use of bacteriophages, enzymes, surface coating agents, pilicides and quorum sensing inhibitors are some of the methods to control biofilm formation. It is challenging in medical science to eradicate infections related to biofilm formation. This is due to the fact that mature biofilms exhibit tolerance towards immune response and antibiotics. Further studies are required to know the mechanism of antibiotics resistance and their gene expression biofilm for better health care improvement.

8.4.1 Introduction of Biofilms

Biofilms are defined as group of microbes in which cells adhere to each other or substratum irreversibly. These sticked cells become embedded in extracellular polymeric substance (matrix) produced by microbes themselves. Biofilms can be present everywhere in environment, industrial and hospital settings and may form on living or non-living surfaces [78]. The antibiotics and human immune system normally cannot access the bacterial biofilms. These biofilms have the potential to neutralize antibiotics and result in prolonged treatment. Due to its resistant properties to antimicrobials and infections related with indwelling devices poses a problem for public health. Biofilm-forming capacity has been found in number of bacterial species such as *Escherichia coli*, *Staphylococcus aureus*, *Pseudomonas aeruginosa*, *Staphylococcus epidermidis*, *Enterobacter cloacae*, *Klebsiella pneumonia* [79].

8.4.2 Composition of Biofilms

Biofilms are community of microbes that produce matrix (extracellular polymeric substances (EPS) which consist of exopolysaccharides, proteins and nucleic acids. Water (97%) is the major component of biofilm which is responsible for the flow of nutrients inside the biofilm matrix. The other component of biofilms are proteins (<1–2%), DNA (<1%), polysaccharides (1–2%) and RNA (<1%) [80]. Various components of biofilms are shown in Table 8.6.

8.4.3 Biofilms Formation

The formation of biofilm is a multi-step process in which adaptation occurs during a series of events under diverse conditions such as nutritional and environmental. During this process, microbes transform from planktonic to the sessile mode of growth. It is a complex process that includes: (a) adherence to a surface (b) growth of colonies (formation of micro-colony and three-dimensional structure formation) (c) detachment (dispersal) as shown in Fig. 8.9 [81].

8.4.3.1 Attachment

When a microorganism cell reaches to surface, the interface of solid–liquid can provide a suitable environment for microbes to attach and grow. Hydrophilic, rough and coated surfaces will provide better environmental attachment and

Table 8.6 Biofilm composition

Constituents	Percentages of matrix
Water	Up to 97%
Microbial cells	2–5%
Polysaccharides	1–2%
Nucleic acid (RNA and DNA)	<1–2%
Proteins	<1–2%

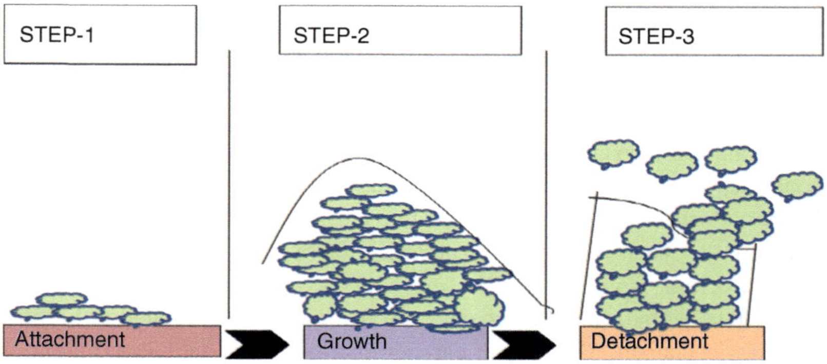

Fig. 8.9 Showing steps of biofilms formation

formation of biofilm. Increase in temperature of the water, flow velocity or nutrients, locomotor organelle can further increase the attachment process.

8.4.3.2 Growth of Colonies

After attachment, chemical signals lead to the process of multiplication of bacteria in the biofilms. The bacterial cell divisions occur within the embedded matrix by using such signals which results in micro-colony formation. After the stage of micro-colony formation, expression of certain biofilms related genes helps in the formation of matrix. The water-filled channel formation takes place after EPS formation for the transport of nutrients within the biofilms. These water channels help in distributing nutrients and removing waste materials from the micro-colonies of the biofilms.

8.4.3.3 Detachment

After micro-colonies formation, occasionally under some mechanical stress bacteria are detached from the communities into the environment. But in most cases, some microbes stop EPS production and are detached into environment. The detachment of new formed cells from growing cells or dispersion of biofilm communities occurs through a mechanism called quorum sensing.

8.4.4 Biofilms and Antibiotic Resistance

The key factors responsible for antimicrobial resistance may vary among different sitting. The following mechanisms have been explored for high resistance nature of biofilms: (1) low penetration of antibiotics, (2) neutralization by enzymes, (3) heterogeneous functions, (4) cells slow growth rate, (5) existence of persistent cells, (6) biofilm phenotype and (7) efflux pump and membrane alteration as shown in Fig. 8.10 [82, 83].

8.4.5 Role of Biofilms in Human Infections

Biofilms have been found to be associated with wide variety of microbial infections in the body. Recently, it has been observed that biofilms can also impair wound healing by reducing topical antimicrobial activity in treating wounds. Association between various human infections and biofilms are shown in Table 8.7 [84, 85].

8.4.6 Biofilms Detection Methods

The biofilms are significantly resistant to antibiotic and infection associated with them is difficult to eradicate. Microbiological diagnosis is important for the diagnosis of biofilms. The traditional methods like microscopy, culture techniques are not always suited for the understanding of biofilm science and are less sensitive for detection. Therefore, there is need of newer methods for the detection of biofilms. Proper sonication of indwelling devices from the patients can significantly improve the detection of biofilms. The development of molecular and imaging techniques leads to a better understanding of biofilm science. Classical and newer biofilm detection methods are shown in Table 8.8 [86].

8.4.7 Methods to Control Biofilms [87]

(A) Pilicides—Small synthetic compounds inhibit the synthesis of pili which further inhibit binding and colonization on epithelial cells.
(B) Enzymes—The enzymes have the capability to degrade the biofilm matrix. Further, degradation of biofilm results in the release of components that are easily clear by immune systems.
(C) Quorum sensing inhibitors—Using quorum sensing inhibitors is another effective way in control of biofilm.

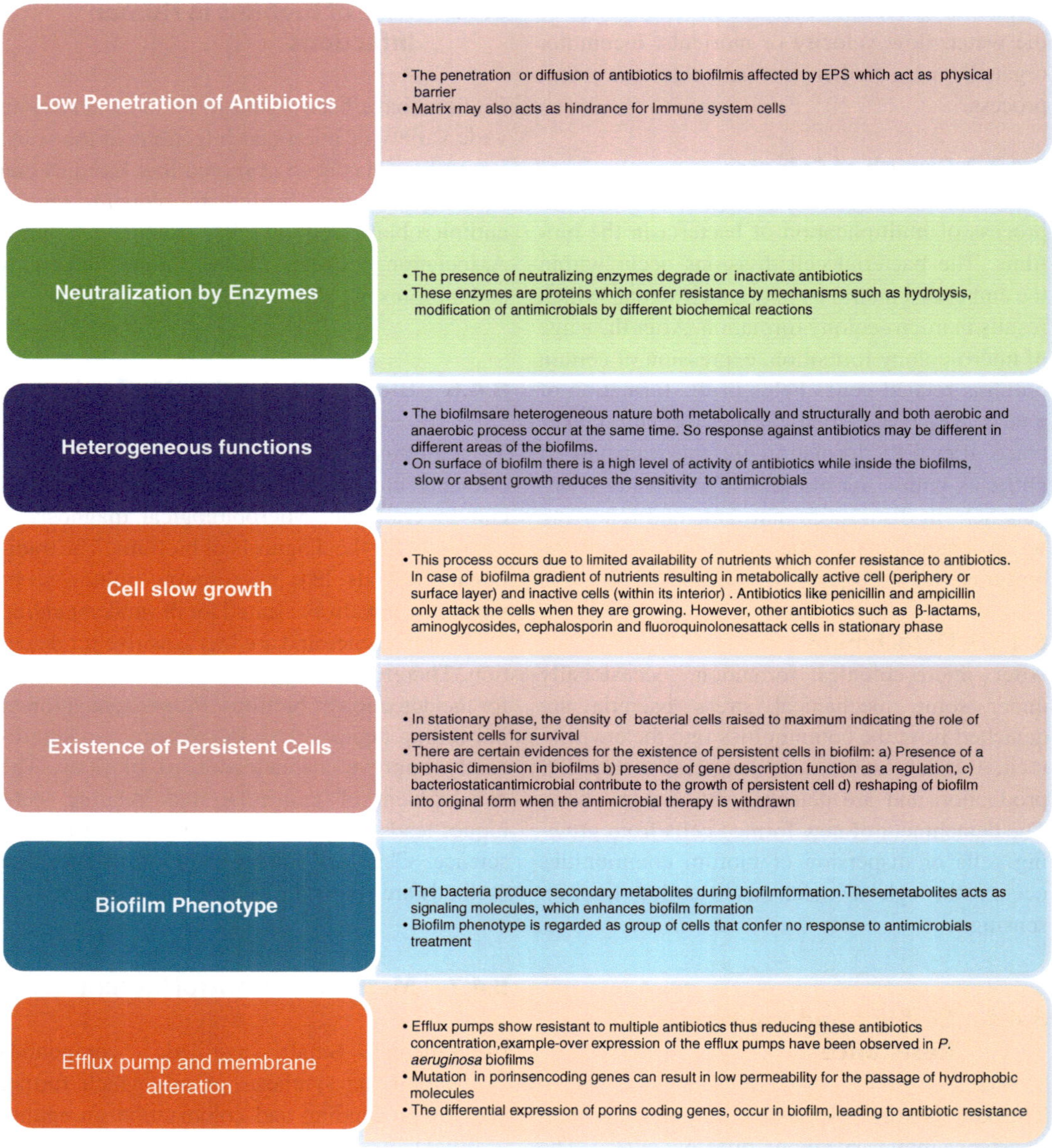

Fig. 8.10 Showing factors responsible for antibiotic resistance in biofilms

(D) Surface Coatings—Another effective way for the eradication of biofilm is coating the indwelling devices with antimicrobials.

(E) Bacteriophages—It has been observed that bacteriophages have the ability to inhibit or reduce formation of biofilm. Phage cocktail can also be used for removal of biofilm.

8.4.8 Future Aspects of Biofilm

It is challenging to eradicate infections related to biofilm formation in medical science. This is due to the fact the mature biofilms exhibit tolerance towards immune response and antibiotics. Further studies are required to know the mecha-

Table 8.7 Showing association between various human infections and biofilms

Condition	Salient features
Acute wound	Biofilm formation in wounds has been investigated *in-vivo* model (murine and porcine) for *S. aureus, P. aeruginosa* and *Streptococcus* biofilm
Chronic wound	In chronic wound, antibiotic treatment is considered to be effective in initial stages but after formation of biofilm, antibiotic therapy is least effective. Because biofilm can be up to 1000 times resistant to antimicrobials
Infectious kidney stones	The interaction between bacteria and mineral substances derived from urine results in formation of kidney stones, which are responsible for urinary tract infections. This result in the formation of biofilm
Bacterial endocarditis	The interaction between bacteria and host components lead to formation of biofilm which is known as vegetation. This vegetation can cause disease by different mechanisms: Disrupting the function of valve by creating leakage, turbulence, causes bloodstream infections or break down the vegetation which is then carried into the circulation (embolization)
Infections in Cystic fibrosis	These patients are most commonly infected with *P. aeruginosa*. The permanent infections in such cases with *P. aeruginosa* biofilm take place which last for the rest of the patient's life
Other Biofilm Diseases	
Otitis media with effusion	• The patient speech development and learning capability will be affected
Acute osteomyelitis	• Necrosed bone produced favourable conditions for biofilm development

Table 8.8 Detection methods of biofilm

Classical methods	Newer methods
Microtiter plate assay	Photobioreactor
Tube adherence method	Ultrasound
Congo red agar method	Sequencing Technologies
Biofilm bioreactor	PCR techniques
Biofilm Ring test	Spectrometry
	Confocal laser scanning microscopy
	Fluorescent in situ hybridization
	Nuclear magnetic resonance imaging

nism of antibiotics resistance and their gene expression biofilm. For better health care improvement, better understanding is needed for the development of novel, effective control strategies against biofilm.

8.5 Part DB: Biofilms: Surgeon's Aspect

Biofilms are increasingly recognized as a cause for persistent otorhinolaryngologic infections. About 75% of the microbial infections in humans are believed to be due to the formation and persistence of biofilms [88, 89]. These biofilms are highly resistant to treatment with antimicrobials and are capable of shedding bacteria into the bloodstream which leads to recurrent bouts of infection [90]. It has been noted that the presence of bacterial biofilms can be the reason for some forms of recalcitrant chronic rhinosinusitis. Biofilms that form on the surface of airway mucosa are known as mucosal biofilms. These are different from those that form on inert devices because these have to overcome the normal airway mucociliary clearance [91]. Inadequate doses of antibiotics for the treatment of rhinosinusitis can lead to biofilm formations and chronic infections. The most common cause of CRS refractory to medical treatment is the opportunistic infection with biofilm-forming *Pseudomonas aeruginosa*. Also implicated are *Staphylococcus aureus*, *Streptococcus pneumoniae*, *Haemophilus influenzae* and *Moraxella catarrhalis* [92, 93]. Fungal elements are also seen in biofilms. *Candida albicans* is the most common cause of biofilm formation among pathogenic fungi [94].

In children suffering from chronic otitis media and CRS, adenoidectomy is considered beneficial. Biofilm covered adenoids in nasopharynx of children with chronic rhinosinusitis, biofilms act as reservoir for reinfection. 95% of the adenoids and 70% of tonsils removed from children suffering from CRS have been found to be covered with biofilms.

It is a potential cause or persistent symptoms in some patients after ESS [95]. Frontal recess stents, stenting for choanal atresia, intranasal tubes are highly likely to be covered with biofilms and this can worsen the prognosis of surgery.

8.5.1 Treatment

Bacteria associated with biofilms behave differently from platonic bacteria, particularly in terms of antibiotic sensitivity. Biofilm cells are about 500 times more resistant to antimicrobial agents [87]. The structure of the biofilm along with the extracellular matrix prevents the drug from reaching the cells. Systemic treatment may require very high doses of antibiotics which may be intolerable and may not be effective at all.

Genetic resistance to antibiotics could be due to decreased penetration, decreased metabolic activity of biofilms, increase in the number of efflux pumps and presence of different subpopulations of bacteria within a biofilm [96]. Interfering in the various stages of biofilm formation like the interruption of quorum sensing or the genes involved in cellular attachment can be used as a strategy to inhibit biofilm formation.

Variety of techniques has been evaluated for managing and treating biofilms including surgery, topical antimicrobials and adjuvant therapies. Newer treatments are aimed at disrupting the life cycle of biofilms, preventing their attachment on to the surfaces and to disrupt the quorum sensing. With topical treatment, there are three strategies for eradication of biofilms.

1. Specific antibiotics against the causative microorganism.
2. Mechanical force for the detachment of the biofilm from the surface. E.g Surfactants, irrigation, surgery.
3. Quorum sensing inhibitors shift the bacterial phenotype from sessile to platonic form.

Various antibiotics have been tested for topical treatment of biofilms.

- Mupirocin has been found effective against the *Staphylococcus aureus* biofilms. It is effective because of its broad spectrum of action.
- Honey was effective against *S. aureus* and *P. aeruginosa* biofilms in vitro. It was found to eradicate 73% of MRSA biofilms and 91% of pseudomonas biofilms [97].

Surfactants break up the biofilm and allow the bacteria to be removed by irrigation.

- Baby shampoo has been used as a chemical surfactant to disrupt biofilms [98].
- Citric acid/zwitterionic surfactant solution by means of pressurized jet lavage is effective in breaking up biofilms in vitro [99].
- Surgical ventilation of the affected sinus helps against biofilm infections. It increases the oxygen tension and mechanically disrupts the biofilms [100].

Quorum sensing inhibitors increase the susceptibility of the biofilms to antibiotics and phagocytosis. Systemic long-term low dose macrolide therapy has been found to decrease the virulence of the bacteria and prevents the formation of biofilms [101]. For medical indwelling devices, ion bombarded silicone ventilation tubes have been found to be better than other silicone tubes.

Preventive Measures:

Biofilm can be prevented by vaccination against organisms that can cause chronic infections like pneumococci. Antibiotic prophylaxis and aggressive antibiotic therapy can prevent biofilm formation.

Newer Advances:

The detection of intercellular signalling system, lasR-lasI and rhlR-rhlI, involved in the development of *P. aeruginosa* biofilms, indicate signal manipulation as a possible target to control biofilms [102].

8.6 Part E: Empty Sinus Syndrome

Empty Nose syndrome (ENS) is a distinct clinical entity, which has been highlighted, in the recent few years because of the increasing incidence of Turbinate Surgeries. Since there are no set diagnostic criteria, so the diagnosis of these patients is based on combination of clinical examination, standardized questionnaires, CT scan and few objective tests. Treatment mainly consists of medical measures, with the surgical options only to be offered once the medical management fails and psychosomatic component is ruled out. In ideally selected candidates, surgery can provide extremely satisfying results by augmenting the volume of the lost tissues of the turbinates, thus channelling the airflow patterns. Research is underway worldwide to restore the function of the turbinates by injecting Platelet-Rich plasma, Platelet-rich lipotransfer and extracellular matrix components, which have shown initial promising results.

8.6.1 Introduction

Eugene Kern from Mayo clinic first described this entity in 1994. Empty Nose Syndrome (ENS) is an iatrogenic disorder characterized by the presence of paradoxical nasal obstruction, despite an objectively visible wide nasal cavity. It occurs few months to years after partial/total resection of the turbinates and sometimes even after turbinate surface cauterization. The basic pathology of this condition stems from changes in nasal physiology after volume reduction of turbinates. Exact incidence is not known, because of the paucity of literature and poor reporting of this entity.

There are various subtypes of ENS described by Houser SM [103], depending on the turbinate tissue, which is involved.

(A) ENS—IT type (Inferior Turbinate), which occurs after various surgeries for Inferior turbinate (IT) reduction (Fig. 8.11a).
(B) ENS—MT type (Middle Turbinate)—Symptoms occur after excessive resection of the middle turbinate (MT). In addition to paradoxical nasal obstruction, patients have pain on breathing.
(C) ENS-both—Refers to patients who have resection of both IT and MT tissues and lastly.
(D) ENS-Type—Patients who seem to have adequate normal tissue volume of the turbinate, yet they have ENS like symptoms. This is because of mucosal changes, which have occurred because of surface cauterization (Fig. 8.11b).

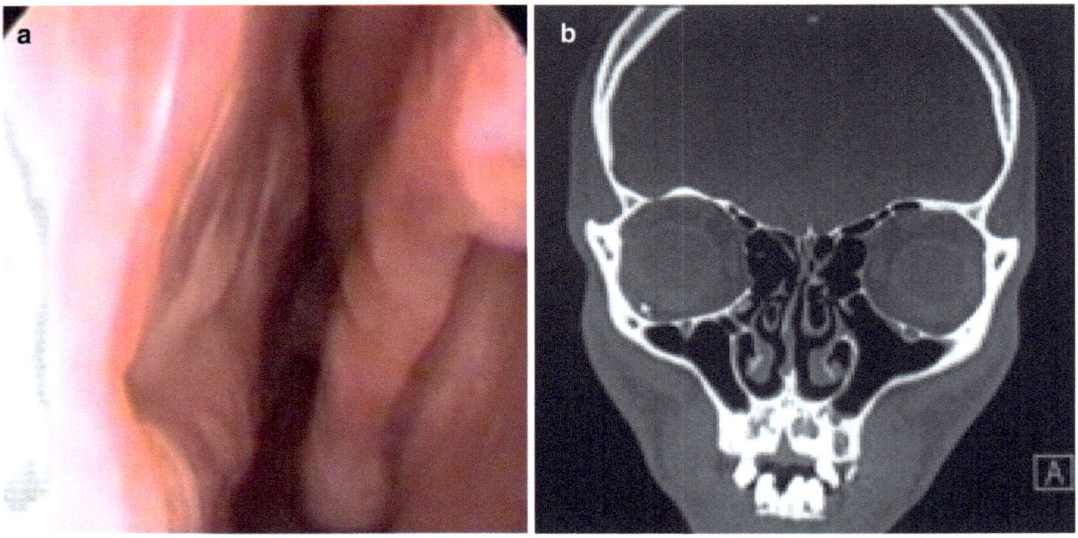

Fig. 8.11 (**a**) ENS is IT TYPE and (**b**) ENS is TYPE 1B

8.6.2 Pathophysiology

Extensive studies on understanding the pathophysiology of ENS have been done by Steven Houser [103]. The perception of the nasal patency has an underlying neuro-sensory mechanism. Activation of trigeminal 'cool' thermoreceptors by nasal mucosal cooling produces the sensation of nasal patency. These receptors are located in abundance in the inferior turbinate tissues, especially the superficial mucosal layers, which if damaged because of turbinate loss—produce sense of suffocation. Also, alteration in the airflow pattern is causative for paradoxical nasal obstruction.

In addition to altering the receptors and the airflow pattern, turbinate surgery also causes nerve damage and aberrant growth of the nerves due to scarring [104, 105] which fails to carry the message of nasal breathing, causing nasal obstruction.

8.6.3 Diagnosis

There are no set criteria for the diagnosis of this condition. Combination of classical patient symptoms, with history of prior surgeries clinches the diagnosis of ENS. The common nasal symptoms include—paradoxical airway obstruction, nose feels too open, sensation of suffocation, unable to feel the breathing from the nose, nasal and pharyngeal dryness, dyspnea, hyposmia and the common extra-nasal symptoms include facial pain, headaches and excessive preoccupation of the patient with the nasal issues affecting the quality of life, sleep patterns and causing severe depression and anxiety [106].

Nasal endoscopy reveals volume loss/scarring with pale and dry looking mucosa with occasional crusting. Houser has devised the Cotton test, which serves dual purposes. It acts as a confirmatory diagnosis for Empty nose Syndrome and also aids in surgically planning the site of sub-mucosal implantation. Moistened cotton with isotonic sodium chloride solution is placed in the nasal cavity for 20–30 min and the patient is asked to breathe comfortably and report the change in symptoms [106]. Patients with ENS will report marked improvement in symptoms with the cotton test (Fig. 8.12). In addition to this, patient's symptoms can be gauged by administering modified SNOT 25 questionnaire and ENS6Q questionnaire [107]. This also acts as a baseline to compare the post-operative surgical outcome. Another objective test to measure nasal obstruction by calculating the peak nasal inspiratory flow rate (PNIFR). Since patients with ENS have paradoxical nasal obstruction, their scores of PNIFR are always in the normal range. Thus the protocol that can be handy for the diagnosis of this entity includes the following

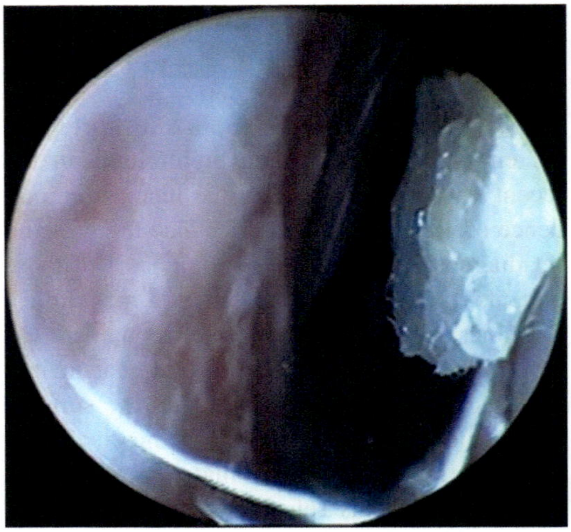

Fig. 8.12 Cotton Test

1. Thorough History taking with symptom evaluation
2. History of prior nasal surgeries
3. Nasal Endoscopy
4. Cotton Test
5. CT—PNS (plain)
6. Administering modified SNOT 25 questionnaire and ENS6Q questionnaire
7. Calculating the PNIFR
8. Psychological evaluation to rule out psychosomatic disorder

8.6.4 Management

Since this is a recently recognized entity, definitive treatment options are still being explored. Preventive strategies will go a long way to prevent this condition. Utmost gentleness and carefulness while handling the turbinate tissues is essential and turbinectomy should be done only in malignant cases when required. Allergy and other reversible factors should be taken care of in cases of turbinate hypertrophy, and if there is non-respondence to these, only sub-mucosal techniques should be used for turbinate reductions.

Conventional medical management is the first line of management. It comprises nasal moisturization with vaseline/lubricants, nasal irrigation and lavage, using cool mist humidifiers at home, increased fluid intake, intermittent nose pinching and cognitive behavioural therapy—for somatic complaints. Surgical options if there is failed medical management, ENS6Q score >11 and positive cotton test with ENS6Q score falling more than 7 points [108]. Aim of the surgery is to restore the nose geometry and function. Various reconstructive options can be used to restore the geometric contours of the nasal passage like sub-mucosal implantation of various alloplastic materials such as hydroxyapatite· Teflon, Gore-Tex and Plastipore, Allograft materials like Alloderm, [109] Autologous cartilage harvested from the septum or the concha to create a neoturbinate [110].

Regenerative medicine options are being explored in few centres worldwide to restore the mucosal function by injecting adipose-derived stem cells(ADSCs), Growth factors from PRP (Platelet-rich plasma), PRL (platelet-rich lipotransfer) [111, 112] and a cell (extracellular matrix components) which is used by Dr. Subinoy Das (USA).

8.6.5 Conclusion

ENS is a complex condition difficult to anticipate and treat. It is essential to be empathetic while dealing with ENS patients. It is imperative to do a detailed psychosomatic evaluation and offer a multimodality treatment to these patients. There are still unanswered questions as to why all patients after turbinectomies not suffer from ENS. Further studies and research are necessary to understand the disease better.

References

1. Silva MP, Baroody FM. Allergic fungal rhinosinusitis. Ann Allergy Asthma Immunol. 2013;110(4):217–22. https://doi.org/10.1016/j.jaip.2016.03.010.
2. Chakrabarti A, Denning DW, Ferguson BJ, et al. Fungal rhinosinusitis. Laryngoscope. 2009;119(9):1809–18. https://doi.org/10.1002/lary.20520.
3. Fokkens WJ, Lund VJ, Mullol J, et al. EPOS 2012: European position paper on rhinosinusitis and nasal polyps 2012. A summary for otorhinolaryngologists. Rhinology. 2012;50(1):1–12. https://doi.org/10.4193/Rhino50E2.
4. Kennedy JL, Hubbard MA, Huyett P, Patrie JT, Borish L, Payne SC. Sino-nasal outcome test (SNOT-22): a predictor of postsurgical improvement in patients with chronic sinusitis. Ann Allergy Asthma Immunol. 2013;111(4):246–251.e2. https://doi.org/10.1016/j.anai.2013.06.033.
5. Kosugi EM, Chen VG, da Fonseca VMG, Pellogia Cursino MM, Mendes Neto JA, Gregório LC. Translation, cross-cultural adaptation and validation of SinoNasal Outcome Test (SNOT) - 22 to Brazilian Portuguese. Braz J Otorhinolaryngol. 2011;77(5):663–9. https://doi.org/10.1590/S1808-86942011000500021.
6. Lund VJ, Kennedy DW. Staging for rhinosinusitis. Otolaryngol Head Neck Surg. 1997;117(3 Pt 2):S35–40. https://doi.org/10.1016/S0194-59989770005-6.
7. Philpott CM, Clark A, Javer AR. Allergic fungal rhinosinusitis – a new staging system. Rhinology. 2011;4:1–7. https://doi.org/10.4193/Rhino10.121.
8. Low T-HH, Woods CM, Ullah S, Carney AS. A double-blind randomized controlled trial of normal saline, lactated Ringer's, and hypertonic saline nasal irrigation solution after endoscopic sinus surgery. Am J Rhinol Allergy. 2014;28(3):225–31. https://doi.org/10.2500/ajra.2014.28.4031.
9. Lilic N, Waldvogel-Thurlow S, Douglas RG. Physical characteristics of commercial and home-made nasal lavage solutions. J Laryngol Otol. 2014;128(S1):S40–3. https://doi.org/10.1017/S0022215113001291.
10. Lee VS, Humphreys IM, Purcell PL, Davis GE. Manuka honey sinus irrigation for the treatment of chronic rhinosinusitis: a randomized controlled trial. Int Forum Allergy Rhinol. 2017;7(4):365–72. https://doi.org/10.1002/alr.21898.
11. Welch KC, Thaler ER, Doghramji LL, Palmer JN, Chiu AG. The effects of serum and urinary cortisol levels of topical intranasal irrigations with budesonide added to saline in patients with recurrent polyposis after endoscopic sinus surgery. Am J Rhinol Allergy. 2010;24(1):26–8. https://doi.org/10.2500/ajra.2010.24.3418.
12. Neubauer PD, Schwam ZG, Manes RP. Comparison of intranasal fluticasone spray, budesonide atomizer,

and budesonide respules in patients with chronic rhinosinusitis with polyposis after endoscopic sinus surgery. Int Forum Allergy Rhinol. 2016;6(3):233–7. https://doi.org/10.1002/alr.21688.
13. Bartle J, Millington A. How to perform nasal douching. Nurs Stand. 2017;31(49):41–5. https://doi.org/10.7748/ns.2017.e10683.
14. Bastier P-L, Lechot A, Bordenave L, Durand M, de Gabory L. Nasal irrigation: from empiricism to evidence-based medicine. A review. Eur Ann Otorhinolaryngol Head Neck Dis. 2015;132(5):281–5. https://doi.org/10.1016/j.anorl.2015.08.001.
15. Biel MA, Pedigo L, Gibbs A, Loebel N. Photodynamic therapy of antibiotic-resistant biofilms in a maxillary sinus model. Int Forum Allergy Rhinol. 2013;3(6):468–73. https://doi.org/10.1002/alr.21134.
16. Huang Z, Hwang P, Sun Y, Zhou B. Steroid-eluting sinus stents for improving symptoms in chronic rhinosinusitis patients undergoing functional endoscopic sinus surgery. Cochrane Database Syst Rev. 2015;6:CD010436. https://doi.org/10.1002/14651858.CD010436.pub2.
17. Gan EC, Thamboo A, Rudmik L, Hwang PH, Ferguson BJ, Javer AR. Medical management of allergic fungal rhinosinusitis following endoscopic sinus surgery: an evidence-based review and recommendations. Int Forum Allergy Rhinol. 2014;4(9):702–15. https://doi.org/10.1002/alr.21352.
18. Campoy S, Adrio JL. Antifungals. Biochem Pharmacol. 2017;133:86–96. https://doi.org/10.1016/j.bcp.2016.11.01.
19. Gallis HA, Drew RH, Pickard WW. Amphotericin B: 30 years of clinical experience. Rev Infect Dis. 1990;12:308–29.
20. Carr M, Dismukes WE. Antifungal drugs. In: Gorbach SL, Bartless JG, Blacklow NR, editors. Infectious diseases. Philadelphia: WB Saunders; 1992. p. 306.
21. Groll AH, Piscitelli SC, Walsh TJ. Clinical pharmacology ofsystemic antifungal agents in clinical use, current investigational compounds and putative targets for antifungal drug development. Adv Pharmacol. 1998;44:343–501.
22. Barton CH, Pahl M, Vaziri ND, et al. Renal magnesium wasting associated with amphotericin B therapy. Am J Med. 1984;77:471–4.
23. Luna B, Drew RH, Perfect JR. Agents for treatment of invasive fungal infections. Otolaryngol Clin N Am. 2000;33:277–99.
24. Kauffman CA, Carver PL. Use of azoles for systemic antifungal therapy. Adv Pharmacol. 1997;39:143–89.
25. Sheehan DI, Hitchcock CA, Sibley CM. Current and emerging azole antifungal agents. Clin Microbiol Rev. 1999;12:40–79.
26. Benitez LL, Carver PL. Adverse effects associated with long-term administration of azole antifungal agents. Drugs. 2019;79(8):833–53. https://doi.org/10.1007/s40265-019-01127-8.
27. Van Burik JA, Hare RS, Solomon HF, Corrado ML, Kontoyiannis DP. Posaconazole is effective as salvage therapy in zygomycosis: a retrospective summary of 91 cases. Clin Infect Dis. 2006;42:e61–5.
28. Garey KW, Rege M, Pai MP, et al. Time to initiation of fluconazole therapy impacts mortality in patients with candidemia: a multi-institutional study. Clin Infect Dis. 2006;43:25–31.
29. Upton A, Kirby KA, Carpenter P, Boeckh M, Marr KA. Invasive aspergillosis following hematopoietic cell transplantation: outcomes and prognostic factors associated with mortality. Clin Infect Dis. 2007;44:531–40.
30. Mora-Duarte J, Betts R, Rotstein C, et al. Comparison of caspofungin and amphotericin B for invasive candidiasis. N Engl J Med. 2002;347:2020–9.
31. Herbrecht R, Denning DW, Patterson TF, et al. Voriconazole versus amphotericin B for primary therapy of invasive aspergillosis. N Engl J Med. 2002;347:408–15.
32. Perlin DS, Rautemaa-Richardson R, Alastruey-Izquierdo A. The global problem of antifungal resistance: prevalence, mechanisms, and management. Lancet Infect Dis. 2017;17(12):e383–92. https://doi.org/10.1016/S1473-3099(17)30316-X.
33. Zhang M, Yang X, Wang D, Yu C, Sun S. Antifungal activity of immunosuppressants used alone or in combination with fluconazole. J Appl Microbiol. 2019;126(5):1304–17. https://doi.org/10.1111/jam.14126.
34. Wiederhold NP. The antifungal arsenal: alternative drugs and future targets. Int J Antimicrob Agents. 2018;51(3):333–9. https://doi.org/10.1016/j.ijantimicag.2017.09.002.
35. Robbins N, Wright GD, Cowen LE. Antifungal drugs: the current armamentarium and development of new agents. Microbiol Spectr. 2016;4(5) https://doi.org/10.1128/microbiolspec.FUNK-0002-2016.
36. Saafan ME, Ragab SM, Albirmawy OA, Elsherif HS. Powered versus conventional endoscopic sinus surgery instruments in management of sinonasal polyposis. Eur Arch Otorhinolaryngol. 2013;270:149–55.
37. Manji J, Habib AR, Amanian AA, Alsaleh S, Thamboo A, Javer AR. Potential risk factors associated with the development of synechiae following functional endoscopic sinus surgery. Eur Arch Otorhinolaryngol. 2018;275(5):1175–81. https://doi.org/10.1007/s00405-018-4936-1.
38. Lee JM, Grewal A. Middle meatal spacers for the prevention of synechiae following endoscopic sinus surgery: a systematic review and meta-analysis of randomized controlled trials. Int Forum Allerg Rhinol. 2012;2:477–86.
39. Vlastarakos PV, Iacovou E, Fetta M, Tapis M, Nikolopoulos TP. How effective is postoperative packing in FESS patients? A critical analysis of published interventional studies. Eur Arch Otorhinolaryngol. 2016;273(12):4061–71. https://doi.org/10.1007/s00405-015-3863-7.

40. Friedman M, Landsberg R, Tanyeri H. Middle turbinate medialization and preservation in endoscopic sinus surgery. Otolaryngol Head Neck Surg. 2000;123:76–80.
41. Boezaart AP, van der Merwe J, Coetzee A. Comparison of sodium nitroprusside - and esmolol-induced controlled hypotension for functional endoscopic sinus surgery. Can J Anaesth. 1995;42:373–6.
42. Mortuaire G, Bahij J, Maetz B, Chevalier D. Lund-Mackay score is predictive of bleeding in ethmoidectomy for nasal polyposis. Rhinology. 2008;46(4):285–8.
43. Hwang SH, Seo JH, Joo YH, Kang JM. Does the preoperative administration of steroids reduce intraoperative bleeding during endoscopic surgery of nasal polyps? Otolaryngol Head Neck Surg. 2016;155(6):949–55. https://doi.org/10.1177/0194599816663455.
44. Günel C, Başak HS, Bleier BS. Oral steroids and intraoperative bleeding during endoscopic sinus surgery. B-ENT. 2015;11(2):123–8.
45. de Vasconcellos SJA, do Nascimento-Júnior EM, de Aguiar Menezes MV, Tavares Mendes ML, de Souza Dantas R, Martins-Filho PRS. Preoperative tranexamic acid for treatment of bleeding, edema, and ecchymosis in patients undergoing rhinoplasty: a systematic review and meta-analysis. JAMA Otolaryngol Head Neck Surg. 2018;144(9):816–23. https://doi.org/10.1001/jamaoto.2018.1381.
46. Kang H, Hwang SH. Does topical application of tranexamic acid reduce intraoperative bleeding in sinus surgery during general anesthesia? Braz J Otorhinolaryngol. 2020;86(1):111–8. https://doi.org/10.1016/j.bjorl.2019.08.006.
47. Ko MT, Chuang KC, Su CY. Multiple analyses of factors related to intraoperative blood loss and the role of reverse Trendelenburg position in endoscopic sinus surgery. Laryngoscope. 2008;118:1687–91.
48. Abdullah B, Lim EH, Husain S, Snidvongs K, Wang Y. Anatomical variations of anterior ethmoidal artery and their significance in endoscopic sinus surgery: a systematic review. Surg Radiol Anat. 2019;41(5):491–9. https://doi.org/10.1007/s00276-018-2165-3.
49. Wynn R, Har-El G. Recurrence rates after endoscopic sinus surgery for massive sinus polyposis. Laryngoscope. 2004;114:811–3.
50. Zhang X, Ye T, Huang Z, et al. Clinical predictors of frontal ostium restenosis after draf 3 procedure for refractory chronic rhinosinusitis. Am J Rhinol Allergy. 2018;32(4):287–93. https://doi.org/10.1177/1945892418773625.
51. Amonoo-Kuofi K, Lund VJ, Andrews P, Howard DJ. The role of mitomycin C in surgery of the frontonasal recess: a prospective open pilot study. Am J Rhinol. 2006;20(6):591–4. https://doi.org/10.2500/ajr.2006.20.2917.
52. Luong A, Ow RA, Singh A, et al. Safety and effectiveness of a bioabsorbable steroid-releasing implant for the paranasal sinus ostia: a randomized clinical trial. JAMA Otolaryngol Head Neck Surg. 2018;144(1):28–35. https://doi.org/10.1001/jamaoto.2017.1859.
53. Benkhatar H, Khettab I, Sultanik P, Laccourreye O, Bonfils P. Mucocele development after endoscopic sinus surgery for nasal polyposis: a long-term analysis. Ear Nose Throat J. 2018;97(9):284–94.
54. Vaezeafshar R, Hwang PH, Turner JH. Commentary on "How to avoid mucocele formation under pedicled nasoseptal flap". Am J Otolaryngol. 2014;35(4):547. https://doi.org/10.1016/j.amjoto.2014.03.009.
55. Lee DH, Jang WY, Yoon TM, Lee JK, Jung S, Lim SC. Sphenoid sinus mucocele caused by complications after transsphenoidal pituitary surgery. J Craniofac Surg. 2018;29(7):1859–61. https://doi.org/10.1097/SCS.0000000000004693.
56. Simmen D, Veerasigamani N, Briner HR, Jones N, Schuknecht B. Anterior maxillary wall and lacrimal duct relationship - CT analysis for prelacrimal access to the maxillary sinus. Rhinology. 2017;55(2):170–4. https://doi.org/10.4193/Rhin16.318.
57. Ali MJ, Nayak JV, Vaezeafshar R, Li G, Psaltis AJ. Anatomic relationship of nasolacrimal duct and major lateral wall landmarks: cadaveric study with surgical implications. Int Forum Allergy Rhinol. 2014;4(8):684–8. https://doi.org/10.1002/alr.21345.
58. Song XC, Sun Y, Zhang H, et al. Zhonghua Er Bi Yan Hou Tou Jing Wai Ke Za Zhi. 2011;46(10):818–24.
59. Rodriguez MJ, Dave SP, Astor FC. Periorbital emphysema as a complication of functional endoscopic sinus surgery. Ear Nose Throat J. 2009;88(4):888–9. https://doi.org/10.1177/014556130908800414.
60. Shameer A, Pushker N, Lokdarshi G, Basheer S, Bajaj MS. Emergency decompression of orbital emphysema with elevated intraorbital pressure. J Emerg Med. 2017;53(3):405–7. https://doi.org/10.1016/j.jemermed.2016.10.021.
61. Ikeda K, Ito S, Homma H, et al. Orbital injury in endoscopic sinus surgery for sinonasal inflammatory disorders: Juntendo's ten-year experience. Int J Otolaryngol Head Neck Surg. 2017;6:65–70.
62. Stankiewicz JA. Blindness and intranasal endoscopic ethmoidectomy: prevention and management. Otolaryngol Head Neck Surg. 1989;101(3):320–9. https://doi.org/10.1177/019459988910100305.
63. Khanna A, Sama A. Managing complications and revisions in sinus surgery. Curr Otorhinolaryngol Rep. 2019;7:79–86. https://doi.org/10.1007/s40136-019-00231-3.
64. Rene C, Rose GE, Lenthall R, Moseley I. Major orbital complications of endoscopic sinus surgery. Br J Ophthalmol. 2001;85(5):598–603. https://doi.org/10.1136/bjo.85.5.598.
65. Mohammadi F, Rashan A, Psaltis A, et al. Intraocular pressure changes in emergent surgical decompression of orbital compartment syndrome. JAMA Otolaryngol Head Neck Surg. 2015;141(6):562–5. https://doi.org/10.1001/jamaoto.2015.0524.

66. Cetinkaya EA, Koc K, Kucuk MF, Koc P, Muluk NB, Cingi C. Calculation of an optic nerve injury risk profile before sphenoid sinus surgery. J Craniofac Surg. 2017;28(1):e75–8. https://doi.org/10.1097/SCS.0000000000003239.
67. Kim JY, Kim HJ, Kim CH, Lee JG, Yoon JH. Optic nerve injury secondary to endoscopic sinus surgery: an analysis of three cases. Yonsei Med J. 2005;46(2):300–4. https://doi.org/10.3349/ymj.2005.46.2.300.
68. Seredyka-Burduk M, Burduk PK, Wierzchowska M, Kaluzny B, Malukiewicz G. Ophthalmic complications of endoscopic sinus surgery. Braz J Otorhinolaryngol. 2017;83(3):318–23. https://doi.org/10.1016/j.bjorl.2016.04.006.
69. Kassam AB, Prevedello DM, Carrau RL, et al. Endoscopic endonasal skull base surgery: analysis of complications in the authors' initial 800 patients. J Neurosurg. 2011;114(6):1544–68. https://doi.org/10.3171/2010.10.JNS09406.
70. Daele JJ, Goffart Y, Machiels S. Traumatic, iatrogenic, and spontaneous cerebrospinal fluid (CSF) leak: endoscopic repair. B-ENT. 2011;7(Suppl 17):47–60.
71. Liu HS, Chen YT, Wang D, et al. The use of topical intranasal fluorescein in endoscopic endonasal repair of cerebrospinal fluid rhinorrhea. Surg Neurol. 2009;72(4):341–6. https://doi.org/10.1016/j.surneu.2009.03.034.
72. Hadad G, Bassagasteguy L, Carrau RL, et al. A novel reconstructive technique after endoscopic expanded endonasal approaches: vascular pedicle nasoseptal flap. Laryngoscope. 2006;116(10):1882–6. https://doi.org/10.1097/01.mlg.0000234933.37779.e4.
73. D'Anza B, Tien D, Stokken JK, Recinos PF, Woodard TR, Sindwani R. Role of lumbar drains in contemporary endonasal skull base surgery: meta-analysis and systematic review. Am J Rhinol Allergy. 2016;30:430–5.
74. Conger A, Zhao F, Wang X, et al. Evolution of the graded repair of CSF leaks and skull base defects in endonasal endoscopic tumor surgery: trends in repair failure and meningitis rates in 509 patients. J Neurosurg. 2018;130(3):861–75. https://doi.org/10.3171/2017.11.JNS172141.
75. Borg A, Kirkman MA, Choi D. Endoscopic endonasal anterior skull base surgery: a systematic review of complications during the past 65 years. World Neurosurg. 2016;95:383–91. https://doi.org/10.1016/j.wneu.2015.12.105.
76. Shelesko EV, Kapitanov DN, Kravchuk AD, Okhlopkov VA, Zaytsev OS, Chernikova NA. Taktika lecheniia defektov osnovaniia cherepa, soprovozhdaiushchikhsia pnevmotsefalieĭ [Management of complex skull base defects accompanied by pneumocephalus]. Zh Vopr Neirokhir Im N N Burdenko. 2019;83(2):85–92. https://doi.org/10.17116/neiro20198302185.
77. Banu MA, Szentirmai O, Mascarenhas L, Salek AA, Anand VK, Schwartz TH. Pneumocephalus patterns following endonasal endoscopic skull base surgery as predictors of postoperative CSF leaks. J Neurosurg. 2014;121(4):961–75. https://doi.org/10.3171/2014.5.JNS132028.
78. Hall-Stoodley L, Costerton JW, Stoodley P. Bacterial biofilms: from the natural environment to infectious diseases. Nat Rev Microbiol. 2004;2(2):95–108. https://doi.org/10.1038/nrmicro821.
79. Parsek MR, Singh PK. Bacterial biofilms: an emerging link to disease pathogenesis. Annu Rev Microbiol. 2003;57:677–701. https://doi.org/10.1146/annurev.micro.57.030502.090720.
80. Fux CA, Costerton JW, Stewart PS, Stoodley P. Survival strategies of infectious biofilms. Trends Microbiol. 2005;13(1):34–40. https://doi.org/10.1016/j.tim.2004.11.010.
81. Costerton JW, Stewart PS, Greenberg EP. Bacterial biofilms: a common cause of persistent infections. Science. 1999;284(5418):1318–22. https://doi.org/10.1126/science.284.5418.1318.
82. Nickel JC, Costerton JW. Bacterial localization in antibiotic-refractory chronic bacterial prostatitis. Prostate. 1993;23(2):107–14. https://doi.org/10.1002/pros.2990230204.
83. Hogan D, Kolter R. Why are bacteria refractory to antimicrobials? Curr Opin Microbiol. 2002;5(5):472–7. https://doi.org/10.1016/s1369-5274(02)00357-0.
84. Edwards R, Harding KG. Bacteria and wound healing. Curr Opin Infect Dis. 2004;17(2):91–6. https://doi.org/10.1097/00001432-200404000-00004.
85. Sims JN, Isokpehi RD, Cooper GA, et al. Visual analytics of surveillance data on foodborne vibriosis, United States, 1973-2010. Environ Health Insights. 2011;5:71–85. https://doi.org/10.4137/EHI.S7806.
86. Azeredo J, Azevedo NF, Briandet R, et al. Critical review on biofilm methods. Crit Rev Microbiol. 2017;43(3):313–51. https://doi.org/10.1080/1040841X.2016.1208146.
87. Xavier JB, Picioreanu C, Rani SA, van Loosdrecht MCM, Stewart PS. Biofilm-control strategies based on enzymic disruption of the extracellular polymeric substance matrix--a modelling study. Microbiology. 2005;151(Pt 12):3817–32. https://doi.org/10.1099/mic.0.28165-0.
88. Davies D. Understanding biofilm resistance to antibacterial agents. Nat Rev Drug Discov. 2003;2(2):114–22. https://doi.org/10.1038/nrd1008.
89. Richards JJ, Melander C. Controlling bacterial biofilms. Chembiochem. 2009;10(14):2287–94. https://doi.org/10.1002/cbic.200900317.
90. Vlastarakos PV, Nikolopoulos TP, Maragoudakis P, Tzagaroulakis A, Ferekidis E. Biofilms in ear, nose, and throat infections: how important are they? Laryngoscope. 2007;117(4):668–73. https://doi.org/10.1097/MLG.0b013e318030e422.
91. Parsek MR, Greenberg EP. Quorum sensing signals in development of Pseudomonas aeruginosa biofilms. Methods Enzymol. 1999;310:43–55. https://doi.org/10.1016/s0076-6879(99)10005-3.

92. Prince AA, Steiger JD, Khalid AN, et al. Prevalence of biofilm-forming bacteria in chronic rhinosinusitis. Am J Rhinol. 2008;22(3):239–45. https://doi.org/10.2500/ajr.2008.22.3180.
93. Ramage G, Mowat E, Jones B, Williams C, Lopez-Ribot J. Our current understanding of fungal biofilms. Crit Rev Microbiol. 2009;35(4):340–55. https://doi.org/10.3109/10408410903241436.
94. Le T, Psaltis A, Tan LW, Wormald PJ. The efficacy of topical antibiofilm agents in a sheep model of rhinosinusitis. Am J Rhinol. 2008;22(6):560–7. https://doi.org/10.2500/ajr.2008.22.3232.
95. Costerton JW, Lewandowski Z, Caldwell DE, Korber DR, Lappin-Scott HM. Microbial biofilms. Annu Rev Microbiol. 1995;49:711–45. https://doi.org/10.1146/annurev.mi.49.100195.003431.
96. Alandejani T, Marsan J, Ferris W, Slinger R, Chan F. Effectiveness of honey on Staphylococcus aureus and Pseudomonas aeruginosa biofilms. Otolaryngol Head Neck Surg. 2009;141(1):114–8. https://doi.org/10.1016/j.otohns.2009.01.005.
97. Chiu AG, Palmer JN, Woodworth BA, et al. Baby shampoo nasal irrigations for the symptomatic post-functional endoscopic sinus surgery patient. Am J Rhinol. 2008;22(1):34–7. https://doi.org/10.2500/ajr.2008.22.3122.
98. Desrosiers M, Myntti M, James G. Methods for removing bacterial biofilms: in vitro study using clinical chronic rhinosinusitis specimens. Am J Rhinol. 2007;21(5):527–32. https://doi.org/10.2500/ajr.2007.21.3069.
99. Zhang Z, Han D, Zhang S, et al. Biofilms and mucosal healing in postsurgical patients with chronic rhinosinusitis. Am J Rhinol Allergy. 2009;23(5):506–11. https://doi.org/10.2500/ajra.2009.23.3376.
100. Tré-Hardy M, Vanderbist F, Traore H, Devleeschouwer MJ. In vitro activity of antibiotic combinations against Pseudomonas aeruginosa biofilm and planktonic cultures. Int J Antimicrob Agents. 2008;31(4):329–36. https://doi.org/10.1016/j.ijantimicag.2007.12.005.
101. Tatar EC, Unal FO, Tatar I, Celik HH, Gursel B. Investigation of surface changes in different types of ventilation tubes using scanning electron microscopy and correlation of findings with clinical follow-up. Int J Pediatr Otorhinolaryngol. 2006;70(3):411–7. https://doi.org/10.1016/j.ijporl.2005.07.005.
102. Davies DG, Parsek MR, Pearson JP, Iglewski BH, Costerton JW, Greenberg EP. The involvement of cell-to-cell signals in the development of a bacterial biofilm. Science. 1998;280(5361):295–8. https://doi.org/10.1126/science.280.5361.295.
103. Sozansky J, Houser SM. Pathophysiology of empty nose syndrome. Laryngoscope. 2015;125(1):70–4. https://doi.org/10.1002/lary.24813.
104. Wu X, Myers AC, Goldstone AC, Togias A, Sanico AM. Localization of nerve growth factor and its receptors in the human nasal mucosa. J Allergy Clin Immunol. 2006;118(2):428–33. https://doi.org/10.1016/j.jaci.2006.04.037.
105. Sofroniew MV, Howe CL, Mobley WC. Nerve growth factor signaling, neuroprotection, and neural repair. Annu Rev Neurosci. 2001;24:1217–81. https://doi.org/10.1146/annurev.neuro.24.1.1217.
106. Chhabra N, Houser SM. The diagnosis and management of empty nose syndrome. Otolaryngol Clin N Am. 2009;42(2):311–ix. https://doi.org/10.1016/j.otc.2009.02.001.
107. Velasquez N, Thamboo A, Habib AR, Huang Z, Nayak JV. The Empty Nose Syndrome 6-Item Questionnaire (ENS6Q): a validated 6-item questionnaire as a diagnostic aid for empty nose syndrome patients. Int Forum Allergy Rhinol. 2017;7(1):64–71. https://doi.org/10.1002/alr.21842.
108. Thamboo A, Velasquez N, Habib AR, Zarabanda D, Paknezhad H, Nayak JV. Defining surgical criteria for empty nose syndrome: validation of the office-based cotton test and clinical interpretability of the validated empty nose syndrome 6-item questionnaire. Laryngoscope. 2017;127(8):1746–52. https://doi.org/10.1002/lary.26549.
109. Houser SM. Surgical treatment for empty nose syndrome. Arch Otolaryngol Head Neck Surg. 2007;133(9):858–63. https://doi.org/10.1001/archotol.133.9.858.
110. Jang YJ, Kim JH, Song HY. Empty nose syndrome: radiologic findings and treatment outcomes of endonasal microplasty using cartilage implants. Laryngoscope. 2011;121(6):1308–12. https://doi.org/10.1002/lary.21734.
111. Xu X, Li L, Wang C, et al. The expansion of autologous adipose-derived stem cells in vitro for the functional reconstruction of nasal mucosal tissue. Cell Biosci. 2015;5:54. https://doi.org/10.1186/s13578-015-0045-7.
112. Friji MT, Gopalakrishnan S, Verma SK, Parida PK, Mohapatra DP. New regenerative approach to atrophic rhinitis using autologous lipoaspirate transfer and platelet-rich plasma in five patients: our experience. Clin Otolaryngol. 2014;39(5):289–92. https://doi.org/10.1111/coa.12269.

Septum, Adenoid, and Epistaxis

9

Ravneet Singh, Hitesh Verma, Shashikant Paul, Sanjeev Bhagat, and Vishal Sharma

Contents

R. Singh
ENT, GMCH, Chandigarh, India

H. Verma (✉)
ENT, AIIMS, New Delhi, India
e-mail: drhitesh10@gmail.com

S. Paul
ENT, JIPMER, Pondicherry, India

S. Bhagat · V. Sharma
ENT, Rajindra Hospital Patiala, Patiala, Punjab, India

9.1 Part A: Nasal Septum, Septal Correction, and Septal Perforation

9.1.1 Introduction

The nasal septum is a midline structure that separates the nasal cavity into two parts and forms the medial part of the nasal valve bilaterally. It supports the nasal dorsum and maintains the nasal tip. It is formed from the posterior midline

H. Verma, A. Thakar (eds.), *Essentials of Rhinology*, https://doi.org/10.1007/978-981-33-6284-0_9

growth of the frontonasal process. Initially formed entirely of cartilage, it later ossifies to form the perpendicular plate of ethmoid and vomer. The nasal septum is easily deformed, and a septal deviation can be seen in up to 80% of the population but only a minority is symptomatic. Surgery is the only definitive treatment for symptomatic cases. SMR and Septoplasty are the two classical techniques with a variety of modifications described to tackle the various types of deviations. Septal perforation is a through and through defect of the nasal septum, perforations can be asymptomatic or can cause severe distress to the patient depending upon the size and location of the perforation.

9.1.2 Anatomy

The nasal septum is a midline structure formed by several bony and cartilaginous sources. It can be divided into three parts:

1. Columellar septum—it is the most anterior part and it forms by the medial crura of alar cartilages.
2. Membranous septum—it is double layer of skin with no bony or cartilaginous support.
3. Septum proper (Osseo-cartilaginous framework)—This can be further divided into bony and cartilaginous segments.

The cartilaginous part is formed by the lamina quadrangularis (quadrilateral cartilage). The bony part is formed by the lamina perpendicularis (the perpendicular plate of ethmoid) and the vomer with minor contributions from crest of nasal bones, nasal spine of frontal bone, rostrum of sphenoid, crest of palatine bones, the maxillary crest, and the anterior nasal spine of the maxilla. A widened region of the anterior nasal septum containing an increased amount of venous sinusoids is called the nasal septal swell body. The concentration of sinusoids suggests that it has the capacity to alter nasal airflow, like the inferior turbinates.

9.1.2.1 Blood and Nerve Supply

Septum receives blood supply from both external and internal carotid artery. The external carotid artery supplies via the braches of facial and internal maxillary artery and internal carotid artery via the branches of the ophthalmic artery. Kiesselbach's plexus (Little's area) is an area of anastomosis within the branches of internal and external carotid artery systems (Fig. 9.1). It lies in the anterior part of the septum and due to the

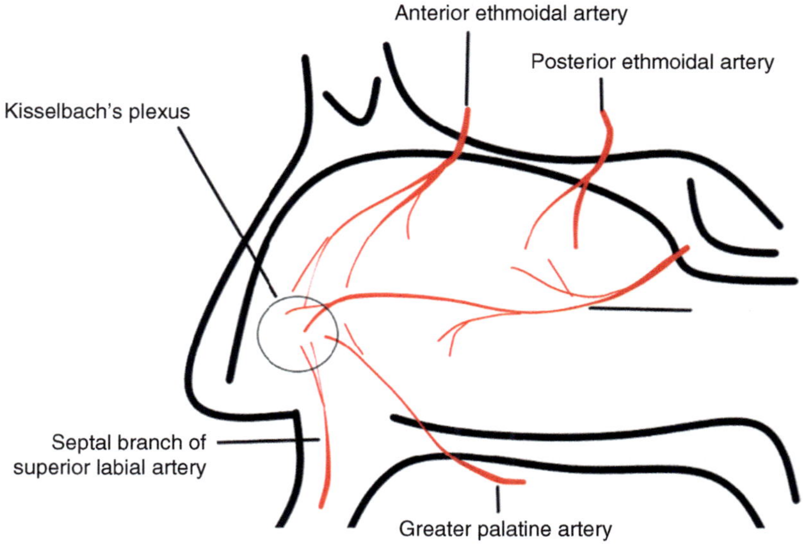

Fig. 9.1 Anterior and posterior ethmoid arteries are the braches of ophthalmic artery. Superior labial is the branch of facial artery. Sphenopalatine and greater palatine are the branches of the internal maxillary artery. Kesselbach's plexus (little area) lies in the anterior part of septum

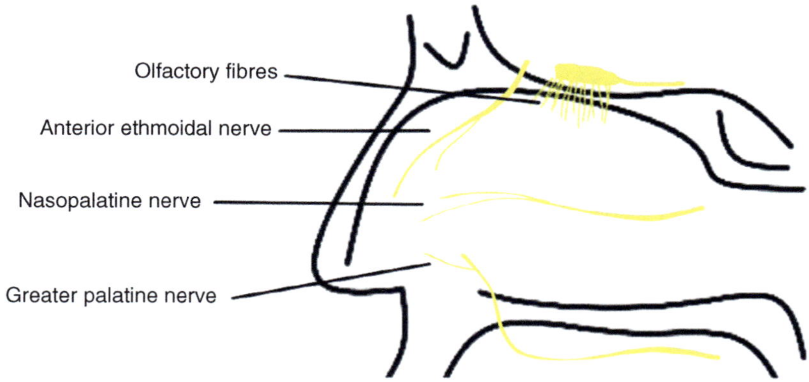

Fig. 9.2 The line diagram is showing the nerve supply of nasal septum

rich blood supply, is a common site of significant bleeding. The posterior septal artery is a branch of the sphenopalatine artery which supplies the posteroinferior septum. The nasoseptal flap (Hadad-Bassagasteguy flap) is the workhorse for endoscopic skull base reconstruction, is based on this artery (Fig. 9.1). The nerve supply of the nasal septum is derived mainly from ophthalmic (Anterior ethmoidal nerve) and maxillary (Greater palatine and Nasopalatine nerves) divisions of the trigeminal nerve (Fig. 9.2).

9.1.3 Development

The neonatal nose is completely cartilaginous, and the cartilaginous septum extends from the columella to the sphenoid. The perpendicular plate of ethmoid is formed by enchondral ossification while the vomer is formed as a result of intramembranous ossification. Premaxillary bone contributes to the nasal septum via the anterior nasal spine and the premaxillary wings. Vomeronasal cartilage is a small portion of cartilage that appears along the lower edge of the septal cartilage and is connected to a small blind pouch called the Vomeronasal organ. The vomeronasal organ is vestigial in humans but functions as an accessory olfactory organ in some mammals, amphibians, and reptiles. The cartilaginous nasal septum acts as a dominant growth centre in the developing mid face. The expanding septum produces mechanical forces that facilitate the separation of facial sutures (Nasal septal traction model). Loss of septal cartilage can lead to abnormal development of the nose, maxilla, and orbit. Septal deviation has been correlated with external nasal deformities as well as facial asymmetries as is evident in children with cleft palate. The deviation of the nasal septum has been shown to affect the thickness of the nasal bones as well as the size of the maxillary sinus and its propensity for inflammation.

9.1.4 Pathology

Pathological deviation is described as a septum deviation with nasal obstruction, i.e., a subjective reduction of nasal breathing.

Etiology: Septal deviations can be caused by (Fig. 9.3) [1].

- Trauma/injury
- Mass lesions—polyposis, neoplasia
- Genetic factors
- Congenital defects or
- Growth differences of the facial bones surrounding the nasal septum

9.1.5 Classification of DNS

Many classification systems have been proposed by authors according to severity, location, or type of deviation.

A. Cottle had classified septal deviations into three types according to severity:
   1. Simple Deviations: mild deviation of nasal septum without any nasal obstruction.

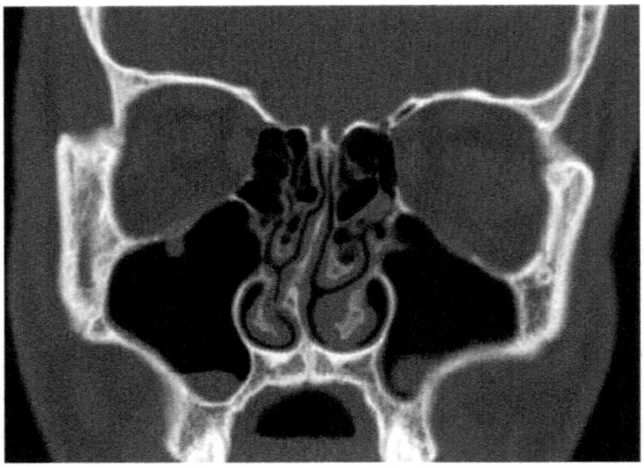

Fig. 9.3 CT Scan Nose and PNS (Coronal view): Deviation of the Nasal septum to the right side and enlarged turbinates on the left sides

This is the commonest and needs no treatment.
2. Obstruction: more severe deviation of the nasal septum. On vasoconstriction, the turbinates shrink away from the septum and obstruction is relieved. Hence surgery is not indicated.
3. Impaction: There is marked angulation of the septum and space is not increased even on vasoconstriction. Surgery is indicated in these patients.

B. DNS can be classified according to the shape
   1. C-shaped
   2. S-shaped
   3. Septal spur
   4. Anterior dislocation

C. Mladina Classification is a more comprehensive system based on the precise location of the deviation.
   - Type 1—Unilateral vertical ridge in the area of the nasal valve.
   - Type 2—Similar to Type 1 but more severe obstruction and disturbance of the nasal valve.
   - Type 3—Unilateral vertical ridge at the level of the head of the middle turbinate.
   - Type 4—Combination of type 3 with either type 1 or 2.
   - Type 5—Horizontal septal crest in contact with the lateral nasal wall.
   - Type 6—Prominent maxillary crest contralateral to the deviation with a septal crest on the deviated side.
   - Type 7—Combination of previously described septal deformity types.

9.1.6 Surgical Management

In patients with symptomatic septal deviation, removal, or correction of the deformity can lead to significant relief. It is vital to select the patients carefully before undertaking surgery on the septum [2]. Classically there are two techniques described:

1. Sub-mucosal Resection (SMR)
2. Septoplasty

While the basic principles of the surgery remain the same, each surgery needs to be modified to tackle different types and degrees of deviation and it may not confirm to the description of any one technique described. This has led to the surgery being commonly referred to as "Septal correction." With any septal surgery, it is important to remember that the dorsal and caudal ends of the septum (Struts) need to be preserved or reconstructed, failing of which, an external nasal deformity can occur. Whenever the area of the strut needs to be tackled, septoplasty is chosen over SMR.

Indications:

1. Nasal airway obstruction.
2. Chronic sinusitis secondary to septal deviation.
3. Epistaxis by septal vessels.
4. Obstructive sleep apnea.
5. In conjunction with other nasal and sinus procedures, such as cosmetic rhinoplasty, functional endoscopic sinus surgery (FESS), and skull base surgery.
6. As an access procedure in Skull base surgery.
7. Rhinological headache, caused by the contact of the septum with the lateral nasal wall.

An ideal surgical correction should satisfy the following criteria:

1. Should relieve the nasal obstruction.
2. Should be conservative.

3. Should not produce iatrogenic deformity.
4. Should not compromise the osteomeatal complex.
5. Should relieve all the contact areas.
6. Must have the scope for a revision surgery if required later.

Contraindications:

1. Acute URTI
2. Bleeding/Clotting disorders
3. Uncontrolled DM/HTN

9.1.6.1 Steps of Surgery

1. Sub-Mucosal Resection (SMR)
   A Killian incision is placed- about 1 cm cephalad from the caudal end of the septum. Mucoperichondrial and the mucoperiosteal flap is elevated on the side of the incision. Cartilage is incised just posterior to the mucosal incision and flaps are elevated on the opposite side. Septal cartilage removed leaving a dorsal and caudal strut. The deviated part of the bony septum is freed from its attachments and removed. The flaps are replaced and sutured at the incision site. Nasal packing, nasal splints, or trans-septal suturing can be used to support the flaps (Fig. 9.4).
2. Septoplasty
   Hemi-transfixation incision is placed at the caudal end of the septum. The mucoperichondrial flap is raised on the concave side. The degree of mucoperichondrial flap elevation depends upon the location and extent of the deviation. The bony osseo-cartilaginous junction is disarticulated to reach the opposite side of the bony septum. The mucoperiosteal flaps on both sides are elevated. The quadrilateral cartilage is disarticulated from the maxillary crest. A piece cartilage is removed to allow for the straightening and lengthening of the quadrilateral cartilage. Deviated part of the bone is also removed.

   The rest of the cartilage is straightened in-situ by (Fig. 9.5):

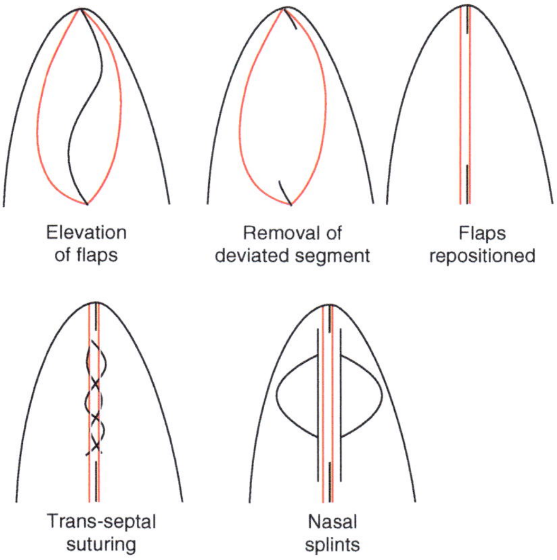

Fig. 9.4 The line diagram is showing different stage of submucosal resection with suturing technique and nasal splint placement

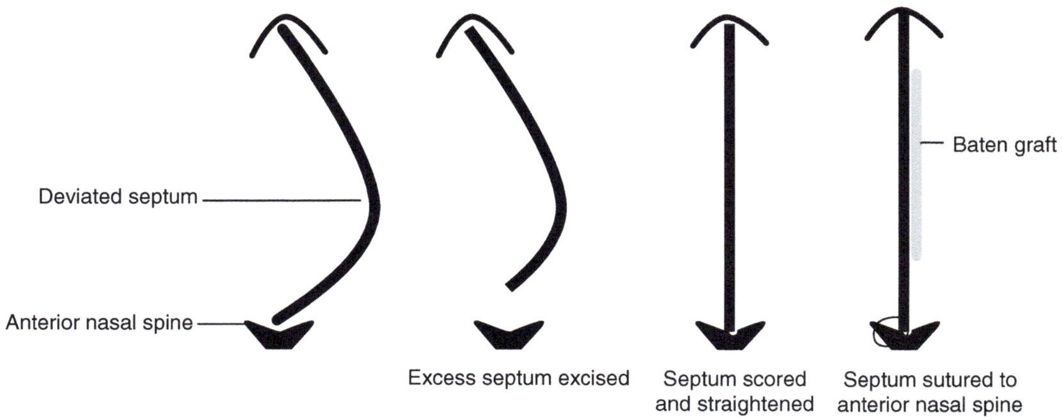

Fig. 9.5 The diagram is depicting ways of septal correction in the septoplasty technique

(a) Scoring of the cartilage.
(b) Scoring and suturing—sutures are tightened till septum is straight.
(c) Scoring and splinting—a batten graft is used to support the scored cartilage.

Tackling the septal spur is performed by mucoperichondrial flap elevation over the quadrilateral cartilage and the bony septum making an anterior tunnel over the spur. A subperiosteal tunnel is raised posterior to the septal spur. The mucosa left attached to the spur is then elevated by sharp dissection (Fig. 9.6).

Modifications

Historical Overview:

1. Metzenbaum (Swinging Door) technique: Technique was used to correct the caudal deviation of septum. The deviated cartilage is removed, the septum is swung into midline and inferior end of the cartilage is anchored with sutures to the anterior nasal spine.
2. Doorstop technique: The excess caudal nasal septum is transposed over the nasal spine and fixed.
3. Peer: Complete removal of the caudally deviated cartilage and reinsertion of the cartilage as a free graft.
4. Galloway: Single free autograft after removal of entire nasal cartilage, fixed with traction sutures.
5. Vilar Sancho: L shaped cartilage graft to support back and tip of nose.

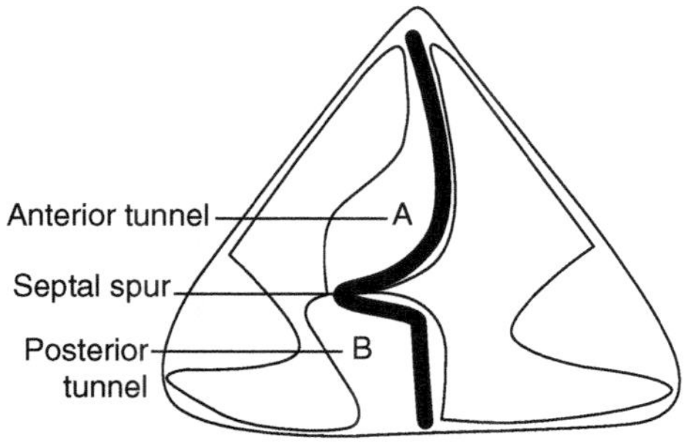

Fig. 9.6 The figure is showing the creation of tunnel anterior and posterior to spur follow by joining of both tunnels so that chances of mucosal perforation is reduced

6. Rees: Relocate entire quadrangular cartilage.
7. Gubisch: Used in combination with closed rhinoplasty. Entire quadrangular cartilage is removed, and the septum is re-created by using cartilage pieces.

Endoscopic Septoplasty:

The advent of the endoscope ushered in a new era in nasal surgery. Endoscopes may be used in nasal septal surgery as the primary or as an accessory tool. They are extremely useful in more cephalic and isolated deviations which can be directly visualized. It allows for localized incisions to be made, obliterating the need for excessive flap elevation. It can also be used along with a conventional technique to tackle the posterior part of the septum which is not otherwise visible. It can be used along with endoscopic sinus and skull base surgery and is also an effective teaching tool for residents.

External Approach Septoplasty:

This is a favorable approach for dorsal L-strut deformity and in complex septal reconstructive cases. Incision is made over the columella and the anterior end of the septum is exposed. This technique can be used along with a rhinoplasty procedure.

Extracorporeal Septoplasty:

Intact septum is excised and replaced by either:

1. Re-orientation: L-strut is harvested from the excised septum and it is reinserted in place.
2. Reconstruction: Pieces of the septum are splinted against the perpendicular plate of the ethmoid and then reinserted into its position. Grooves are made onto the maxillary crest and the anterior nasal spine where the septum is secured.

Pediatric Septoplasty:

The age and extent of septal surgery in the pediatric population is still controversial. Delaying surgery can affect nasal and facial growth and lead to prolonged nasal obstruction. Early intervention carries the risk of disturbance of the ossification centers leading to nasal and facial deformity. A range of techniques from closed reduction to the extracorporeal technique has been used. Resection of the cartilage should be conservative, and disruption of the endochondral ossification plates needs to be avoided [3].

Complications [4]
1. Bleeding
2. Infection
3. Saddle deformity
4. Columellar retraction
5. Supratip deformity
6. Adhesion
7. Septal Perforation
8. Septal hematoma/abscess
9. Sensory changes including upper dental anesthesia

9.1.7 Nasal Septal Perforation

It is defined by through and through defect of the nasal septum which may be more than one in number. It may be asymptomatic, especially if the perforation is small and located in the posterior part of the septum. It can lead to crusting, blockage, epistaxis, whistling sound while inhaling air, a feeling of dryness, emptiness in the nose, or a general feeling of discomfort. Huge perforations may cause rhinolalia aperta [5].

Causes:

1. Traumatic causes—nasal surgery, nose picking, nasal packing for epistaxis, septal hematoma/abscess, foreign body, etc.
2. Surface irritants—cocaine insufflation, heroin inhalation, lime, cement, glass, salt, dust, nasal decongestants, etc.
3. Infections—syphilis, TB, typhoid, diphtheria, rhinoscleroma, leprosy, mucormycosis, aspergillosis, etc.
4. Neoplastic—melanoma, adenocarcinoma, squamous cell carcinoma, lymphoma, etc.
5. Inflammatory—sarcoidosis, Crohn's disease, rheumatoid arthritis, SLE, dermatomyositis, etc.

The prevalence after submucous resection operations is higher (17–25%) compared to septoplasty procedures (1.4–5%). Septal perforations may also be surgically created in complex nasal and skull base endoscopic surgeries to provide a bi-nostril approach.

Management:

Conservative/Medical—The aim is to reduce drying, crusting, and epistaxis. Alkaline nasal douches, saline sprays, and petroleum-based ointments are commonly used.

Obturator—The principle of obturation is to cover the inflamed mucosal margin. It helps by controlling whistling and epistaxis.

Surgical—Variety of techniques and materials has been described to close the perforation.

- Free Grafts:
  - Autografts
  - Allografts
- Pedicle Flaps:
  - Local nasal mucosal
  - Buccal mucosal
  - Composite cartilage and mucosa or cartilage and skin
- Rotation/advancement of mucoperichondrial or mucoperiosteal flaps.

The selection of surgical approach is based on the size of perforation. Endonasal approach is good for small size perforation (5 mm to 1 cm). Medium size perforation (1 to 2 cm) requires wider exposure and approach is external rhinoplasty. Large size (more than 2 cm) can be managed by midfacial degloving approach.

Factors that affect the outcome are:

1. The amount of mucosa available in the nasal cavity can be mobilized.
2. The use of an interposition graft to support the mucosal repair.

9.2 Part B: Adenoid Hypertrophy and Management

William Meyer coined the term Adenoid for vegetations in the nasopharyngeal cavity in 1870. It is also called as pharyngeal tonsil. It forms the central part of the inner Waldeyer's ring.

Embryology The adenoid develops as a midline structure by the fusion of two lateral primordial that become visible during early fetal life. Adenoid tissue is fully developed by the seventh month of gestation and continues to grow until the fifth year of life often causing some airway obstruction then it gradually atrophies with airway improvement. It is lined by respiratory ciliated epithelium.

Function The function of adenoid is to produce antibodies like IgG and IgA. It also plays vital role in the development of immunological memory in younger children [6].

Etiology Adenoid hypertrophy is mainly caused by infections which includes

1. Coronavirus, Cytomegalovirus, EBV, HSV, Rhinovirus, etc.
2. Infection—Alpha, Beta, Gamma Haemolytic Streptococci, *Haemophilus influenza*, *Moraxella catarrhalis*, *Staphylococcus aureus*, *Corynebacterium diphtheriae*, etc.
3. Infectious causes that can lead to adenoid hypertrophy are GERD, allergy, etc.
4. Lymphoma, Sinonasal malignancy.

Blood Supply Arterial supply is mainly derived from ascending palatine artery, ascending pharyngeal artery, the pharyngeal branch of internal maxillary artery, ascending cervical branch of thyrocervical trunk. Venous drainage usually drains into the pharyngeal plexus, pterygoid plexus of veins, and also into the internal jugular vein. Lymphatic drains to upper jugular nodes directly or via retropharyngeal nodes.

Clinical Features Chronic nasal obstruction is the commonest symptom which leads to nasal discharge, sinusitis, open mouth breathing, an elongated face, dental malocclusion [7]. Aural symptoms include otitis media with or without effusion, decreased hearing, otalgia, etc. Other symptoms include sleep apnea, hyposmia, failure to thrive, excessive daytime sleepiness, impairment of cognitive functions, poor school performance, and psychosocial problems [8]. Adenoid faces is the term used to denote certain features in prolonged cases which include dull looks, pinched nostrils, open mouth, narrow maxillary arch, retracted upper lip, high arch palate (Fig. 9.7).

Diagnosis Clinical examination including examination of the external nose, anterior rhinoscopy,

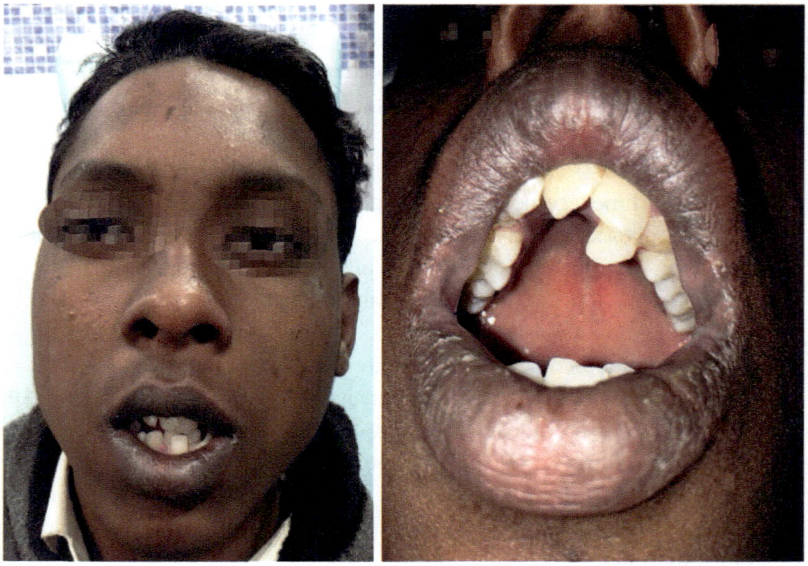

Fig. 9.7 The clinical photograph is showing features of adenoid faces (Courtesy—Dr. Hitesh Verma, Associate Professor, AIIMS, New Delhi, India)

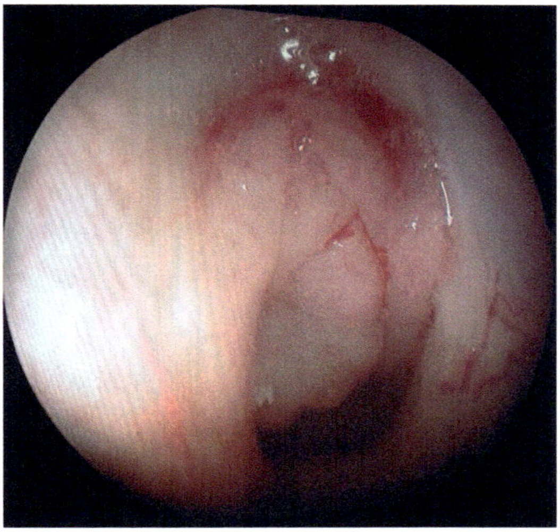

Fig. 9.8 Endoscopic view is shwoing grade 2 adenoid hypertrophy

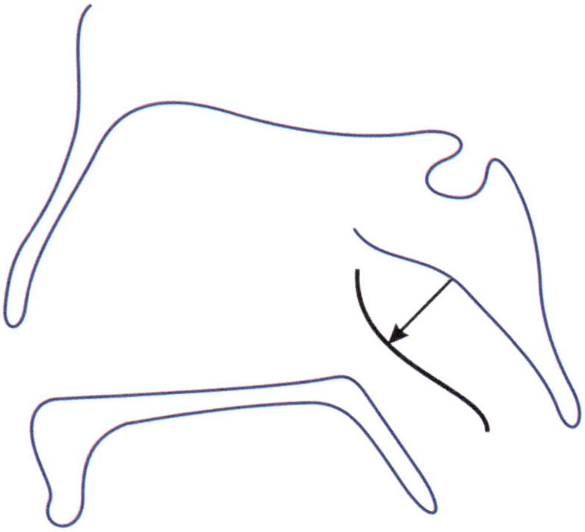

Fig. 9.9 Adenoid hypertrophy is assessing by measuring distance at maximum convexity from skull base (Courtesy—Dr. Hitesh Verma, Associate Professor, AIIMS, New Delhi, India)

oral and ear examination with the neck. Posterior rhinoscopy is relatively uncomfortable for young children. Hence imaging is helpful in making diagnosis which includes lateral neck radiography. Computerized scan or magnetic resonant imaging is indicated in doubtful diagnosis. Nasal endoscopy is the gold standard in the modern era for diagnosis and grading of adenoid hypertrophy (Fig. 9.8). Rhinomanometry and polysomnography are indicated in OSA patients. For reflex associated adenoid hypertrophy, pH monitoring is indicated.

9.2.1 Clinical Grading of Adenoid

Clinical grading system is based on part of choana is fill by adenoid tissue on endoscopic examination.

- Grade I—adenoid tissue filling one-third of the vertical portion of the choana.
- Grade II is when adenoid tissue filling one-third to two-thirds of the choana.
- Grade III fills from two-third to nearly complete obstruction of the choana.
- Grade IV there is complete choanal obstruction.

9.2.2 Radiological Staging

1. Johanneson proposed in the year 1968. Adenoid hypertrophy is assessed by measuring the distance from skull base at maximum convexity (Fig. 9.9).
2. Cohen and Konak method: The airway-to-soft-palate ratio is a comparison between the width of the airway immediately behind the soft palate and the width of the soft palate 1 cm below the hard palate (Fig. 9.10). Patients then were categorized into one of three groups:
   (A) Normal (airway-to-soft-palate ratio $\geq$1)
   (B) Mild-to-moderate hypertrophy (airway-to-soft-palate ratio between 0.5 and 1)
   (C) Severe hypertrophy (airway-to-soft-palate ratio <0.5) [9]

   2-A-N ratio: This ratio is calculated by measuring the maximal thickness of adenoid tissue and distance measured along the line from posterior–superior to spheno-occipital synchondrosis on skull base (Fig. 9.11) [10]. AN ratio greater than 0.80 can be the indicator of enlarged adenoids.

3. Crepeau et al. [11] graded adenoid hypertrophy by measuring maximum thickness of adenoid tissue and the shortest distance between the anterior aspect of adenoid with the posterior wall of maxillary antrum (Fig. 9.12).

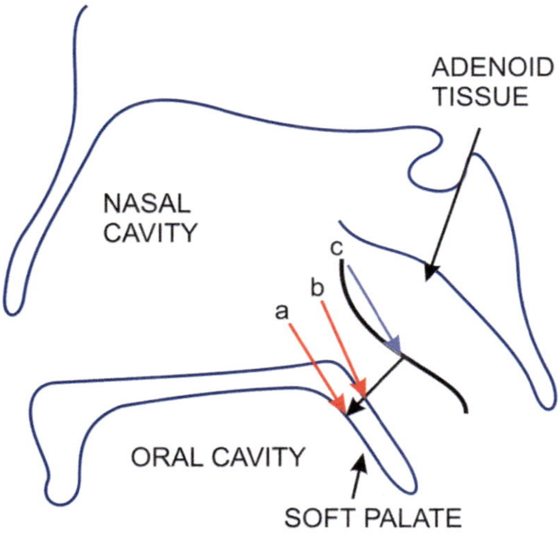

Fig. 9.10 The distance between point a to b is soft palate thickness and in between b to c is airway width (Courtesy—Dr. Hitesh Verma, Associate Professor, AIIMS, New Delhi, India)

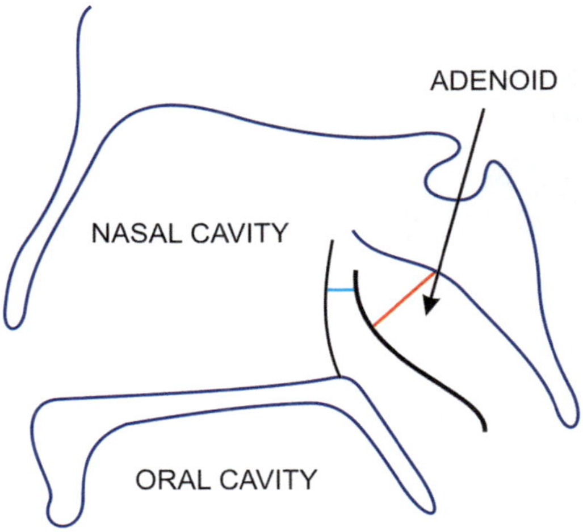

Fig. 9.12 The red line representing adenoid thickness and the blue line is showing distance between anterior aspects of the adenoid with choana. (Courtesy- Dr. Hitesh Verma, Associate Professor, AIIMS, New Delhi, India)

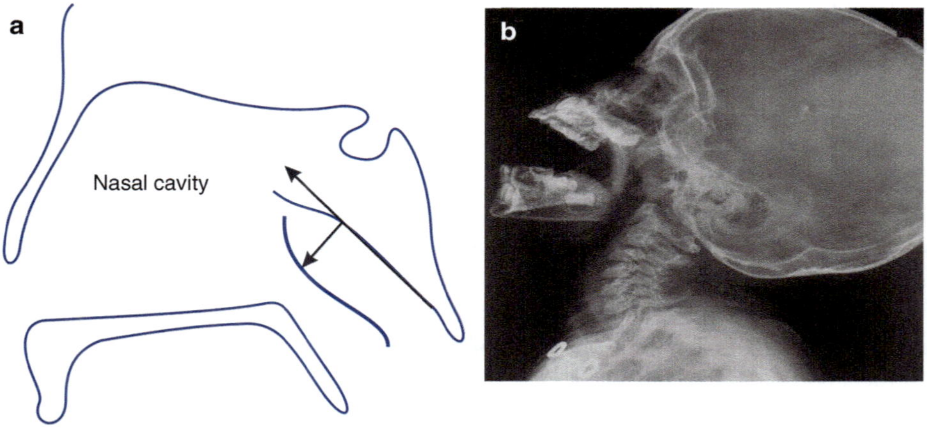

Fig. 9.11 The line diagram is showing assessment of the nasopharynx (posterior–superior edge of the hard palate to spheno-occipital synchondrosis on skull base—black line). Spheno-occipital synchondrosis point can also define by the uppermost point of posterior margin of the pterygoid plate (red line). Adenoid is measure by assessing from point of maximum convexity to right angle point from the imaginary line from anterior border of basi-sphenoid and basi-occipit. X-ray lateral view of the neck showing enlarged grade 3 adenoids (A-N radio) blocking the nasopharyngeal airway (Courtesy—Dr. Hitesh Verma, Associate Professor, AIIMS, New Delhi, India)

9.2.3 Management

Medical Management Breathing exercises, steam inhalation, regular nasal douches and Valsalva or reverse Valsalva maneuver are the conservative method. Lifestyle modification such as regular exercise and avoidance of preserved food for reflux induced adenoid hypertrophy. The selection of pharmacotherapy is based on the history of the patient. Anti-inflammatory treatment (antihistaminic, steroid nasal spray, etc.) is indicated in recurrent or persistent rhinosinusitis. Steroid based nasal spray is the usual prescription for allergic and persistent nasal obstruction secondary to adenoid hypertrophy. Mometasone based nasal spray is approved above 2 year of age whereas the majority of other spray is approved above 5 years of age. Decongestant nasal drops can be advice for both acute and chronic cases for not more than 7 days. Antibiotics are reserved for patient with purulent nasal discharge and for complicated adenoiditis. Proton pump inhibitors and antacids are indicated in reflux cases. Leukotriene receptor antagonist (montelukast) has shown to be effective in reducing the size of adenoids and respiratory-related sleep disturbances in children with mild OSA.

Surgical Management Adenoidectomy is mainly indicated when there is no response to conservative treatment. But surgery should be done early in grade 3 and grade 4 obstruction cases and also when adenoid hypertrophy induces sequelae because of its mass effect. Up to grade 2 adenoid hypertrophy, the surgical selection is based on the response to medical management.

9.2.4 Indications

A. **Infection**—Purulent adenoiditis, adenoid hypertrophy associated with complications such as otitis media with effusion, chronic recurrent otitis media, chronic otitis media with perforation.
B. **Obstruction**—Adenoid hypertrophy associated with excessive snoring and chronic mouth breathing, sleep apnea or sleep disturbances, adenoid hypertrophy associated with cor pulmonale, failure to thrive, dysphagia, speech abnormalities, craniofacial growth abnormalities, occlusion abnormalities.
C. **Other**—Suspected neoplasia, adenoid hypertrophy associated with chronic sinusitis.

Contraindications Cleft palate, velopharyngeal insufficiency, and bleeding diathesis. Systemic review in cases of palatal abnormality showed partial adenoidectomy is safe and effective procedure in problematic cases [12].

9.2.5 Surgical Techniques

1. **Conservative (Cold) Technique:** For cold technique, the patient should be placed in Rose's position after induction of general anesthesia and Boyles Davis mouth gag is applied for oropharyngeal exposure. Red rubber tube or catheter can be used to retract the soft palate for better visualization of the nasopharynx. The size of the adenoid can be assessed either by nasopharyngeal mirror or by digital palpation. Use of endoscopes increases visualization by both trans-nasal and per-oral route. For the appropriate selection of curette, the width of incisors needs to be assessed. Curette is held in dagger-like fashion and placed high in the nasopharynx, abutting the posterior aspect of the nasal septum and neck is flexed in the neutral position to avoid injury to posterior pharyngeal wall and dens. Then adenoid pad can be curetted with care taken not to penetrate deeply into the prevertebral region. Care needs while removing tissue far laterally to avoid trauma to eustachian tube. Endoscopic assessment can be done in between procedure to conform tissue excision and for prevention of injury to normal structures. Packs can be placed into the nasopharynx for hemostasis [13]. Other techniques include suction diathermy ablation of the adenoid, radiofrequency adenoidectomy. Suction diathermy ablation is safe with minimal blood loss however it is slow and has the risk of cicatrization and burns to surrounding tissue [14].
2. **Endoscopic Powered Technique** includes adenoidectomy by microdebrider. Power-

assisted adenoidectomy allows more precise, rapid, safe, and it achieves complete removal of adenoid tissue. It is especially useful in removing adenoid tissue that extends through the choana and into the nasal cavity. It can be done with multiple blades with different angles ranging from 30 to 90° either through the nasal cavity or through the oral cavity. Due to the suction and shaving action of microdebrider, it can remove the tissue down to the less vascular fascial plane. Oscillation cutting action of the blade minimizes the bleeding [15].
3. **Coblation Adenoidectomy:** It utilizes a system of radiofrequency bipolar electrical current that passes through a medium of normal saline, which results in the production of plasma field of sodium ions. These ions break down intercellular bonds and effectively vaporize tissue at a temperature of only 60°C. The coblator consists of a handpiece with a suction irrigation tip that transmits the radiofrequency current and dissects tissue. It also has cautery for hemostasis. With this technique, separate suction cautery device is not necessary. It also ensures the complete removal of adenoid tissue with minimal bleeding. Coblation has advantages like very limited depth of penetration, minimal collateral tissue damage, localized effect, controlled volumetric tissue removal, low surface temperature. To reduce the operating duration, the surgeon combines microdebrider with coblator.

Among all technique, simultaneous use of nasal endoscopes reduces complication to great extent and conventional technique is rapid as compared to other techniques. Powered instruments are more precise, less traumatic to surrounding structures [16].

9.2.6 Complications of Adenoidectomy

1. Bleeding
2. Dental trauma
3. Infection
4. Grisel syndrome
5. Velopharyngeal dysfunction
6. Regrowth of adenoids

Bleeding is mainly reactionary with the rate of 0.7%. It can be managed by proper hemostasis. Rarely, post nasal packing is required. Secondary hemorrhage is very rare. It may be due to bleeding from the aberrant ascending pharyngeal artery or by infection in the postoperative cavity. Unusual reactionary or secondary bleeding raises the possibility of clotting or coagulation defect. Nasopharyngeal blood clot may get pooled in the nasopharynx during the procedure. Failure to clear this clot may cause fatal acute airway obstruction which is called Coroner's clot. Infection is relatively uncommon and rarely retropharyngeal and mediastinal abscesses may occur. Grisel Syndrome is non-traumatic atlantoaxial subluxation seen more commonly with curette adenoidectomy. Velopharyngeal dysfunction is rare but can cause significant problems with hypernasal speech and swallowing. It is mandatory to assess the palate and uvula for submucous cleft prior to surgery. Regrowth of adenoid is usually seen more commonly with curettage adenoidectomy.

9.3 Part C: Epistaxis and Management

Epistaxis, or bleeding from the nose, is the commonest emergency in ENT practice. It affects up to 60% of the population in their lifetime, and in 6%, it requires medical attention. It can be life threatening in elderly patients and can cause major concern in parents of young children. Nasal cavity mucosa is supplied by the terminal branches of the internal and external carotid artery (Fig. 9.13). Nasal bleeding most commonly occurs from Kiesselbach's plexus or Little's area, which is supplied by both systems. Woodruff's plexus lying in the posterior part of nasal cavity just inferior to posterior-most end of the inferior turbinate. It is generally responsible for posterior epistaxis.

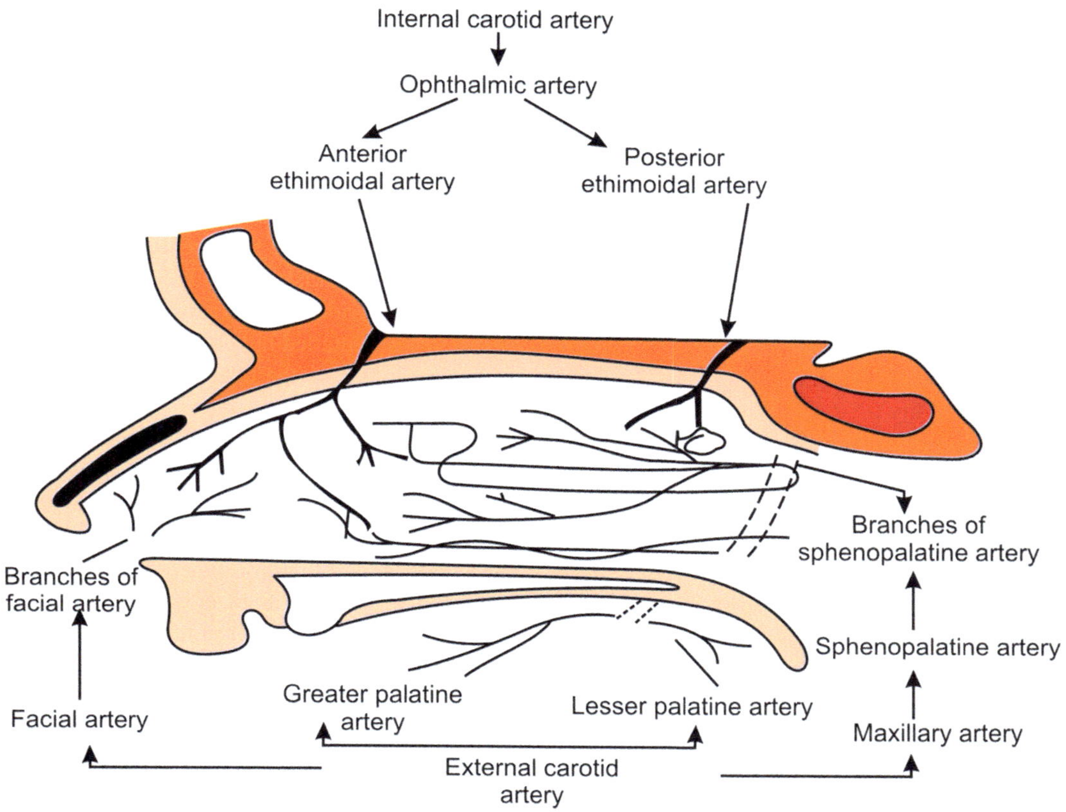

Fig. 9.13 The line diagram is showing the nasal cavity blood supply

9.3.1 Causes

The etiology of epistaxis can be divided into local and general causes; however 80–90% of cases are idiopathic.

9.3.1.1 Local

1. Trauma
   (a) Nasal fracture
   (b) Nose picking
   (c) Foreign body
   (d) Continuous positive airway pressure
2. Inflammatory Conditions
   (a) Allergic rhinosinusitis
   (b) Bacterial rhinosinusitis
   (c) Common cold
3. Neoplasia
   (a) Septal and turbinate hemangioma
   (b) Nasal papilloma
   (c) Juvenile nasopharyngeal angiofibroma
   (d) Squamous cell carcinoma
   (e) Inverted papilloma
4. Granulomatous disorder
   (a) Sarcoidosis
   (b) Wegener's granulomatosis
   (c) Tuberculosis
5. Structural
   (a) Septal Spurs
   (b) Septal perforation
6. Iatrogenic
   (a) Functional endoscopic sinus surgery
   (b) Septoplasty
   (c) Turbinate reduction
   (d) Nasogastric tube insertion
   (e) Nasotracheal intubation
7. Drugs
   (a) Nasal steroids
   (b) Cocaine abuse

9.3.1.2 General

1. Hematological
   (a) Coagulopathies
   (b) Thrombocytopenia
   (c) Platelet dysfunction, e.g., Von Willebrand's disease
   (d) Hemophilia
   (e) Aplastic anemia
   (f) Hereditary hemorrhagic telangiectasia/ Osler Weber Rendu disease
2. Hypertension
3. Environmental factors
   (a) Humidity
   (b) Altitude
   (c) Temperature
   (d) Pollution
4. Drugs
   (a) Anticoagulants like heparin, warfarin
   (b) Antiplatelets like ecosprin, clopidogrel
5. Organ failure
   (a) Uremia
   (b) Cirrhosis
6. Atherosclerosis
7. Alcoholism

Epistaxis can be classified on the basis of etiology. Epistaxis is called primary when no cause is identify whereas secondary when cause is available. When the site of bleeding is visible on anterior rhinoscopy or anterior to pyriform aperture, it is called anterior epistaxis. When the site of bleeding is not visible by anterior rhinoscopy or behind the pyriform aperture, it is called posterior epistaxis.

9.3.2 Risk Factors

Risk factors for recurrent epistaxis include the following:

1. Hypertension and diabetes mellitus are minor risk factors for recurrent epistaxis as both these conditions are known to induce atherosclerotic changes in the vasculature system [17].
2. Congestive heart failure is the cause of recurrent epistaxis because of the increased venous pressure in the nasal vessels.
3. Anatomical abnormalities like septal deviations and spurs are also responsible.

9.3.3 Management

The initial most management is resuscitation. It includes correction of volume loss by intravenous fluid administration. Blood transfusion should be considered if hemoglobin levels fall below 9 g/dl. Detailed history and examination is helpful to diagnose the cause of bleeding. After primary resuscitation, necessary blood investigation is advised on the basis of history. Blood grouping and cross-matching is must for moderate to severe epistaxis cases. For anterior epistaxis, the patient should be asked to pinch the lower cartilaginous part of the nose while leaning forward over a bowl as bleeding into the nasopharynx is more uncomfortable. Also, the blood will not be swallowed causing subsequent nausea. The treatment policy is followed in the form of four line of management. First line of management is indicated when the site of bleeding is visible either by anterior rhinoscopy or by nasal endoscopy. Bleeding point can be cauterized by electric or by chemical application and it is known as the direct method. Chemical cautery with silver nitrate is more useful for bleeding points in anterior part of the nose. Bipolar or monopolar suction cautery is an alternative if bleeding is more posterior, rigorous, or if refractory to chemical cautery (Fig. 9.14) [18]. Simultaneous bilateral cautery on the nasal septum should be avoided to minimize the risk of septal perforation.

When the site of bleeding is not visible or it is generalized, then second line of management is applicable. It is an indirect method and nasal packing is done to control bleeding. The different kinds of packing materials are mentioned in Chap. 1. In this chapter, we are discussing packing technique. Newer absorbable and non-absorbable packing materials are generally effective in low to moderate amount of epistaxis. Absorbable packs offer greater patient comfort and are more desirable in patients with thrombocytopenia or coagulopathy. They create less injury to the surrounding mucosa. Three fourth inch width Roller Gauze is helpful in almost all kind of anterior epistaxis. It is applicable when, newer packing material failed, in moderate to severe epistaxis and recurrent epistaxis. Roller gauze is soaked in Vaşeline or petroleum jelly to prevent surrounding adhesion and to minimized insertional/removal trauma. Pack can be placed in vertical and horizontal manner (Fig. 9.15). Horizontal manner is relatively easy and most followed. Gauze is generally kept for 48–72 h. If required for more than 72 h, then it should be changed to prevent toxic shock syndrome. Newer

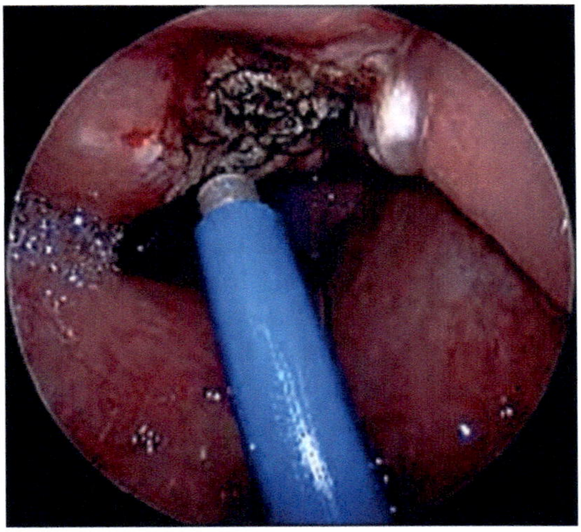

Fig. 9.14 The suction monopolar cautery is used to control epistaxis

commercial packs can be kept for 4–5 days. The alarming signs for toxic shock syndrome are purulent foul smelling discharge from pack, fever, tachycardia, etc. In such situation, the pack should be removed immediately and broad-spectrum antibiotics should start.

Posterior Packing is indicated for posterior epistaxis. It can be achieved by high volume, low-pressure balloon packs. **Brighton Balloon** is specifically manufactured for epistaxis. It has a postnasal balloon and immobile anterior balloon that are independently inflated. **Epistat Nasal Catheter** has two independently inflatable bulbs for precise control of bleeding. The hollow catheter allows nasal breathing. Conventionally posterior nasal pack is prepared with gauze material. The volume of the nasopharynx should be kept in mind while preparing it. Incisor width is the rough estimation of nasopharynx width. Foley's catheter is generally available in operation theaters. It is more in use for posterior packing. Ten to fifteen ml of water is sufficient to obliterate the nasopharynx. It can hinge over columella with umbilical tap. Columella should be secured to prevent necrosis. When both anterior and posterior nasal packing is required, the posterior should be placed first.

Studies have shown the benefit of warm water irrigation in posterior epistaxis as compared to nasal packing. A modified bladder catheter that seals the choana can be inserted. Water at 50 °C is irrigated through the catheter with the help of a

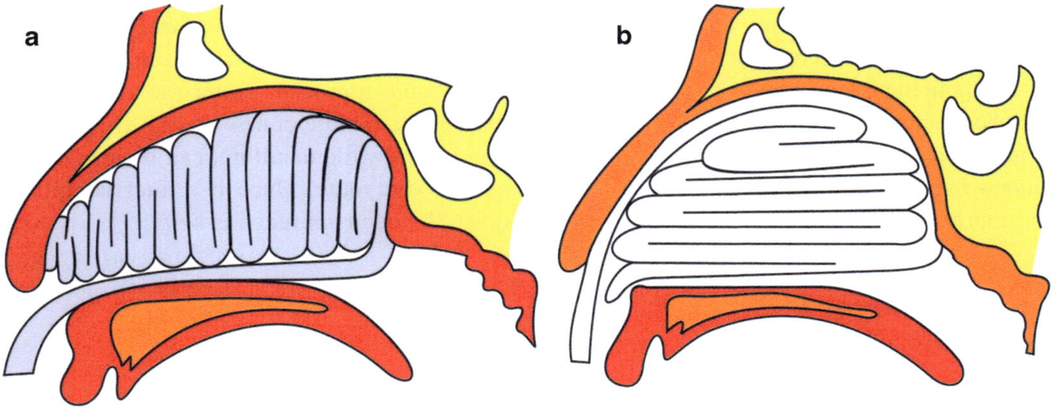

Fig. 9.15 The diagram is depicting the vertical and horizontal way of nasal cavity packing with gauze material

caloric stimulator and will exit the catheter through a hole proximal to the inflated balloon. It is believed that the warm water causes edema of the nasal mucosa thereby compressing the bleeding vessels in addition to possibly stimulating the coagulation cascade. Tranexamic acid and epsilon aminocaproic acid are useful as adjuvant systemic therapy for recurrent and refractory epistaxis [19].

9.3.4 Surgical Management

If all the above methods fail to control the bleeding, definitive surgical procedures have to be performed. It is the third line of management. Sphenopalatine is the major blood supply for nasal mucosa [20]. It can ligate by endoscopic or by sub-labial transmaxillary approach.

9.3.4.1 Endoscopic Sphenopalatine Artery (SPA) Ligation

The SPA is the last branch of the internal maxillary artery and it enters the nasal cavity through the sphenopalatine foramen. Foreman lies in the posterior lateral nasal wall in the posterior-most part of the middle meatus, just inferior to the lateral attachment of middle turbinate. Sphenopalatine foramen is lying behind and inferior to the ethmoid crest (Fig. 9.16). Clipping or diathermy of the sphenopalatine artery is currently the accepted treatment. 97% of individuals have two or more branches medial to the ethmoid crest. Failure to identify these branches can lead to the recurrence of bleeding. If no bleeder identified, SPA ligation can be done as it has the widest supply in the nasal cavity.

Sphenopalatine bleed can also control by identification in pterygopalatine fossa by creating window in posterior wall of maxilla by Caldwell-Luc approach in difficult case scenario.

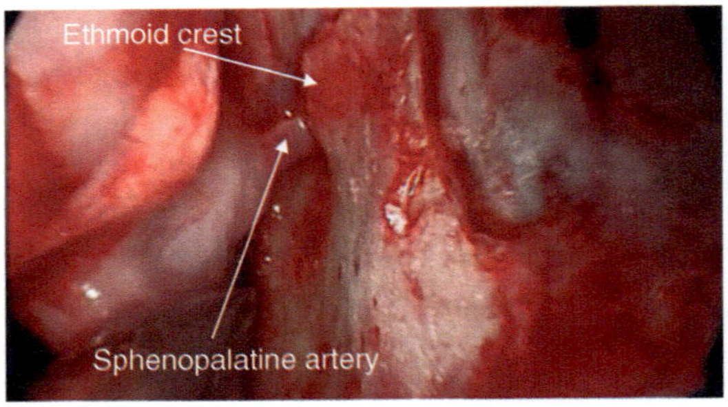

Fig. 9.16 The endoscopic picture is showing the relationship of the left sphenopalatine artery and ethmoid crest

9.3.4.2 Anterior Ethmoidal Artery Ligation

Anterior ethmoid artery is branch of ophthalmic artery. It enters into nasal cavity via anterior ethmoid foreman. It runs with in ethmoid roof bone in 90% of cases. In 10% it runs deep within nasal cavity just posterior to frontal recess. Anterior Ethmoidal artery can be injured in naso-ethmoid fractures or during sinus surgery. It can lead to severe epistaxis. Injury to the artery can also lead to intraorbital or intracranial bleeding [21]. Retro-orbital hemorrhage is an emergency as it can lead to blindness. Its management requires ligation of the artery either by an external approach or endoscope approach. Open approach is preferred over endoscopic approach in traumatic cases. Lynch Howarth's incision is the incision made in the region of the medial cantus (Fig. 9.17). Lacrimal sac requires lifting from its bed for better access. Artery is locating 24 mm deep to the anterior lacrimal crest. In endoscopic approach, cauterization of artery is done in its middle course so that if any bleeding occurs while handling, can be managed by endoscopic route. Once it retract laterally in orbit, the open approach is better.

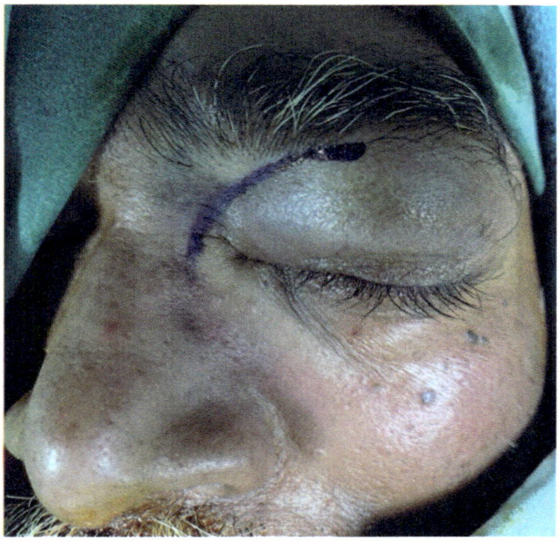

Fig. 9.17 Lynch incision is marked on the left side of medial and supra canthal region (Courtesy—Dr. Hitesh Verma, Associate Professor, AIIMS, New Delhi, India)

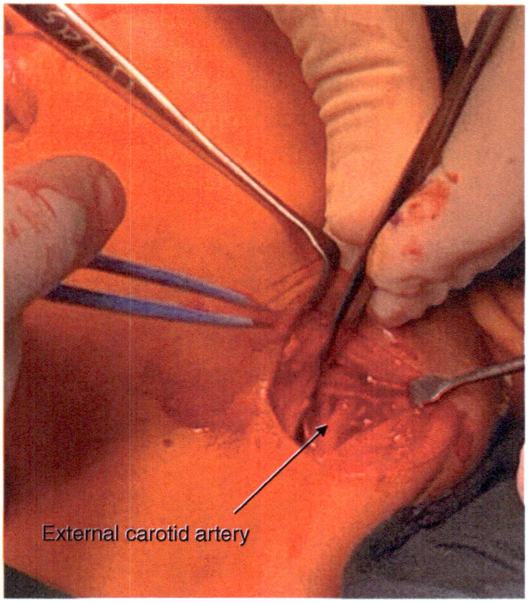

Fig. 9.18 The clinical photograph is showing the left side of the external carotid artery and its branches (Courtesy—Dr. Hitesh Verma, Associate Professor, AIIMS, New Delhi, India)

9.3.4.3 Maxillary Artery Ligation

Internal maxillary artery runs behind maxilla in infratemporal fossa and pterygopalatine fossa. It may bleed while handing of nasal tumor extending in retromaxillary space via trans-nasal approach. Caldwell-Luc approach, endoscopic Denker's or posterior sub-labial approaches are useful to get access in retromaxillary space [22, 23].

9.3.4.4 External Carotid Artery Ligation

External carotid artery ligation is advised in extreme cases and when intervention radiologist is not available. The horizontal incision is made at the level of the hyoid bone. Sternocleidomastoid muscle is retracted laterally. Carotid space is entered and the external carotid artery is conformed with its branches in the neck. The external carotid artery is ligated above its first branch (Fig. 9.18).

Angiography assisted embolization is the fourth line of management. It is advocated in patients of refractory epistaxis who are unfit for surgery or in whom surgery has failed to stem the bleeding. Technique entails cannulation of the external carotid artery and location of the bleeding point by water-soluble contrast. Coils, gel foam, and polyvinyl alcohol can then embolize the causative artery [24]. The success rate has been reported to be as high as 87%, which is similar to arterial ligation. Complication includes cerebrovascular accidents when material dislodges into the internal carotid system but it is relatively rare in recent scenario due to upgradation of material, technique, and expertise.

9.3.4.5 Internal Carotid Bleeding

1. The carotid artery can injure by accidental trauma and during skull base surgery. It is rare but life threatening. Proper identification of sphenoid sinus ostia and sphenoid ostium should be widened in inferomedial direction to prevent this catastrophe. If it occurs while surgery, immediate compression of the CCA in the neck and tight packing of the sphenoid sinus is needed. Small rent can be managed by mashed muscle piece but it is challenging. Clipping of injured site and direct vessel closure can be attempted if there is adequate exposure of the vasculature during surgery otherwise patient should be shifted to the intervention radiology Department. Endovascular occlusion or stenting is performed by localizing the site of injury. The selection of technique is verified by balloon occlusion test to check the adequacy of collateral circulation [25]. Flow diversion is indicated in complex and recurrent aneurysm cases. Silk flow, pipeline embolization, flow redirection endoluminal devices are the recent therapy for the persistent aneurysm. These devices reconstruct the artery by creating thrombosis at the aneurysm site [26]. The pack should be removed after conformation with angiography.

9.3.4.6 Medical Management for Epistaxis

Topical decongestants like oxymetazoline can be useful in mild epistaxis and when the mucosa is congested. Steam inhalation, nasal douches, liquid paraffin nasal drops, and ointments are helpful in hydration of dehydrate nasal mucosa. Topical tranexamic acid can be used in patients taking anti-platelet drugs. Avoidance of warfarin, aspirin, and other nonsteroidal anti-inflammatory drugs (NSAIDs) is required as these medications can affect platelets function. The correction of clotting factor derived from the liver, can be done by administration of vitamin K injection. The choice of clotting factor correction is based on deficit parameter. Literature is controversial for prescribing prophylactic antibiotics in anterior nasal packing [27].

9.3.4.7 Hereditary Hemorrhagic Telangiectasia

It is an inherited autosomal dominant disorder that is characterized by malformations of various blood vessels (vascular dysplasia), potentially resulting in recurrent bleeding. The surgical management varies from the coagulation of vessel by laser to complete closure of the nasal cavity (Fig. 4.5, Chap. 4). In septal dermoplasty, the nasal mucosa is replaced with autologous skin grafts. The nasal cavity is closed by modified Young's operation and it is indicated in moderate to severe epistaxis that has proved unresponsive to other treatment options. Antifibrinolytic drugs such as tranexamic acid have been found to have mixed results in treating nosebleeds. Bevacizumab (Avastin) has been used experimentally to reduce the number and severity of nosebleeds in persons with HHT [28].

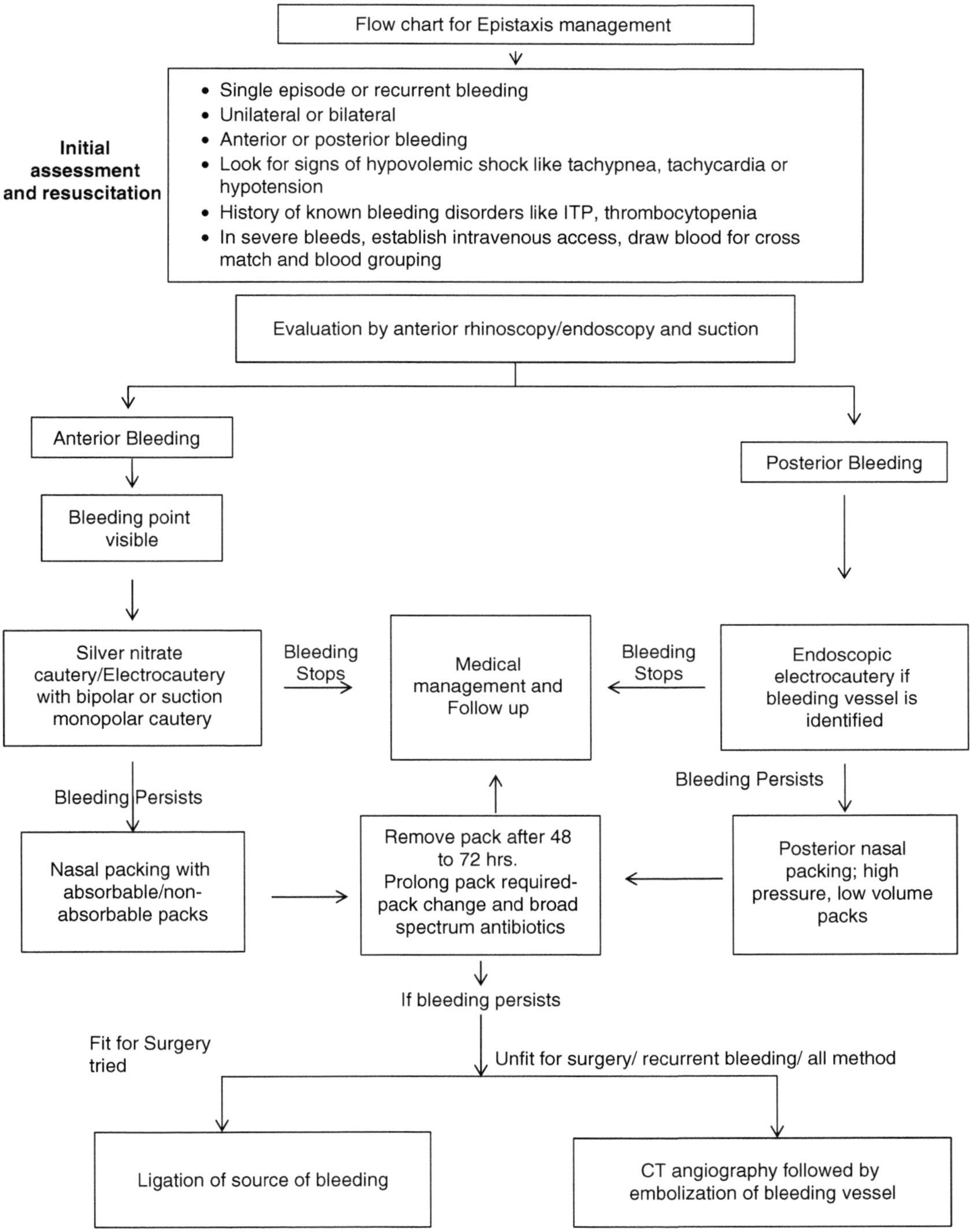
Flow chart for Epistaxis management
Initial assessment and resuscitation
• Single episode or recurrent bleeding
• Unilateral or bilateral
• Anterior or posterior bleeding
• Look for signs of hypovolemic shock like tachypnea, tachycardia or hypotension
• History of known bleeding disorders like ITP, thrombocytopenia
• In severe bleeds, establish intravenous access, draw blood for cross match and blood grouping
Evaluation by anterior rhinoscopy/endoscopy and suction
Anterior Bleeding
Posterior Bleeding
Bleeding point visible
Silver nitrate cautery/Electrocautery with bipolar or suction monopolar cautery
Bleeding Stops
Medical management and Follow up
Bleeding Stops
Endoscopic electrocautery if bleeding vessel is identified
Bleeding Persists
Bleeding Persists
Nasal packing with absorbable/non-absorbable packs
Remove pack after 48 to 72 hrs. Prolong pack required- pack change and broad spectrum antibiotics
Posterior nasal packing; high pressure, low volume packs
If bleeding persists
Fit for Surgery tried
Unfit for surgery/ recurrent bleeding/ all method
Ligation of source of bleeding
CT angiography followed by embolization of bleeding vessel

References

1. Takahashi R. The formation of the nasal septum and the etiology of septal deformity. The concept of evolutionary paradox. Acta Otolaryngol Suppl. 1987;443:1–160.
2. Fettman N, Sanford T, Sindwani R. Surgical management of the deviated septum: techniques in septoplasty. Otolaryngol Clin N Am. 2009;42:241–52.
3. Verwoerd CDA, Verwoerd-Verhoef HL. Rhinosurgery in children: surgical and developmental aspects. In: Nolst Trenité GJ, editor. Rhinoplasty. 3rd ed. Amsterdam: The Hague; Kugler; 2005. p. 201–8.
4. Ketcham AS, Han JK. Complications and management of septoplasty. Otolaryngol Clin N Am. 2010;43:897–904.
5. Kridel RW. Septal perforation repair. Otolaryngol Clin N Am. 1999 Aug;32(4):695–724.
6. Wysocka J, Hassmann E, Lipska A, Musiatowicz M. Naïve and memory T- cells in hypertrophic adenoids in children according to age. Int J Pediatr Otorhinolaryngol. 2003;67:237–41.
7. Bluestone CD. Current indications for tonsillectomy and adenoidectomy. Ann Otol Rhinol Laryngol Suppl. 1992;155:58.
8. Peter JR. The adenoid and adenoidectomy. In: Michael G, George GB, Martin JB, Ray C, John H, Nicholas SJ, et al., editors. Scott-Brown's otolaryngology, vol. 1. 7th ed. London: Hodder Arnold; 2008. p. 1095–101.
9. Cohen D, Konak S. The evaluation of radiographs of the nasopharynx. Clin Otolaryngol. 1985;10:73–8.
10. Fujioka M, Young L, Girdany B. Radiographic evaluation of adenoidal size in children: adenoidal-nasopharyngeal ratio. Am J Radiol. 1979;133:401–4.
11. Crepeau J, Patriquin H, Poliquin J, Tetreault L. Radiographic evaluation of the symptom—producing adenoid. Otolaryngol Head Neck Surg. 1982;90:548–54.
12. Salna I, Jervis-Bardy J, Wabnitz D, et al. Partial adenoidectomy in patients with palatal abnormalities. J Craniofac Surg. 2019 Jul;30(5):e454–60.
13. Clemens J, McMurray JS, Willging JP. Electrocautery verses curette adenoidectomy: comparison of post-operative results. Int J Pediatr Otorhinolaryngol. 1998;43:115–22.
14. Owens D, Jaramillo M, Saunders M. Suction diathermy adenoid ablation. J Laryngol Otol. 2005;119(1):34–5.
15. Stanislaw P, Koltai PJ, Feustel PJ. Comparison of power assisted adenoidectomy vs adenoid curette adenoidectomy. Arch Otolaryngol Head Neck Surg. 2000;126(7):845–9.
16. Ferreira MS, Mangussi-Gomes J, Ximendes R, et al. Comparison of three different adenoidectomy techniques in children - has the conventional technique been surpassed. Int J Pediatr Otorhinolaryngol. 2018;104:145–9.
17. Payne SC, Feldstein D, Anne S, Tunkel DE. Hypertension and epistaxis: why is there limited guidance in the nosebleed clinical practice guidelines? Otolaryngol Head Neck Surg. 2020;162(1):33–4.
18. Tunkel DE, Anne S, Payne SC, et al. Clinical Practice Guideline: nosebleed (Epistaxis). Otolaryngol Head Neck Surg. 2020;162(1_Suppl):S1–S38.
19. Kamhieh Y, Fox H. Tranexamic acid in epistaxis: a systematic review. Clin Otolaryngol. 2016;41(6):771–6.
20. Kitamura T, Takenaka Y, Takeda K, et al. Sphenopalatine artery surgery for refractory idiopathic epistaxis: systematic review and meta-analysis. Laryngoscope. 2019;129(8):1731–6.
21. Turri-Zanoni M, Arosio AD, Stamm AC, et al. Septal branches of the anterior ethmoidal artery: anatomical considerations and clinical implications in the management of refractory epistaxis. Eur Arch Otorhinolaryngol. 2018;275(6):1449–56.
22. Polev GA, Carrau RL, Golbin DA, et al. Intraoral Endoscopic Ligation of Maxillary Artery in the Infratemporal Fossa. J Craniofac Surg. 2019;30(1):137–40.
23. Huyett P, Jankowitz BT, Wang EW, Snyderman CH. Endovascular embolization in the treatment of epistaxis. Otolaryngol Head Neck Surg. 2019;160(5):822–8.
24. Cheng CL, Lee BJ, Chen WH, Hu SY. Epistaxis from ruptured pseudoaneurysm of the internal carotid artery. Br J Hosp Med (Lond). 2019;80(4):iv.
25. Zhang Z, Lv X, Yang X, Shiqing MU, Wu Z, Shen C, et al. Endovascular management of giant aneurysms: an introspection. Neurol India. 2015;63:184–9.
26. Tran QK, Rehan MA, Haase DJ, et al. Prophylactic antibiotics for anterior nasal packing in emergency department: a systematic review and meta-analysis of clinically-significant infections. Am J Emerg Med. 2020;38(5):983–9.
27. Hsu YP, Hsu CW, Bai CH, et al. Medical treatment for epistaxis in hereditary hemorrhagic telangiectasia: a meta-analysis. Otolaryngol Head Neck Surg. 2019;160(1):22–35. https://doi.org/10.1177/0194599818797316.
28. Stokes P, Rimmer J. Intranasal bevacizumab in the treatment of HHT-related epistaxis: a systematic review. Rhinology. 2018;56(1):3–10. https://doi.org/10.4193/Rhin17.166.

Radiotherapy, Chemotherapy, and Quality of Life

10

Bharti Devnani, Suman Bhasker, Raja Pramanik, Surya Prakash Vadlamani, and Suresh Mani

Contents

B. Devnani · S. Bhasker (✉)
Radiotherapy, AIIMS, New Delhi, India
e-mail: drsumanbhasker@gmail.com

R. Pramanik · S. P. Vadlamani
Medical Oncology, Dr.B.R.A-IRCH, AIIMS, New Delhi, India

S. Mani
ENT, CMC, Vellore, Tamil Nadu, India

H. Verma, A. Thakar (eds.), *Essentials of Rhinology*, https://doi.org/10.1007/978-981-33-6284-0_10

The decision needs to be made in a multidisciplinary clinical team. Para-nasal sinus malignancies are rare aggressive tumors. Radiotherapy is an integral part of management either as single modality or in combination. There is wide range of histo-pathological entities in this subtype with varying radiation sensitivity. Local failure is the major pattern of relapse. Lymph nodal involvement is less frequent in nasal and para-nasal sinus malignancies although in cases of nasopharyngeal cancers it is present in up-to 90 % of the cases. Advent of advanced technologies in the form of IMRT and particle therapy substantially improved the clinical outcome. Conformal treatment provides high rates of local control with decreased toxicities. Margin positivity & extra-capsular spread in Lymph nodes are the indication for chemotherapy. Chronic rhinosinusitis negatively affects quality of life (QoL) by disturbing the physical, social, and emotional well-being of patients. It also reduces economic productivity and can increase the risk of depression and sleep dysfunction. EuroQol 5D, Rhinosinusitis outcome measures (RSOM), McGill Pain Questionnaire, Short Form-36 Health Survey and Short Form-12 Health Survey Rhinosinusitis Disability Index, Chronic Sinusitis Survey Score, Sinonasal Outcome Test-20, -16, and -22 are the scoring systems used to assess the quality of life.

10.1 Part A: Radiation Therapy in Nasal Cavity, Paranasal Sinus, and Nasopharyngeal Tumors

10.1.1 Introduction

Management of sinonasal region tumors is challenging in view of the close proximity of the tumor to adjacent critical structures. Radiation therapy (RT) plays a pivotal role in the multimodality treatment of these tumors. Technological advancements in the form of Intensity-modulated radiotherapy (IMRT) has given an advantage of steep radiation dose gradients to achieve more conformal treatment and better sparing of normal tissues.

10.1.2 Radiation in Nasal Cavity Tumors

Radiation therapy is an important treatment modality in the management of nasal cavity cancers. For small tumors of vestibule radical radiotherapy alone provides excellent cosmetic outcomes, especially in small anterior septal tumors and nasal ala region tumors. In locally advanced tumors of the nasal cavity, RT can be used as an adjuvant treatment modality in the postoperative setting or in the preoperative setting to debulk the tumor in surgically challenging cases. Indications of postoperative RT include advance stage T3 or T4 tumor, close or positive margin in early stage, high tumor grade, and involvement of lymph nodes or perineural invasion. In cases of unresectable disease, a combined modality approach with concurrent chemotherapy and radiotherapy is advocated. Palliative radiation is offered to control the symptoms of pain, nasal obstruction, proptosis, epistaxis and for tumor growth restrain in ulcerative or fungating lesions.

Radiation can be delivered by external beam radiotherapy, brachytherapy, or a combination of both. In a study by Allen et al. [1], 32 patients with nasal cavity tumors were treated by a median EBRT dose of radiation of 65 Gy. At a median follow-up of 11 years, 5-year locoregional control was 81% and OS was 94%, with few serious adverse events. Brachytherapy is used for small lesions using interstitial brachytherapy catheter implants or intracavitary mold using ^{192}Ir radioactive sources. Anterio-inferior septal lesions (<1.5 cm) are suitable for interstitial brachytherapy [2]. Tumor volume is an important prognostic factor for regional recurrence following brachytherapy. Tumor volume <2.3 cc is associated with a 3-year locoregional control of 96%. Nasal Appearance and Function Evaluation Questionnaire (NAFEQ) is a 14-questions questionnaire to assess patient satisfaction with esthetic and functional outcomes following brachytherapy. It consists of two parts, including seven questions regarding nasal function and seven items to assess satisfaction with nasal appearance.

10.1.3 Indications of Radiotherapy in Paranasal Sinus Tumors

Surgery followed by postoperative radiation therapy (PORT) is the mainstay of treatment in advanced paranasal sinus tumors. Other indications of PORT include high tumor grade or high-risk histology, perineural invasion, lymphovascular space invasion, positive lymph nodes, margin positivity, and inadequate resection or tumor spillage. Radical radiotherapy with chemotherapy is used in locally advanced T3, T4 tumors especially in ethmoid sinus tumors where extensive surgery may lead to structural and functional deficit. Patients who are not fit for surgery due to medical comorbidities are also candidates for radiotherapy. In cases of borderline resectable tumors with anterior soft tissue or skin infiltration, minimal preorbital invasion or pterygopalatine invasion preoperative radiation is indicated [3, 4].

10.1.4 Radiation Therapy for Nasopharyngeal Cancer

Radiation therapy is the mainstay of treatment for nasopharyngeal malignancies. Surgery is typically limited to biopsy for histological confirmation and in cases of salvage therapy. Early-stage nasopharyngeal cancer can be successfully treated with RT alone. In a study by Chua et al. [5], 10-year recurrence-free survival (RFS) was more than 96% with radiation therapy. Concurrent chemotherapy needs to be added with radiation in case of locally advanced nasopharyngeal cancer (T3, T4, or N+ disease). A precision radiotherapy technique like IMRT is the standard of care to achieve a higher therapeutic ratio. Particle beam therapy with proton beam and carbon ion therapy is an emerging modality due to its physical characteristics of the Bragg's peak. Proton beam therapy is especially useful in cases of reradiation in recurrent disease [5]. Radiation workflow is mentioned in Fig. 10.1.

10.1.5 External Beam Radiotherapy Planning

Meticulous radiotherapy planning is very crucial to achieve higher control rates. MRI of the nasopharynx and neck is an important diagnostic investigation and is very useful for radiation planning as clivus and nerves are best seen on MRI. Figure 10.2 shows the various steps of radiation therapy workflow from preplanning to delivery of radiation. Target volume delineation involves contouring of tumor volumes and organs at risk. Gross tumor volume (GTV) consists of the entire visible gross tumor clinically or radiologically. Clinical target volume (CTV) encompasses GTV, postoperative bed in cases of postoperative cases, regions of positive margin, and regions with nodal extracapsular extension and regions at higher risk of micrometastasis. A 3–5 mm margin is given to CTV to account for inter- and intrafraction set-up errors to create a planning target volume (PTV) [6, 7].

10.1.6 Time, Dose, and Fractionation

A radiation dose of 70 Gy in 35 fractions delivered over 7 weeks is recommended to gross

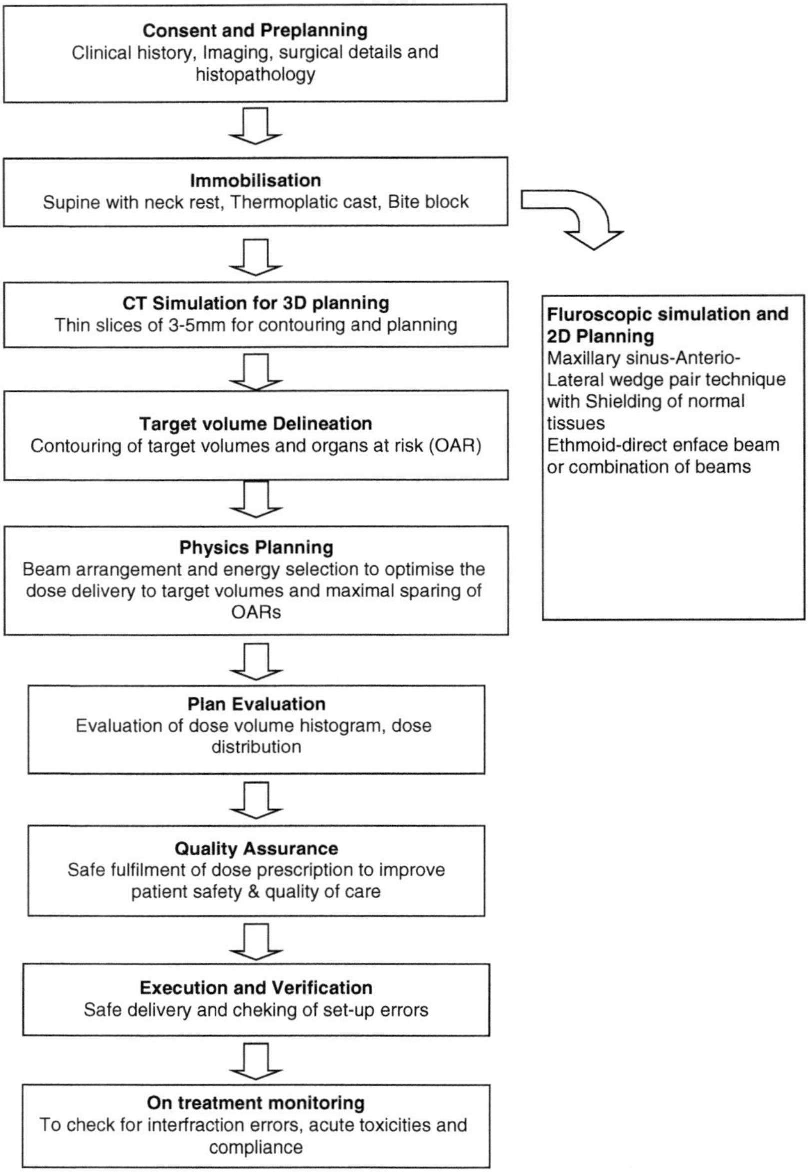

Fig. 10.1 Radiation therapy workflow

tumor volume along with a 50–60 Gy to the areas of micrometastasis. In cases of pre-op RT where debulking is the primary aim, an RT dose of 50Gy/25# is given. There are different fractionation schedules for palliative RT ranging from 8Gy in a single fraction to 30Gy in 10 fractions. 20 Gy over 5 fractions is one of the commonly followed palliative dose fractionations.

10.1.7 Techniques of Radiation

In two-dimensional conventional radiotherapy, the volume of irradiated tissue is simply determined by anatomical field borders that are based on radiological bony landmarks. There are more chances of excess normal tissue toxicity and beam arrangements are limited to orthogonal

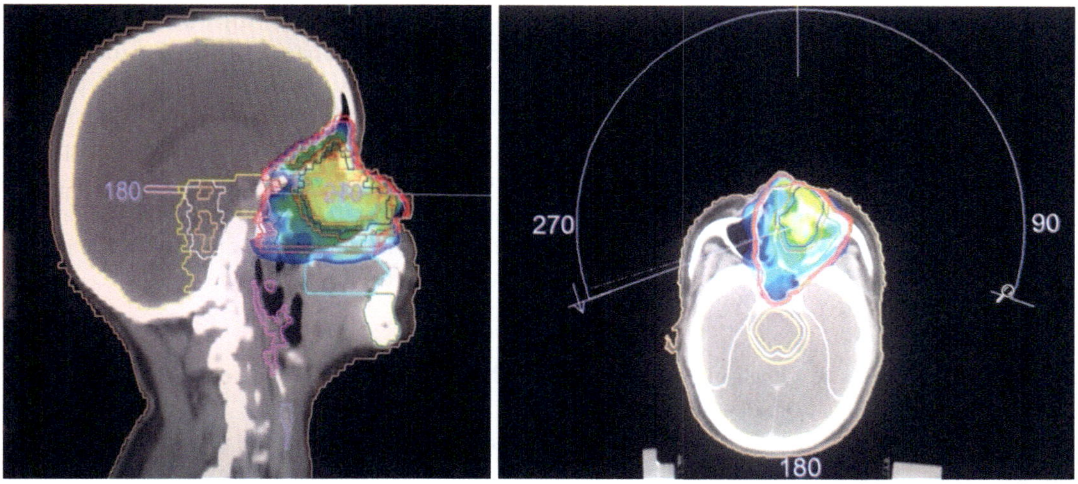

Fig. 10.2 A case of esthesioneuroblastoma showing radiation dose distribution in targets and organs at risk (**a**) Sagittal section (**b**) Axial section

placements with crude shielding techniques. The advantage of conformal radiotherapy is a steep dose gradient close to the target. Conformal radiotherapy includes 3D-Conformal radiotherapy (3D-CRT), Intensity-modulated radiotherapy (IMRT), and Image-guided radiotherapy (IGRT) techniques. 3D-CRT technique shapes the beams based on 3D reconstructions of the tumor size and shape and the location of nearby normal tissues. IMRT changes the intensity of each small beamlet to obtain even more conformal dose distribution and avoidance of normal tissue damage. IMRT is the standard technique for definitive radiation therapy for nasopharyngeal cancer. *IGRT* is a method of radiation therapy that incorporates imaging techniques during each treatment session. Conformal radiotherapy offers precise dose shaping, minimizes the dose to critical normal tissues thereby decreasing the radiation toxicities.

10.1.8 Radiation Toxicities

Skin erythema, mucositis, dryness, dysgeusia, bleeding from the nose, and fatigue are some of the common acute radiation toxicities. Nasal cavity mucositis and dryness of mucous membranes is common following RT and should be managed by saline nasal sprays. Nasal cavity synechiae is prevented by regular nasal dosches and by proper cavity management. Xerostomia is a common sequelae post RT and parotid sparing IMRT should be used wherever feasible based on tumor extension. Decaying of teeth commonly follows xerostomia for which prophylactic fluoride toothpaste should be prescribed and loose or decayed teeth should be removed prior to starting RT to further prevent osteoradionecrosis. Ocular symptoms in the form of chronic keratitis can occur in the RT of paranasal sinus malignancies. Sensorineural hearing loss is prominent with concurrent use of chemotherapy for which mean cochlea dose should be kept below 48 Gy to minimize damage. Carotid artery stenosis is a potentially fatal complication in reradiation cases. Routine duplex ultrasound scanning can be done in cases of higher-risk patients.

10.1.9 Radiotherapy in Specific Histological Subtype

Squamous cell carcinoma is the most common histopathological type of nose and paranasal sinus tumor. The treatment policy is mentioned above. Esthesioneuroblastomas, Kadish A tumors can be treated with the single modality treatment in the form of primary RT alone. The rest of the tumors can be best treated by a combination of surgery and radiotherapy. It tends to invade the cribriform plate and anterior cranial fossa, and therefore, these regions should be encompassed in the target volume. Elective nodal radiation is generally not required. In terms of radiotherapy techniques, it is evident that 3D radiotherapy significantly improves local control compared to the 2D technique (74% vs. 59%).

Adenoid cystic carcinoma originates mostly from the minor salivary glands. In view of the highly neurotropic nature of adenoid cystic carcinomas, radiotherapy volumes must encompass the afferent and efferent local nerves to the skull base. Adenocarcinoma is a locally aggressive tumor that occurs almost exclusively in the ethmoid sinus. Conformal radiation should be used for this location of the tumor. Combination chemotherapy with cisplatin, fluorouracil, and leucovorin has been shown to be efficacious. Mucosal melanoma of the paranasal sinuses is a rare form of melanoma (0.2–4%) and is notoriously resistant to conventional chemoradiotherapy. Hypofractionated RT, combined immuno-IMRT that may potentially enhance the therapeutic ratio is investigational. Radiotherapy is an important role in the curative treatment of patients with Nasal Natural Killer T Cell Lymphoma. Yang et al. reported that definitive radiation therapy with or without chemotherapy was more effective than strategies that used induction or primary chemotherapy. RT dose of >50 Gy is recommended in contrast to other lymphomas [8].

10.1.10 Radiotherapy in Benign Tumors

Radiotherapy is also helpful in some benign conditions especially in cases of medically inoperable or locally recurrent tumors. RT is used in advanced inoperable or recurrent tumors juvenile nasopharyngeal angiofibroma. Recommended RT dose is 30–50 Gy @2 Gy per fraction. Local control rates are around 85–100%. In cases of ameloblastoma, RT helps in achieving local control in cases of multiple recurrences and preventing recurrences in cases of positive margins after surgery. Radiation therapy in chordoma is challenging due to the intrinsic radio-resistance of these tumors coupled with the increased sensitivity of the adjacent critical neural structures. Charged particle therapy has an established role and increases control rates. The role of radiation therapy for inverted papillomas is seen in patients with carcinoma in situ or invasive features found after resection.

10.1.11 Future Directions

Particle beam therapy with proton beam and carbon ion therapy is an emerging modality due to its physical characteristics of the Bragg's peak. There are ongoing randomized prospective trials evaluating the efficacy of the same. Although data for charged particles are encouraging, the lack of widespread access and high cost associated with these facilities limit their routine use.

10.2 Part B: Chemotherapy Perspectives in Nasal and Paranasal Sinus Tumors

10.2.1 Summary

Cancers arising primarily from the nasal cavity and paranasal sinuses are fairly uncommon. The most common histology encountered is squamous in nature, yet one is more likely to see other histologies like adenocarcinomas, lymphomas, sarcomas, plasmacytomas, etc. (Fig. 10.3) in this region than elsewhere in the head and neck, thereby making things challenging. Each of these distinct etiologies needs to diagnose accurately for optimal management. This requires an experienced head–neck pathologist. The paradigm for the management of each of these tumors is histologically driven. For each histological type of tumor, the plan of management depends on the stage, location, age, comorbidities, performance status, and previous therapies received. Traditionally treated by chemotherapy, surgery, and radiotherapy, the advent of immunotherapy and targeted therapy in these malignancies has

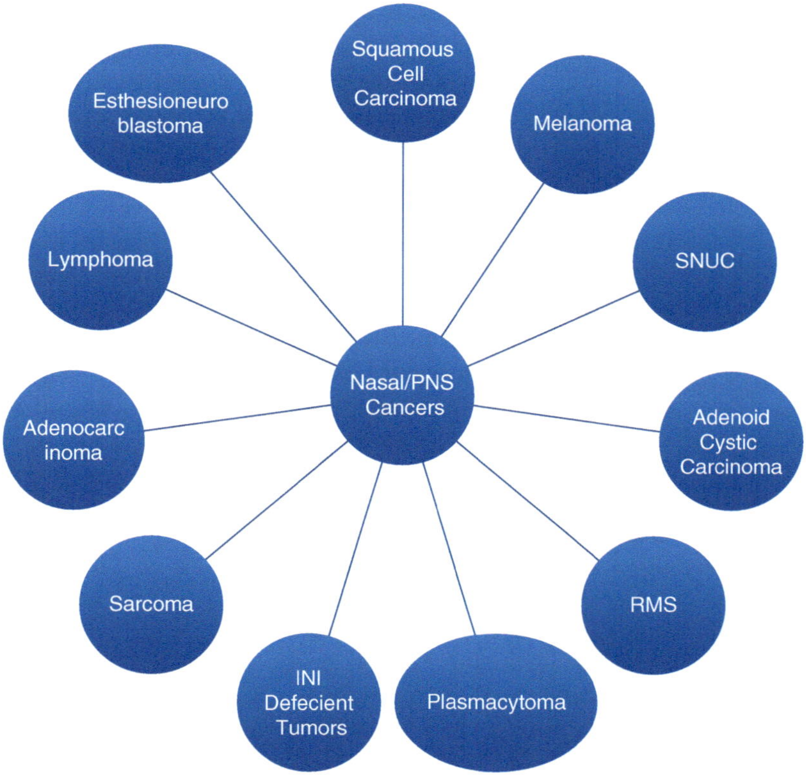

Fig. 10.3 Spectrum of tumors in nose and PNS

opened up new vistas in the management of squamous cell head–neck carcinoma. The recent most addition is the use of combined immunochemotherapy as the first-line palliative therapy in recurrent metastatic settings. PDL1 combined positive score (CPS) has emerged as a predictive biomarker in the clinic. For those R/M HNSCC, where the combined positive score of PDL1 >20%, single-agent pembrolizumab has arrived as the standard of care.

10.2.2 Strategies for Chemotherapies in Head and Neck Cancers

1. **Neoadjuvant/induction**: Chemotherapy given prior to definitive surgical or radiation therapy.
2. **Adjuvant**: Chemotherapy given after radical curative surgery. Mostly given as concurrent chemo + radiotherapy.
3. **Definitive or radical chemoradiotherapy**: CTRT done with a curative intent. Usually for surgically inaccessible sites.
4. **Palliative**: Chemotherapy given in metastatic disease with a noncurative intent, to palliate symptoms, prolong life with good quality.
5. **Sequential therapy**: Induction chemotherapy followed by definitive CTRT.

10.2.3 Chemotherapy in Different Tumors of Nose and Paranasal Sinuses

1. **Squamous Cell Carcinoma:**
   (a) **Adjuvant setting:** After surgery for SCC, adjuvant chemotherapy concurrent with radiotherapy (CTRT) is indicated in the following situations:
      (i) Margin positivity.
      (ii) Extracapsular spread in lymph nodes.

(iii) Two types of concurrent regimens are used worldwide. The optimum cumulative dose of cisplatin is 200 mg/m^2. The weekly cisplatin regime till 7 weeks period and the dose is 40 mg/m^2. For a 3-weekly cisplatin regime, the dose is 100 mg/m^2 per dose and 3 doses advised at day 1, day 22, day 43. Three-weekly cisplatin is associated with better locoregional control (LRC) but increased toxicity profile [9]. In cisplatin-ineligible patients (renal dysfunction, SN Hearing loss), cetuximab is indicated only in trial settings. Carboplatin (50 mg/m^2 or AUC 1.5–2) is often used but is not evidence-based [10].

(b) **Definitive setting:** SCC may be definitively treated with (concurrent chemoradiotherapy) CTRT. Dosage is cisplatin weekly at 40 mg/m^2 for 7 doses along with RT. Nimotuzumab (anti-EGFR antibody) added to weekly cisplatin (30 mg/m^2) during CTRT improves DFS (disease-free survival) [11]. Cisplatin-ineligible patients may be treated with concurrent cetuximab (400 mg/m^2 loading 1 week before RT, then 250 mg/m^2 weekly).

(c) **Neoadjuvant setting:** Chemotherapy may be used in specific cases to downsize tumors and increase resectability (skin involvement, low ITF, induration above zygoma). Preferred regimens:
   (i) Three-drug regimen (q 3 weekly): DCF (Docetaxel 75 mg/m^2D1, CDDP 75 mg/m^2 day 1, 5FU-750 mg/m^2/day continue intravenous infusion over 96 h from day 2–5).
   (ii) Two-drug regimen (q 3 weekly): CDDP+5FU (CDDP 75 mg/m^2 D1, 5FU-750 mg/m^2/day continue intravenous infusion over 96 h from day 2–5).
   (iii) Two-drug regimen (q 3 weekly): T + P (Paclitaxel 175 mg/m^2 day 1, Carboplatin AUC6 day 1).

(d) **Sequential setting:** NACT followed by definitive CTRT is occasionally used in locally advanced tumors not amenable to surgical resection.

(e) **Palliative setting:** Indications: Recurrent and metastatic HNSCC (not amenable to salvage surgery or re-irradiation). The extent of treatment is till progression of disease control by management.
   (i) Standard of care:
      - Firs Line: KEYNOTE 048
        If rapid tumor response is not needed, when PDL1 CPS is more than 20% than single-agent pembrolizumab and when PDL1 CPS is less than 20%, cisplatin+5FU+ pembrolizumab is the combination of drug. If rapid tumor response is needed, the regimes are cisplatin +5FU+ cetuximab (EXTREME trial) [12, 13]/Cisplatin +5FU + pembrolizumab (if PDL1 CPS >1%).
      - Second line:
        If immune-oncology is used as first line then cetuximab + chemo is the regime and if immune-oncology is not used previously then nivolumab (240 mg q 2 weeks)/pembrolizumab 200 mg iv q3 weekly is the treatment regime [14].
        Other treatment options in resource limited settings are CDDP +5FU, Paclitaxel + Carboplatin, Single-agent Methotrexate i.v (40 mg/m^2 weekly) and Oral metronomic therapy: Gefitinib (500 mg/day), Erlotinib (150 mg/day), Oral weekly Methotrexate (15 mg/m^2) + Celecoxib (200 mg BID) [15].

2. **Nasopharyngeal carcinoma:**
   (a) Definitive treatment—Standard of care for Stage II and above is Concurrent CTRT (weekly CDDP) + 3 cycles of adjuvant chemotherapy (3 weekly CDDP+5FU).
   (b) Neoadjuvant setting—In cases of T4 or bulky tumors, treatment may start with

NACT (e.g., 3 cycles of CDDP+ 5FU or DCF) followed by CTRT.

(c) Palliative setting: Following regimens may be used in cases of metastatic disease:
   (i) Gemcitabine (1 g/m^2 on day 1, day 8) + CDDP (80 mg/m^2 day 1) (first Line) [16]
   (ii) CDDP+ 5FU
   (iii) Paclitaxel + Carboplatin

3. **Esthesioneuroblastoma:** Doubtful role of adjuvant chemotherapy after craniofacial resection and RT. NACT (Cisplatin 30 mg/m^2 D1,2,3 + Etoposide 100 mg/m^2 D1,2,3) is often used in Kadish C, D tumors based on institutional experiences to downsize the tumor and make it amenable to resection. Cisplatin + Etoposide are used in palliative therapy of relapsed or metastatic disease.
4. **Adenoid cystic carcinoma**: In the adjuvant setting, the treatment policy is the same as HNSCC. Wait and watch policy is indicated in asymptomatic metastatic cases. For symptomatic disease, the options include CAP (Cisplatin [50 mg/m^2, D1], doxorubicin [50 mg/m^2, D1], and cyclophosphamide [500 mg/m^2, D1]) q 28 days.
   (a) **NK-T Cell lymphoma:** These tumors are resistant to CHOP chemotherapy due to the expression of P-glycoprotein. Preferred regimens in early stage (IE/IIE contiguous):
      (i) Concurrent CTRT, where chemotherapy regime is DeVIC [Dexamethasone, Etoposide, Ifosfamide, Carboplatin]).
      (ii) Another regime is radiotherapy followed by 3 cycles of DeVIC/VIPD (etoposide, ifosfamide, cisplatin, dexamethasone).
      (iii) In the third form of regime, 3 cycles of SMILE regime followed by RT and then again 3 cycles of SMILE regime. The detail of the SMILE regime is:

Methotrexate 2 g/m^2	Day 1 (Leucovorin Rescue)
Ifosfamide 1500 mg/m^2	Days 2 to 4
Etoposide 100 mg/m^2	Days 2 to 4
Dexamethasone 40 mg PO or IV	Days 2 to 4
L-asparaginase 6000 units/m^2 IM	Days 8, 10, 12, 14, 16, 18, 20

   (b) Advanced stage (II non-contiguous, III, IV): the treatment policy is 6 cycles of the SMILE regime.

5. **DLBCL (Diffuse Large B cell Lymphoma):** For early-stage (I, II) non-bulky lesion, 3 cycles of R-CHOP+IFRT whereas for early bulky lesion (>7.5 cm), 6 cycles of R-CHOP +IFRT. For advanced stage (III, IV), 6 cycles of R-CHOP regime (Table 10.1).
6. **Sinonasal Adenocarcinoma:** They may be salivary gland type, intestinal type (ITAC), or non-intestinal type. The treatment policy is similar to HNSCC.
7. **Sarcoma (STS):** Radiotherapy is the mainstay of treatment in all high-grade tumors. The role of adjuvant chemotherapy in H&N sarcomas is unknown. In metastatic disease, performance status and histology is the guide for the choice of drugs. Commonly used regimens are:
   (a) Doxorubicin-based chemotherapy (IA: Ifosphamide+ doxorubicin)
   (b) Angiosarcoma: weekly paclitaxel, Gemcitabine + Docetaxel, Pazopanib, Trabectedin

Table 10.1 The list of drugs comes under the R-CHOP regime, their doses, and the day of administration

R-CHOP	Drug	Dose	Schedule
	Rituximab	375 mg/m^2 i.v	Day 1
	Cyclophosphamide	750 mg/m^2 iv	Day 1
	Doxorubicin	50 mg/m^2 iv	Day 1
	Vincristine	1.4 mg/m^2 (2 mg max) iv	Day 1
	Prednisolone	100 mg po	Day 1–5

Table 10.2 Risk categories, chemotherapy schedule, and doses

Risk category	Chemotherapy schedule	Drug regimen
Low risk		**VA:**
Subset A Subset B	VA X 15 cycles (45 weeks) VAC × 14 cycles (40 weeks)	V = Vincristine 1.5 mg/m^2 (max 2 mg) q week A = Actinomycin-D (0.045 mg/kg) (Max 2.5 mg) q 3 week
Intermediate risk	VAC × 14 cycles (40 weeks)	**VAC:** V = Vincristine 1.5 mg/m^2 (max 2 mg)q week A = Actinomycin-D (0.045 mg/kg) (Max 2.5 mg) q 3 week C = Cyclophosphamide (1200 mg/m^2 with Mesna) q 3 week
High risk	VAC × 14 cycles (40 weeks)	Same as intermediate risk regime

 (c) Chondrosarcoma: Low grade (well-differentiated): no role. Poorly differentiated (doxorubicin-based chemotherapy)

8. Rhabdomyosarcoma: It usually occurs in children. It commonly involves three subsides of head and neck region, orbit (25%) [favorable], Para-meningeal (paranasal sinuses, nasopharynx, nasal cavity, middle ear, mastoid) (50%) [non-favorable], non-orbital non-para-meningeal (25%) [favorable]. The choice of adjuvant therapy (RT/chemo) and selection of chemotherapy is based on various clinical factors such as TNM stage, clinical group after surgery, site, size (>/<5 cm), age, histology (embryonal/alveolar), and FOXO1 fusion. Combining these information, we define three risk categories as in Table 10.2.

9. **Osteosarcoma (OS):**
 Head and Neck OS is notorious for local recurrence and less commonly distant metastases than limb OS. Adjuvant chemotherapy is given to all cases (although evidence exists only for extremity OS). Cisplatin + doxorubicin are most commonly used. Adjuvant RT is for R1 resections even after re-resection. Cisplatin may be added concurrent to RT, although evidence is limited. Regimens for metastatic disease: Cisplatin + doxorubicin, high-dose methotrexate, ifosphamide+ etoposide [17].
10. **Mucosal Melanoma:** It has a poorer prognosis and response compared to skin melanomas. There is no established role of chemotherapy or immunotherapy in an adjuvant setting. In metastatic cases, treatment is extrapolated from that of skin melanomas.
 (a) BRAF V600E mutated: Dabrafenib, Vemurafenib
 (b) Kit mutated: Imatinib, dasatinib, sorafenib
 (c) No mutation: Nivolumab, Nivolumab + Ipilimumab
11. **SNUC (sinonasal undifferentiated Carcinoma):** It has a very poor prognosis. It has no clinical trial evidence. Trimodality therapy is the maximum surgical resection followed by concurrent CTRT is standard.
12. **INI-deficient carcinoma:** It is a recently recognized entity (SMARCB1/INI deficient) with a very poor prognosis. Surgery with adjuvant chemoradiation is used.
13. **Plasmacytoma:**
 If it is a solitary disease, then radiotherapy alone is sufficient. If multiple, then treatment is the same as multiple myeloma: VRd regime, 6 cycles followed by autologous transplant (eligible pts) [V = Bortezomib 2 mg subcutaneous injection on days 1, 8, 15, 22; R = Lenalidomide 25 mg once daily from day 1 to day 15, d = Dexamethasone 40 mg weekly].

10.3 Part C: Perioperative and Postoperative Measures to Improve Quality of Life After Nasal Surgery

Chronic rhinosinusitis (CRS) is a common disease that can be managed either medically or surgically with ongoing medical management.

Around 20–30% of patients who undergo sinus surgery for CRS do not experience significant improvement. Physical, social, emotional, psychological, sexual, cognitional, and economic aspects of life can be integrated in a general term of well-being and it is commonly known as health-related QoL (HRQoL). Chronic rhinosinusitis negatively affects quality of life (QoL), reduces economic productivity, and can increase the risk of depression and sleep dysfunction. In the last few decades, quality of life has represented the development of patient-oriented assessment of health status and it is being increasingly perceived by researchers and physicians as a significant outcome measure. Questionnaires, visual scales, and grading systems are just some of the instruments used in quantitatively measuring HRQoL. Many such instruments are available at present to measure the QoL in CRS. Functional outcome following sinus surgery is determined by preoperative, intraoperative, and postoperative management. Careful analysis of these measures results in an improvement in surgical outcome which in turn improves the quality of life.

10.3.1 Quality Indicators

Generally, questionnaires allow the patient to rate the impact of the disease alongside a number of other areas of healthcare interest. Every question is scored according to the severity or repercussion of the disease and individual domain scores are combined to produce an overall score. EuroQol 5D, Rhinosinusitis outcome measures (RSOM), McGill Pain Questionnaire, Short Form-36 Health Survey and Short Form-12 Health Survey Rhinosinusitis Disability Index, Chronic Sinusitis Survey Score, Sinonasal Outcome Test-20, -16, and -22 are the most widely used specific questionnaires in clinical trials. Of these, the 22-item Sinonasal Outcome Test (SNOT-22) has been widely adopted in clinical practice and has been proved to be the most suitable sinonasal outcome scoring system [18]. The SNOT-20 was developed from the 31-item Rhinosinusitis Outcome Measure (RSOM-31) by removing 11 items thought to be redundant. The addition of two items of interest (nasal obstruction and olfaction) formed the SNOT-22, which has been demonstrated to be reliable, valid, and responsive [19, 20]. In SNOT-22, the domains are broke down into three sinus-specific symptom domains (Rhinologic, Extra-rhinologic, and Ear/facial symptoms) and two general health-related QoL domains (Psychological and Sleep dysfunction).

10.3.2 Preoperative Measures

There are no clinical trials of immediate preoperative medication. Many surgeons have preferred to use oral steroids and antibiotics in the preoperative period to improve the outcome of surgery. Oral systemic steroids (preferably Prednisolone) for 10–14 days preoperatively and 7–14 days postoperatively (1 mg/kg) follow by tapering of therapy in 1–2 weeks is the commonly followed therapy. The dose used is around 30 mg which is taken as a single daily dose in the morning. Since there is no solid evidence on which to base this choice of dose, the clinical experience of the surgeon is used to inform this choice. The moderate dose chosen (30 mg) is believed to be sufficient for effective clinical activity and to mitigate the potential undesirable short-term side effects associated with higher doses (e.g., 50–60 mg). Topical corticosteroids (commonly fluticasone propionate, mometasone furoate, ciclesonide, and fluticasone furoate) are of use in the primary treatment of nasal polyps when they are of a small or medium size but surgery is generally required for larger polyps because of the resultant nasal obstruction and limited access for topical preparations. Maximal medical therapy for patients with nasal polyposis included prolonged trials of topical therapy for more than 3 months. Topical therapy was defined as intranasal steroids given twice daily and saline irrigations. No statement can be made regarding a specific length of treatment in CRS without polyposis and the decision should be individualized based on the degree of symptom relief, patient preference, and clinician experience.

Clinical experience suggests that oral antihistamines may provide symptomatic relief of excessive secretions and sneezing although there are no clinical studies supporting the use of antihistamines in CRS. In the preoperative period, antibiotics may decrease inflammation by minimizing infection and so improve the operative field. Culture-specific antibiotics may prevent antibiotic resistance in most of these cases. Smoking can severely affect the outcome of sinus surgery. Smoking causes increased scar tissue and poor healing that lead to failure of endoscopic sinus surgery. Cessation of smoking 3–4 weeks before surgery and avoidance of smoking for an additional month after surgery is an absolute must to achieve good results. There are certain medications that can increase the risk of bleeding during and after sinus surgery. These medications include Aspirin, NSAIDs, anticoagulants and they should be stopped at least 1 week prior to surgery. Vitamin E and herbal medicines such as ginkgo biloba, ginseng, and garlic tablets can also increase the risk of bleeding and should be stopped prior to surgery.

Asthma, prior paranasal surgery, nasal polyps, aspirin-exacerbated respiratory disease, depression or anxiety disorder, and poor preoperative QoL have been linked with poorer QoL outcomes after ESS. Preoperative screening of undiagnosed psychological disorders may allow for improved patient counseling and psychology/psychiatry referral and initiation of complementary therapies [21].

10.3.3 Perioperative Measures

Surgical technique has developed with improvements in instrumentation, optics, and mucosal preservation techniques. Psychological and sleep dysfunction were significantly more likely to have a greater relative influence on patients electing surgical therapy than any of the sinus-specific symptom domains (Rhinologic, Extra-nasal rhinologic, Ear/facial symptoms). Surgical and medical treatment modalities result in improvement across all domains of SNOT-22 but subjects opting for surgical interventions experience greater relative improvement. Patients with recurrent sinusitis with prior sinus surgery having poorer QoL and more radical surgery may require eradication of the disease. Failed endoscopic sinus surgery continues to be a significant problem both in terms of its economic consequences and also with respect to significant patient quality of life issues.

Increased nasal hair density decreases the development of asthma in those who have seasonal rhinitis, possibly due to an increased capacity of the hair in the nostrils to filter out pollen and other allergens. Moffett's solution is a popular choice for the preparation of the surgical field in sinonasal surgery due to its efficacy. It decreases intraoperative bleeding by vasoconstriction and allows improved operative access and visualization by decongesting the nasal mucosa. Cocaine also exerts its analgesic effects by blocking sodium channels along the axons of sensory nerves, dampening pain signal generation and propagation but a long list of side effects limits its uses.

10.3.4 Postoperative Measures

Antibiotics are widely used by surgeons both before and after sinus surgery. Used following sinus surgery, they may facilitate healing by preventing infection. This generally pertains to macrolide agents, which have been suggested to possess significant anti-inflammatory attributes. The most duration still recommend is 4–6 weeks of uninterrupted therapy for CRS. Postoperative fibrin clot debridement and granulation removal are thought to be necessary to prevent scar tissue formation. This is achieved by postoperative office debridement and nasal douching [22].

Postoperative daily use of nasal douching with hypertonic saline alone for a period of 6 months has shown comparable outcomes in terms of symptom scores and prevention of synechiae. The best way of nasal irrigation should follow these steps:

1. Stand with head over a sink and tilt head to one side.
2. Using a squeeze bottle or bulb syringe, pour or squeeze the saline solution slowly into the

upper nostril, allow the solution to pour out of the other nostril and into the drain.
3. Breathe through the mouth, not the nose.
4. Repeat on the opposite side.
5. Try not to let the water go down the back of the throat.
6. Gently blow nose into a tissue to clear out any mucus.

Despite the widespread use of steam inhalations and nasal decongestants, there is no available evidence as to their efficacy in improving outcomes after sinus surgery. Despite significant postoperative improvements, the elevated prevalence of symptoms of psychological dysfunction following sinus surgery underscores the difficulties in treating patients with recalcitrant CRS. Causes for persistent psychological dysfunction are likely multifactorial and include persistent sinonasal inflammation, unmeasured patient factors including healthcare satisfaction, postoperative response shifts, and comorbid psychological factors such as undiagnosed anxiety and depressive disorders.

10.3.5 Follow-Up

Early detection of worsening lesions in the sinonasal area is of great importance in the successful treatment of chronic rhinosinusitis. Postoperative endoscopic evaluation is a simple and cost-effective method to assess the nasal mucosa following surgery. Several postoperative endoscopic scores have been developed such as the Lund and Kennedy score and its modification, Perioperative Sinus Endoscopy scoring system and operating score.

The operating score reflects the course following Functional Endoscopic Sinus Surgery (FESS). Patients with more severe operative findings require longer postoperative treatment. The operating score is based on the operative findings in the sinuses (sinus score) and olfactory clefts (olfactory cleft score) on both sides [23, 24]. The operating score ranges from 0 to 60 points. According to the operating score, the severity of operative findings was classified in terms of three grades: mild (0–20 points), moderate (21–40 points), and severe (41–60 points). Patients with younger age, accompanying asthma, severe eosinophilia, severe chronic rhinosinusitis, polyps in the frontal sinus, and olfactory disorders in the preoperative stage are adverse predictors. Such people should be carefully treated for a longer time after FESS [25–28].

10.4 Conclusion

Although rhinosinusitis is not a life-threatening condition, it impairs daily functioning and quality of life (QoL). The measurement of sinus specific quality of life is perhaps the most commonly utilized outcome measure for CRS. Surgical and medical treatment modalities result in improvement across all domains but subjects electing surgical interventions experience greater relative improvement. The decision to undergo surgical intervention is best predicted by health-related QoL domains pertaining to psychological impairment and sleep dysfunction. Previous sinus surgery, asthma, smoking, and aspirin intolerance may affect the results of surgical treatment. Functional outcome following sinus surgery is determined by preoperative, intraoperative, and postoperative management which facilitates mucosal healing, minimizes scar tissue, and ensures rapid return of nasal mucosa to normal function. Adjuvant medical therapy such as oral steroids, leukotriene antagonists, immunotherapy, and monoclonal antibodies also play a vital role in resulting overall improvement in the quality of life.

References

1. Allen MW, Schwartz DL, Rana V, et al. Long-term radiotherapy outcomes for nasal cavity and septal cancers. Int J Radiat Oncol Biol Phys. 2008;71:401–6.
2. Czerwinski MD, Van Leeuwen R, Kaanders J, Zwijnenburg EM, Lipman D, Takes RP, et al. Image guided brachytherapy for cancer of the nasal vestibule: local control and cosmesis. Int J Radiat Oncol Biol Phys. 2018;103:913–21.
3. Liang ZG, Kusumawidjaja G, Kazmi F, Wee JTS, Chua MLK. Intensity-modulated radiotherapy for

paranasal sinuses and base of skull tumors. Oral Oncol. 2018;86:61–8.
4. Wang K, Zanation AM, Chera BS. The role of radiation therapy in the management of sinonasal and ventral skull base malignancies. Otolaryngol Clin N Am. 2017;50(2):419–32.
5. Chua DT, Sham JS, Kwong DL, et al. Treatment outcome after radiotherapy alone for patients with stage I-II nasopharyngeal carcinoma. Cancer. 2003;98:74–80.
6. Halperin EC, Brady LW, Wazer DE, Perez CA. Perez and Brady's principles and practice of radiation oncology. 7th ed. Philadelphia: Wolters Kluwer Health/ Lippincott Williams & Wilkins; 2018.
7. Lee NY, Lu JJ. Target volume delineation and field setup-a practical guide for conformal and intensity-modulated radiation therapy. Springer; 2015.
8. Yang Y, Zhu Y, Cao JZ, et al. Risk-adapted therapy for early-stage extranodal nasal-type NK/T-cell lymphoma: analysis from a multicenter study. Blood. 2015;126:1424–32.
9. Noronha V, Joshi A, Patil VM, Agarwal J, Ghosh-Laskar S, Budrukkar A, et al. Once-a-week versus once-every-3-weeks cisplatin chemoradiation for locally advanced head and neck cancer: a phase III Randomized Noninferiority Trial. J Clin Oncol Off J Am Soc Clin Oncol. 2018;36(11):1064–72.
10. Racadot S, Mercier M, Dussart S, Dessard-Diana B, Bensadoun R-J, Martin M, et al. Randomized clinical trial of post-operative radiotherapy versus concomitant carboplatin and radiotherapy for head and neck cancers with lymph node involvement. Radiother Oncol J Eur Soc Ther Radiol Oncol. 2008;87(2):164–72.
11. Patil VM, Noronha V, Joshi A, Agarwal J, Laskar SG, Budrukkar A, et al. Results of a randomized phase III study of nimotuzumab in combination with concurrent radiotherapy and cisplatin versus radiotherapy and cisplatin alone, in locally advanced squamous cell carcinoma of the head and neck. J Clin Oncol. 2018;36(15_suppl):6000.
12. Vermorken JB, Mesia R, Rivera F, Remenar E, Kawecki A, Rottey S, et al. Platinum-based chemotherapy plus cetuximab in head and neck cancer. N Engl J Med. 2008;359(11):1116–27.
13. Burtness B, Harrington KJ, Greil R, et al. Pembrolizumab alone or with chemotherapy versus cetuximab with chemotherapy for recurrent or metastatic squamous cell carcinoma of the head and neck (KEYNOTE-048): a randomised, open-label, phase 3 study. Lancet. 2019;394:1915.
14. Ferris RL, Blumenschein G, Fayette J, Guigay J, Colevas AD, Licitra L, et al. Nivolumab for recurrent squamous-cell carcinoma of the head and neck. N Engl J Med. 2016;375(19):1856–67.
15. Patil VM, Noronha V, Joshi A, Pinninti R, Dhumal S, Bhattacharjee A, et al. Metronomic chemotherapy in platinum-insensitive failures and/or early failures postmultimodality management in oral cancers. Indian J Med Paediatr Oncol. 2015;36(3):161.
16. Zhang L, Huang Y, Hong S, Yang Y, Yu G, Jia J, et al. Gemcitabine plus cisplatin versus fluorouracil plus cisplatin in recurrent or metastatic nasopharyngeal carcinoma: a multicentre, randomised, open-label, phase 3 trial. Lancet Lond Engl. 2016;388(10054):1883–92.
17. Vermorken JB, Mesia R, Rivera F, et al. Platinum-based chemotherapy plus cetuximab in head and neck cancer. N Engl J Med. 2008;359:1116.
18. Soler ZM, Jones R, Le P, et al. Sino-nasal outcome test-22 outcomes after sinus surgery: a systematic review and meta-analysis. Laryngoscope. 2018;128(3):581–92.
19. Quintanilla-Dieck L, Litvack JR, Mace JC, Smith TL. Comparison of disease-specific quality-of-life instruments in the assessment of chronic rhinosinusitis. Int Forum Allergy Rhinol. 2012;2(6):437–43.
20. Lehrer-Coriat E, Mariño-Sánchez F, Alobid I, Mullol J. Quality of life measures in patients on rhinosinusitis trials. Clin Invest. 2013;3(3):251–63.
21. Levy JM, Mace JC, DeConde AS, Steele TO, Smith TL. Improvements in psychological dysfunction after endoscopic sinus surgery for patients with chronic rhinosinusitis. Int Forum Allergy Rhinol. 2016;6(9):906–13.
22. Alakarppa AI, Koskenkorva TJ, Koivunen PT, Alho O-P. Quality of life before and after sinonasal surgery: a population-based matched cohort study. Eur Arch Otorhinolaryngol. 2017;274:795–802.
23. Kohli P, Naik AN, Farhood Z, Ong AA, et al. Olfactory outcomes after endoscopic sinus surgery for chronic rhinosinusitis: a meta-analysis. Otolaryngol Head Neck Surg. 2016;155(6):936–48.
24. Bugten V, Nilsen AH, Thorstensen MW, Moxness MHS, et al. Quality of life and symptoms before and after nasal septoplasty compared with healthy individuals. BMC Ear Nose Throat Disord. 2016;16:13.
25. Alakärppä AI, Koskenkorva TJ, Koivunen PT, Alho O-P. Predictive factors of a beneficial quality of life outcome in patients undergoing primary sinonasal surgery: a population-based prospective cohort study. Eur Arch Otorhinolaryngol. 2018;275:1139–47.
26. Le PT, Soler ZM, Jones R, Mattos JL, et al. Systematic review and meta-analysis of SNOT-22 outcomes after surgery for chronic rhinosinusitis with nasal polyposis. Otolaryngol Head Neck Surg. 2018;159(3):414–23.
27. Rosenfeld RM, Piccirillo JF, Chandrasekhar SS, et al. Clinical practice guideline (update): adult sinusitis. Otolaryngol Head Neck Surg. 2015;152(2S):S1–S39.
28. Tsuzuki K, Hashimoto K, Okazaki K, et al. Postoperative course prediction during endoscopic sinus surgery in patients with chronic rhinosinusitis. J Laryngol Otol. 2018;132:408–17.

GPSR Compliance

The European Union's (EU) General Product Safety Regulation (GPSR) is a set of rules that requires consumer products to be safe and our obligations to ensure this.

If you have any concerns about our products, you can contact us on ProductSafety@springernature.com

In case Publisher is established outside the EU, the EU authorized representative is:

Springer Nature Customer Service Center GmbH
Europaplatz 3
69115 Heidelberg, Germany

Batch number: 10732809

Printed by Printforce, the Netherlands